Child Abuse and Neglect
A Clinician's Handbook

Commissioning Editor: Maria Khan
Development Editor: Rachel Robson
Project Supervisor: Mark Sanderson
Typeset by Saxon Graphics Ltd, Derby
Printed in Hong Kong

Child Abuse and Neglect
A Clinician's Handbook

Christopher J. Hobbs

BSc MB BS FRCP DObstRCOG FRCPCH
Consultant Community Paediatrician, St James's University Hospital and
Senior Clinical Lecturer, Leeds University, Leeds, UK

Helga G. I. Hanks

BSc MSc DipPsych AFBPsS
Consultant Clinical Psychologist, St James's University Hospital and
Honorary Senior Lecturer, Leeds University, Leeds, UK

Jane M. Wynne

MB ChB FRCP MRCPCH
Consultant Community Paediatrician, Leeds General Infirmary and
Senior Clinical Lecturer, Leeds University, Leeds, UK

SECOND EDITION

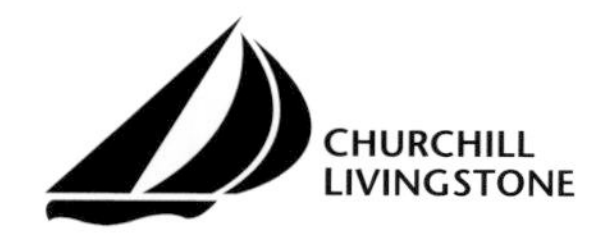

Edinburgh • London • New York • Oxford • Philadelphia • St Louis • Sydney • Toronto 1999

CHURCHILL LIVINGSTONE
An imprint of Elsevier Science Limited

ISBN 0-443-05896-2

First edition published 1993
Second edition 1999
Reprinted 2000, 2002

British Library Cataloguing in Publication Data
A catalogue record for this book is available from the British Library

Library of Congress Cataloging in Publication Data
A catalog record for this book is available from the Library of Congress

Medical knowledge is constantly changing. As new information becomes available, changes in treatment, procedures, equipment and the use of drugs become necessary. The authors and publishers have, as far as it is possible, taken care to ensure that the information given in this text is accurate and up to date. However, readers are strongly advised to confirm that the information, especially with regard to drug usage, complies with latest legislation and standards of practice.

The publisher's policy is to use **paper manufactured from sustainable forests**

Printed in China by RDC Group Limited
C/03

Contents

Preface

Even as this is written, news comes of greater commitment to controlling children in schools amid the crescendo of criticism of their behaviour, their tendencies toward crime, substance abuse and more. The President of the United States can it seems be forgiven but our children must be blamed.

In 1993 we made our first attempt to write a book which was clinically useful. It contained sufficient information and summarised and referenced enough of the available research to support a sustainable paediatric opinion so as to move away from anecdotal testimony. Inevitably the second edition is longer and more fully illustrated, reflecting the rapidly growing knowledge in child abuse and neglect but continuing to highlight sadly, the damage done to our children.

Where do the origins of abuse lie? We fail to prevent abuse, when recognised we fail to prevent further abuse and we look for scapegoats and someone to blame. The older abused child, the maladjusted child, the adolescent with conduct disorder, the young feckless parent are all named in causality.

Child rearing is made more difficult by poverty – a fate that one in three children suffer in the UK. We exclude children from school, we lock them up, and parents may hit them. As children's professionals we respect children but cannot begin to provide them with the nurture needed by each and every child, as well as by many of their parents.

The task is clear, but our best response is to acknowledge the urgent requirement to prevent abuse whilst attempting to recognise abuse early and attempt to mitigate the worse effects. Children need adults and it is the adults who must take responsibility to redress the inadequacies in parenting with the support of society (which includes financial support). Perhaps we may then move on to leave later generations to wonder at the cruelties of the twentieth century.

1999
Leeds

C.J.H.
H.G.I.H.
J.M.W.

Preface to first edition

The origins of our interest in child maltreatment lie with our good friends and colleagues Dr Michael Buchanan and the late Jill McMurray. For many years Jill was a social worker who developed an understanding and interest in protecting children that was well ahead of her time. Michael Buchanan's interest started around the time that Henry Kempe described 'battered babies' in the 1960s. The authors joined the team later, towards the end of the 1970s, by which time procedures for handling physical abuse and neglect were being established. The idea of working as a team appealed to all of us because we recognised at an early stage in this work the importance of sharing information, concerns and above all our anxieties about the children and families who we were seeing. Being able to talk about a subject which has its own taboos, stigma and secrecy was an important part of getting to grips with the broad issues which surround it and which can make this work so difficult. We also recognised that our training only equipped us in part for dealing with this problem and that we needed to talk to others who held different perspectives if we were to progress. Increasingly the developmental view of child maltreatment is offering the most valuable insights into its pathways and patterns, its prevention and treatment.

This book sets out to be a clinical handbook for clinicians who find themselves confronted by child maltreatment in their work with children and families and wish to read more widely. We recognise that individual cases present some of the most difficult problems encountered in clinical practice with children and that a sound knowledge base is vital.

The book comprises separate chapters on all the various major forms of abuse and neglect which come under the broad umbrella of child maltreatment. Their recognition, assessment, management and treatment are all described. We have also attempted to explain the wider context in which maltreatment occurs in order to give a broader understanding of the nature and origins of maltreatment. However, there remain many unsolved problems and unanswered questions in this field, which has been growing rapidly in recent years.

The high mortality of children at the beginning of this century has now been replaced by an expectation that children will survive. This has focused child care on the quality of children's lives, their rights as human beings and inevitably child maltreatment. As a result child maltreatment is now being recognised as a major morbidity for children and therefore indirectly for society. The scientific, humanistic and compassionate study of the complex relationship between parents and their offspring is fraught with resistances of every kind.

If this book appears to have all the answers, then this is folly on our part as there is much that is not known or understood. Nor is this a book for bedtime reading or casual voyeurism. It is a book about the suffering and sadness of children and the hope and expectation that things may be a little better in the future for the generations to come.

1993 C.J.H
Leeds H.G.I.H.
J.M.W.

1

Introduction: a theoretical perspective

THE EXTENT OF THE PROBLEM

THEORETICAL VIEWS OF CHILD ABUSE

VIOLENCE AND CRIMINALITY

HUMAN AGGRESSION

The purpose of writing this book is to present the current thinking of a group of professionals who are actively interested and working in the field of child abuse, or *child protection* as it is now more often described. The book is written for practitioners by practitioners, but we hope that in our active and deliberate preoccupation with practice we have nevertheless had time to stand back and reflect more widely on the many issues for everyone which child abuse raises. We hope, therefore, that others with a greater interest in developing a theoretical understanding will study this text because theory should learn from practice just as practice must have a sound theoretical basis.

There are as many definitions of child abuse as there are viewpoints of the problem. Even the terminology varies and evolves. The term *battered baby* (or *battered child*) *syndrome* was deliberately used to focus attention on a previously concealed problem. The less emotive term *non-accidental injury* was later adopted by professionals who strove to work with the clinical problems. As other forms of ill-treatment were appreciated, the term *child abuse* became more widely used and accepted. When sexual abuse was acknowledged in the 1970s and 1980s, for some the term child abuse virtually became synonymous with sexual abuse and it was then necessary to add the prefix 'physical' to describe abused children who had been battered. With the wider and global perspective, the term *child maltreatment* has been more often used. In seeking to focus on prevention, the National Commission of Inquiry into the Prevention of Child Abuse (Childhood Matters 1996) adopted an all-inclusive definition:

> 'Child abuse consists of anything which individuals, institutions, or processes do or fail to do which directly or indirectly harms children or damages their prospects of safe and healthy development into adulthood.'

For clinicians this definition is too all-inclusive and the working definition quoted by Helfer (1987) is preferable for our needs:

> Child abuse and neglect is 'any interaction or lack of interaction between family members which results in non-accidental harm to the individual's physical and/or developmental states.

Obviously abuse by unrelated individuals is important, but our main focus as childcare professionals remains with the family.

Defining child abuse can be difficult and itself raises other issues relating to the purpose for which the definition is to be used and how narrow or wide the definition should be made. It should be sufficient to say that there are definitions, many of which are embodied within the legal framework of child protection practice (see Ch. 17), and that these will be referred to in the various chapters on the major kinds of abuse. These definitions are essential as starting points in understanding, and they provide clear statements at an early stage of dealing with a problem which is still emerging in societal consciousness.

This book is written from the perspective of those in health professions and presents to some extent a medical model for the understanding of abuse. In no way should this diminish any other model or perspective on the subject, a full understanding of which requires that views are shared and that we seek to combine different ideas rather than seeing them as mutually exclusive or as inherently affording more or less insight than other views.

The extent of the problem

Statistical information on child abuse is never more than a reflection of the problem. Changes in figures over time are as likely to reflect changes in awareness, recognition and reporting as changes in the epidemiology of abuse. Nowhere is this demonstrated more clearly than in the differences between reported rates in different countries. Much child abuse remains invisible and uncounted. Even the apparently more obvious cases are regularly missed.

In a recent study (Ewigman et al 1993), as many as half of all childhood deaths under 5 years due to abuse could not be recognised as such from the death certificate. In the UK there is no formal system for quantifying the scale of child abuse. Our current knowledge derives from various sources, including officially registered children and supplemented by various surveys. On 31 March 1995, there were 34 954 children on child protection registers in England. The registered categories were:

physical abuse	37%
neglect	32%
sexual abuse	26%
emotional abuse	13%
more than one category	9%

These figures do not reflect accurately patterns of abuse but rather administrative convenience. For example many more children are emotionally abused in addition to being physically or sexually abused, but the trend toward single registration obscures this.

Other research has lead to much greater estimates of the extent of child abuse in the UK. These have been summarised in Childhood Matters (1996):

- at least 150 000 children annually suffer severe physical punishment
- up to 100 000 children each year have a potentially harmful sexual experience
- 350 000–400 000 children live in an environment which is consistently low in warmth and high in criticism. This group have been defined as being in need of services and as children who are being emotionally neglected.

The figures for severe physical punishment and sexual abuse are derived from research sponsored by the Department of Health (Smith 1995 and Kelly et al 1991 respectively).

In support of these figures, many more children are reported to the statutory agencies than those whose names appear on the child protection registers. According to Department of Health research in 1992:

- 160 000 children were referred to the child protection process
- 120 000 of these received a family visit
- some 40 000 child protection conferences were held
- 24 500 children were registered as a result.

The research concludes that probably only a small proportion of the 160 000 referrals are ill-founded, and that the majority of the families from which these children come are multiply disadvantaged.

Despite these findings, the figures and rates in the UK are considerably lower than those in the USA, where 1.7 million reports annually involving 2.7 million children indicate a referral rate of three times that of the UK. The figure for children in state care is also considerably higher.

Theoretical views of child abuse

In the jigsaw puzzle approach to child maltreatment, various perspectives from different disciplines and professional viewpoints are combined to provide an overall picture. This can be compared, for example, to the complex process which is involved in individual case diagnosis where information from a variety of individuals and agencies covering many aspects of the child and family is put together to obtain a comprehensive record. The individual pieces in our theoretical jigsaw overlap or fit together, but in themselves do not purport to provide the 'answer' or solution to our understanding. Table 1.1 illustrates 12 areas which have provided valuable understanding, and some of these are described below.

Table 1.1 The jigsaw approach to a theoretical understanding of child abuse

Historical perspective	Medical model	Psychological theory
Sociological theory	Legal standpoint	Education
Societal beliefs and attitudes	Violence and criminality	Children's rights
Power and political theory	The family as a system.	Biological views of aggression
	Family violence	

Historical perspective

The historical approach is dealt with in more detail in Chapter 2. History not only informs us that child abuse has happened in many cultures examined closely over the time of recorded history but also shows how social history has been reflected in the evolution of child-rearing practice. As societies have become more tolerant and respectful of the individuals within them, so it seems that children have enjoyed greater protection and better care. Recent experience from Romania has demonstrated the relationship between wider social and political pressures and child maltreatment. In the past widespread practices which would now be termed maltreatment were either condoned or found to be socially acceptable. History suggests that societies have struggled at times with the problem of child abuse, although not always with great success or effect.

The medical model

The adoption of non-accidental injury by the medical profession as a diagnostic category of disorder has arguably been the single most important step in catalysing the recent progress in understanding child abuse. Caffey's 'parent–infant stress disorder' (1946) and Kempe's 'battered baby syndrome' (Kempe et al 1962) did much to focus attention on the problem of child abuse and at the same time implied that, with the adoption of a medical model, a therapeutic approach might be useful.

In the medical world, the disorder lies primarily with the child whose condition requires to be recognised, diagnosed and treated. Fortunately medicine has been less willing to apply loose pathological or psychiatric diagnoses to the parents who have abused their children, recognising the inherent difficulties in that approach. This is not to say that there has been no acknowledgement of the perpetrators' difficulties and need (often denied) for help.

Psychological theories including the stress model

There is no single psychological theory to explain child abuse. Theories have focused on an understanding of the broad area of parent–child behaviour and incorporate developmental psychological thinking. A recognition that infants born prematurely appeared to be at greater risk of abuse suggested that if attachment or bonding was impaired, e.g. by separation in the special care or neonatal unit, then abuse was more likely (Lynch & Roberts 1977). This coincided with strenuous attempts to promote early attachment in hospital with breast-feeding and the focus shifting onto parents' emotional health after birth (Klaus & Kennell 1976). Other insights from the psychological approach have emphasised that abusers are not recognisable as different within society and do not suffer from psychiatric disorders. They are characterised principally by the fact of their abusing behaviour. It has also been established that abuse is not simply an occurrence in situations where everything is going badly (e.g. unemployment; poverty; bad housing; history of maltreatment as a child; unintelligent, uneducated or depressed parents; or where society condones brutal treatment of children). These formulations do not work out in practice and therefore theoretically form a doubtful basis for our understanding of child abuse. There appears to be more to this problem than the insights afforded to us by the stress model; a predisposed or deviant parent plus an at-risk child plus a stressful situation does not produce child abuse in a predictable way.

Crittenden & Ainsworth (1989) remind us that more sophisticated and comprehensive ecological models such as those of Garbarino (1977) and Belsky (1980) provide us with infinite complexity, but we are still left wondering what it is that determines when abuse will take place. They suggest that it is necessary to focus on the critical causes of maltreatment and propose that anxious or insecure attachment is a critical concept in regard to both the origin of family maltreatment and the rehabilitation of families.

Attachment theory

Attachment theory is a recent development which grew out of the work of Bowlby (1969). He proposed that survival of humans, especially infants, was best ensured by proximity to an attachment figure or figures. Infants are able to emit signals which lead to responses in the attachment figure; this draws the pair together when the situation requires. The process of attachment develops in phases in the early part of life and is closely linked to maternal behaviour and responsiveness. Carers who are inaccessible, unresponsive, or inappropriately responsive to the child's behaviour are likely to produce children who are insecure or anxious in their attachments to them.

In maltreatment it has been postulated (and there is observational work to support this by Ainsworth et al 1978) that the children are anxiously attached and that this can be demonstrated in the testing construct of the 'strange situation'. In this manoeuvre the child is briefly placed with a stranger while the mother leaves the room. The child's reactions are then observed under the standardised situation. It appears that it is not the absence of a 'bond' that is important in situations of child abuse, but rather the nature of the bond. Children who were neglected also appeared to show similar patterns of anxious attachment, although they tended to be passive rather than either difficult or compulsively compliant (Crittenden 1981). This is discussed further in Chapter 3.

Sociological theory

Sociologists view child abuse as an aspect of much wider social issues. For example, they point out that it was only because of the challenges of judicial policy relating to sex crimes and rape against women that the scene was set for the sexual abuse of children to be confronted. Sociologists see the family as a microcosm of society. The power struggles between men and women in the family reflect the wider issues of women's rights in society. Research work on prevalence, which is discussed more widely in Chapter 8, suggests that sexual abuse is a far more common occurrence than previously imagined. This in itself raises issues which cannot easily be addressed by reference only to personal or individual factors. Wider forces are at work.

Goodwin (1988) provides another interesting example of the importance of social attitude in this field when she analyses the decision process which occurs when societies, individuals and families consider intervention in childhood sexual abuse. She points out that in doing so they are simultaneously taking positions along at least five axes of beliefs and attitudes which are based on society's values and rules (Fig. 1.1)

Sociologists would further wish to point out that other issues of social justice are involved in child abuse. Poverty, unemployment, racism and inequality place individuals, including children, at risk of neglect and abuse as individuals within that society.

Legal standpoint

Kempe said that child abuse is what the law says it is. Most countries have developed a legal framework for handling the problem of child abuse. This framework does not in itself prevent child abuse but provides a formal structure for dealing with the problem. Those who argue for the decriminalisation of child abuse are asking for a less punitive and more therapeutic response to the problem. However, even where more radical therapeutic solutions have been introduced, as in Holland's 'confidential doctor' programme, there is also a legal framework to be used as appropriate. In English law it is still permissible for a parent to hit a child, but only to use reasonable force. The law reflects societal views – for example the recommended sentence for in-decent assault of a male child is greater than that for a female child.

Violence and criminality

Violence has been defined as 'behaviour by people against people liable to cause physical or psychological damage' (Children and Violence 1995).

There is a great deal of information to link child abuse with other violent and criminal behaviour in the parents. The NSPCC statistics indicate that of cases reported to their system from 1983 to 1987 (Creighton & Noyes 1989), 15% of the mothers and 41% of the fathers had criminal records prior to the abuse being diagnosed. Among the recorded crimes, violent offences are over-represented, particularly in the case of the fathers where crimes of assault against both children and adults outnumbered non-violent criminal records; this contrasts with national data where non-violent crimes heavily outnumber violent crimes. Interestingly, when the recorded abuse was broken down into categories (physical

Preference for informal social controls	⇔	Preference for legal controls
Viewing the child as parental (mainly paternal) property	⇔	Viewing the child as an autonomous individual
The need for inviolate family privacy	⇔	The need for the community overseeing child-rearing
Viewing the child as a sensual expert	⇔	Viewing the child as a virginal innocent
Viewing sexuality as dangerous and secret	⇔	Viewing sexuality as harmless or natural

Fig. 1.1 Axes of belief and attitudes.

injury, sexual abuse, neglect, failure to thrive, emotional abuse), the highest rate for criminal records for all offences was encountered amongst both mothers and fathers in the neglect cases. However, the highest number of crimes of violence against adults was recorded for the fathers of physically injured children (18%). Finally, the data also indicate that in cases of physically injured, sexually abused and neglected children, parents with a criminal record of any kind were significantly more likely to be implicated in the abuse or neglect of their child.

Much is known about the origins of violent behaviour. Negative, violent and humiliating forms of discipline are significant factors in the development of violent attitudes and actions from a very early age (Children and Violence 1995). Further, there is good evidence that aggressive children become violent teenagers who become violent adults. Television and media influences play a minor part in comparison to experiences in the family. If people have violent tendencies, violent films can make them worse. It seems that there is a link between abuse and offending in general, particularly violent offending against adults, although the NSPCC data are undoubtedly biased as they represent cases that have come to professional attention, and this is more likely when the parents have criminal records.

From another standpoint, Lewis et al (1989) believe that a high proportion of violent delinquents have been severely abused. There are several American studies which have found that 80% or more of juvenile offenders had been abused or neglected, often as pre-school children. Other studies (Welsh 1976, Feshback 1979) have linked the severity of corporal punishment received as a child with the degree of aggressiveness shown by delinquents. Similar findings have emerged from the work of the Newsons (Newson & Newson 1968) in Nottingham who found a 'very clear association' between the frequency of physical punishment at age 11 and the child's perceived delinquency.

Similar associations have been claimed for adult violent offenders. In one particularly disturbing study (Feldman et al 1986) of 15 death row inmates awaiting execution for murder, eight had been victims of potentially filicidal assaults as children. Others had been physically and/or sexually abused by their parents.

Of course, some would pose the question the other way round: perhaps these individuals as children invited and deserved such treatment in view of their inherent badness? However, the view which blames the children grossly misrepresents the situation. The existence of neurological, psychological and behavioural difficulties in these individuals has been reported with greater frequency than in the population as a whole. Whether these have resulted from abusive head injury or other causes remains speculative, although there is some evidence to implicate the former (Oliver & Buchanan 1978).

Family violence

In the USA today it has been said that people are more likely to be killed, physically assaulted, hit, beaten up, slapped or spanked in their own homes by other family members than anywhere else or by anyone else (Gelles & Cornell 1990). Some observers have proposed that violence in the family is more common than love (Strauss et al 1980). These statements apply not only to American families but are also accurate assessments of family life in the UK, western Europe and many other countries and societies around the globe (Gelles & Cornell 1990).

This view is in conflict with the traditional idealised view of the family as a safe haven to which one can flee from the dangers of the hostile outside world. Much of the violence is denied, ignored and not seen. Traditionally 'domestic' violence was often viewed as outside the province or interest of the law, but these attitudes have now been challenged. This is reflected in the reorganisation of the police and the establishment of family violence units.

There has been a tendency for the categories of family violence listed in Table 1.2 to be viewed and studied in isolation. However, the family functions as a system and it is common to observe more than one type of abuse occurring within the family. Browne (1989) suggests that abuse be categorised into 'active' and 'passive' forms:

Table 1.2 Categories of family violence

Adult perpetrator	Child perpetrator
Child abuse	Sibling abuse
Spouse abuse	Parent abuse
Elder abuse	Elder abuse
Courtship abuse	

- active abuse involves violent acts in a physical, emotional or sexual context
- passive abuse refers to neglect which can only be considered violent in a metaphorical sense as it does not involve physical force. Neglect can, of course, result in both physical and emotional injury.

Spouse abuse

Spouse abuse (Bowder 1974, Gayford 1975, London 1978, Walker 1979, Andrews & Brown 1988, Dickstein 1988) denotes physical and/or psychological violence by a man or woman towards an intimate partner (Browne 1989), whether married or unmarried. Clearly there is a spectrum of violence from slaps, pushes, shoves and spanking to punches, kicks, bites, chokings, beatings, shootings and stabbings where the injury clearly may be severe or fatal. Psychological violence is more difficult to define but includes verbal or non-verbal threats against a person or their belongings, e.g. threatening suicide, punching walls, destroying pets and throwing things (Gelles & Cornell 1990). Spouse abuse also includes material deprivation, emotional and sexual abuse, marital rape and pornography.

Traditionally spouse abuse is considered to be a male to female directed behaviour but Strauss et al (1980) observed in a US National Incidence Survey of 2143 families that 4.6% of wives had engaged in abusive violence towards their husbands.

The lifetime incidence of marital violence has been estimated to lie between 11% and 28% of all marriages, making this the second most common form of interpersonal violence reported to police in Scotland in one study (Dobash & Dobash 1987). Between 20% and 40% of all homicides in the USA are domestic murders, 9% of women in one study (Hall 1985) in London reported forced sex by spouses and in San Francisco 4% experienced forced sex, 14% were raped and battered and 12% battered but not raped (Russell 1982).

There are also various accounts in the literature of husband abuse (e.g. Steinmetz 1978), refuting the view that women are the only victims of violence in the home. However, men are typically stronger, have more physical and social resources to hand and rarely suffer as much damage as women. Careful studies of the homicides within marriage have revealed that where a wife kills a husband this usually follows years of physical violence by the husband and is motivated by self defence. However, violence in general remains a predominantly male issue. Men are responsible for over 90% of convicted cases of violence against the person.

Recent changes in the law have acknowledged the crime of marital rape.

Refuges

Erin Pizzey, who established a refuge in Chiswick, in 1974 wrote a book entitles 'Scream quietly or the neighbours will hear'. In the UK refuges for women seeking a place of safety from violence for themselves and their children are now widespread. By the end of the 1970s it was estimated that 11 400 women and 20 850 children used 150 refuges in a 12-month period. The women reported physical and mental cruelty, including being kept prisoner, verbally tormented and threatened as well as the batterings. Sadly, those who have worked with battered women report the difficulties that some women have in breaking the bonds of these violent, dangerous and symbiotic relationships (Pizzey & Shapiro 1982). Sometimes it seemed almost as though there was an addiction to the violence, although there was very real fear as well as excitement accompanying the violent interactions. However, difficulty for a woman in separating and protecting herself frequently relates to the social, legal and material entrapments of marriage.

Children of course are frequently witnesses to this violence which is often chronic, lasting for years before the woman moves out or away from her husband or partner.

It is also important to acknowledge that family violence, although reported more often from lower social classes, also occurs in middle-class and upper-class homes. Levinger (1966), in studying the reasons cited for divorce, found that while 40% of working-class applicants named abuse as the reason for the divorce, 23% of middle-class applicants mentioned violence as the reason for wanting to end the marriage. It occurs within every culture and refuges have been opened for women and teenage girls from ethnic minorities in Britain. There are also 'safe houses' for children.

It is beyond the scope of this text to discuss in detail the causes of spouse violence. Understandably cultural values and exposure to models of aggression which are sanctioned and unpunished are factors. Social structural explanations emphasise the importance of the existence of asymmetric social relationships within society (as in poverty, unemployment, homelessness) and in the family (authoritarian, wife dominance). Domestic violence is then a means of improving low status and low self-esteem. Finally, psychological explanations have focused on personality characteristics, psychiatric history and alcohol and drug use (e.g. the explosion of 'crack'-related violent crime in the USA). Many women describe drunkenness as a factor contributing to violence in their husbands. For further details the reader is referred to Browne (1989) and Gelles & Cornell (1990).

Elder abuse

Information on elder abuse is increasingly becoming available; there are obvious parallels with child abuse. Cloke (1983) defined 'granny battering' as the systematic and continuous abuse of an elderly person by the carer – who is often, although not always, a relative on whom the elderly person is dependent for care. The abuse may involve physical violence, threats of physical violence, sexual abuse including rape and pornography, neglect, abandonment, psychological abuse and exploitation (Eastman 1989). The incidence of elder abuse is difficult to ascertain, but in the USA it is estimated that 7% of the elderly population is abused. With increasing numbers of elderly persons dependent on relatives or institutional care, it is likely that this form of abuse will become more prevalent. It is associated with the stress and frustration of the care-giver faced with the elderly person's increasing age and continual presence. Other factors similar to those described in other aspects of family violence may also apply, e.g. alcohol, personality characteristics.

Courtship violence

Researchers in this country and in North America have drawn attention to courtship violence as a form of interpersonal violence (Browne 1989, Gelles & Cornell 1990). Studies have found that between 10% and 67% of dating relationships involve violence of some kind. The violence ranges from mild (pushing, shoving, slapping) to severe, which is surprisingly common (Gelles & Cornell 1990). Interestingly attitudes frequently included an acceptance of the violence as a protective sign of the romantic illusion of dating. In addition to physical violence, sexual violence in the form of 'date rape' is also described.

Both men and women report being the victims in the situation of courtship violence and there is considerable evidence of the interactive nature of the behaviour. It is not surprising that courtship violence is frequently continued into the marital relationship and that 20% of battered women claim that the first violent assault occurred prior to marriage or cohabitation (Dobash et al 1978).

Human aggression

Lorenz (1966) wrote 'what is the significance of all this fighting?' He had started by looking at coral fish and found that some species, particularly some of the brightly coloured ones, were very fierce and very willing to fight. In the animal kingdom aggression is either interspecific (between members of different species) or intraspecific (between members of the same species). In a sense interspecific aggression and fighting seem to make some sense within the Darwinian construct of the struggle for existence, although it is successful competition which determines species survival rather than the results of the more active struggles in which aggression plays a part. Clearly some species prey on others and all animals have some capacity for self-defence. The predator–prey relationship is a classic one in the history of evolution, each species changing under the influence of the other's evolution in a process which leads to a balance so that neither party has too much of an upper hand. Predators do not necessarily or usually exhibit aggression in their predation but predators are frequently counterattacked by their prey and in this situation aggression can be clearly defined. Crows may mob a bird of prey or a cat if they see it in the day when its advantage is less. Aggression is therefore useful and has survival value. Within species, aggression is encountered in fights over territories leading to spacing out of the individuals and in sexual selection of the strongest by rival fights and in defence of the young. In all these situations it is functional and serves to assist in the preservation of the species. It is not surprising therefore that the aggressive drive in animals is a vital and essential part of their make-up and is a major motivation in much behaviour.

Lorenz reasons that in considering human behaviour from a distant position where one could look at the broad patterns such as migration, wars, historical events, one would not gain an impression that such behaviour was dictated by intelligence, still less by moral responsibility. It is difficult to make sense of much human behaviour if one assumes that it is determined by reason and cultural tradition alone. Lorenz suggests it continues to be subject to the laws prevailing in all phylogenetically adapted instinctive behaviour.

Is there any help in understanding child abuse from this perspective? Certainly it helps us to understand the role of aggression in human behaviour (Storr 1974) and how it can become adapted in destructive ways towards other members of the species. In social animals (of which humans are a good example) there are inhibitions controlling aggression to other members of the species but because humans are not predators or carnivores as such, these inhibitions are not as well developed as in species where there is a much greater risk from a single act of aggression. Rapid changes in human ecology and sociology by cultural development may disrupt phylogenetically adapted behaviour mechanisms and lead to dysfunctional patterns.

Child abuse, as described in twentieth-century Britain, is clearly an extreme form of dysfunctional behaviour between members of the human species. There are no clear parallels within the animal kingdom and it is difficult to discern any survival or functional value in such behaviour.

Summary

1. It is not possible to provide a single comprehensive and simple theory by which to understand child abuse.
2. There are as many viewpoints as there are disciplines and each individual has a personal and differing perspective.
3. Child abuse appears to be a uniquely human problem embedded in psychological and social factors in the complex societies in which people live. Attitudes and beliefs are fundamental to an understanding, and politics, morality and religion also seek to be heard in this debate.
4. The stakes are high. It is not just the health, well-being and happiness of generations of children as they grow up into adults but more than this, the future of the society which the children will construct out of their childhood experiences.
5. There is little doubt that aggression is a central part of much abusive behaviour and it seems likely that it is linked in some way to perceived or

imagined threats upon the individual who perpetrates the abuse. However, the complex way in which aggression is directed towards an individual's offspring remains incompletely understood.

6. The mechanisms in the human for managing and coping with trauma, including psychological as well as physical injury, also begin to suggest the special problems which confront the highly developed human mind. Thus, for example, whilst the immediate effects of emotional dissociation which may follow extremely traumatic situations may provide acute survival value, in the long term these very effects may present challenges of adaptation for the individual. The increased likelihood of abusive behaviour to be 'handed on' from generation to generation suggests that long-term adaptations are playing a part in these processes (Widom 1989).

REFERENCES

Ainsworth M O, Blehar M C, Waters E, Wall S 1978 Patterns of attachment: a psychological study of the strange situation. Erlbaum, Hillsdale, NJ

Andrews B, Brown G W 1988 Marital violence in the community: a biographical approach. British Journal of Psychiatry 153:305–312

Belsky J 1980 Child maltreatment: an ecological integration. American Psychologist 3:320–335

Bowder B 1974 The wives who ask for it. Community Care 1:18–19

Bowlby J 1969 Attachment and loss. Vol 1: Attachment. Basic Books, New York

Browne K D 1989 Family violence: spouse and elder abuse. In: Howells K, Hollin C R (eds) Clinical approaches to violence. J Wiley, Chichester

Caffey J 1946 Multiple fractures in the long bones of infants suffering from subdural haematoma. American Journal of Roentgenology 56:163–173

Childhood Matters 1996 The report of the National Commission of Inquiry into the Prevention of Child Abuse Volume 1. Stationery Office, London

Children and Violence 1995 Report of the Gulbenkian Foundation Commission. Calouste Gulbenkian Foundation, London

Cloke C 1983 Old age abuse in the domestic setting: a review. Age Concern, England (cited in Eastman 1989)

Creighton S J, Noyes P 1989 Child abuse trends in England and Wales 1983–87. NSPCC, London

Crittenden P M 1981 Abusing, neglecting, problematic and adequate dyads: differentiating by patterns of interaction. Merrell-Palmer Quarterly 27:210–218

Crittenden P M, Ainsworth M D S 1989 Child maltreatment and attachment theory. In: Cicchetti D, Carlson V (eds) Child maltreatment. Cambridge University Press, Cambridge

Dickstein L J 1988 Spouse abuse and other domestic violence. Psychiatric Clinics of North America 11(4): 611–628

Dobash R E, Dobash R P 1987 Violence towards wives. In: Coping with disorders in the family. Guildford Press, Surrey, pp 169–193

Dobash R E, Dobash R F, Kavanagh K, Wilson M 1978 Wifebeating: the victims speak. Victimology 2(3/4): 608–622

Eastman M 1989 Old age abuse. In: Archer J, Browne K (eds) Human aggression: naturalistic approaches. Routledge, London

Ewigman B, Kivlahan C, Land G 1993 The Missouri Child Fatality Study: under reporting of maltreatment fatalities among children younger than five years of age 1983 through 1986. Pediatrics 91(2):330–337

Feldman M, Mallouh C, Lewis D O 1986 Filicidal abuse in the histories of 15 condemned murderers. Bulletin of the American Academy of Psychiatry and Law 14(4): 345–352

Feshback N D 1979 The effects of violence in childhood. In: Gil D G (ed) Child abuse and violence. AMS Press, New York

Garbarino J 1977 The human ecology of child maltreatment: a conceptual model for research. Journal of Marriage and the Family 39:721–727

Gayford J J 1975 Wife battering: a preliminary survey of 100 cases. British Medical Journal i:194–197

Gelles R J, Cornell C P 1990 Intimate violence in families, 2nd edn. Sage, London

Goodwin J M 1988 Obstacles to policy making about incest. In: Wyatt G E, Powell G J (eds) Lasting effects of child sexual abuse. Sage, London

Hall R 1985 Ask any woman. Falling Wall Press, Bristol

Helfer R E 1987 The developmental basis of child abuse and neglect: An epidemiological approach. In: Helfer R E and Kempe R S (eds) The battered child. University of Chicago Press, Chicago, ch 4

Kelly L, Regan L, Burton S 1991 An exploratory study of the prevalence of sexual abuse in a sample of 16–21-year-olds. University of North London

Kempe C H, Silverman F N, Steele B F, Droegmuller W, Silver H K 1962 The battered child syndrome. JAMA 181:17–24

Klaus M, Kennell J 1976 Maternal-infant bonding. C V Mosby, St Louis, MO

Levinger G 1966 Sources of marital dissatisfaction among applicants for divorce. American Journal of Orthopsychiatry 26:803–897

Lewis D O, Mallouh C, Webb V 1989 Child abuse, delinquency and violent criminality. In: Cicchetti D, Carlson V (eds) Child maltreatment. Cambridge University Press, Cambridge, p 707

London J 1978 Images of violence against women. Victimology 2:510–524

Lorenz K 1966 On aggression. Methuen, London
Lynch M, Roberts J 1977 Predicting child abuse: signs of bonding failure in the maternity hospital. British Medical Journal 1:624–626
Newson J, Newson E 1968 Four years old in an urban community. Allen & Unwin, London
Oliver J E, Buchanan A 1978 Maltreatment of children as a cause of impaired intelligence. In: Smith S M (ed) The maltreatment of children. MTP Press, Lancaster
Pizzey E 1974 Scream quietly or the neighbours will hear. Penguin, Harmondsworth
Pizzey E, Shapiro J 1982 Prone to violence. Hamlyn, London
Russell D 1982 Rape in marriage. Macmillan, New York
Smith M A 1995 A community study of physical violence to children in the home and associated variables. Poster presented at International Society for the Prevention of Child Abuse and Neglect: V. European Conference, May 1995, Oslo, Norway
Steinmetz S K 1978 The battered husband syndrome. Victimology 2(3/4):499–509
Storr A 1974 Human aggression. Penguin, Harmondsworth
Strauss M A 1978 Wife-beating: how common and why? Victimology 2(3/4):443–458
Strauss M A, Gelles R J, Steinmetz S K 1980 Behind closed doors: violence in the American family. Anchor Press, New York
Walker L E 1979 The battered woman syndrome study. In: Finkelhor D, Gelles R, Hotaling G, Strauss M (eds) The dark side of families: current family violence research. Sage, London
Welsh R S 1976 Severe parental punishment and delinquency: a developmental theory. Journal of Clinical Child Psychology 5:17–21
Widom O S 1989 The cycle of violence. Science 244:160–166

2

Child abuse and neglect: a historical perspective

The lessons of history

This chapter relies heavily on the now classic contributions on the history of child abuse of Lloyd De Mause (1980), Margaret Lynch (1985) and Samuel Radbill (1987). These authors and others have shown us that there is nothing new about child abuse. Its existence has been recognised for a very long time. What is new is the recent willingness to address its existence and to look for ways of preventing its occurrence.

The historical perspective allows us to stand back from the everyday experience of confronting the battered or neglected child and to reflect on the wider issues of what has been presented to us as a single incident in time. Those who have sought to uncover evidence of child abuse in the past have had to collect their material widely, often reading between the lines and recognising indirect messages of what was happening. There is much to support a view of history that 'the things that really matter are hardly ever committed to paper'. Thus wrote Lloyd De Mause in the Preface of his history of childhood. William Langer, Professor of History at Harvard University, wrote:

> The direction of human affairs has never been confided to children, and historians, who have concerned themselves primarily with political and military affairs and at most with the intrigues and rivalries of royal courts, have paid almost no attention to the ordeals of childhood. Even the students of education have, on the whole, devoted themselves to

the organisation and curriculum of schools, and with theories of education with only occasional reference to what happened to the pupils at home and in the world at large.

Yet the history of childhood must be of major importance to any study of human society, for if, as it is said, the child is the father of the man, it should be possible, with an understanding of any individual's or any group's past, to form a more intelligent judgement of their performance as adults.

Unhappily, the results of these investigations are most depressing. They tell a long and mournful story of the abuse of children from the earliest times even to the present day. We need not assume that the generalisations here advanced apply to all people at all times. No one can doubt that there have always been parents who loved and cherished their children and that such mistakes as they may have made in the upbringing were due to ignorance rather than to ill will.

Although the true frequency of child abuse today remains unknown, it is clearly altogether a common occurrence, but it must be said that since the eighteenth century a more humanitarian attitude has gradually emerged (De Mause 1980).

Langer comments that much of the wanton abuse of children related to the fact that humans produced more babies than they could possibly care for, or have room or employment for. Hence the widespread practice of infanticide existed in one form or another, the chief victims usually being the female infants because it was they who would eventually produce yet more souls. From this probably also arose the notion that sexual relations were sinful and that the resultant offspring was, from the moment of birth, evil. How else could one explain the cruel practices designed to exorcise the evil and make children less of a nuisance than they were?

So it is not an exaggeration when de Mause (1980) said that 'The history of childhood is a nightmare from which we have only recently begun to awaken'. The further back in history one goes, the lower the level of child care and the more likely children were to be killed, abandoned, beaten, terrorised and sexually abused.

Where the historians usually look to the sandbox battle of yesterday for the causes of those of today, we instead ask how each generation of parents and children creates those issues which are later acted out in the arena of public life. These links have been recognised for centuries. St Augustine's cry of 'give me other mothers and I will give you another World' was quoted by De Mause to indicate the importance of parent–child relations in the process of social change. Links between parents and the development of personality of the child were recognised in the seventeenth century, when it was considered that traits might be transmitted in breast milk from mother to baby. Much attention was therefore given to the choice of a suitable wet nurse for the offspring of the affluent. Such was the advice given by Burton in 1651 to parents:

> that they make choice of a sound woman of good complexion, honest, free from bodily diseases, if it be possible, and all passions and perturbations of the mind, as sorrow, fear, grief, folly, melancholy. For such passions corrupt the milk and alter the temperature of the child which now being moist and pliable clay, is easily seasoned and perverted. (Fomon 1974)

However, it was Freud who more clearly changed our view of childhood. Now at case conferences we are interested to know of the parents' childhoods to understand their present actions. History, in the same way, must turn itself towards childhood if it is to understand some of the upheavals of the societies which it studies.

De Mause's studies draw together two important threads:

- Parent–child relationships are undergoing a process of constant evolutionary change. Each generation is able to regress to the psychic stage of their children and work through the anxieties of that age so as to manage them better the next time.
- The history of childhood suggests that there is a general improvement in child care, i.e. the further back, the worse things seemed to be. Therefore, although today in the USA there may be as many as a million abused children, one could imagine a time earlier in

history when most children would, by today's standards, be considered abused.

The present day, so different?

It would, however, be unwise to distance ourselves too much from the past. Samuel Radbill (1987) reminds us that, in 1895, the NSPCC summarised many of the ways that London children were battered: 'by boots, crockery, pans, shovels, straps, ropes, thongs, pokers, fire and boiling water'. In the Newsons' studies (1968, 1986), they found that by the age of 7, 26% of boys and 18% of girls had been hit with an implement and a further 53% (65% boys and 41% girls) threatened with an implement, so perhaps change should be seen as gradual and faltering. Neglected children in 1895 were described as miserable, vermin infested, filthy, shivering, ragged, nigh naked, pale, puny, limp, feeble, faint, dizzy, famished and dying. One hundred years ago, begging was common but children begging in the streets of London has become a common occurrence in the 1990s.

It was not assumed in ancient times that children automatically had a right to live. This right was ritually bestowed and if it was withheld the child could, with little compunction, be disposed of as a nonentity. Usually it was the father who had to acknowledge the child, proclaiming him or her for his own. In some cultures, until nourishment had passed the child's lips, the child was not really of this world.

Radbill comments that the fitness to live could also be tested. The Germans would plunge the child into icy cold water, the Greeks would leave the child on a mountain top, North American Indians threw children into a pool of water to see if they floated. Naming of the child is another important way of recognising the child's existence. Christian children required to be christened and given a name before their soul could go to heaven. Without christening, they would have to be buried in unhallowed ground along with the dogs and cats. Children born out of wedlock have long been outlawed and especially liable to abuse and infanticide. William Blake expressed this as 'the youthful Harlot's Curse Blasts the newborn Infant's tear'. In 1917, of 4–5000 illegitimates born in Chicago, 1000 disappeared without trace (Radbill 1987).

Exposure and infanticide

Exposure and infanticide (or filicide) are the time-honoured methods of lethal child abuse (Hobbs 1991). Weak, premature or deformed infants were frequently disposed of in ancient times. However, although infanticide was common in many cultures, the Egyptians would sentence parents who killed their children to hug the corpse continuously for 72 hours. The Greeks actually encouraged the disposal of handicapped children, believing that they would pass on defects to the next generation. It is interesting to note how even today the handicapped are at greater risk of abuse than other groups of children. The existence of the practice of infanticide is reflected in the passing of laws, e.g. the Chinese in 1654 banned the drowning of little girls, but laws have never stopped infanticide, which continues to exist to the present day in our society. While it is clear today that most 'cot deaths' do not arise from abuse, a small proportion – certainly less than 10% – arise from infanticide (Emery 1985).

If children are seen as the property of parents, or more usually their fathers, then it is not surprising that the owners are given a fairly free hand in how they treat them. In Roman law, *patriae potestia* was the concept which meant children were property and fathers were in charge.

Child labour

Child labour remains another major way in which children have been abused and misused over the centuries. The statute of artificers in 1562 gave the government regulatory controls over apprentices, binding children to their masters by indenture for seven years (Radbill 1987). This produced a situation of enslavement which lasted until 1815. The stories of children being beaten in clothing mills in England in the 1800s are well known, and the child chimney sweeps were described as England's disgrace. 'Little black things among the snow crying "weep", "weep" in notes of woe', wrote William Blake (quoted by Radbill 1987). The children were intentionally kept small and thin (failure to thrive) so that they could clamber up the soot-clogged flues. The major causes of child labour today in developing countries are poverty and inequality (Naidu 1986). Development is inversely related worldwide to the incidence of child labour. High illiteracy rates, backwardness in economic development, and poor environmental resources encourage child labour. In developing countries today, child labour remains a major issue.

Estimates of the number of children worldwide in the official workforce vary. A United Nations report (Bouhdiba 1982) estimated that there were 145 million children, aged between 10 and 14, most of them in developing countries, and younger children may also be involved. Child work is exploitative when it prevents access to education, leaves no time for recreation or is hazardous to health. In addition, the physical and emotional stresses of work can produce psychosocial hazards.

Sexual abuse

There is little doubt that sexual abuse of children has been recorded as long as human beings have kept records. De Mause (1980) wrote 'the child in antiquity lived his earlier years in an atmosphere of sexual abuse'. Growing up in Greece or Rome often included being used sexually by older men. In Rome, boy brothels were common and there was a rent-a-boy service in Athens. The abuse involved not only boys over 11 or 12, but also much younger children.

Girls were also involved, as well as women. Petronius described the rape of a 7-year-old girl with women clapping in a long line around the bed, suggesting that women were not exempt from playing a role in the process. Aristotle commented that homosexuality often becomes habitual in 'those who are abused from childhood'. The Jews attempted to eradicate adult homosexuality with severe punishments but were more lenient in the case of young boys. The penalty for sodomy or, as we would know it, buggery, with children over 9 years of age was death by stoning. Despite Moses' injunction against corrupting children, copulation with younger children was not, however, considered a sexual act and was punishable only by whipping 'as a matter of public discipline'.

There are remarkable parallels between the patterns of abuse in ancient Greece and what is being witnessed in England in the present day (Hobbs & Wynne 1986). Martial said the favourite sexual use of children was not oral sex but anal intercourse. There has always been an awareness of the harmful effects of sexual abuse of children. The concept of children's innocence was well accepted, but there were dangers in this because it was suggested that children would not suffer from abuse because they could not be corrupted.

In the Renaissance moralists warned against sexual use of children, but in the eighteenth century the moral view took an unusual turn. Children were punished for touching their genitals. Prohibitions against masturbation are generally unusual in primitive societies, and this seems to be a late development in the historical sequence of rejecting child abuse. The sinfulness of masturbation was supported by the medical profession, who advised that it could cause insanity, epilepsy, blindness and death. Mutilation, circumcision, and infibulation were sometimes used as punishments, and casts and cages used to restrain the child.

In the eighteenth century, sexual abuse was widespread amongst servants and others acting in parent roles. Cardinal Bernis, who was himself sexually abused as a child, warned that

> there is nothing so dangerous for morals and perhaps for health as to leave children too long under the care of chambermaids or even of young ladies brought up in the Chateaux. I

> will add that the best among them are not always the least dangerous. They dare with a child that which they would be ashamed to risk with a young man.

Freud said he was seduced by his nurse when he was two.

Discovery and denial

In more modern times, there have been various attempts to bring the issue of the continued existence of the sexual abuse of children out into the open (Summit 1989). Ambrose Tardieu, the Dean of Forensic Medicine in France, published in 1860 a startling exposé (Tardieu 1860 cited by Masson 1984) entitled: 'a medico-legal study of cruelty and brutal treatment inflicted on children'. In his book on rape, reviewing an 11-year period from 1858 to 1869, he cited 11 576 people accused of completed or attempted rape in France. Of these cases, 9125 (or almost 80%) involved child victims, mostly girls aged 4–12 years. Tardieu's work encouraged a transient interest in the publication of a new journal – *Archives of Criminal Anthropology and Penal Science* – which encouraged studies of child sexual abuse. Soon after Tardieu's death, Fournier in 1880 (quoted in Masson 1984) proclaimed that children were faking sexual abuse and that respectable men were targets of extortion by perfidious children and their lower-class parents.

Brouardel, a student of Tardieu, also attacked the treachery of children, asserting that 60–85% of their complaints were unfounded. He used an attractive argument to blame the victims. In his address in the 1880s, 'The causes of error in expert opinion with respect to sexual assault', he asserted that:

> The child comforts herself by touching herself, fantasies that she knows are false on every point . . . This child, to whom one ordinarily paid only the most minor attention, finds an audience that is willing to listen to her with a certain solemnity and to take cognisance of the creations of her imagination. She grows in her own esteem, she herself becomes a personage and nothing will ever get her to admit that she deceived her family and the first people who questioned her. (Brouardel, quoted in Masson 1984).

Freud also became aware of child sexual abuse, not only from his work with his adult patients in psychotherapy, but also from visits to the mortuary in Paris where he observed signs of rape in children (Masson 1984). On this latter point, it is interesting to note that Tardieu said that if doctors are called in they should tell the police, and the pathologists should not be surprised at anything they see. Freud made the link between early sexual assault of a child and emotional illness in the victims in later life – particularly from his studies of patients with hysteria. The story of his recantation of the seduction theory in favour of the Oedipus complex – children are traumatised by projection of their own wishful masturbatory fantasies and not by actual sexual assault – is well known (Masson 1984). Freud found that he was alienated and isolated and in danger of rejection. He had discovered the stuff of our nightmares, a lost world of hidden pain, and society did not wish to join him in his discovery. By diverting his awareness into more acceptable channels he kept face and was accepted back into the fold of his professional colleagues. Only one of his followers, Sandor Ferenczi, continued to accept his original theory.

Ferenczi (1932) wrote of his experience of abused children:

> The overpowering force and authority of the adult makes them dumb and can rob them of their senses. The same anxiety, however, if it reaches a certain maximum compels them to subordinate themselves like automata to the will of the aggressor to divine each one of his desires and to gratify these; completely oblivious of themselves, they identify with the aggressor.

Lynch reviews the nineteenth- and twentieth-century literature up to the time of Kempe et al. (1962). The way in which medicine gradually accepted the traumatic nature of the bony lesions in babies is well described.

Tardieu also described battered children, but it was John Caffey (1946), Silverman (1953) and others working in the 1940s and 1950s who identified multiple fractures and subdural haematoma and suggested that they resulted from trauma and were not due to previously unrecognised disease. The papers were largely ignored. In 1961 Henry Kempe presented his paper, 'The battered child', and people listened (Kempe et al 1962). In that paper he estimated that there could be as many as 447 cases of the battered child syndrome in the USA. Krugman (1986) declared the above figure to be an 8-hour total, for in 1983 there were 1 007 658 reported cases and in 1985 1 700 000. A rise in reported cases involving sexual abuse is also included in these figures. In 1984 200 000 new cases were reported to the child protective services in 19 states, with 100 000 cases substantiated – 22% involving a male child, 78% a female child.

We need not, however, look to reported cases for estimates of the size of the present-day problem. Over the last 15 years a number of prevalence studies of sexual abuse have examined the lifetime rates for at least one incident having occurred before age 18 years and found a range of 6–62% for females and 3–31% for males in the USA (Peters et al 1986). The wide ranges relate to methodological variations, especially data collection, sampling techniques and differences as to how child sexual abuse is defined (see Ch. 8).

Despite all this, society still moves slowly to acknowledge the existence of the problem. In the UK reported rates are rising (Creighton 1988) but the discovery of over 100 children over a few months in 1987 in Cleveland led to widespread disbelief and a formal inquiry took place (Butler-Sloss 1988). Even now there are many who believe that the problem of sexual abuse was grossly exaggerated despite the clear message of the report. Will the present be historically yet another episode that is buried and passed over, leaving children much as before – unprotected, abused and harmed – or is this the dawning of an era of new social justice for children and society?

Evolution of social and legal protection

If within people's minds child abuse remains the unthinkable, then progress cannot be made. Advances in the sociolegal mechanisms have been occurring in the past 150 years in both Britain and America. The story of Mary Ellen (Williams 1980) is worth recounting. Mary Ellen was born in the USA in the 1860s and was found starved and physically abused by her adoptive parents – the abuse included being chained to a bed. In 1874 publicity for her plight reached national awareness but there was no child protection agency in existence to handle her case. The founder of the Society for the Protection of Animals, Henry Berg, invoked action when the New York police refused to do anything. This led to the foundation of the Society for the Prevention of Cruelty to Children in 1875. Interestingly, in 1876 a photograph of the abused, neglected and starved child was displayed alongside specimens of abused members of the animal kingdom as part of the Society for the Prevention of Cruelty to Animals' exhibit at the Philadelphia Centennial Exhibition to mark the nation's centenary. The Society for the Prevention of Cruelty to Children (SPCC) was organised by the leadership of the SPCA and modern American child protection was born. Mary Ellen grew up to be married, and had two children. She died aged 92 years but bore the scars of her injuries for life (Lazoritz 1990).

Societies such as the NSPCC and Speedwell Society, actively promoted children's causes at the turn of the century. There was a gradual shift in child-rearing methods from punitive to more sensitive ones. Radbill (1973) reminds us that child welfare was recorded as long ago as 6000 years in Mesopotamia, where orphans had a patron goddess to care for them. Institutional care has a long history going back to ancient Greece and Rome and then, in Europe, in the seventh century in France.

Unfortunately, the foundling hospitals and homes, who aimed to rescue abandoned and unwanted children, offered minimal care in many cases, and death from exposure and malnutrition was the fate of many children (Chapin 1915). Because of the failings of institutional care, children were readily fostered, although the mortality in London in the nineteenth century was 80% from abuse or neglect (Radbill 1987). Nurses who were skilled baby killers were called 'angel makers' or 'harpies' and could earn profits from insurance benefits on dead infants. In Germany, giving the baby nothing but a dummy soaked in brandy usually saw it off. A report in 1881 estimated that 31% died in foster-care in Germany (Radbill 1987).

An article in the British Medical Journal (BMJ 1903) criticised systems of baby farming and urged licences for foster-parents and inspectors. Although fostering has improved in modern times, it should come as no surprise that children are occasionally abused in the system which is designed to protect them.

Child protection laws

There have been many laws which have as their central concern the protection of children. In 1224 overlaying was so prevalent that the Statutes of Winchester penalised women for keeping infants in bed with them. Infanticide is still viewed as a lesser crime than murder, but murder in the first year of life remains 5–10 times higher than at any other age, with a rate of 66 per million of population.

Most countries have laws prohibiting incest. Incest became a criminal offence in England in 1908, although it was briefly a criminal offence from 1650 to 1660. Prior to 1909 it was punishable by ecclesiastical courts.

The legal age of consent varies from country to country and between states of the USA. It is 16 years in the UK and theoretically serves to reduce sexual abuse and exploitation. Mrazek (1982) noted that anthropologists have documented that all societies have some kind of incest taboo with or without formal criminal sanctions or punishments. This suggests that all human societies have a tendency to encounter incest.

Much of the present law and new law incorporated in the Children Act (1989) is based on experience accumulated in childcare practice in the latter half of this century. A series of inquiries following on from the Inquiry into the death of Maria Colwell (DHSS 1974) have led to changes in practice and legislation.

Conclusion

De Mause suggests that parent–child relations have evolved historically through various key modes or stages. His sequence is shown in Table 2.1. In the infanticidal mode, parents routinely resolved their anxieties about caring for their children by killing them. Gradually, as parents accepted the notion of the child possessing a soul, the only way they could escape from the difficulties with their children was through abandonment, either physically to wet nurses or foster families or by severe emotional abandonment at home. Between the fourteenth and seventeenth centuries parents allowed children more into their emotional lives and saw themselves as having a task to mould the child who was seen as clay or soft wax to be beaten into shape. Child instruction manuals first appear around this time. As the eighteenth century was reached, parents became more intrusive in their child care, punishing the child with threats and guilt but also developing more understanding and empathy with the child. During the socialisation mode, which is still prevalent today, the child was seen as someone to be trained, guided and taught to conform. This grew with a behaviourist and sociological function. The father started to become more involved in childcare for the first

Table 2.1 Evolution of parent–child relations

Mode	Historical era
Infanticidal	Antiquity–4th century AD
Abandonment	4th–13th century
Ambivalent	14th–17th century
Intrusive	18th century
Socialisation or training	19th–mid-20th century
Helping	Mid-20th century

time. The helping mode judges that the child must be supported and helped through his development, which he can explore for himself. There is more tolerance, the child is not struck or scolded, and the process requires great emotional and time commitment from the parents. The reader is referred to De Mause (1980) for further details.

Obviously there are considerable overlaps and ranges of parental behaviour within and between different societies. However, the study of European culture in particular suggests that child-rearing practices have gradually evolved for the better. Recently we have seen six European countries outlaw the hitting of children altogether, and in Great Britain corporal punishment has been prohibited in state schools since 1987.

History gives us a perspective which helps us understand our shortcomings towards children better. Humanity strives to do better by its children and thereby to secure a future for itself and generations to come. This history of childhood is one which should not deter us or depress us too much. The good old days were surely the bad old days but we should not pretend that the lives of children are always so different, even now, and be aware that change is often painfully slow and faltering.

Summary

1. History informs us that child abuse has existed as long as there are records of human societies.
2. Child-rearing practices are evolving over time.
3. Violence to children has been outlawed in some countries in the twentieth century.
4. Humanity strives to do better for its children although this is only achieved by constant effort and determination to improve their care and welfare.

REFERENCES

BMJ 1903 British Medical Journal, 17 January:154–155

Bouhdiba A 1982 Exploitation of child labour. Report, United Nations, New York

Butler-Sloss E 1988 Report of the inquiry into child abuse in Cleveland 1987. HMSO, London

Caffey J 1946 Multiple fractures in the long bones of infants suffering from chronic subdural haematoma. American Journal of Roentgenology 56(2):162–173

Chapin H D 1915 Are institutions for infants necessary? Journal of the American Medical Association 64:1–3

Creighton S J 1988 The incidence of child abuse and neglect. In: Browne K, Davies C, Stratton P (eds) Early prediction and prevention of child abuse. J Wiley, Chichester, ch 3, pp 31–41

De Mause L 1980 The history of childhood. Souvenir Press, London

DHSS 1974 Report of the Committee of Inquiry into the care and supervision provided in relation to Maria Colwell. HMSO, London

Emery J L 1985 Infanticide, filicide and cot death. Archives of Disease in Childhood 60:505–507

Ferenczi S 1932 Confusion of tongues between adults and the child: the language of tenderness and of passion. In: Balint M (ed), Mosbacher E (trans) Final contributions to the problems and methods of psychoanalysis 1955. Basic Books, New York. See also International Journal of Psychoanalysis 1949;30:225–230

Fomon S J 1974 Infant nutrition, 2nd edn. Saunders, Philadelphia

Hobbs J 1991 Infanticide and the battered baby. Current Paediatrics 1:116–122

Hobbs J, Wynne J M 1986 Buggery in childhood – a common syndrome of child abuse. Lancet ii:792–796

Kempe J, Silverman F N, Steele B F, Droegmueller W, Silver H K 1962 The battered child syndrome. Journal of the American Medical Association 181:17–24

Krugman R 1986 Child maltreatment and its presentation in industrialised countries. In: Battered children and child abuse. Proceedings of XIXth Council of the International Organisation of Medical Sciences Round Table Conference. Council of the International Organisation of Medical Sciences, Switzerland, pp 14–21

Lazoritz S 1990 Whatever happened to Mary Ellen? Child Abuse and Neglect 14:143–149

Lynch M A 1985 Child abuse before Kempe: a historical literature review. Child Abuse and Neglect 9:7–15

Masson J N 1984 The assault of truth: Freud's suppression of the seduction theory. Farrar, Strauss & Giroux, New York

Mrazek P B 1982 Definition and recognition of sexual child abuse. Historical and cultural perspective in sexually abused children and their families. In: Mrazek P B, Kempe H (eds) Sexually abused children and their families. Pergamon, Oxford, pp 5–16

Naidu U S 1986 Exploitation of working children. Situation analysis and approaches to improving their

conditions. In: Battered children and child abuse. Council of the International Organisation of Medical Sciences, Switzerland, pp 70–80
Newson J, Newson E 1968 Four years old in an urban community. Allen & Unwin, London
Newson J, Newson E 1986 The extent of parental physical punishment in the UK. Available from Child Development Research Unit, University of Nottingham, University Park, Nottingham NG7 2RO
Peters S D, Wyatt G E, Finkelhor D 1986 Prevalence. In: Finkelhor D (ed) A sourcebook on child sexual abuse. Sage, London, pp 15–59
Radbill S X 1973 Mesopotamian paediatricians. Episteme 7:283
Radbill S X 1987 Children in a world of violence: a history of child abuse. In: Helfer R E, Kempe R S (eds) The battered child, 4th edn. University of Chicago Press, London, pp 3–22
Silverman F 1953 The roentgen manifestations of unrecognised skeletal trauma. American Journal of Roentgenology 69:413–426
Summit R C 1989 Hidden victims, hidden pain: societal avoidance of child sexual abuse. In: Wyatt G E, Powell G J (eds) Lasting effects of child sexual abuse. Sage, London, pp 39–60
Tardieu A 1860 Etude medico-legale sur les services et mauvais traitments exercés sur des enfants. Ann Hyg Pub Med Leg 13:361–398
Williams G J 1980 Cruelty and kindness to children: documentary of a century, 1874–1974. In: Williams J G, Money J (eds) Traumatic abuse and neglect of children at home. Johns Hopkins University Press, Baltimore, pp 68–77

3

Failure to thrive

The term *failure to thrive* is used with reference to children who are growth-retarded secondary to malnutrition. The use of the term 'failure to thrive' rather than 'malnutrition' is preferable not only because it is less emotive but also because it allows us to consider a wider range of pathways and mechanisms in its causation. The subdivision of children who fail to thrive into two broad groups, *organic* and *non-organic*, has been criticised because of its oversimplification of a complex area. Clearly there are many patterns of failure to thrive – as many as there are individual cases.

It is useful, however, to differentiate physical from psychosocial factors, albeit with the acknowledgement that both can exist in a single child and that physical factors can have profound effects on psychological functioning such that one is bound to feel that these factors are almost primary in causation.

In the USA, paediatricians who have written much about this problem mention that the term 'failure to thrive' was used at the beginning of this century to describe the sad and pathetic state of infants living in institutions or hospitals (Spitz 1945). Radbill (1987) referred to

> children who failed badly under the dismal routine of institutions. They suffered from deprivation and starvation with little consideration for their recreational needs. A visitor to a foundling asylum was dejected by the sight of children sitting all day long bound to potty chairs. Few survived.

Interestingly, in more recent times, Izuora & Epigbo (1983) found similar reactions among adult Africans who were looking after children with severe kwashiorkor in Nigeria in the 1980s. In this study, the effects of such children not only on their parents but also on the staff caring for them was found to be marked. Adults tended to become depressed, apathetic and unresponsive to the needs of the children, thus perpetuating the cycle. Kwashiorkor, a prevalent form of malnutrition in the developing world, has also been described elsewhere, for example in the USA.

The recognition of the importance of institutional factors in the aetiology of failure to thrive was the first time attention had been focused on this problem and links made between 'depression' (usually termed *anaclitic depression*), malnutrition and growth failure. With the interest after the Second World War in the wider welfare of the family and children, and the beginning of official acknowledgement of physical abuse, it became recognised that failure to thrive could also occur within the family (Coleman & Provence 1957).

However, non-organic failure to thrive has received little attention until recently. In one British paediatric textbook (Ellis & Mitchell 1965), although the battered baby syndrome was beginning to be recognised, marasmus or infantile atrophy received only brief mention, the authors acknowledging that

> whilst it may arise simply from underfeeding, it is more often due to a variety of other causes, e.g. chronic infection of any type, chronic diarrhoea, coeliac disease, mental defect, parasitic infection, metabolic disorder or even prolonged hospitalisation.

There is no discussion of psychosocial factors or what is meant by 'underfeeding'. Similarly, in the chapter on growth, dwarfism is linked to various skeletal, endocrine, metabolic and other problems or referred to as 'simple hereditary' – racial and familial.

However, the proof of any hypothesis must be in its testing and so it is with the theoretical basis of failure to thrive. The clinical trials reported by Whitten et al (1969) confirmed that failure to thrive resulted from a lack of food and could be largely resolved by feeding adequate calories. Supernormal calorie intake was required in order for the underweight children to grow if they were admitted to hospital and simply fed without providing additional stimulation or affection. What Whitten et al's studies showed was that it was basically a deficiency of calories which caused the clinical picture and that if the calories could be replaced then the child would recover. However, not all the children responded by taking extra food and growing. This observation does not detract from the main hypothesis that these children are primarily short of calories. However, it does indicate that the situation is more complex for some of the children than simply withholding of food: the child becomes part of the process, i.e. it is interactional, and there are important additional factors in operation in many cases.

In summary, therefore, although failure to thrive in the absence of organic disease was originally regarded as an outcome of emotional deprivation, it is now clearly accepted that it results from inadequate nutrition and nurturing, though the causes of poor feeding practices may well have origins in psychological difficulties of the parents and are ultimately contributed to by the child. This formulation is vitally important. The fact that treatment is possible through improvement in the child's nutritional intake provides strong support to this view.

Definition of failure to thrive

- Failure to thrive occurs when an infant or child fails to achieve the expected growth as assessed by measurements of weight and height. The child may also fail to achieve full potential in other parameters of development

In a sense failure to thrive is best considered a symptom of a wider disorder, in psychosocial terms, usually involving the parents and the family situation. In practice, it is best not to spend too much time debating on the grounds of growth criteria whether the child is failing to thrive or not, but instead to stand back and look at the wider situation surrounding the child. Failure to nourish an infant usually occurs amidst a range of parenting difficulties and these become apparent as the picture of the family emerges over time.

Failure to thrive is defined as a failure to achieve the normal potential for growth and is related to undernutrition and insufficient calories. This may come about simply by the infant or child not having enough food or being fed on an unusual diet, for instance a vegan diet. Adults may do well on a strict vegetarian diet but infants and small children simply do not.

Failure to thrive undoubtedly persists throughout childhood into adolescence, and patterns of poor feeding may be found in adults who have failed to thrive as infants. However, the term is most usually applied to babies and toddlers, although it is quite legitimate to use it with older children.

As the problem most often comes to notice through deviations of growth from the normal expected pattern, it should be said that the definition of failure to thrive must start with an understanding of the nature of normal and abnormal growth within populations of children. Failure to thrive includes not only failure to grow but also failure to develop intellectually and emotionally. These other aspects are equally important in the whole problem of failure to achieve potential. Figure 3.1 demonstrates the theoretical model of failure to thrive described in this chapter.

Consequences of failure to thrive

Mortality and morbidity

Failure to thrive is linked with an increased risk of death. In developed countries death following failure to thrive may be linked to serious abuse or neglect, but there will also be deaths from infectious disease where failure to thrive must be considered an important contributing factor.

An association with sudden and unexpected death in infancy has also been described. Failure to thrive or poor growth (falling centiles) was identified in 19 out of 37 infants who died unexpectedly (Hobbs et al 1995). They included six whose weight at death was below the third percentile. An association of poor growth and failure to thrive with unexpected infant death including sudden infant death syndrome (SIDS) has been described in other reports (Knowleden et al 1985, Williams et al 1990); see also Chapter 19. Presumably this association reflects poor nutrition secondary to inadequate food intake as organic failure to thrive should be excluded at post-mortem. The major area of concern remains the substantial morbidity that arises from undernutrition at important and critical times in the development of the individual.

Because growth, especially of the brain, is so rapid in the first months of life, particularly up to the second year, this early period is the most vulnerable part of the human life cycle (Fig. 3.2). According to Taylor & Taylor (1976),

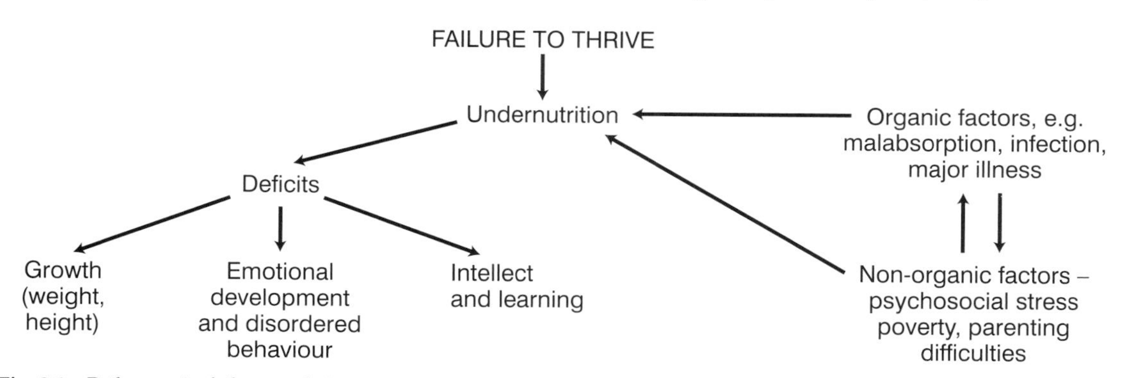

Fig. 3.1 Pathways in failure to thrive.

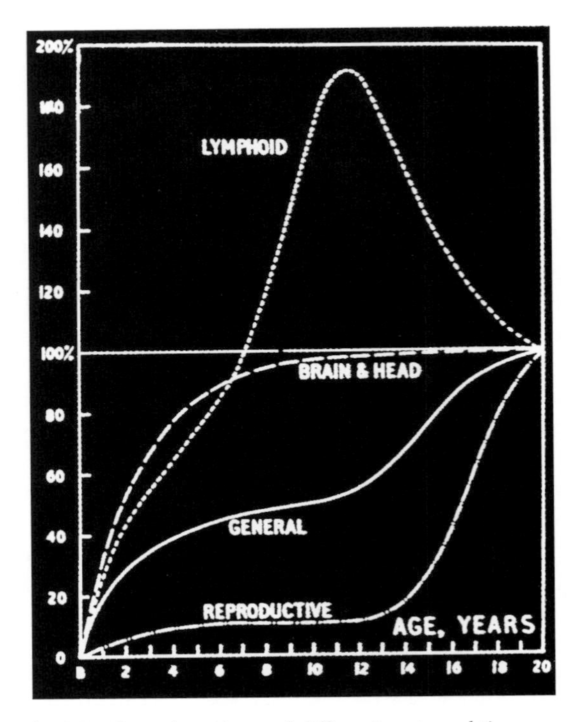

Fig. 3.2 Growth patterns of different parts and tissues of the body, showing the four chief types. All the curves are of size attained and plotted as percentage of total gain from birth to 20 years, so that size at age 20 is 100 vertical scale. (Reproduced with permission from Tanner J. 1962 Growth at adolescence, 2nd edn. Blackwell Scientific Publications, Oxford.)

> The period between the start of weaning and the fifth birthday is nutritionally the most vulnerable segment of the human life cycle. Rapid growth, loss of passive immunity and as yet undeveloped acquired immunity against infection produce dietary needs more specific and inflexible than at later periods.

Undernutrition at this stage rapidly leads to a curtailment of growth in order to preserve other essential body functions vital to survival. The damage inflicted by this is almost certainly likely to be permanent, related to both the severity of growth retardation, its duration and the age at which it occurs. Illingworth (1983) indicated that

> . . . studies all over the world have shown that severe growth retardation in the first year retards later mental development, and the longer the duration of the growth retardation, the greater is the effect on mental development.

We now appreciate that catch-up growth is possible, leading to improved growth and development, but how far potential can be permanently reduced remains unclear and certainly unquantifiable at present (Figs 3.3–3.5).

Continued poor growth

Although all children with failure to thrive have the potential for catch-up growth, it is a feature of this condition that poor growth continues in many cases once it has begun; there are children who do not catch up satisfactorily or do so only in part. Skuse (1988) studied a cohort of 200 children born in an inner city population and identified failure to thrive in 39 cases. Interestingly the majority (over 70%) of these children had not been referred for a specialist opinion for their failure to thrive. He successfully followed up 34 of the children noting that 15 (44%) remained below the third centile for weight on their third birthday. McIntyre & Collinson (1997) reported that 9.4% (out of 15 100 children) under the age of 5 years attended with a growth pattern that required a health plan. They also confirmed that this was probably an underestimate because some of the more vulnerable children had failed to attend child-health clinics and the children who attended local authority day nurseries had not been included.

Even with hospitalisation and outreach programmes, Sturm & Drotar (1989) found significant continuing growth problems in 59 3-year-olds hospitalised as infants. When children are followed up for longer, fewer children are likely to remain below the third centile. Oates et al (1985) found that on follow-up of 14 children admitted to hospital 13 years earlier, none were below the third centile for weight and only one was below the third centile for height, although

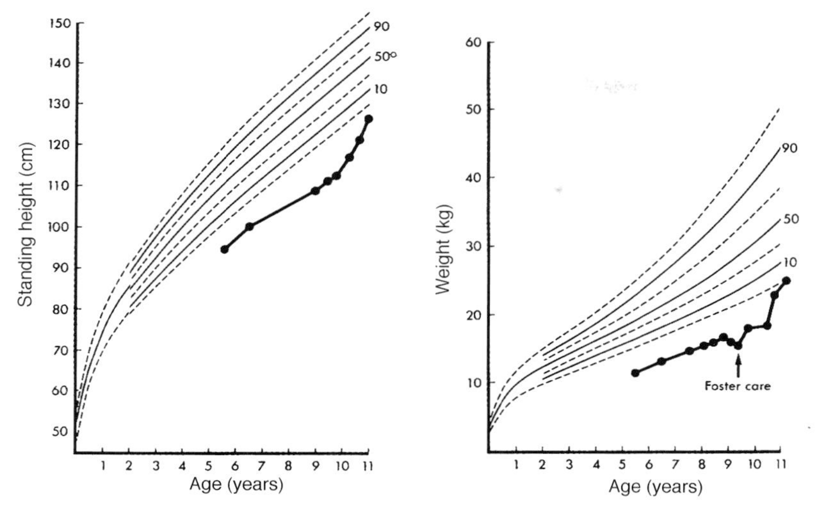

Fig. 3.3 Growth charts (height and weight) of a girl suffering from severe and long-standing social deprivation and failure to thrive. Admission to foster care at age 9 years resulted in improvement in growth, general well-being and emotional development and behaviour but educational attainment remained poor with moderate to severe learning difficulties.

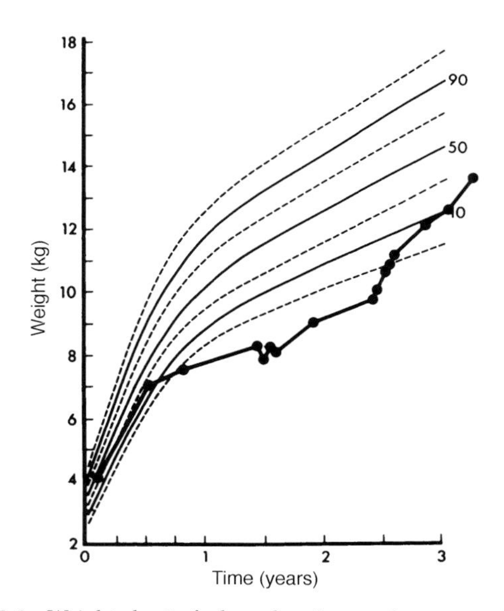

Fig. 3.4 Weight chart of a boy showing catch-up growth from age 2½ years when a diagnosis of neglect was made and conveyed to the parents. The boy remained at home, showing that his normal growth potential could be reached. Same case as Plate 2.

six were one or more years below their chronological age for height and also for weight.

Reduced developmental attainment

Although it is clear that some improvement in growth can be expected with or without intervention in some children over time (Mitchell et al 1980), it is not so clear how their neurodevelopmental attainment progresses. Developmental scores on follow-up of these children have shown a high frequency of being depressed (Elmer et al 1969, Chase & Martin 1970, Hufton & Oates 1977, Skuse 1988). Children who have failed to thrive show reduced scores on tests of language development, reading age, social maturity and verbal intelligence on follow-up in school (Hufton & Oates 1977). Furthermore, Skuse (1988) suggests from his data that late improvement of growth by age 4 for children who have severely failed to thrive is not correlated with any better neurodevelopmental attainment in comparison to

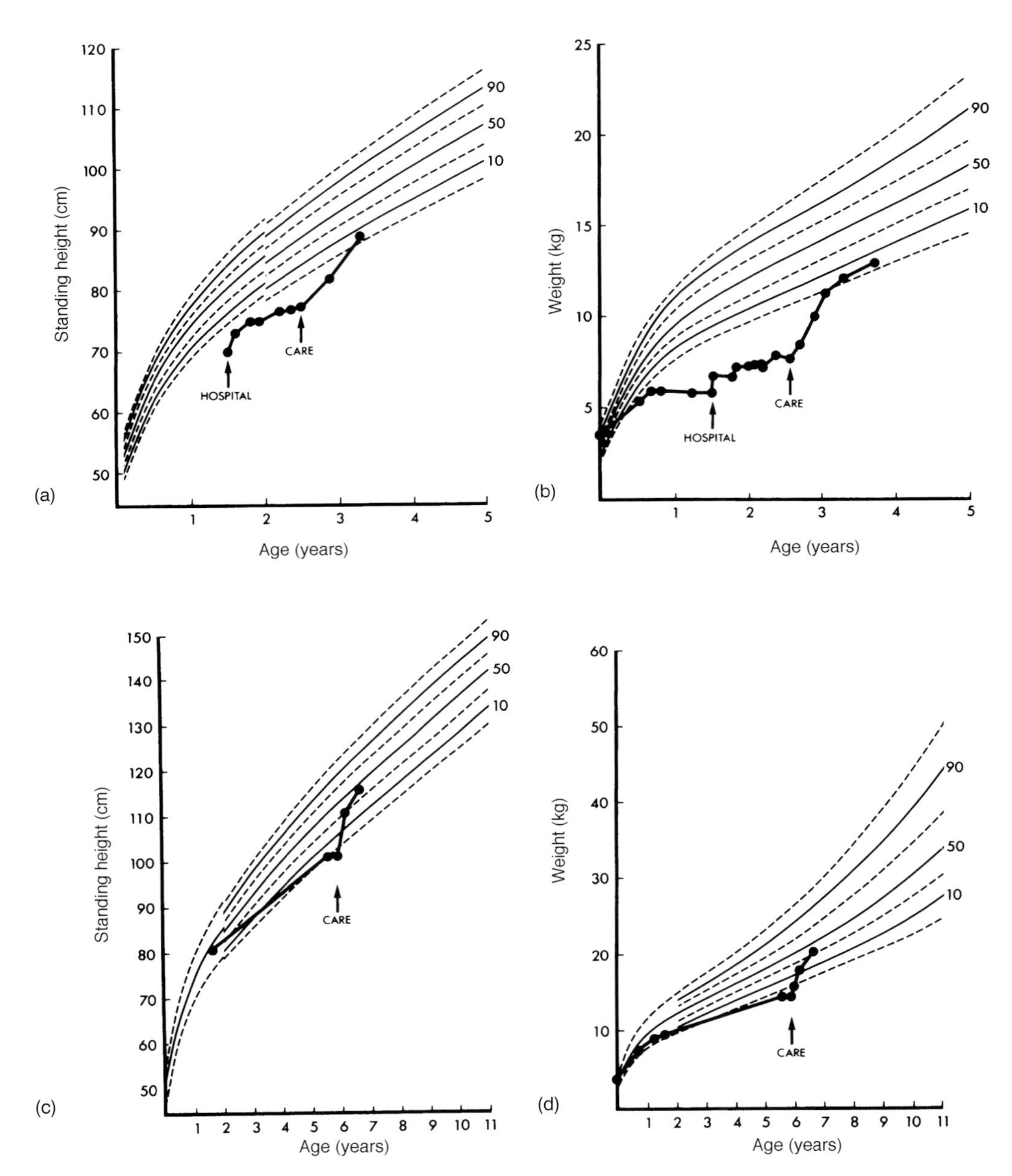

Fig. 3.5 (a),(b): Height and weight charts of index child failing to thrive who shows two episodes of catch-up growth. (c),(d): Height and weight charts of older sibling whose failure to thrive was unrecognised prior to admission to foster care but recognised retrospectively when she showed accelerated growth.

those children who persist in poor growth. It is beyond the scope of this text to discuss in detail the relationship between intellectual development and nutrition. However, there is evidence to show that brain growth is maximal up to the end of the second year of life and that the adult number of neurones is achieved quite early in brain development, perhaps as early as 20 weeks after conception (Frank & Zeisel 1988). A further period of cellular multiplication commences at about 25 weeks and probably ends in the second year of postnatal life. The difficulties of disentangling the direct effect of nutrition from the concomitant effects of poor social environment which are usually also present in families with malnourished children pose a problem for research. However, studies such as that of Evans et al (1980) support the view that improved nutrition in malnourished children early in life may improve verbal intelligence.

For the same reason, children who show poor brain growth (linked to head circumference) should theoretically command our increased concern as potentially they are at greater risk of intellectual retardation. This may necessitate more aggressive and early intervention.

Mackner et al (1997) undertook research comparing children who were neglected and failed to thrive. Their research showed that when children were neglected and failed to thrive their cognitive performance was significantly below those children who were 'only' neglected or failed to thrive. They indicated that comparing these children with those from low-income families showed comparatively little difference in their cognitive performance. However, accumulation of risk factors is detrimental to cognitive functioning.

Personality and behaviour problems

Behavioural disturbance is commonly associated with failure to thrive. On follow-up, children who fail to thrive score lower on tests of ego strength and emotional stability. Behavioural difficulties may persist even after recovery in growth. The psychological consequences are discussed throughout the chapter. However, two studies substantiate some of the concerns for these children. Whereas Mitchell et al (1980) reported that children failing to thrive in an outpatient sample did not show more behavioural problems when compared with a control group, Oates et al (1985) showed clear differences in their clinical group of children failing to thrive. There was a high prevalence of reported behavioural problems in the children who failed to thrive when they were followed up at 12 years of age. Both Mitchell and Oates in the same studies found that those children who failure to thrive showed long-term intellectual deficits.

CASE HISTORY 3.1

A mother was informed from the antenatal observations of her doctors that her first infant had congenital heart block. She was very carefully monitored both before and during labour and her baby was taken to the special care unit for management after birth. She remembered vividly when visiting her baby an overwhelming feeling that her infant had died and it was a great shock to find that she was alive. The infant required no initial treatment and had good circulatory function maintained with a bradycardia of around 50–60 beats/min.

The mother was intelligent but from a poor family, her husband unemployed and their housing in poor condition and damp. She soon became pregnant again and her first child started to fail to thrive. There were difficulties with in-laws who tended to use the couple to sort out their arguments. The mother continued to believe that the child would eventually die and was sure that the obvious malnutrition was directly caused by the congenital heart block although she was strongly advised to the contrary by the doctors. Observations of the mother and child revealed little physical contact and generally negative patterns of interaction. The child was hyperactive, attention seeking and resorted to difficult and 'naughty' behaviour to get her mother's generally 'hostile' attention.

At about 2 years of age, a pacemaker was inserted because of persisting bradycardia without any signs of cardiac failure. The pacemaker worked well and the mother was able to check for herself that the heart was beating faster. The child started to thrive, her behaviour improved, the second child was born and thrived and the mother spontaneously commented that she felt closer to her first child. An air of optimism surrounded the situation and she had arranged a holiday – the first she had had since the child had been born.

This case illustrates the complexity of the problem of failure to thrive. Clearly the serious anxieties surrounding the child's condition before and after birth had affected the mother–child relationship. The insertion of the pacemaker had changed the situation and the mother had allowed the relationship to become more secure and herself to feel closer to her child.

It is therefore better to understand what is happening in the processes surrounding the child's nutrition than to have an over-inclusive categorisation.

CASE HISTORY 3.2

The parents had brought baby Emma to the clinic because both the health visitor and the general practitioner had told the parents that they were concerned that Emma was not putting on weight as she should and that her growth was falling behind. The health visitor had paid extra attention to the case and given the mother help and advice. During this time she had noted that the mother found it hard to hold Emma when she was feeding her and was much inclined to prop her up with cushions and resting the bottle in such a way that Emma could feed by herself. Emma was inclined to go to sleep during the feed. If father was around during the feeding he did not attempt to intervene, leaving the childcare to his wife. When he was asked whether he would take over feeding Emma at those times he was at home, he said that he felt this would interfere with his wife's routine and that he did not wish to 'meddle' in what she was doing in the home.

It is important to pay particular attention to what contributes to the failure to thrive of the child both from the parental and the child's points of view. The case of the mother and child described in Case History 3.1 highlights a number of issues relevant to the relationship of mother and child, father and child and mother and father, as well as the fact that the child is not growing. Discussions with the parents can bring in issues to do with the feeding, with mother's difficulties about holding Emma, and what thoughts the couple have on why this might be so. At the next stage it might be feasible to explore what holds father back from feeding his child and – as he put it – 'meddle' in his wife's business. When the health visitor asked what Emma's sleeping pattern was like, she was informed that Emma had previously been a poor sleeper, that she would wake and scream in the night, but that during the last 3 months this had disappeared and Emma had her last feed at 20:00 to 20:30 and did not make a noise until 7:00 the following day. The sequence of events is often not 'visible' to the parents and a discussion about what has been noted, particularly if it can be undertaken in a neutral and non-blaming way, can frequently have a positive effect.

Assessment of growth

Normal infants and children never remain static in their physical and mental characteristics, because of the continuing process of growth and development. Understanding the normal patterns of growth and development is essential if the problem of failure to thrive is to be addressed. Data from populations of children relating to growth and development is widely available (for example in Buckler 1979).

Centile distributions

For any given measurement, for example weight or height, the distribution of values within a defined population is conveniently shown on a centile chart. The position on the chart indicates the proportion (or percentage) of the population with values greater or smaller than that of the particular individual measured. Therefore, if the individual lies on the 25th percentile, 25% of individuals will have smaller values and 75% greater values at a given age. Relationships between centiles and standard deviations for a Gaussian distribution are shown in Figure 3.6.

From this, it can be seen that –2 SD from the mean lies at 2.28% and +2 SD at 97.72%, i.e. roughly corresponding to the 2nd and 98th percentiles.

The relationship of a particular measurement to the concept of normality is complex and various factors need to be considered, best summarised in the following statements:

- We should be less interested in the terms 'normal', 'mean' or 'average' and more

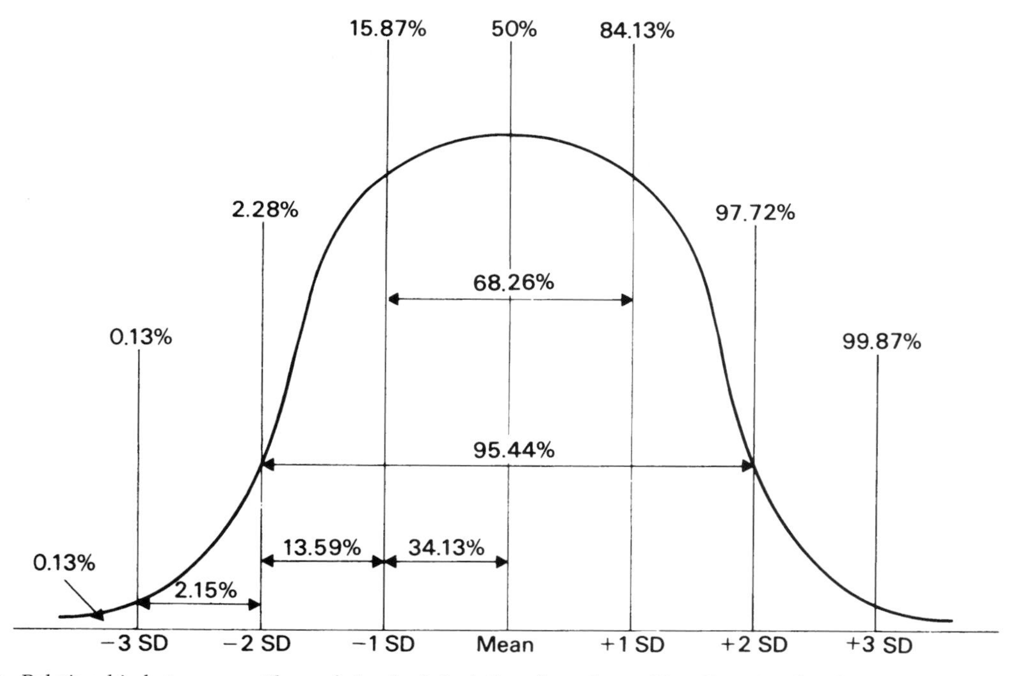

Fig. 3.6 Relationship between centiles and standard deviations for values with a Gaussian distribution. (Reproduced with permission from Buckler J M H 1979 A reference manual of growth and development. Blackwell Scientific, Oxford.)

interested in *optimal* measurements. For example, in some developed countries, there are large numbers of overweight individuals and this has the effect of skewing the distribution. Optimal values relate to those associated with good general health and appropriate development.

- Although it is generally true that the closer one is to the mean value the greater the probability of 'normality', there may be situations – for example when a child has tall parents – where a mean value represents a failure to achieve optimum growth.
- It is necessary to consider a wide range of information when making judgements about growth data.

New centile charts

New centile charts based on the 1993 United Kingdom Child Growth Standards were introduced by the Child Growth Foundation in 1994, replacing the charts compiled by Tanner and Whitehouse in 1965. They reflect increasing size overall of the population and earlier entry into puberty for girls. The standards are based on the indigenous population and do not include centiles for ethnic communities. The charts use nine centiles arranged as shown in Table 3.1.

Common measurements in failure to thrive

Weight

A baby should be weighed nude, an older child in underclothes only. Because instrumental variation is possible, the same scales should be used for serial measurements. The baby is laid on a cloth or paper towels whose weight has been adjusted for. Older children stand on scales, not touching anything or anybody. If a child is fretful or refuses to be weighed, subtraction weight can be obtained with the child being held in an adult's arms.

Table 3. 1 New centile charts

Centiles	SD
99.6th	+2.66
98th	+2.00
91st	+1.33
75th	+0.66
50th	
25th	–0.66
9th	–1.33
2nd	–2.00
0.4th	–2.66

It is reasonable to record weight in kilograms with an accuracy to 0.1 kg (100 g). There is little to be gained from any greater degree of accuracy as minor fluctuations with state of bowel or bladder occur in normal circumstances from day to day. Growth charts usually only permit charting to 100 g. Imperial units (stones and pounds) are now obsolete in professional practice but parents will probably want to know the weight in these units so conversion charts should be available.

Assessing changes in weight; frequency of weighing

Regular weighing of babies is valued by parents and acts as a focus of visits to a clinic or doctor's surgery. Mothers vary in the frequency which they choose for this but, in the first months, the more anxious or less experienced mother may visit weekly whilst others may come less often, perhaps only 2–3 times in the first year of life (Hall 1989).

Guidelines for weight increases are traditionally taught. The average weight gain in the first 3 months is 200 g (7 oz) per week, and 150 g (5.3 oz) in the second 3 months, falling to 40 g (1.5 oz) per week in the second year (Illingworth 1981). According to Illingworth, there is a strong correlation between birth weight and subsequent weight and height in the years up to puberty. If weight gain becomes erratic, static or negative, it will be necessary to follow the child more closely at regular intervals, depending on the situation. It is usually sufficient to weigh the child no more often than weekly and, in many cases, less often, say every 2–4 weeks, in order to check for subsequent growth.

Height and length

Up to the age of 2 years, length is conventionally measured with the infant horizontally extended and firmly held by two persons. A measuring table or infantometer is most accurate, but cheaper alternatives, e.g. Pedobaby, are now widely in use. Measurements (metric) up to 0.1 cm accuracy are made with the feet at 90° and the legs straight. Infants do not particularly enjoy this manoeuvre and poor cooperation can lead to inaccuracies.

Height is measured using a stadiometer or a microtoise fixed to a wall with the child's feet together, without shoes and with the child standing as straight as possible. The child's head should not be tilted and the lower margin of the eye socket should be on the same horizontal plane as the external auditory meatus. Height is usually about 1 cm less than length. It is not customary to measure length or height routinely in clinics or surgeries but the recent working party on Child Health Surveillance (Hall 1989) recommended a single height measurement at age 3 or sooner if the opportunity occurs. If, however, there is concern about a child's weight, and failure to thrive is being considered, measurement of height or length is essential both at assessment and for serial growth monitoring.

Head circumference

Routine measurement of head circumference is used to detect an excessively large or small head. In severe failure to thrive, poor growth of the head may also be observed with head circumference measurements falling across the centiles. The measurement should represent the maximum measurement around the head in the horizontal plane. The tape-measure should be of a non-stretch material and the child's head may need to be held firmly by an assistant or parent.

Mid-upper arm circumference

This measurement of mid-upper arm circumference has been widely used for nutritional screening in the developing world but much less commonly in the UK or USA (Burgess & Burgess 1969, Jellife & Jellife 1969a,b, Frisancho 1974, McDowell & King 1982). There are no readily available centile charts. We have used the measurement most often from the age of 9–12 months as an adjunct to other measurements.

Between the ages of 12 and 60 months, there is only a small increase in the values for the 50th percentile – 15.9 cm at 1 year, 17.0 cm at 5 years for boys and 15.6–16.9 cm respectively for girls, based on Burgess & Burgess (1969). Cut-off points should be derived from clinical assessments including weight and height. Between the ages of 12 and 60 months, the values shown in Table 3.2 have been found to be useful and are presented as instructions for primary care professionals.

In addition to this use of the arm circumference in complementing weight measurements and helping to sort out small normal children from small malnourished ones, serial measurements assist in detecting improvements in nutritional state in failure to thrive. An increase of 0.5–1.0 cm in mid-upper arm circumference as measured by the same examiner usually correlates with a significant improvement in the general appearance and well-being of the child.

There are various methods for taking this measurement, but the simplest one includes the use of a loop of non-stretched tape-measure in gentle apposition measuring against the 10 cm mark so as to give two tape 'ends' for the examiner to hold. The child's arm should be straight and, if possible, relaxed (down by the side). It is not necessary to measure the mid-point of the upper arm accurately in clinical work.

Table 3.2 Mid upper arm circumference (MUAC)

<14.0 cm	Very likely to be a significantly malnourished child and needs skilled paediatric assessment
14.0–15.0 cm	May be malnourished (likelihood greater if age nearer 5 than 1 year). Useful to make a more detailed assessment and monitor future growth
>15.0 cm	Nutrition likely to be reasonable

At school entry (usual age of examinations between 5 and 6 years) add 1.0 cm to each of the above measurements.

Patterns of growth in failure to thrive

The normal situation

There can be differences of professional opinion regarding what does or does not constitute normality in the growth chart, but it is important that the chart is interpreted in the light of other information relating to the child's circumstances. The closer the child is to the mid-point (50th centile), the more confident one can be of normality. The more closely the child follows such a centile the more likely he or she is to be in good health. Most healthy children match height for weight centiles fairly closely – for example if a child is on the 25th centile for weight, it is usual for the height to be fairly close to or on the 25th centile.

Irregularities in the growth chart of a normal healthy child usually reflect the methodologies of measurement. In general, growth is a smooth and continuous process and the longitudinal growth studies of individual children measured regularly under standardised conditions attest to this fact (Tanner 1978).

Abnormal patterns in failure to thrive

Batchelor & Kerslake (1990) describe several abnormal patterns in failure to thrive (Table 3.3).

Falling centiles

Falling centiles are the classic feature of failure to thrive. A fall of one or definitely two major centile lines should trigger concern that the child is failing to thrive.

Table 3.3 Abnormal patterns in failure to thrive

Falling centiles
Parallel poor centiles
Markedly discrepant height and weight centiles
Discrepant family pattern
Retrospective rise
Saw-tooth – erratic fluctuating pattern (also referred to as dipping)

Parallel poor centiles

Many children who fail to thrive appear to go through a situation when their centile position falls and they then take a position of continuing to grow, sometimes rather erratically but parallel to centile line for both weight and height but at a much lower level.

Very often there is a small difference between centile position for height and weight, with the height generally the greater centile. It is now thought that these children adapt to an abnormal situation of poor nutrition and the situation becomes chronic. This is common in medicine where a homeostasis is established in an abnormal situation. These children are undernourished, their growth compromised and there are usually other developmental and educational deficits. Behavioural and feeding patterns also change but the children grow, albeit at a slower rate and the absolute deficit from the 50th centile becomes gradually greater. Only if there is a change in the child's circumstances, for example nutrition, social relationships or environment, will there be a significant change in the growth velocity; sometimes if the child is well adapted to the original environment the change will be slow and gradual. For others, it is more dramatic and allows one to perceive the abnormality of the previous situation. This is the so-called retrospective pattern and is seen when children are taken into care, often for reasons other than growth, and then show a growth spurt in a foster home.

Markedly discrepant height and weight centiles

Other situations where failure to thrive should be suspected include discrepancies in the centile ranking between height and weight and between the individual child and other family members.

Tanner (1978) states that at most ages a person at the 50th centile for height should be within the limits of the 10th and 90th for weight. A person at the 75th centile for height should be within somewhat higher limits for weight, very roughly estimated by moving all the centile lines in the weight chart upwards so that the 50th lies at the printed 75th and then taking the 10th and 90th in this position. It is possible that smaller differences in centile ranking for height and weight may be significant, but Tanner's guidelines are useful. Rate of growth in height in some children appears better preserved than weight, and indeed many of the anthropometric measures of malnutrition depend on assessing the percentage expected weight for height. These deficits are of course more pronounced in children who are not growth retarded but who are malnourished. The relationship between height and weight is complex and its intricacies not within the scope of this text. However, one system found useful in practice is the Cole's slide rule (Cole et al 1981) which enables a weight for height ratio to be calculated, standardising for age. Cole has validated his method and provides a centile ranking for percentage weight for height up to and during puberty. The third centile is at 85%, and figures of 80% or below normally indicate wasting. However, not all children who fail to thrive show height and weight discrepancy, particularly those children who appear to be both nutritionally and emotionally abused. Skuse (1989) discusses these children and suggests that growth hormone secretion is probably dysfunctional, leading to a child who is proportionately stunted and has a low linear growth rate. Such children may appear not to be particularly thin and certainly not wasted but their bone age is likely to be significantly retarded. The child may be growing well but below the lowest centiles and the body proportions remain infantile. There are other behavioural and developmental associations well described in the literature.

Discrepant family pattern

Calculation of mid-parental height is theoretically useful, but this calculation is based on parental attainment of height which is itself influenced by a number of factors including whether the parents themselves failed to thrive as children.

Children who fail to thrive frequently show marked discrepancies from the parent's attained height centiles. Ideally one should measure parents' heights and weights, not just relying on parents' estimates. Certain patterns seem to us to be prominent. Many 'failure to thrive mothers' are thin, underweight and have poor eating habits. These mothers can be seen as representing a generational pattern of failure to thrive. Obviously dismissal of the significance of the child's failure to thrive because the mother (and sometimes father) is also small on the grounds of a genetic predisposition would be unwise if there are other indicators of poor parenting and deprivation in the parent's past. At the other end of the spectrum, some mothers of children who fail to thrive are obese and are frequently trying to diet. This is another manifestation of eating difficulty, and the contrast in these cases between the mother's body build and that of her child is startling.

In some families there is a single child who fails to thrive and stands out from the growth pattern of the siblings and parents; it is always worth measuring and plotting all the children. However, in other families, all the children may show a period of poor growth, sometimes with recovery as they grow older. It is always important, therefore, to look at the whole family in assessing the significance of findings in an individual child.

Retrospective rise

Improvement in a child's centile position may occur if nutrition is improved (Fig 3.6c,d). Children who fail to thrive have a capacity to demonstrate catch-up growth. This was described by Prader et al in 1963 and occurs following recovery from severe illness or malnutrition. Children showing catch-up growth have supernormal rates of increase of weight and height during recovery. During these periods enormous food intakes have been described and foster-mothers have commented that several sizes of shoes and clothes have been outgrown at relatively short intervals. Occasionally brain growth is so rapid that it outstrips growth of the skull, leading to widening of the sutures and confusion with increased intracranial pressure in infants (Capitanio & Kirkpatrick 1969).

Figures 3.7 and 3.8 show periods of catch-up growth in an emotionally abused and malnourished girl. Between the ages of 1 year and 2 years and between 3 years and 4 years there is rapid growth – up to 3–4 times the normal rate.

Saw-tooth pattern

In the saw-tooth pattern, also referred to as dipping (Batchelor & Kerslake 1990), the weight goes up and down, crossing and re-crossing centile positions. Dips may be related to episodes of intercurrent illness, usually infection, but commonly reflect family stress around life events, e.g. parents experiencing difficulty in their relationship, mother feeling depressed, difficulty with childcare or just having a good week or a bad week. 'Ups' often coincide with support being given (e.g. by the general practitioner, health visitor, grandparents); dips indicate when help is withdrawn. Sometimes an association can be seen in some children with physical injury and other forms of abuse, as is well demonstrated in Figure 3.9.

Dips tend to be associated with incidents of injury and improvements in weight with active

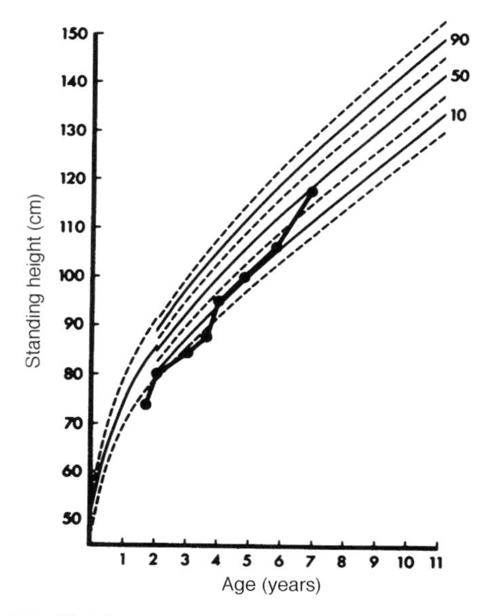

Fig. 3.7 Height chart demonstrating gradual catch-up of height to 50th centile at age 7 years in an emotionally abused child. Same case as Fig. 3.8.

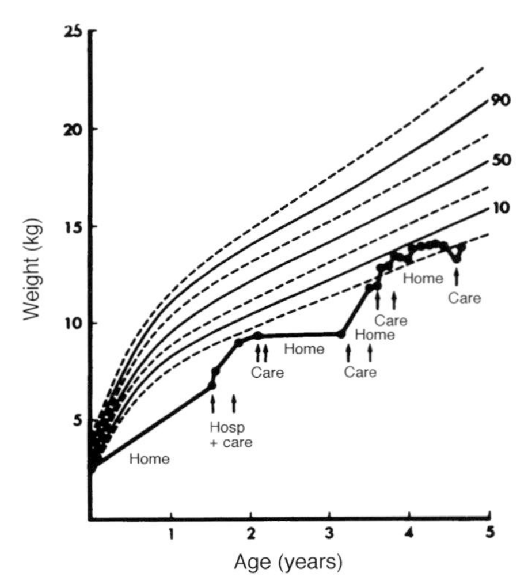

Fig. 3.8 Weight chart demonstrating the use of weights and life events to chart progress in a child with severe emotional abuse and failure to thrive. Prolonged efforts at rehabilitation to parents' care have failed but the child repeatedly shows catch-up growth in substitute care.

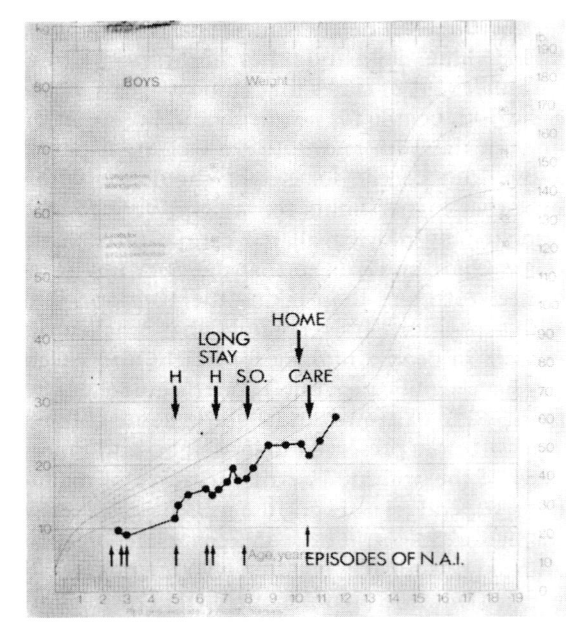

Fig. 3.9 Growth chart of a boy with a long history of failure to thrive and physical abuse demonstrating life events, growth pattern and recorded episodes of physical injury. H, hospital; S.O., Supervision Order; CARE, foster care.

intervention. Actual loss of weight over several weeks is a warning sign that acute intervention is required.

Plate 6b shows this point clearly. This girl started to fail to thrive at around 4 months of age when care was transferred from grandmother to aunt but failure to thrive became more severe at about 11 months when she moved to her natural mother's care. She experienced actual weight loss which culminated in injury at 14 months. She demonstrates catch-up growth in foster-care, in both weight and linear growth. The absence of earlier measurements of length is usual in clinical practice in this area and needs further consideration.

Clinical approach to failure to thrive

Primary identification

Recognition that a child is failing to thrive may be parental, professional or both. Sometimes it is a member of the extended family or a friend who comments that the child is small and/or lagging behind in development. Active denial by parents or professionals is common, making intervention difficult. Initially, assessment may involve regular weighing until a growth pattern has been established and it is clear whether there is a problem or not. Many cases have been missed but with the routine use of growth charts for all children from birth, active health visiting and a greater willingness to comment on the kind of abnormal patterns discussed previously, more cases of failure to thrive will come to attention and before patterns of poor nutrition and growth become firmly entrenched.

Various approaches have been tried to improve detection of failure to thrive in the community. In Newcastle in 1991 a screening service was set up to identify children with poor weight gain (Wright 1995). The criteria used in Newcastle were based on growth velocity calculated using a baseline weight within the first 6 weeks (rather than birth weight which is less reliable) and later weight. The slowest growing

5%, in terms of weight gain, were identified by obtaining weights in the first year of life. This method is preferable to using centile position alone because it identifies more children and earlier. Formal programmes based on routine weighing of all children of this kind are not essential for early identification of failure to thrive as 80% of the children so found were already known by health visitors to be growing poorly (Wright 1996).

Batchelor & Kerslake (1990) discovered that there was widespread failure of health professionals to discover failure to thrive even when they had collected the necessary measurements of growth. In two studies in which they focused on the work of health visitors they found that one in three children whose weight had fallen below the third centile were not recognised by health professionals as children who had failed to thrive.

Reasons for non-recognition of failure to thrive

- a general lack of awareness of the problem.
- Social class: a child under the third centile from an owner-occupying, two-parent family was more likely to be considered 'small'.
- Well cared-for child: a child who shows no signs of being physically neglected in addition to low weight is less likely to be diagnosed as failing to thrive.
- No reported feeding difficulties: if there are feeding difficulties, it is more likely that a child will be identified as failing to thrive.
- Under-use of growth charts: the significance of single or unplotted measurements is less likely to be appreciated than where growth charts are routinely plotted.
- Lack of treatment facilities: where there is little treatment on offer, it is less likely that a child will be recognised and referred.

Batchelor (1996) reported, in a more recent study in the same area, that some improvement in recognition had occurred over a 5 year period. She found that four out of five children under the third centile were recognised as failing to thrive. However, in acknowledging more recent definitions of failure to thrive, a half of all children whose weight had deviated by crossing major centile lines for 3 consecutive months, were not picked up by health professionals.

Paediatric referral and assessment

The paediatrician faced with a child who is failing to thrive must decide how to proceed. Conscious that organic disease can contribute, he or she is faced with the question of whether to investigate for occult organic pathology or not. Goldbloom (1982) reviewed the literature on this question and concluded that

> with no exceptions, the differentiation between organic and psychosocial causes of failure to gain, grow or develop, can and should be based on positive findings, not on exclusion.

In both instances, the history, physical examination and simple observation of family interaction usually suffice to point to appropriate investigation and management. In expressing this view, he quoted Glaser et al (1968) and Sills (1978), and to these can be added Rosenn et al (1980), Homer & Ludwig (1981) and Berwick et al (1982) .

Sills (1978) found, for example, that many laboratory tests had been performed in 185 children with failure to thrive but that out of 2067 tests only 1.4% were of positive assistance and in every case there was a specific indication from the history and physical examination that there was an organic component to the failure to thrive. It is therefore perfectly reasonable and sound practice not to undertake laboratory or other investigations unless there is an indication from the history and examination. Medical investigations which are used to search for occult conditions where the clinical history indicates failure to thrive have been suggested (Hobbs 1994, Wright & Talbot 1996). Of all the investigations shown in Table 3.4, the haemoglobin is the one most likely to produce abnormal results. Raynor and Rudolf (1996) found that 35% of

Table 3.4 Medical investigations in failure to thrive

Test	Condition
Haemoglobin and full blood count	Iron deficiency, coeliac disease
Urinalysis, microscopy and culture	Urinary tract infection, kidney disease
Urea and electrolytes, creatinine	Kidney failure
Liver function tests	Liver disease
Antibodies for coeliac disease	Coeliac disease
Stool for ova and parasites	Giardiasis
Other investigations include:	
Sweat test	Cystic fibrosis
Thyroid function test	Hypothyroidism
Mantoux test	Tuberculosis
Jejunal biopsy	Coeliac disease, giardiasis

their sample of children who failed to thrive were anaemic. This is usually the result of dietary iron deficiency and should be corrected by dietary advice.

The subdivision of failure to thrive into organic and non-organic is somewhat arbitrary and artificial. The boundaries are not clear and there are many cases where the aetiology is complex and multifactorial. It is far better to think of the child who fails to thrive as having a nutritional deficiency and then set about trying to understand the factors responsible. This will then avoid the kind of compartmentalised thinking that says that all children with cerebral palsy who fail to thrive must have chewing and swallowing difficulties and that the only reason that children from poor families fail to thrive is because there is no food in the house.

The next section will briefly indicate the main points to be considered in checking for organic factors and then proceed to discuss non-organic failure to thrive.

Organic factors in failure to thrive

The list of organic factors in Table 3.5 is not exhaustive. Almost any paediatric condition, if severe enough, may interfere with normal growth. Organic factors exist in some children and in a small number of cases may be the principal reason for the failure to thrive. They need to be recognised and treated, but details are not included here.

Table 3.5 Organic factors in failure to thrive

Group 1	
Adequate intake with poor weight gain	Malabsorption, e.g. coeliac disease, cystic fibrosis, occasionally cow's milk intolerance
Group 2	
Inadequate intake due to swallowing difficulties, inability to eat large quantities or vomiting or regurgitation	Central nervous system disease Oesophageal or oropharyngeal malformation Gastro-oesophageal reflux Severe cardiopulmonary disease Chronic infections, e.g. tuberculosis Inflammatory bowel disease, e.g. Crohn's disease Intestinal obstruction, e.g. pyloric stenosis
Group 3	
Conditions interfering with appetite	Metabolic disease, e.g. methylmalonic acidaemia Renal failure Diabetes mellitus and insipidus

Finally, caution must be exercised in the diagnosis of poor growth. A good example is the Russell–Silver syndrome. In this syndrome, which has at its centre failure to thrive, other features described include intrauterine growth retardation, postnatal growth deficiency, normal psychomotor development and various 'soft' dysmorphic features including body asymmetry, clinodactyly and triangular facies. Such patients are presumed to have a genetically based condition which impairs long-term growth potential and is truly an organic cause for failure to thrive. Catch-up growth is not expected and parenting is not a significant issue. The temptation to label a child with failure to thrive as suffering from an organic syndrome is understandable where the parents may reject a non-organic diagnosis as a criticism of themselves.

Saal et al (1985) reviewed previously diagnosed cases of Russell–Silver syndrome and found a heterogeneous picture including cases with global developmental delay as well as those who had shown catch-up growth. The danger of an incorrect diagnosis is that it may prevent further search for treatable conditions including non-organic failure to thrive.

Assessment in non-organic failure to thrive

While the history is being taken (Table 3.6) there should be an assessment including the following points:

- Both parents present: assess the family as a whole, parents' relationship, father's involvement and position of siblings.
- Schedule more than one session: in failure-to-thrive cases the parents are often reluctant to talk about the difficulties.
- Observe parents with child using a positive and respectful stance: valuable information can be obtained by watching patterns of relationships and the way parents and child manage the situation (e.g. who is the child most/least attached to).

Physical examination of child

Measurements to be taken and associated signs of failure to thrive are indicated in Tables 3.7 and 3.8 respectively.

Behavioural and emotional signs

Certain characteristics may be more apparent in children who fail to thrive than in those who do not. Noting these behaviours over a number of years has produced some interesting results. The checklist of common signs (Table 3.9) shows that children in situations such as failure to thrive may hold opposing behaviours in their repertoire which can be puzzling as well as informative for the parents, the observer and the child. In some ways this is of course perfectly ordinary; most human beings are fairly complex and can hold opposing thoughts, feelings and behaviours. As will be clear from the lists shown here this is nevertheless sometimes surprising, though for the purpose of establishing how to intervene it is most helpful.

Observations such as those in Table 3.10 can be made either in the clinical setting or the home, or by video recording the child in either situation. As already indicated, these checklists are included to help to establish a pattern relating to the child who is failing to thrive, not to make a diagnosis of failure to thrive.

Parents of children who fail to thrive

Parents of children who are failing to thrive may present as

- depressed
- mourning, having lost someone close
- in ill health
- stressed
- having eating problems
- neglectful of themselves and children
- having poor maternal attachment to the child
- maternal rejection
- having difficulties in parenting
- having distorted and unrealistic expectations of the child
- lacking in education/knowledge about child care
- too poor to have adequate food in the house.

Iwaniec et al (1988) pointed out that the mothers of these children in particular had recognisable difficulties when they were compared with a group of mothers whose children did not fail to thrive. Others have pointed to difficult histories in the childhoods of mothers whose children fail to thrive. In one study 80% of mothers of children failing to thrive reported that they were victims of abuse as children, significantly higher than the comparison group (Weston et al 1993).

Mothers of failure to thrive children (Iwaniec et al 1988)

- often reported a disturbance in their sense of the child belonging to them
- report that they have little or no pleasure in the baby
- spend less time interacting (talking, cuddling, etc.) with these children
- pick up failure-to-thrive babies/children less often
- smile and talk less to these babies/children
- play less often with the child
- report that they get on better with their other children who do not fail to thrive.

Table 3.6 History in failure to thrive

Feeding history (supplement with diary card, videotaped or direct observation as necessary)	How much, what food, how often? Any difficulties in feeding Refusal, vomiting, spitting or ruminating Who feeds and how successfully? Do parents give up or force?
Pregnancy and birth history	Helps to establish the emotional climate surrounding this child, e.g. was he/she wanted or planned for? Have there been miscarriages or cot deaths? Is this a replacement child?
What kind of child?	Is he/she the wrong sex, appearance, personality? What is easy or difficult about her/him? Contrast with other children in and out of the family
Child's health	Illnesses – infections, hospital admissions Immunisation Physical symptoms, e.g. diarrhoea, vomiting Behaviour – sleeping, crying, tantrums, irritability Developmental history, particularly language and social delay Review of growth chart Identification of major dips and rises in the growth chart
Sibling(s)	Failure to thrive? Health, development, growth (measurements if possible) How is the family spaced?
Parents' history	Other recognised maltreatment Are they married, – if so, happily? What is the quality of their relationship? Are there stresses or tensions, anger? What is their psychological well-being? Do the parents agree the child is too small? Is the parenting good enough?
Mother's history	Health, eating difficulties, depression, good/low coping, energetic/tired, overworked, frustrated, poor self-care Is mother underweight, overweight, dieting?
Father	Present or absent, supportive or rejecting? Caring or distant? Doing the feeding?
Social history	Is this a well-functioning household? Evidence of family dysfunction? Arguments, violence Support systems, relations, friends Alcohol, drugs Bereavement, loss Economic situation – employment, income, debts, expenditure on food Housing, overcrowding, poverty or social exclusion, stress
Professionals and others	Their views, advice, attitudes Names, telephone numbers Who can help? Nursery or playgroups Childminders What is the parent's view of professional advice?

Table 3.7 Measurements in children who are failing to thrive

Weight	Calculate weight and height age (i.e. age at which child's actual height or weight reaches 50th centile) and inform parents
Height	Demonstrate and explain growth chart Assess severity of failure to thrive and pattern: improving, worsening, acute, chronic Comment on nutritional status
Head circumference	
Arm circumference	
Other measurements, e.g. skin-fold thickness, velocity of weight gain or height gain may occasionally be useful	

Table 3.8 Associated signs of failure to thrive

Skin folds, hair, wasting, prominent bones, musculature, e.g. back	Pinch up abdominal skin between finger and thumb Hair fine, scruffy, alopecia Wasted buttocks, thighs Ribs and spinal musculature may appear prominent and outlined
Posture (Krieger & Sargent 1967)	Persistent flexed or folded, especially arms Floppy
Hands and feet	Cold and red 'deprivation' hands and feet
Face	Pale, apathetic, lack of expression
Mouth	Check teeth, dental caries, delayed eruptions, signs of injuries, e.g. traumatic ulcers on palate, torn frenulum
Abdomen	Protuberant
Signs of neglect	Nappy rash, bald patch on back of head, dirty, ungroomed, poorly dressed
Signs of abuse	Bruises, scars, other injury
Behaviours	Quiet, sad, withdrawn, pathetic, overfriendly, attention seeking, indiscriminate, overactive, constantly 'on the go', poor communication
Development	Delay variable Social and language, if severe, gross and fine motor
Signs of organic disease	Depends on nature of condition. General effects on nutrition similar regardless of cause

Table 3.9 Common signs of failure to thrive

Behavioural signs	Emotional signs
Attention seeking	Frantically searching
In perpetual motion	Confused
Restless	Stillness
Overactive	Expressionless
Lethargic	Unresponsive
Withdrawn	Not inquisitive
Going rigid	Diminished vocalisation
Crying	Minimal or no smiling
Noisy	Demanding
Screaming	Sadness
Over-friendly	Depression
Clinging or whining	Detached
Poor language	Insecure
Absence of appropriate play	Anxious
Impaired concentration	Angry
Disturbed sleeping patterns	Frustrated
Destructive (self/others)	Tearful
Poor eating patterns	Rejecting
Fussy or reluctant eater	
Ruminating	
Food fads	
Vomiting	
Fast eater	
Diarrhoea	

Note: It is important to establish both the behaviour and date of onset.

Table 3.10 Observations of child who is failing to thrive

Child	Parents
Poor feeding/eating	Poor interaction with child
Fear of feeding situation	Distant from child
Fear of sitting down	Over-protective and over-intrusive
Fear of food entering the mouth (too hot, too harsh, etc.)	Inability to play with child
Fear of adults	
Poor sleeping patterns	
Note periods without food	
Poor attachment	
Inability to play with others or self	

A mother's perception of her child can be a crucial aspect of how the child is growing. One study (Stratton & Swaffer 1988) investigated the causal beliefs of mothers whose children had been physically abused and found consistent patterns of perception. The mothers tended to see themselves as helpless, and the child as being to blame when anything went wrong. In the same paper a case study of a mother whose child was failing to thrive revealed a remarkably strong tendency to believe that nothing would change in the future. The mothers' attitudes to food and feeding is recognised as influencing how their children grow. Food and eating are used to express much about ourselves and the relationships with other people. When observing children who do not eat well, one can recognise that a child that refuses to eat food a mother has prepared is rejecting so much more than just the food on the plate. The attitudes flowing between parents and children are crucial and it needs to be recognised that the child's refusal is a response to something in the relationship. Sturm & Drotar (1991) reported that in their study 47% of the mothers with children who failed to thrive believed that this related to a physical problem in the child whereas only 6% of the doctors believed that these same children had a physical problem.

It is well worth knowing what mothers and fathers believe their children to be capable of. Sometimes parents have very high expectations which their children cannot fulfil, but parents may believe that if only the child tried he or she would manage to do what the parents wanted. This can happen to the most experienced parents at times and, although the child will not suffer from an occasional misunderstanding about his ability, when the pattern is repeated over and over again and the demands possibly even escalate, the child cannot cope and may show distress (see also Ch. 7). Refusing to eat may be the channel through which the child expresses anxiety.

Overweight or underweight mothers and fathers

The parents' struggle with their weight can have profound consequences on their children. Body image is an issue for both men and women, from the point of view of fashion as well as health. If a parent has a distorted image of his or her body shape this may not only result in difficulties for the parent but may also affect how the parent sees the child and how the parent teaches the child about size and shape.

Because women are usually the ones who prepare food and feed the children, their influence is most often crucial in the feeding situation. The mother's health may be at risk from obesity and she may have specific difficulties feeding her child. In treatment the problems of both mother and child must be addressed. Body & Skuse (1994) reported that children both in the failure-to-thrive and control groups were left to sleep through feeds, but infants who failed to thrive were less often woken to be fed. Why this is happening is an important question to be addressed.

It is well recognised that a mother may feel resentment while preparing food for the child alone. Her own efforts to avoid thinking about food may deny the child's needs. This is not to say that these mothers are harsh or uncaring, though some can be, but to indicate the complexity of the interactions between parents and children. The father's role is essential and if the father is also dieting the difficulties may be multiplied. Parents may also believe that children will grow on minimal food intake – low calorie food and salads, for instance. Also, in our society women's ideal figures are thin and mothers may attempt to reproduce this ideal shape in their child. Under such circumstances children simply may not get enough food as well as receiving the message that they are causing their mother psychological discomfort and putting her under pressure.

Thin and underweight mothers

Another group of mothers whose children may fail to thrive are those who are very thin; they may also diet to keep thin or they may be very thin for other reasons such as poverty, worry, stress and distress. However, these mothers too may use their thinness as a yardstick for the children's growth. Distorted body images can be a result of dieting and a woman who is either very thin or overweight may have a distorted view not only of her own body but also of those around her, including her children. It is hard for those mothers to recognise what is happening and an 'outsider' such as a doctor or health visitor can, in a supportive but firm way, point this out and help the mother to achieve a more balanced image both of her children and of herself. In one study (McCann et al 1994) 26 mothers of children attending paediatric clinics for failure to thrive were compared with 26 individually matched controls. The mothers showed a significantly higher level of dietary restraint. Despite their child's low weight, 50% were restricting the child's intake of sweet foods and 30% restricted foods they considered fattening or unhealthy.

None of the mothers were suffering from clinical eating disorders but their response to their child being underweight appeared paradoxical and raised the question that there may be a causal link between their behaviour and the failure to thrive.

Management of failure to thrive

There can be little doubt that effective intervention is required in failure to thrive. As has been demonstrated, failure of growth and development primarily follows deprivation of calories and food. The thrust of the treatment programme must therefore be to address the nutritional problem, although inevitably there will be other issues arising during the course of treatment which will need to be addressed.

Aims of treatment

- To correct malnutrition and induce catch-up growth.
- To address general issues of parenting to provide the optimal environment for the nurture and care of the child and his or her developmental needs.
- To provide support and care for the parents to assist them in achieving the first two aims, except where it has been decided to seek alternative care for the child.

Two important principals have guided this work:

- The management and treatment is rarely effective if dealt with by single professional input.
- When the medical and psychological aspects of failure to thrive are combined into a single central focus on food and feeding the treatment and management becomes more effective.

Research findings which have influenced management

The most important findings include:

- Deficiency of calories, not protein or other specific dietary deficiency, is the issue that needs addressing, i.e. it is the inadequate quantity rather than quality of the food which is the problem.
- Reduced blood growth hormone levels are in most cases a secondary phenomenon rather than the primary cause of the poor growth.
- Mood changes and difficult behaviours can be the result of chronic lack of food or starvation.
- Children can recover if given supernormal calorie diets, sometimes as much as 50% to 100% above the normal requirements of a healthy child of similar age of normal weight and height. Parents, foster-parents and professionals are often very surprised about the quantity of food the children can consume when they are in a phase of catch-up growth.
- Children can occasionally demonstrate temporary increase in head growth resulting in cranial suture splitting in infants. Benign intracranial hypertension has also been described during phases of rapid catch-up

growth on nutritional rehabilitation in older children and associated with increased growth hormone secretion.
- Catch-up growth was described by Prader et al (1963) and occurs when children who have been growing poorly are given increased calories and make up the growth deficit.
- Psychological issues, particularly the relationship between parents and the child, are paramount in developing a treatment approach.
- Discussion and advice about food and feeding is acceptable to parents and can yield important changes.
- A multidisciplinary team when professionals with knowledge and skills with children work together enhances the chances of bringing about change for the child (Bithoney et al 1991, Hobbs & Hanks 1996).
- Professionals who may be involved in the failure to thrive team are:
  - health visitor
  - clinical psychologist
  - community paediatrician
  - community dietitian
  - nursery nurse
  - social worker.

A clinic for children failing to thrive

The clinic runs for a half day every week. Families are given 30–60 minute appointments with a maximum of 6–7 families attending each week. Many families contain more than one child with difficulties. Two professionals work directly with each family while the others observe and work from behind a screen with the family's full cooperation. Parents, grandparents, other relatives and first-line professionals including social workers and health visitors are variably involved. This model is widely used in complex treatment work with families. A full paediatric assessment is done and clinical investigations organised on the basis of clinical need. Routine laboratory and radiological investigation are undertaken as required.

Difficult cases are referred on the basis of lack of progress from home visiting support by a health visitor. Feeding history and mealtime observation is routinely performed. A parent is asked to complete a 3-day diet diary at home (see Fig. 3.10). This gives an idea of the food and drink, with estimated quantities of what the child consumed during this period. The child's feeding behaviour is often observed in the clinic consultations. A plate of biscuits will often provide a practical way of illustrating a child's hunger to professionals and parents alike.

Weight, height, head and arm circumferences are routinely measured. In addition to standard growth charts which are kept for every child, charts in the parent held record are completed for the parents.

Liaison with primary care professionals – health visitors, social workers, GPs and others – is done by letter, telephone or when they attend the clinic either with the family or for a consultation with the team. The health visitor has a lead role in liaison although all professionals take a part. Good team cohesion and support are vital for this work. High attendance rates can be achieved in a traditionally difficult area of child health. Improvements in the children's growth hopefully reflect real changes in the parent's ability to cope with this difficult problem. Every case is different and success can be achieved with only a proportion. Child protection agencies may need to be involved if real danger to the child is perceived through parents' ability to cope with the problem.

Hospitalisation versus outpatient treatment

The vast majority of children who fail to thrive can be very adequately treated as outpatients. Work with the parents in the home, during visits to outpatient clinics in hospital, in community-based clinics, health centres and other facilities such as nurseries is most helpful.

Hospital treatment is useful when:

- severe failure to thrive, especially in an infant, makes treatment urgent

- extreme anxiety in the parents renders them in need of greater support and some transfer of responsibility for the child
- there is coexistent physical abuse which requires investigation and treatment whilst the child is in a safe environment
- there is concurrent infection or illness.

Advantages of hospitalisation

In theory, at least, the calorie intake of the child can be closely monitored and a carefully prescribed diet administered, having been calculated on the basis of that required for a healthy child of normal weight for the particular child's length, plus an amount for catch-up growth. This will vary, but it is usual to calculate to a figure of 50% on top of the basic requirement (Kempe & Goldbloom 1987).

Energy requirements for catch-up growth

- Usual calorie requirement for healthy child of normal weight for length + 50% extra

or

- 120 kcal/kg body weight × median weight for current length/current weight

The infant's weight can be monitored daily if necessary and signs of associated physical illness monitored. Investigations can be ordered as required and samples such as stool cultures more readily obtained. The parents' responses to the child and their approach to feeding can also be observed, although some parents find the hospital situation threatening and may feel that it serves to emphasise their feelings of inadequacy. However, a supportive and caring ethos can do a great deal to assist parents who are desperate and feel that they are failing in the care of their child. This can provide the initial boost to their confidence and rehabilitation with the child if approached in a way that does not 'take over' the feeding and care of the child. Naturally facilities for resident parents and a welcoming approach to their presence are taken for granted, but parents should also be encouraged at times to get away from the sometimes dreary and boring hospital routine, and attend to their own needs. During the admission the parents' practical involvement in their child's care will increase and they will have an active role in discussions about the time for discharge.

Children with serious feeding difficulties who are slow or at times resistant to feeding may often fare best being fed by a particular member of staff and this can be a highly personal situation. Often the particular nurse for whom the child eats and feeds best is also most able to help the parents. It is usually advantageous for the child to have few carers, especially at feeding times, although in a busy paediatric ward this may not always be possible.

Hospital admission can at best be viewed as the beginning of any treatment programme and a launch for the crucial part of treatment which involves the parents taking full responsibility for their child's nutrition (Haynes et al 1984).

Disadvantages of hospitalisation

If the hospital takes over the parents' role successfully, in that the infant thrives, or unsuccessfully (toddlers in particular may not thrive), this may only serve to reinforce the parents' feelings of hopelessness, frustration or powerlessness to nurture their child. When the child returns home the situation may return to that before the admission or even deteriorate further. If investigations (laboratory tests, radiography) are undertaken and found negative, a false reassurance that all is well may be transmitted to the parents who may feel that the child 'has been treated'. Similarly, children should be on an ordinary diet without high-density calorie supplements. Failure of the child to gain weight in hospital (not uncommon if wards are very busy with seriously ill children), may provide a reason for acceptance of continuing failure to thrive and discourage further intervention.

The reasons, aims and conduct of hospital admission must therefore be clearly considered and discussed with the parents and staff on the ward if useful outcomes are to be achieved from the short-term manoeuvre.

Hospital practice in failure to thrive

- Assemble a detailed weight chart from birth. Height and head circumference measurements should also be included. Parental height should be recorded and, if applicable, parental weight.
- A detailed medical history should be taken including relevant symptoms, feeding difficulties, behavioural problems and a social history.
- Physical examination must include:
  - full system examination
  - description of child's appearance
  - any signs of neglect (clothing, cleanliness, hair and nails,
  - nappies/rash, infestation, pallor, dental caries.
  - assessment of whether child appears 'ill' or not.
- Developmental assessment.
- Dietary assessment should take place in every case ideally by a paediatric dietitian in conjunction with medical and nursing staff.
- Nursing observations should include:
  - food intake chart
  - identity of feeder
  - description of how fed
  - qualitative and quantitative intake
  - regular weighing including admission and discharge weight.
- Investigations
  - every child to have Hb, FBC, U & E, MSU
  - other investigations as indicated by clinical symptoms and examination findings, and after discussion with senior team members.
- A clear diagnostic formulation must be made (organic and non-organic factors) and written in the records.
- Management plan: a clear plan should be formulated involving hospital staff and parents and communicated to community staff (health visitor, general practitioner, social workers or others) at discharge. The plan should describe:
  - what the problem is
  - what needs to be done
  - who will help
  - what the follow-up is.
- Clear arrangements for follow-up must be made before discharge and contingency plans should planned follow-up fail.

Outpatient treatment

For detailed discussions of outpatient treatment see for example Iwaniec & Herbert (1982), Iwaniec et al (1985), Hanks et al (1988), Ayoub et al (1989), Schmitt & Mauro (1989).

Methods for assessing nutritional intake, including assessment in the home (Moores 1996), are shown in Table 3.11. An assessment of the food intake of the child can be made in the home by the parents and forms an integral part of the programme. The parents are provided with an open diary card (see Fig. 3.10) with an instruction sheet which requests that they record as accurately as possible what the child eats and drinks, providing times, quantities and brands, if appropriate, of manufactured food. It is reasonable to ask for this to be completed over 2–3 days and then to be returned for analysis. If the services of a paediatric dietitian are available then a detailed analysis can be undertaken.

Information from the daily dietary diary

- Total calorie intake (can be expressed as a proportion of the estimated average requirement (EAR) for a child of that age as stated in Dietary Reference Values (DoH 1994)
- Range and variety of foods given
- Frequency of food/drink intakes and the length of intervals between them, giving a pattern of feeding
- Variation from day to day

Table 3.11 Methods for assessing nutritional intake

Method	Comments
Weighed food intake	Difficult, needs high motivation, equipment expensive, precise results
Dietary history	Takes time and skill
24-hour recall	Quick, limited, inaccurate
Food diary	Used by parent, gives additional information to food intake

A dietary record can be a helpful source for discussion and the development of advice on a practical level as well as a baseline instrument which can show positive as well as negative results of feeding a failure-to-thrive infant or child.

A diet diary can be very simple, and may be repeated at intervals and comparisons made. Records may of course at times be falsified, and 'food lies' appear on the record sheet. There are ways of detecting this. A diet sheet which is placed in the kitchen usually comes into contact with food; through its use it becomes creased and the handwriting is neither even nor the same and differences from meal to meal can be spotted. The reasons for under-reporting and over-reporting can form the basis for important hypotheses:

- Why should this have occurred?
- Is the parent feeling uneasy and why?
- Has the parent an inkling that the child requires more food and that they should provide it?
- Could under-reporting point to listlessness, tiredness, helplessness and possibly depression in the parent?
- Could over-reporting indicate that the parent/s are concerned lest they be seen as not feeding their child adequately and are therefore now overcompensating?
- Are they hiding something, if so what and why?

It is well recognised that parents whose children are failing to thrive often have low self-esteem and the fact that they cannot give their children adequate nourishment is another blow to their psychological well-being. Bringing these issues out in the open has been found to be a turning point in many cases.

A suitable dietary record and guidelines to accompany it are shown in Figures 3.10 and 3.11.

The help of the dietitian can be invaluable at this point. Once a diary has been kept, the items of food can be converted into calorie and energy units and form another discussion point with the parents, including giving them advice on how much children need at any given time in their development to grow adequately. Parents rarely find this threatening and usually manage to contribute considerably. It quite often stimulates their curiosity and a dietitian is then able to make helpful suggestions as to how diet can be varied, what foods are over-represented or under-represented in the existing diet, etc. This discussion adds a different dimension to the whole issue and can be made to be therapeutic for both parents and child.

Child's name:
Date of birth:
Date record started:
Where is the child (home, hospital):

Time (o'clock)	Day 1	Day 2	Day 3
1 a.m.			
2 a.m.			
3 a.m.			
4 a.m.			
5 a.m.			
6 a.m.			
7 a.m.			
8 a.m.			
9 a.m.			
10 a.m.			
11 a.m.			
12 (midday)			
1 p.m.			
2 p.m.			
3 p.m.			
4 p.m.			
5 p.m.			
6 p.m.			
7 p.m.			
8 p.m.			
9 p.m.			
10 p.m.			
11 p.m.			
12 (midnight)			

Fig. 3.10 Dietary record.

Many mothers, and it is usually the mothers who fill in the diet sheets, will record what the children have eaten. However, as already indicated, this is emotionally a taxing task; it can lead to the mother having to face the feeding difficulty and this can be very upsetting. Some mothers find it very hard because on one hand they genuinely wish to cooperate with the task but on the other they cannot face up to the stark realities of their child's food intake. This may lead to the mother filling in the record sheet just

Keeping a food chart will help me to get a good idea of which foods your child enjoys eating.
Please follow these guidelines when filling in the chart:

- Record everything that your child eats and drinks on all three days, including anything during the night.
- Record the time, type and amount of food eaten.
- Use handy measures to give an idea of quantity, e.g. 1 cup/mug, number of tablespoons/dessert spoons/teaspoons.
- Only record what food is eaten or drunk even if you have offered more. e.g. 1 slice of toast – ate only half.
- Record the brand name of the food if using ready-made meals or foods, e.g. Findus Fisherman's Pie.
- Record as you go along as it is difficult to remember at the end of the day.

Fig. 3.11 Food chart guidelines.

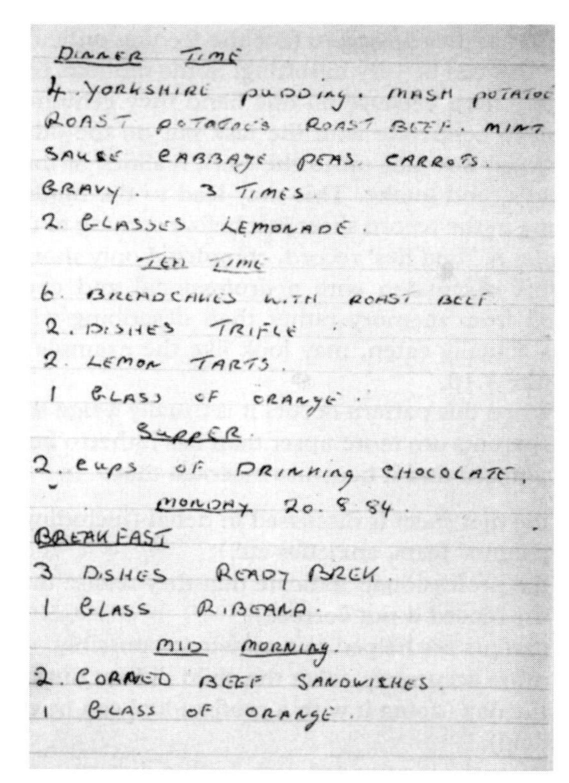

DINNER TIME
4. YORKSHIRE PUDDING. MASH POTATOE
ROAST POTATOE'S ROAST BEEF. MINT
SAUSE CABBAGE PEAS. CARROTS.
GRAVY. 3 TIMES.
2. GLASSES LEMONADE.
TEA TIME
6. BREADCAKES WITH ROAST BEEF.
2. DISHES TRIFLE.
2. LEMON TARTS.
1 GLASS OF ORANGE.
SUPPER.
2. CUPS OF DRINKING CHOCOLATE.
MONDAY 20. 8. 84.
BREAKFAST
3 DISHES READY BREK.
1 GLASS RIBEANA.
MID MORNING.
2. CORNED BEEF SANDWISHES.
1 GLASS OF ORANGE.

Fig. 3.12 'Food lies' – one page out of a diary kept by a mother of her child's eating habits. All the pages were in the same hand and pen. The child was seriously underweight.

before coming to the clinic. A 'food lies' record, completed only shortly before discussion with a professional and compiled from memory rather than describing what was actually eaten, may look like the example in Fig. 3.12.

When this pattern occurs it is usually a sign that the parents are more upset than has hitherto been recognised and it becomes essential that:

- the diet sheet is discussed in detail (including parents' fears, anxieties, etc.)
- the professionals indicate that they realise that the record is not correct
- parents are helped to reconstruct, possibly more accurately, what the child did eat during the day (doing it with a professional can be of help)
- parents are provided with further dietary information if this is required
- enquiry is made about their cooking facilities (Have they got a cooker, gas, electricity? How much money is available for food during the week? Is this a problem?)
- the professional enquires whether mother filled in the sheet or did she have to ask someone else to do this because she cannot read or write, or has difficulties with such tasks?

Depending on the circumstances of the family, there may be further issues which are relevant and need further exploration. Such interventions can be powerful and help the mother/parents to develop ways and means to feed the child in such a way that the child gains weight.

Common patterns revealed by the diet diary

- Reduced total daily calorie intake. This is the most usual finding, as expected, and results from infrequent meals and low total intake.
- Strict 'three meals per day'. There are few opportunities for the child to feed between meals, with long intervals and no intake. 'Night starvation' is frequently a feature. Drinks may also be limited. Intervals of between 12 and 15 hours between intakes of food are not uncommon.
- 'Healthy' diet. Food consists of low fat, low energy, density foods. This has also been termed the 'muesli belt syndrome' as it tends to occur in those sections of society who are health conscious about what they eat. Dietary fibre may be high, leading to satiation, but total energy intake is too low (Roberts et al 1979, Sinatra & Merritt 1981).
- Chaotic pattern. This is characterised by little pattern and wide variation between the individual days. The child may receive sufficient on one day but substantially less on another.
- Over-optimistic or 'food lies'. Occasionally parents express what they would like to think the child is eating or what they think the doctor or health visitor wishes to hear. Two Weetabix for an 18-month-old child for breakfast is a lot – some adults find this difficult to manage.
- Refusal pattern. Parents repeatedly record that the child refuses what food is offered.

Time-spans between meals

Children who are already failing to thrive do not manage well on three meals a day and need to have food offered more frequently. This can often conflict with what the parents have been taught to do, which is not to give children food between meals because it spoils their appetite for the main meals. Rigid frameworks and feeding schedules are still much more likely to be applied, particularly when one or both parents experience difficulties around the topic of eating. It is interesting to note how hard it can be for a mother to feed her child between mealtimes if she feels this is outside her normal routine.

The diary of food intake gives a clear view of the eating pattern for the child. It also shows the actual time-spans between food intake. As illustrated in the case material, children who fail to thrive often cannot manage without food for the entire night. This is more easily recognised for small neonates and babies in the first few months, but not for the child as he grows older. Two- or three-hourly feeding schedules are acceptable for the baby but may also have to be thought of when an older child is not managing to eat and grow.

There may be worries that the child might become spoilt and not give up the little meals and frequent feeding, spoiling the child's appetite for the main meals. However, once children gain weight and catch up, they themselves are more satisfied, less restless or listless and manage to learn new things, including the fact that mealtimes will eventually become more spaced and fit into a routine which suits the whole family, not only the child. Both parents and professionals are often concerned with this 'spoiling' aspect and may need reassurance that children are adaptable and will learn to eat at different times.

Observation of feeding practice

An important aspect of management is observation of the child being fed (Table 3.12). Where possible it is best to do this in the child's home and in the usual situation in which the child is fed. Recording of observations on videotape, if available, is also acceptable to many parents and enables the session to be played back and viewed and discussed with the parents if they wish. Sometimes additional information is available on reviewing which was not noticed when the

Table 3.12 Observation of feeding practice
Feeding behaviour
Interactions between parents and child
Hierarchy of family members, i.e. who is served first
Position and social arrangements for eating
Type and presentation of food
Quantity of food offered (including differences between members of the family)

feeding took place. Feeding observation allows information to be obtained on feeding behaviour, parent–child interactions and the emotions surrounding feeding. It also allows assessment of the child's eating patterns, intake, hunger and interest and any abnormal or unusual behaviour. How the child is held, whether he or she is allowed to participate, how hot or cold the food is, its appearance and presentation to the child are also noted. The parents should be asked to feed the child in the usual circumstances and setting which would occur if the observation was not being made.

In order to carry out observations from feeding we have developed a way of analysing certain aspects of the child's and carer's feeding (see Table 3.13). These observations can be altered so that they fit a specific feeding situation.

CASE HISTORY 3.3

After seeing a 4-year-old girl who was failing to thrive in the outpatient clinic for some months without improvement, it was decided to visit the child's home and observe her feeding.

She was the middle child of five and her other four sisters appeared to be thriving well. The children ate in the kitchen, the food was distributed by the father and then eaten with the parents sitting apart in another room. The food was distributed in quantity according to a well-established formula which the father knew and could explain. The oldest child, aged 9, received the most, about 2–3 times that which the child who was failing to thrive received. The other three children, including a 2-year-old, also received more than her. The father explained that it was pointless to give her more food because she would not eat it and it would probably land on one of the other children's plates. The child confirmed the father's prediction and ate very little in comparison to her sisters.

Table 3.13 Mealtime and presentation of food

Is there a table?
Is there a chair?
Is it fun for everyone there?
Where is the TV?
Is there a plate?
Is there a spoon, a fork, a cup to eat and drink with?
Is the food too hot or too cold?
Is there too much or too little?
Is the food in too-large pieces or is it in liquid form?
Is it too spicy?
Is the child fed by mother, father or siblings or others (what relationship to child)?
Does the child eat alone?
Does the child eat with mother?
Does the child eat with father?
Does the child eat with siblings?
Does the child eat with others (and their relationship to child)?

CASE HISTORY 3.4

A boy of 15 months had been failing to thrive from about 4 months of age. He had had many infectious illnesses including bacterial meningitis but it was felt that his failure to thrive was primarily the result of inadequate feeding. His mother was a slim, unsupported single parent who negated most of the advice which had been offered, predicting that nothing would work. She said that he usually refused much of what was given him.

A feeding session was recorded in the home. The child was fed a large bowl of stew by spoon, initially with him standing with a toy in his hand. He started to refuse but his mother then held him tightly and encouraged him, eventually giving him a good-sized portion. Towards the end of the feeding both she and the child appeared to become more relaxed and she interacted in a warm and encouraging way with him. On viewing the film later, it was noticed that steam was rising from the food and it could be seen quite clearly that the child pulled back as the first mouthfuls of food touched his mouth. The mother said she did not wish to see the film but the temperature of the food was discussed. Shortly after this the child started to thrive quite dramatically after a long period with little weight gain. The reasons, however, were not clear.

CASE HISTORY 3.5

A 3-year-old girl was brought by her parents because she was failing to thrive and because there were a number of behaviours which made it difficult for the parents to care for her. The girl would not sleep, was restless day and night, clinging to her mother and generally a miserable little girl. The parents, from a middle-class background, had an older child who had never presented them with such difficulties. The girl had recently begun to refuse food altogether and would go for long periods of time (e.g. from breakfast to teatime) without taking nourishment. The mother had a difficult relationship with the child and she felt that this child did not give her half the pleasure the older one gave her at the girl's age or now. It was agreed that the child would be videotaped during feeding and her behaviour discussed with the parents. A suggestion to offer the child small amounts of food on an hourly basis for a short time was an easier task for father than for mother. The child went to bed at about 19:30 but would regularly wake up and cry. The father had begun to give the child food and drink if she woke up during the night, despite the fact that this caused disagreement between the parents. However, they came back with the girl and reported that she was sleeping better when father was there to feed her at night. The child had indeed put on weight.

Sometimes the interventions seem unorthodox, as in this case, but what can also be observed is that behavioural and physical changes take place. The little girl in this case was reported to sleep better, demand food, allow father to feed her, smile and play with her mother and other children. Mother in turn found the child easier and said that she had become a little more patient with her and no longer felt so helpless.

Most parents have no difficulties in recognising what kind of food children need at certain ages, even when they are failing to thrive. However, it is important to check with the parents that they are aware of the dietary needs of their children and that they have adequate facilities to meet their children's needs. Again, a checklist can assist the practitioner and parents to look at what might be missing. Not every family has a cooker or electricity and gas, so it is important to know whether food can be cooked (Table 3.13).

Eating is a social activity during which much is learnt and experienced. Children do not often like to eat on their own, however difficult they may find the alternative. Hearing mother and father talking, and watching how the siblings interact with each other and the parents, grandparents and visitors are vital socialising factors. Learning how to eat food and what the rules are in the family makes eating into a very important experience. Children are influenced by this in many ways and their attachments are shaped during such interactions. Mealtimes are much more crucial than one would at first glance believe, particularly in a family setting, and the ways of doing things are often reproduced in an intergenerational pattern. How mother and father were fed as babies and children, and how they experienced mealtimes while growing up, will be remembered when they are parenting and feeding their children. In order to intervene and help the child to grow when he is failing to thrive, some if not all of these issues need to be understood in order to achieve change.

Type of food

Less emphasis is generally given to what is fed as it is usually quantity that is lacking. However, inappropriate diets, late weaning practice and over-reliance on junk-food snacks, e.g. sweets and the like, will need to be addressed at some stage. What is emphasised is that 'eating to thrive' is necessary for children to catch up. Children thrive if

- they are provided with three meals a day
- have energy-dense foods
- are offered snacks in between meals
- are not forced to eat
- have the opportunity for relaxed mealtimes together with their families or carers.

Parents should be advised to avoid substitute, synthetic or medicalised food supplements. Advice which relates to parent's financial and food preparation resources is essential. Cheap, value-for-money foods such as bread, milk, potatoes, eggs, baked beans, spaghetti, etc. should be emphasised, rather than more expensive meat or manufactured food products. The ability to cook and prepare food must not be taken for granted; gentle exploration of the parents' knowledge and skills should be sought before advice is given. Advice must be coordinated if more than one professional is involved with the family, and networking is crucial. Contradictory statements lead to confusion and resentment.

Cultural issues need to be discussed sensitively and on an informed basis. Parents from different cultures are often only too willing to explain food values, customs and childcare issues practised in their culture.

The use of video recording meal times with the child

As already indicated in the section on observation of feeding practice, video recordings of children and families eating can highlight a wonderful array of interactions and behaviours, which may provide many clues to the child's and family's problems about eating and failure to thrive. As mentioned earlier, mealtimes can be a socially highly rewarding time, and a platform for children to learn and communicate with their parents and each other. It has been recognised over time that the video recording as such can be a therapeutic process if undertaken sensitively.

The issues of recording the child's feeding situation, or the family's mealtime, must be discussed with the parents, and their anxieties about being scrutinised, watched and criticised must be dispelled. The video recording should not serve to criticise parents, but be used to explore aspects of the situation with them sensitively. Often, distraught parents do not realise how difficult mealtimes have become for everyone when a child is failing to thrive, will not eat, and is generally difficult at this time. Food is a powerful psychological weapon between children and their parents at the best of times and mealtimes can escalate into a battleground for all. It may also be important to make video recordings at intervals, so that progress can be noted, particularly when the progress is at first slow.

Watching the video together with the parents and the child can often be a moving experience, particularly when parents recognise their struggle as well as the child's difficulties. Video recordings can produce the same experience as one might have when looking at a painting for the first time, then coming back and looking at it again and discovering that something was simply not seen the first time round; was that apple really on the ground? Did the child really keep the food in her mouth for 3 minutes before spitting it out?

Some patterns of eating which can be observed

- Does the child eat on his/her own or with family?
- Does the child eat off his/her own plate or off others?
- How long does the child take to eat?
- What does the child do when he/she has had enough?
- Does the child like to be fed or eat by him/herself?
- What are the family patterns and rules during mealtimes?
- Does the child use fingers or implements?
- What do the parents prefer?
- What likes and dislikes has the child?

There are many more patterns which can be gleaned from such a recording, both on a micro level (details of interactions, feeding, etc.) and a macro level (family patterns, emotional atmosphere, etc.).

The parents sometimes request a copy of the recording and this can be an important moment. However, it should be stressed here, and explained to the parents, that it can be very painful for all concerned to have only a record of the poor feeding situation and that in such a case another recording showing the child eating when changes have taken place is vital. It might be possible to edit two parts of a video together and show the child at different periods in time. A video recording should not be kept by the parents in order to show how difficult mealtimes have been for parents and child, because this could be used punitively towards the child.

As with all interventions, when taking video recordings in order to help develop interventions and changes for the family, ethical considerations need to be thought through. The filming must be done in the child's and family's interest, and the family must know about it in advance and have the chance to give proper informed consent.

These considerations and the actual videotaping of mealtimes can bring parents and those who are attempting to help them together in a common quest to look at the difficulties and then attempt to work together in order to bring about change. This kind of intervention does not have to be threatening; it can be viewed positively, and even introduce some light-heartedness and fun.

The role of the father in interventions

Increasingly, more fathers wish to be involved when their child is failing to thrive and it cannot be sufficiently stressed how valuable their contribution in the intervention can be. It must be also pointed out that the father can of course be an important contributing factor to the child's failure to thrive. Though we have used the terms 'mother' and 'parents' predominantly, all our thinking applies to fathers as much as to mothers, whether one or the other parent figure is in the primary childcaring role.

Management of denial

Many parents will maintain that the child receives sufficient food and may be angry at the implication that the child's nutrition is inadequate to encourage normal growth. It is as well to emphasise that there is no criticism or blame attached to this situation but that in order for the child to gain weight more quickly he or she will require additional food over and above the present intake. It is quite common, however, for parents to continue to deny the link with food, even when the child begins to thrive. It is important not to be drawn into and accept the parent's denial. 'Everyone in our family is small and he is very healthy, so I don't know what all the fuss is about after all' may be taken as an open invitation to discharge the child from the clinic. It is obviously in the child's interest to resist this and maintain an objective professional view for the parents even if it attracts anger and disbelief.

Iwaniec (1996) pointed out that there is still comparatively little awareness and understanding among professionals. In her experience some mothers who were rightly concerned about their children's poor growth were dismissed 'as worrying about nothing' and told that the child would grow out of it. Parent-held records should improve this situation, but only if professionals are able to respond appropriately.

There are other issues which may fall under this heading and they relate to professionals being at times either enmeshed with the family and, like them, unable to see that a child may fail to thrive, or they may have been brought up on a very strict 'behavioural diet' themselves and so believe that eating between meals will spoil a child and must be avoided. Consequently, our advice of eating to thrive may not fall on fruitful ground. Batchelor (1996) discusses the issues of recognition and points out that though there seems to be a level of improvement in recognising and referring children when they are failing to thrive, there is still much room for improvement.

The use of growth monitoring

An important part of management is the continued monitoring of the child's growth. At the initial assessment the parents will have been shown the child's growth pattern and his or her weight age given – for example a 4-year-old girl whose weight is 12 kg (about 1 kg below the third centile) is said to have the weight of an average 2-year-old girl. Parents can be given their own growth charts, and with the introduction of parent-held records this should become standard practice. At the commencement of treatment, intervals for further measuring should be discussed and agreed with the parents. In the initial stages weekly or fortnightly measurements are usual if the parent's efforts are to be sustained. As the situation improves less frequent weighing may be appropriate. Too much concern about weighing without other aspects of treatment can be counter-productive, and weighing by itself is unlikely to achieve much.

It is useful to give parents some idea of what is a reasonable weight gain so that they can have something to aim at. The improvement which may occur as weight increases provides feedback and further encouragement. The family may come to recognise good weeks and bad weeks and begin to understand how the child's weight fluctuates with the overall situation at home or with how the parents are feeling. Fluctuations in weight in children who fail to thrive are very common and these can be discussed. After a while parents learn to judge whether the weight gain is good or not even before the child is put on the scales and in this they come to feel more in control of the situation.

Targets are very important and the second centile is often a useful one to aim for, although for most children more catch-up is essential. It must be recognised that the second centile is only the lowest point on the centile chart and that for almost all children it does not represent their optimal chances for growth. The height centile can also be a useful guide to produce a target for weight in children with a wide discrepancy.

Although children are often weighed every 2–3 weeks, an opportunity to discuss the child's progress should in general be given every month. Less frequent attendance than this is not as helpful, especially at the most active stage of treatment. Once progress is being made and catch-up is occurring consistently, less frequent appointments can be an encouragement but it is wisest to keep in touch for a while afterwards or ensure that continual help and advice is available from another source, e.g. health visitor, general practitioner.

Education

There are many parents with children who fail to thrive who lack basic information about nutrition and malnutrition. Emphasis is put on the usefulness of teaching cooking skills and how to choose the appropriate food for children according to their age. Self-help groups can be of value, particularly if they can be housed in a community-based centre and supported by a professional such as a dietitian or health visitor. Some of the reading material provided by the National Dairy Council or the Health Visitors Association, for instance, is helpful. However, when one considers the number of people at present who cannot read, who have difficulties reading or do not like reading, it becomes clear that providing information by such means alone will not assist all groups of parents. It simply cannot replace the human contact, modelling and teaching which professionals and some voluntary groups have to offer.

Intervention

'Intervention' in this context is probably a more accurate term than 'therapy' or 'treatment', because it is easier to convey to parents and professionals alike that it is possible to be of help to this group of people, though this can sometimes be quite difficult. Chapter 15 outlines the different therapeutic interventions that can be offered and what is needed in the way of training to carry them out.

From what has been described so far, there is no doubt that complex medical, psychological and social dimensions are at work in cases of non-organic failure to thrive. Intervention is essential for all concerned. The benefits for these children and their families when professionals have worked as a team have been particularly highlighted. Dietitians, health visitors, nursery nurses, doctors, psychologists and social workers all have something useful to offer (see Table 3.14).

Strict or unusual diets

With a far greater acceptance and availability of 'health foods', some parents have turned to vegetarian, vegan or other diets which are very restricting. Although adults may experience no difficulties with such diets, children, particularly small ones, do not manage to thrive.

CASE HISTORY 3.6

Tina was 11 months when her parents, who were both strict vegetarians, realised their daughter was thinner and smaller than other children and was falling below the tenth centile on the weight chart. They were encouraged to feed Tina more food more often and to keep a food diary. It became clear from the food diary that Tina would be given

Table 3.14 Multidisciplinary approach to failure to thrive

Professional group	Involved	Role
Health visitor	All cases	Recognition, prevention, advice re feeding, diet and childcare Empowerment of parents
General practitioner/ Community health doctor	Most cases	Surveillance/recognition, referral Support for family Care of parents' and child's health
Paediatrician	Referred cases (HV/GP)	Assessment, advice re cause and necessary treatment Recognition of illness factors Follow-up coordination
Dietitian	Selected cases Depends on availability	Dietary assessment and advice Support for other professionals and family
Child psychologist/child psychiatrist	Complex cases Disturbed families	Management of complex parent–child relationships Support and encourage positive parenting Psychotherapy for family
Social worker	Where associated with abuse, social deprivation	Child protection, case work, resource finding Statutory function
Others, e.g. nursery, family aide, home care worker, home-start	Selected cases	Promote parenting skills, support parents, assist with child's care

Note: close cooperation between the professionals involved with the family is essential, and joint working is ideal.

cold cooked potato, carrot or other vegetable, which she did not like. She also refused brown bread unless it was spread with jam or honey, which the parents did not keep in the house. The parents reported that Tina did not want the food they were eating, despite the fact that they would mash it and select some of the things she seemed at times to favour. On observation it became clear that both parents brought variety and flavour into their diet by using hot spices, like curry, and it was only when mother cooked totally separate meals for Tina that they realised that Tina did not cope even with lightly curried foods. This caused a dilemma for the parents, because they did not wish to cook totally separate meals for their child.

This is an ongoing problem which is not easy to resolve. As already stated, the self-esteem of parents with children who fail to thrive is often already low and suggestions need to be carefully phrased at times so as not to further demoralise the parents. However it must be stressed that facing the issues is an important aspect of the intervention and professionals must be clear of the likely consequences for the child if there are no changes in management. Denial or thinking that the subject must only be raised very delicately would be detrimental for the child because in cases such as Tina's the weight loss can be rapid and associated behavioural problems quick to follow.

Tina stopped crawling, would demand to be carried all the time, did not sleep easily at night, whined continually and became more miserable and could only be pacified if mother offered her the breast. After a while she would refuse all solid food and only take the breast. Both parents needed considerable support at that time. They had become very angry and felt their daughter was rejecting them. There were times when they could cope more easily if it was suggested by a professional that Tina was probably ill and needed investigation in hospital, rather than accepting that what Tina needed was special food appropriate to her age rather than the food the parents ate. Once the 'deadlock', particularly between Tina and her parents, but also between the parents and professionals, was broken and Tina received ordinary baby food, things eased. The food was vegetarian, but cooked with a baby's taste buds and needs in mind. Tina began to smile again and generally became less clingy as she recovered and put on weight.

The balance of vegetarian or other specialised diets needs careful monitoring. Small children do not thrive on what are irreverently called 'muesli belt diets' or cult diets (Roberts et al 1979). Parents may need considerable help in preparing food for their children when they themselves are on such diets. Parents may often feel criticised if dietary changes are suggested and become defensive in a way that makes it difficult to find a way for their children to grow.

Diets related to failure to thrive in children

- Parental food fads
- Strict vegetarian/vegan or Zen macrobiotic diets
- Diets high in carbohydrates, high in fibre, low in fat, and vitamin deficient
- Breast-feeding at an inappropriate age to the exclusion of other foods

The doctor, dietitian, health visitor or other professional may need considerable skills to discuss these issues with the parents and help them to work out a diet which will suit the child. The experience of grandparents can at times be very valuable, though the dynamics need to be understood by the professionals and great care has to be taken to empower the parents. If the family can be united in the task of helping with the feeding of the child it may relieve much of the tension that can develop in these situations. Not being able to feed one child can undermine the fundamental role of the parents and can lead to considerable lack of self-esteem, particularly in the mother.

Failure to thrive is often experienced as a major crisis which can escalate into a life-or-death situation for many babies, small children and their mothers. Mother's feelings of inadequacy have often reached a low ebb and may be worsened when others – nurse, friend or grandparent – can feed the child adequately. Parents often indicate that they have become demoralised and distressed by the feeding process. Some rally their psychological defences and come to believe that their children are the same as others in the neighbourhood, ignoring the evidence of the weight chart and other signs of their child failing to thrive. Professionals may join in this defensive manoeuvre and strengthen this parental belief, often by pointing out children who are thinner. This may produce comments like 'there are many children thinner in the neighbourhood and little Emma is just taking after her mother, who was small as a child too'. On the other hand, parents realise the seriousness of the situation and recognise the often destructive pattern they are in. These parents are often distraught and feel helpless to effect change in the eating behaviour of their child. A vicious circle is often the outcome for both groups, with an unhelpful preoccupation about food associated with a high level of tension. Neither position is conducive to change.

Attachment

The theme of attachment will emerge throughout this book and will be related to the different forms of child maltreatment. The concept of attachment is integral to any discussion of failure to thrive and parent–child behaviour. Attachment is a certain relationship without which human beings have difficulties to exist. The development of a baby's secure attachment takes place during the first year of life. These attachment figures are usually the main carers for the child and they provide the young child with a base from which to explore the world and helps to ensure that the child's needs are met. Bowlby (1969, 1973, 1980), Ainsworth et al (1978), Crittenden (1988), Crittenden & Ainsworth (1989) and Parkes et al (1990) have researched and written extensively on the attachments between human beings, and specifically about the attachment needs of the infant and child. The small child shows attachment behaviour by insisting on close proximity to a few specific individuals, with mother and father figuring high on the list. Attachment needs relate to close, emotionally powerful relationships between two of more people in which each of them seeks for closeness. Children and adults alike feel more secure when they are close to an attachment figure. Attachment bonds between mother and child are particularly important, and how sensitively or insensitively a mother handles her child will have consequences both in the long and short term. For instance, the quality of attachment in infancy affects play and exploration on the one hand and cognitive, behavioural and social functions on the other. Distorted developments of attachment often lead to the child growing into a distrusting or withdrawn individual who attempts to protect him- or herself, in the present and the future, from the pain of angry or unfulfilling relationships. Attachment behaviours are crucial in the feeding situation and if they are distorted in this context anxiety and/or ambivalence feature strongly in the relationship and may lead to maltreatment or lack of adequate care. Because infants can form attachments to a number of close figures who take part in their early care, the mother is not the only one who shoulders the responsibility for her infant's attachment. However, she is usually the key figure and the patterns of attachment which may develop depend largely on her care. Ainsworth et al (1978) showed that there are very clear patterns of attachment.

Patterns of attachment

- Secure attachment
- Anxious/avoidant attachment
- Anxious/ambivalent attachment
- Anxious/resistant attachment

Any intervention needs to pay attention to the pattern between the infant/child and mother, and attachment figures other than the mother should be included in any assessment. Clearly, if the mother is the sole attachment figure, this can be an important indicator that support for her in her childcare duties is of relevance. How these concepts and the theory fit into our understanding of child abuse and its treatment are discussed in more detail in Chapter 15.

There are other writers and clinicians who have contributed to our understanding of the mother–infant dyad: Winnicott (1964) described beautifully the details in the interaction between mother and infant during the feeding situation in the early days and weeks of life.

Treatment failure

Success of treatment is measured by improvement in growth and development of the child, reduction of behavioural disturbance and a more positive nurturing and caring attitude towards the child. In the experience of the authors success is more likely if children are referred in the first year of life. The prognosis is poorer if the child is referred with a long history of failure to grow, and there may be only moderate or no improvement (Iwaniec 1995). In addition, follow-up has indicated that there is an increased risk of subsequent abuse and or neglect in children identified in the first year of life who were failing to thrive (Skuse 1992). In this study 1 in 12 cases were put on the child protection register for reasons other than poor growth.

Failure of treatment occurs when parents fail to comply, which usually means that they do not keep appointments or cooperate with treatment or the child continues to lose weight or to fall further behind in growth. These children are at risk of death or injury and active approaches must be taken. Removal of a child into substitute care requires statutory legal action in most cases; a case has to be made that the child is being harmed by the parents' continued failure to nourish him. Usually it is sufficient to show that the child's growth is seriously impaired and that there is no other cause that would absolve the parents of responsibility for this.

It is unusual for a court to make the necessary orders until the agencies involved have shown that they have offered all possible available practical help to the parents. This would include, for example, provision of necessary placement, family help and social work support as well as assistance with housing where appropriate (Table 3.14). Only then, and if the parents are either refusing or failing to use help, will an order be made. Sometimes legal proceedings have the effect of encouraging previously refractory parents to confront the situation of their child and provide the necessary intervention for them to start to work at improving matters. Rehabilitation will then need to proceed quickly and without the children being separated from their parents for very long. Use of the legal system to introduce external control in this way has produced significant results in some cases.

In the case of a very young infant who is failing to thrive in the care of an unsupported mother in very difficult social circumstances, early decisions about removal and adoption should be made, if at all possible. The outcome for the child is likely to be better if alternative care is found early.

It is always helpful to impose a time framework on difficult cases where the possibility of termination of parental care is considered. Older children with long-standing failure to thrive sometimes present, not having been diagnosed or treated in infancy. These children frequently have associated behaviour disturbance and may show signs of serious emotional deprivation. They are often short as well as light and have bizarre or unusual eating habits.

CASE HISTORY 3.7

Josephine was aged 9 years when she was referred from school because she had said very little during the time that she had been a pupil. She had daytime wetting and appeared a quite shy child. Her weight of 16 kg corresponded to a weight age of 4 years and her height was 108 cm – also well below the third centile.

She was uncommunicative but cooperated passively. Her mother acknowledged her poor growth and after counselling agreed that Josephine should be given a trial period in foster care. She was fostered as the only child with an older foster mother who gave her a lot of individual attention. Her wetting stopped and she began to communicate. She was moved to a school for children with moderate learning difficulties where she became much happier. She exhibited catch-up growth for both weight and height (Fig. 3.3) which have eventually reached the third centile.

If a child is failing to thrive it is helpful to look at a variety of signs and recognise those behavioural and emotional patterns which are apparent in each individual case. This can be achieved by asking the parents, and/or by observing the child. If there are other professionals involved it is important to talk with them. These patterns are not meant to establish a diagnosis of failure to thrive, rather they are there to help identify the particular difficulties which can accompany the failure to thrive. It is useful to establish when each of the behaviours first appeared. Whether the failure to thrive of the child is primary or secondary can be assessed and will be essential in the formulation and progress of treatment. As illustrated above, the relationship between various family members can be mapped and put together with the medical findings and the social factors that are part of the jigsaw.

Summary

1. Failure to thrive, formerly only recognised in institutions, is now seen as part of the wider syndrome of child maltreatment.
2. Failure to thrive is failure to grow – physically, intellectually, emotionally, socially.
3. To thrive optimally, a child must be well fed and loved.
4. The consequences of failure to thrive are profound and long-lasting on health and development.
5. failure to thrive should be recognised in primary care using standard techniques of growth measurement in a programme of health surveillance.
6. Non-organic failure to thrive should be positively identified through a detailed assessment of the child and family. Laboratory investigations have a minimal part to play in investigation.

7. Treatment aims to improve the child's nutrition and promote satisfactory parenting whilst supporting the family.
8. Management is multidisciplinary and close cooperation is essential.
9. Programmes of management should be developed around the child's home environment; hospitalisation should be seen as a last resort.
10. Intervention focuses on a detailed history of feeding and diet obtained through diaries and direct observation.
11. Parental and professional difficulties in acknowledging failure to thrive may lead to denial, and this should be recognised.
12. Failure to thrive occurs in all sections of society, and can be associated with eating disorders in the parents, cult and unusual diets as well as poverty, ignorance and neglect.
13. Failure to thrive is associated with other forms of abuse and can itself be considered a form of emotional abuse.
14. Eating to thrive is the important message to get over to all concerned.

REFERENCES

Ainsworth M D, Blehar M C, Waters E, Wall S 1978 Patterns of attachment: a psychological study of the strange situation. Erlbaum, Hillsdale, NJ

Ayoub C, Pfeifer D, Leichtman L 1989 Treatment of infants with non-organic failure to thrive. Child Abuse and Neglect 3:937–941

Batchelor J A 1996 Has recognition of failure to thrive changed? Child: care, health and development 22:235–40

Batchelor J A, Kerslake A 1990 Failure to find failure to thrive. Whiting & Birch, London

Berwick D M, Levy J C, Kleinman R 1982 Failure to thrive. Diagnostic yield of hospitalisation. Archives of Disease in Childhood 57:347–351

Bithoney W G, McJunkin J, Michalek J, Snyder J, Egan H, Epstein D 1991 The effect of a multidisciplinary team approach on weight gain in non-organic failure to thrive children. Dev Behav Pediatr. 12:254–258

Body J, Skuse D 1994 Annotation: The process of parenting in failure to thrive. Journal of Child Psychology and Psychiatry 35(3):401-424

Bowlby J 1969 Attachment and loss. Vol I Attachment. Basic Books, New York

Bowlby J 1973 Attachment and loss. Vol II Separation. Basic Books, New York

Bowlby J 1980 Attachment and loss. Vol III Loss. Basic Books, New York

Buckler J M H 1979 A reference manual of growth and development. Blackwell, Oxford

Burgess H J L, Burgess A P 1969 A modified standard for the mid-upper arm circumference in young children. Journal of Tropical Paediatrics 189–192

Capitanio M A, Kirkpatrick J A 1969 Widening of the cranial sutures. Radiology 92:53–59

Chase H P, Martin H P 1970 Undernutrition and child development. New England Journal of Medicine 282:933–939

Cole T J, Donnet M L, Stanfield J P 1981 Weight for height indexes to assess nutritional status – a reminder on a slide rule. American Journal of Clinical Nutrition 34:19–35

Coleman R W, Provence S 1957 Environmental retardation (hospitalisation) in infants living in families. Paediatrics 19:285–292

Crittenden P 1988 family and dyadic patterns. In: Browne K, Davies C, Stratton P (eds) Prediction and prevention of child abuse. J Wiley, Chichester

Crittenden P, Ainsworth M D S 1989 Child maltreatment and attachment theory. In: Cicchetti D, Carlson V (eds) Child maltreatment. Cambridge University Press, Cambridge

DoH 1994 Dietary reference values for food energy and nutrients for the UK. RHSS 41, HMSO, London

Ellis R W B, Mitchell R G 1965 Disease in infancy and childhood, 5th edn. Livingstone, Edinburgh

Elmer E, Gregg G S, Ellison P 1969 Late results of the 'failure to thrive' syndrome. Clinical Paediatrics 8:584–589

Evans D, Bowie M D, Hansen J D L et al 1980 Intellectual development and nutrition. Journal of Paediatrics 97:358–363

Fomon S J 1974 Infant nutrition, 2nd edn. Saunders, Philadelphia

Frank D A, Zeisel S H 1988 Failure to thrive. Pediatric Clinics of North America 35:1187–1206

Frisancho A R 1974 Triceps skin fold and upper arm muscle size norms for assessment of nutritional status. American Journal of Clinical Nutrition 27:1025–1058

Glaser H H, Heagerty M C, Bullard D M et al 1968 Physical and psychological development of children with early failure to thrive. Journal of Paediatrics 73:690–698

Goldbloom R B 1982 Failure to thrive. Paediatric Clinics of North America 29(1):151–166

Hall D M B 1989 Health for all children. A programme for child health surveillance. Oxford University Press, Oxford

Hanks H G I, Hobbs C J, Seymour D, Stratton P 1988 Infants who fail to thrive. An intervention for poor feeding practices. Journal of Reproductive and Infant Psychology 6:101–111

Haynes C F, Cutler C, Gray J, Kempe R S 1984 Hospitalised cases of non-organic failure to thrive: the scope of the problem and short term lay health visitor intervention. Child Abuse and Neglect 8:229–242

Hobbs C J 1994 Child abuse. in Addy D (ed) Investigations in paediatrics. W B Saunders, London, Ch 11

Hobbs C J, Hanks H G I 1996 A multidisciplinary approach for the treatment of children with failure to thrive. Child: care, health and development 22:273–284

Hobbs C J, Wynne J M, Gelletlie R 1995 Leeds inquiry into infant deaths: the importance of abuse and neglect in sudden infant death. Child Abuse Review 4:329–339

Homer C, Ludwig S 1981 Categorisation of etiology of failure to thrive. American Journal of Diseases of Childhood 135:848–851

Hufton I W, Oates R K 1977 Non-organic failure to thrive. A long term follow up. Paediatrics 59:73–77

Illingworth R S 1981 Weight and height. In: The normal child, some problems of the early years and their treatment. Churchill Livingstone, Edinburgh, Ch 5, pp 48–69

Illingworth R S 1983 The development of the infant and young child, 8th edn. Churchill Livingstone, Edinburgh

Iwaniec D 1995 The emotionally abused and neglected child: identification, assessment and intervention. J Wiley, Chichester

Iwaniec D, Herbert M 1982 The assessment and treatment of children who fail to thrive. Social Work Today 13:8–12

Iwaniec D, Herbert M, McNeish A S 1985 Social work with failure to thrive children and their families. Parts I and II. British Journal of Social Work 15:243–259, 375–389

Iwaniec D, Herbert M, Sluckin 1988 Helping emotionally abused children who fail to thrive. In: Browne K, Davies C, Stratton P (eds) Early prediction and prevention of child abuse. J Wiley, Chichester, pp 229–244

Izuora G I, Epigbo P 1983 Emotional reactions of adult Africans to children with severe kwashiorkor. Child Abuse and Neglect 7:351–356

Jellife D B, Jellife E F P 1969a The arm circumference as a public health index of protein calorie malnutrition of early childhood. Journal of Tropical Paediatrics 15:253–260

Jellife E R P, Jellife D B 1969b The arm circumference as a public health index of protein calorie malnutrition of early childhood. Journal of Tropical Paediatrics 15:176–188

Kempe R S, Goldbloom B 1987 Malnutrition and growth retardation ('failure to thrive') in the context of child abuse and neglect. In: Helfer R E, Kempe R S (eds) The battered child. University of Chicago Press, Ch 16, pp 312–335

Knowelden J, Keeling J, Nicholl J P et al (1985) Postneonatal mortality. Report on a Multicentre Study, Department of Health and Social Security, London

Krieger I, Sargent D A 1967 A postural sign in the sensory deprivation syndrome of infants. Journal of Paediatrics 70:332–339

McCann J B, Stein A, Fairburn C G, Dunger D B 1994 Eating habits and attitudes of mothers of children with non-organic failure to thrive. Archive of Diseases in Childhood 70:234–6

McDowell I, King F S 1982 Interpretation of arm circumference as an indicator of nutritional status. Archives of Disease in Childhood 57:292–296

McIntyre C & Collinson M 1997 Failure to thrive: a prevelance audit to aid monitoring. Health Visitor 70

Mackner L M, Starr Jr., R H, Black M M 1997 Effects of neglect and failure to thrive on cognitive functioning. Child Abuse and Neglect 21(7):691–700

Mitchell W G, Gorrell R W, Greenberg R A 1980 failure to thrive. A study in a primary care setting. Epidemiology and follow up. Paediatrics 65:961–977

Moores J 1996 Non-organic failure to thrive – dietetic practice in a community setting. Child: Care, Health and Development 22:251–259

Oates R K, Peacock A, Forrest D 1985 Long term effects of non-organic failure to thrive. Paediatrics 75:36–40

Prader A, Tanner J M, Von Harnack G A 1963 Catch up growth following illness or starvation. Journal of Paediatrics 62:646–659

Radbill S X 1987 Children in a world of violence: a history of child abuse. In: Helfer R E, Kempe R S (eds) The battered child. University of Chicago Press, Chicago, Ch 1, pp 3–22

Raynor P, Rudolph M C J 1996 What do we know about children who fail to thrive? Child: Care, Health and Development 22:241–250

Renoud S S 1993 A legacy of violence in non-organic failure to thrive. Child Abuse and Neglect 17(6):709–14

Roberts I F, West R J, Ogilvie D, Dillon M J 1979 Malnutrition in infants receiving cult diets: a rare form of abuse. British Medical Journal 1:296–298

Rosenn D W, Loeb L S, Jura M B 1980 Differentiation of organic from non-organic failure to thrive syndrome in infancy. Paediatrics 66:689–704

Schmitt B D, Mauro R D 1989 Non-organic failure to thrive: an outpatient approach. Child Abuse and Neglect 13:235–248

Sills R H 1978 Failure to thrive. The role of clinical and laboratories evaluation. American Journal of Diseases in Childhood 132:967–969

Sinatra F R, Merritt R J 1981 Iatrogenic kwashiorkor in infants. American Journal of Diseases in Children 135:21–23

Skuse D H 1988 Emotional abuse and delay in growth. In: Meadow S R (ed) ABC of child abuse. British Medical Journal, London, pp 26–28

Skuse D 1992 The relationship between deprivation, impaired growth and the impaired development of language. In: Fletcher P, Hall D (eds) Specific speech and language disorders in children. Whurr, London

Spitz R A 1945 Hospitalism. Psychoanalytic Study of the Child 1:53–74

Stratton P, Swaffer R 1988 Maternal causal beliefs for abused and handicapped children. Journal of Reproductive and Infant Psychology 6:201–216

Sturm L, Drotar D 1989 Prediction of weight for height following intervention in three-year-old children with early histories of non-organic failure to thrive. Child Abuse and Neglect 13:19–28

Tanner J M 1978 Foetus into man. Open Books, London

Taylor C R, Taylor E M 1976 Multifactorial causation of malnutrition. In: McClaren D (ed) Nutrition in the community. J Wiley, Chichester

Weston J A, Colloton M, Halsey S et al 1993 Sudden infant death syndrome in Hamburg. An epidemiological analysis of 150 cases. Acta Paediatrica Scandinavica 80:86–92

Whitten C F, Pettit M G, Fischoff J 1969 Evidence that growth feeding from maternal deprivation is secondary to undereating. Journal of the American Medical Association 209(11):1675–1682
Williams S N, Taylor B J, Ford R P K, Nelson E A S (1990). Growth velocity before sudden infant death. Archives of Disease in Childhood 65:1315–1318
Winnicott D W 1964 In: Davies, Wallbridge (eds) Boundary and space. Penguin, Harmondsworth
Wright C M 1995 A population approach to weight monitoring and failure to thrive. In: David T J (ed) Recent advances in paediatrics vol 13. Churchill Livingstone, Edinburgh, pp 73–87
Wright C M, Talbot E 1996 Screening for failure to thrive – what are we looking for? Child: Care, Health and Development 22:223–234

4

Physical abuse

Physical abuse, also known as battering or non-accidental injury, refers in this chapter to violence directed towards children. A physically abused child is defined as

> any child who receives physical injury (or injuries) as a result of acts (or omissions) on the part of his parents or guardians.

The definition includes

- actual or likely physical injury to a child
- failure to prevent physical injury (or suffering) to a child including deliberate poisoning, suffocation and Munchausen syndrome by proxy.

Within these definitions, hitting a child does not constitute physical abuse unless it results in injury. The law states that parents may use reasonable force. However, several countries in Europe have passed laws against the hitting of children by parents. In the UK, corporal punishment in state schools is now prohibited, although it is permitted in private schools.

Corporal punishment

'Spare the rod and spoil the child' is firmly embedded in our culture. The use of physical pain for the purposes of discipline is long established. These views are still firmly held by a majority of present-day society. Although physical punishment has been outlawed in most other settings – for example prisons, military establishments – it persists with regard to children. With the banning of corporal punishment in state schools and codes of conduct to prohibit it in day nurseries, childminders' and children's homes and foster-homes, some progress has been made in acknowledging the limitations of this practice. Research, however, continues to show that hitting children is widely practised by parents of all social classes, involving children of all ages (Newson & Newson 1986). More recently Smith and colleagues (1995) found in a sample of 403 families that 90% of children had been smacked, and 75% of 1-year-olds in the year preceding the interview. Most children received mild punishment but 15% were categorised as receiving severe punishment with half the mothers saying the hitting was hard enough to hurt the child. Most smacking was an irritated or angry response rather than a controlled one.

Supporters of corporal punishment claim it is simple, effective and often the only way of maintaining discipline. Opponents say it is associated with higher levels of delinquency, is ineffective and teaches violence (Newell 1989). It may create resentment and a desire in the child to hurt back. The child's self-esteem may be adversely affected. With regard to physical abuse, although there is clearly a difference between corporal punishment and physical abuse, it is obvious that the two are closely linked. Many parents who end up battering their children start out by disciplining them. The injuries resulted when things got out of hand.

Physical abuse varies from fatal to severe or moderate. All abuse is serious, and soft tissue injuries such as bruising involve considerable force in their production. This in turn inflicts pain and is invariably associated with some degree of emotional abuse, including harsh words, threats and rejection. The degree of danger of an injury relates especially to the age of the child. A small bruise in a baby may be a predictor of later serious or fatal abuse whereas a beating in an older child may denote no threat to life.

Failing to protect or deliberately placing in danger is as serious as deliberately inflicting injury. Such passive abuse may reflect a conscious or unconscious urge to be rid of a child. Acts of omission include failing to protect or deliberately placing a child in a dangerous situation (For example, leaving a baby in a bath unsupervised.)

Children are very vulnerable and few parents who shake, hit or slap a child intend to cause serious injury. Many injuries occur when parents lose control under stress, but some are sadistic and premeditated, for example some burns and scalds.

Incidence and prevalence of child abuse

Officially reported cases of child abuse and neglect represent only a fraction of the total number of cases in the population as a whole. Reporting depends on awareness of the problem by the public and professionals including doctors, nurses, social workers, teachers and others in contact with children. Such awareness tends to increase following the reporting of a particularly serious, often fatal, case by the media. Referrals then tend to rise for a while.

In the year up to March 1995 25 000 children were on the child abuse registers in the UK for physical abuse. However, it is estimated that each year 150 000 children are bruised or marked as a result of physical assault (Childhood Matters 1996).

Comparison with earlier figures confirms that although abuse may be getting worse, detection is also likely to be improving. Earlier figures from the NSPCC's annual statistics (Creighton & Noyes 1989), based on a sample of registers covering 9% of the population of England and Wales, suggest that over 8000 cases of physical abuse were registered in England and Wales in 1987: of these 0.6% were classified as fatal, 9% serious and 90% moderate. In Leeds, where cases have been recorded since 1969, Figure 4.1 shows the growth in diagnosed cases over the period 1969–88 (figures by permission of M F G Buchanan, unpublished.) Note the high proportion of serious cases in the earlier part of this study.

It has been estimated (Creighton & Noyes 1989) that between 200 and 230 non-accidental deaths occur each year in Britain and that 1.5–2%

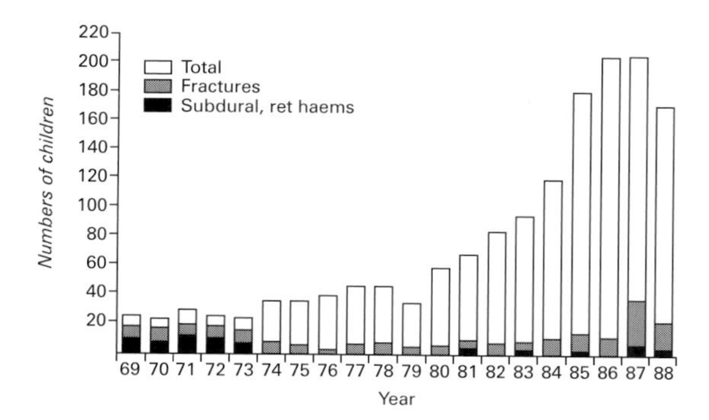

Fig. 4.1 Annual total number of cases of non-accidental injury seen by Leeds paediatricians, 1969–88.

of all children have been physically abused by the age of 17 years, but these are likely to be underestimates. In reported physical abuse, boys outnumber girls – for example, in the NSPCC's series from 1983–87, 55% were boys, 45% girls. Nearly half are aged 0–4 years, with about a quarter each of 5–9 and 10–14 years. Although only 1 in 8 is aged less than a year, 70% of serious head injuries occurred to children less than 1 year old (Creighton & Noyes 1989).

Unlike sexual abuse, there are fewer studies of the prevalence of physical violence and abuse of children and of the general level of physical punishment in the home. Although ultimately the law determines what is and what is not 'abuse', there are clearly links between the use of physical punishment against a child and physical abuse. Most children are occasionally hit by their parents. More than 3 million adults – 1 in 12 of the adult population – said that they had frequently or occasionally suffered bruising or marking following physical punishment as a child and 9% of these felt they had suffered long-term effects (Creighton & Russell 1995).

Recent research on ordinary families in the community (Smith 1995)

- Physical control strategies included:
  - hitting
  - physical restraint/shaking
  - punishment by example
  - forcing child to eat or ingest something
- 9 out of 10 children are hit at some time
- Frequency of hitting declines with age:
  - 38% age 4 years
  - 27% age 7 years
  - 3% age 11 years (hit more than once per week)
- Severe physical punishment – defined as 'intention or potential to cause injury or psychological damage, use of implements, repeated actions or over a long period of time' – affected 15% of all children in sample (88% involved hitting). None were found under 1 year of age
- Severe punishment was linked to poor marital relationship, family variables and mothers described as irritable
- Demographic variables poorly distinguished severely punishing families. No risk is associated with low income, overcrowding or single status
- Mothers hit more than fathers even when childcare equally shared
- Children aggressive to siblings were four times more likely than those rarely aggressive to their sibling to have been severely punished at some time

Physical punishment remains a major strategy for parents in controlling their children. It is an inefficient way of modifying behaviour and also runs the risk of the undesirable side-effects of both fear and learned imitative behaviour in the child (British Psychological Society 1992), but this acts as no deterrent to its continued use.

Physical abuse rarely exists on its own, however, and it is important to recognise links with other forms of abuse (Hobbs & Wynne 1990). One in six physically abused children have also been sexually abused and others have been neglected or are failing to thrive. Emotional abuse coexists in most cases. Physical abuse occurs to children of all ethnic groups, but possibly has different frequency between the groups. Handicapped children are seen to be at increased risk and, in one study (Smith & Hanson 1974),

13.5% of physically abused children had handicaps. In some instances, the abuse may be the cause of the handicap (Buchanan & Oliver 1972).

There is a marked tendency for this as well as other types of abuse to recur after coming to the attention of child protection agencies.

Between a quarter and a third of children diagnosed as abused physically were re-abused in a recent review of current research (Messages from Research 1995).

Social background

Physical abuse is reported more often from conditions of social deprivation and poverty, although it occurs in all social classes. In the NSPCC's figures (Creighton & Noyes 1989), only 4% of mothers and 5% of fathers were in non-manual occupational categories but, more significantly, 67% of mothers and 52% of fathers were unemployed and only 15% of mothers and 35% of fathers reported as being in paid employment.

In that study 15% of mothers and 43% of fathers had criminal records but often these were unrelated to crimes towards children. However, fathers were more likely than mothers to have a record of violence against adults.

There is a greater tendency for families in which there is a physically abused child to be larger than the national average – 25% of such families have four or more children. Very nearly half of the abused children are first-born. Younger siblings also carry a significant risk, although the percentage of injured children falls with each succeeding child after the first.

Poverty

The dehumanising effects of poverty are well understood. People unlucky enough to be poor and not very bright are more likely to adapt to their survival in ways which are unattractive and harmful to others around them. Poverty where the characters are witty, resourceful and courageous is more likely to be found in the novels of Charles Dickens or the plays of George Bernard Shaw. Nelson Algren, an American writer reporting on what he saw of poor and dehumanised Americans with his own eyes, 'day after day, year after year' in the mid-twentieth century said

> Hey, an awful lot of these people your hearts are bleeding for are really mean and stupid. That's a fact. Did you know that?

The harshness of poverty is destructive to human values and child abuse is one of its legacies. That is not to say that all parents who are poor abuse their children, nor is it to say that abuse occurs only among the poor. But there is no denying the link. Low income is associated with a marked increase in violence. Detection rates are also linked to low socio-economic status, many times more cases being found in these groups.

Perpetrators

Natural parents or parent figures are responsible for causing the injury in over 90% of cases. Overall, natural mothers are responsible in one-third and natural fathers in slightly fewer (Creighton & Noyes 1989). If figures are analysed according to who the child was living with at the time, then natural mothers were implicated in 36% but natural fathers in 61% of cases where the child was living with them. Mother substitutes appear much less often in the statistics, whereas stepfathers and father substitutes, including cohabiting boyfriends of mother, account for almost one in five cases. Stepfathers appear to be implicated relatively more often than cohabitees. Occasionally other relatives or babysitters are implicated.

Fewer than half of physically abused children come from families with both natural parents present, but marital difficulties are common when both parents are present.

Bullying

Definition

Bullying is a wilful, conscious desire to hurt another and put him/her under stress (Tattum & Lane 1988). It has also been referred to as 'peer abuse' (Dawkins & Hill 1995).

Children may be the victims of violence and physical abuse perpetrated by other children. A clear relationship to abuse in general is now established. Bullying can be broadly defined to include physical assault and intimidation, theft and extortion, verbal abuse including teasing, racial and sexual harassment or harassment on grounds of religion, gender, sexuality or similar. It may take various forms including physical, verbal, gesture, extortion and exclusion bullying.

Prevalence

Bullying is common: one study of over 6000 pupils in 23 Sheffield schools found that 27% of junior and middle, and 10% of secondary pupils reported bullying that term, sometimes or more often, with 10% and 4% respectively bullied at least once per week (Whitney & Smith 1993). Most had not told either a teacher or parent. A telephone helpline for bullying received 50 000 calls in less than a year, twice as many from girls as boys. Bullying is rife in young offender institutions (Kennedy 1995) and residential care. Both boys and girls bully; boys are more likely to use violence, girls to use more subtle tactics.

The following two quotations are taken from the Gulbenkian Report, (Children and Violence 1995):

> I reckon some kids might bully because their parents are violent and shouting at each other. I also think they do it for fun. A kid by ours got bullied and hung himself in the woods.

> . . . because they are bullied at home. They are very insecure and because they are so weak inside they have to appear strong on the outside.

Effects

Victims of bullying lack confidence, have poor self-esteem and may have poorer school attendance and academic achievement. In addition, symptoms commonly associated with abuse in other situations may lead to clinical presentation, e.g. headache, abdominal pain, sleep disturbance, wetting, fits, faints, vomiting, limb pains, hysteria. It has been reported that more severe symptoms including self-harm and suicide may occur. Adjustment difficulties in adult life may result.

Prevention

Bullying can be significantly reduced by well-planned strategies. Norwegian experience emphasised positive involvement by teachers and parents, setting firm limits on unacceptable behaviour and the use of non-hostile, non-corporal sanctions on rule violations. This was set in the context of prohibition of all physical punishment of children in Norway from 1987 (Children and Violence 1995).

In the UK the Department of Education circulated an anti-bullying pack to schools in 1994 (DES 1994). It is recommended that each school has a formal written anti-bullying policy. These policies must cover:

- arrangements to ensure that everyone in the institution is aware of the importance of reporting bullying and the importance of ensuring that those bullied are not blamed in any way
- specific strategies for preventing bullying
- provision of appropriate protection and support for those who are bullied
- appropriate responses for those who bully, with a strong emphasis on non-stigmatising and non-punitive approaches
- arrangements for responding to those forms of bullying that appear to involve criminal offences.

Training courses are available from Kidscape (Elliott 1991). Rao (1995) supports a more active policy which would include education of children and a response to identifying bullying more along the lines of traditional child protection practice, including holding a case conference and a plan for the prevention of future cases.

Bullying – the clinician's role (Dawkins 1995)

- Ask directly about bullying as a possible cause of a child's symptoms
- Parents should be informed and advised to take the matter up with the school directly

- Simple advice can be given to children including telling the appropriate person
- Keep informed of the policies and procedure
- Approach head teacher to clarify school's policy where appropriate.

Recognition of child abuse

Presentation

Direct report

A report of abuse may be made by a child, a parent or an interested third party. Most such reports are true and should, in general, be believed. Third party reports (often anonymous telephone calls to the NSPCC or social services) should be treated seriously but sometimes are found to have no basis, or to carry malicious intent. Worries by grandparents and other responsible family members also need careful assessment. The reasons for the reports must be identified, even if no obvious abuse is found.

CASE HISTORY 4.1

A boy of 8 told the teacher that he had not been to school because daddy had given him a black eye. The injury had resolved and could not be verified, but there appeared to be no reason for the child to lie. A report was filed with the social services department, who agreed to check any further absences from school through the Education Welfare Officer.

Presentation of an injury

Following abuse, parents frequently take the child for help – to hospital, to a health visitor or general practitioner.

Incidental discovery of injury

Abused children are frequently allowed to go to school, to nursery or to another person's care where injuries may be found and reported. It is not unusual for parents in this situation to deny knowledge of the injury and for there to be no satisfactory explanation.

Some pointers to physical abuse

- Repetitive pattern of injury (but parents may use different hospitals to avoid detection)
- Injuries not consistent with the history, i.e. too many, too severe, wrong kind, wrong distribution, wrong age
- Patterns of injury which strongly suggest abuse, e.g.
  - bruising to a young baby (there are few reasonable explanations)
  - multiple injuries following a moderate fall
  - severe head injuries in babies or toddlers
  - rib fractures
  - subdural haematoma and retinal haemorrhage from violent shaking
  - multiple cigarette burns
  - fractures in infants and toddlers
- Presence of other signs of abuse, e.g. neglect, failure to thrive, sexual abuse
- Unusual behaviour in the parents, e.g. delay in seeking medical advice, refusal to allow proper treatment or admission to hospital, unprovoked aggression towards staff

Features in the history

It is unusual for any one professional to have all the information required in the history. A check-list of important features can be assembled by the various professionals involved. Table 4.1 provides a summary of influencing factors in physical abuse.

Important features in the history

- Discrepant history
  - Does it change with telling or with who tells it?
  - Is it vague or unclear? Exact details of time, place, person and actions are needed. For example, how did the child fall, how far, on to what?

- Compare your account with that of others – social worker, health visitor, policeman. Major differences need explanation.
- Do the father and mother give the same story?

▶ Unreasonable delay in seeking help or care for the child, especially following a fracture or serious burn or scald, is a strong indicator
- Denial that the child was in pain and minimisation of the symptoms are common. Following a serious head injury, a baby may be left tucked up in a cot, only to be brought hours later when he refuses a feed or begins to have seizures. One parent of a child with a serious burn said the doctor's surgery was closed so she didn't do anything for a week.

▶ Family crisis
- There may be a family crisis or a complicated home situation which has precipitated the injury. This could be, a bereavement, break-up of relationship, loss of job or final demand for a debt. These stresses are usually revealed if parents are listened to.

▶ Trigger factors are behaviours in the child which precipitate the parent's violence
- Inconsolable crying in the night, difficult feeding or wetting are common; in older children, stealing or lying may provoke.

▶ Parental history of abuse
- Parent's traumatic experiences as children are important, but may be forgotten or repressed. Parents may admit to being beaten themselves as children. Some may have been in care.

▶ Unrealistic expectations coupled to a poor understanding of child development
- The child is expected to love and accept the parents. When he cries or won't take his feeds, it is because he is rejecting or punishing them. An expectation that a 2-year-old will behave in model and ideal ways is likely to lead to what parents perceive as a failure on the part of the child.
- Obsessional and rigid patterns of child-rearing may be expressed in other ways (e.g. a meticulously clean and tidy home) and can create stresses and tensions.

▶ Social isolation
- Isolation from friends, extended family and professionals is a common finding in parents who abuse. 'Who can you turn to for help?' is a crucial question. As the abuse escalates, the parents find it increasingly difficult to allow anyone into their lives for fear of discovery.
- Abusing parents tend to attribute their problems to external factors rather than to their own difficulties.

▶ Past history of child
- The presence of high levels of parental anxiety, frequent admissions to hospital in the first months of life, frequent 'accidents', 'a tendency to bruise easily' are often found.
- The child's behaviour, growth and development and health may also be sources of anxiety.
- Much of this information will come from sources other than parents, who may minimise their difficulties in their eagerness to present themselves as perfect parents.

Parenting in physical abuse

Waterhouse and colleagues (1993) found in a random sample of physical abuse cases that although the level of injury sustained was often quite slight, the psychological state of the children caused concern. Although the parents' relationship on the face of it appeared favourable and aspects of care such as clothing, feeding and washing acceptable, the parents were remarkably unresponsive to the emotional needs of the children. They spent little time with them in ways which required active engagement, failing to discipline them consistently, resorting instead to spasmodic hitting, shouting or attempts to reason, all to little long-term or even short-term effect. Their parenting was characterised by its passivity and the patterns of control were considered erratic (Messages from Research 1995).

Denial

As with all forms of abuse, denial that the injury arose non-accidentally is commonly encoun-

Table 4.1 Influencing factors in physical abuse

Sociocultural	Attitudes toward physical punishment, values placed on children as individuals versus chattels, property, ownership
Socio-economic	Poverty is a major stress, promoting violence, deprivation and child abuse Not all poor families abuse
Unemployment	A special kind of social stress, linked with poverty
Family breakdown	Unstable marital relationships, spouse violence, separation and divorce Loss of extended family supports from increased social mobility
Health	Poor health in parents, especially mother, reduces coping and tolerance levels Psychiatric illness or poor psychological health including symptoms of stress Alcohol and drug usage including prescribed psychotropic drugs
Handicap	One child factor that is important Difficult children to care for – e.g. screamers, poor feeders – are other examples
Education	Lack of education and the personal resources this brings results in fewer ways of coping Low intelligence is another factor
Poor parenting	From poor childhood experiences, or lack of opportunity to learn
Individual	Youth, immaturity, isolation, criminality are all adverse factors
Generational	Tendency to repeat the cycle of abuse from generation to generation
Environmental	Effects of cold, damp, overcrowded housing, nowhere for the children to play, enforced proximity
Media	On children already predisposed to violent behaviour as a result of home experience, the influence of violent screen images has been estimated to account for around 10% of the problem
Services	Lack of appropriate, accessible services – e.g. day care, nurseries, maternal and child health services

tered. Although it is the parents who are usually most actively involved in the denial, others – including the child, other family members and professionals, especially those who know the family – may also be involved.

Parents may convince themselves that there has been no abuse and may even go as far as claiming that there is no injury. This is to be distinguished from deliberate attempts to conceal or lie which are also commonly encountered. In denial the parents may appear remarkably unmoved, and their simple logic 'If I'd done that to him, would I have been so foolish to have brought him to hospital?' can be quite appealing to the inexperienced. Denial is best seen as a coping mechanism to reduce the distress surrounding the crisis of the diagnosis. The seriousness of denial lies in the way that it very effectively prevents any intervention or change. Professional denial has the same effect.

Procedures

Approaches to investigation

Key figures include:

- social worker
- paediatrician
- police officer.

Vital sources of information are:

- general practitioner
- Accident and Emergency doctor or nurse
- health visitor, school nurse or midwife
- paediatric nurse (if child is in hospital)
- other individuals – e.g. probation officer, obstetrician, adult psychiatrist and staff, pathologist – can occasionally help
- other sources – other hospitals, towns, armed forces units.

It is usual for each team to have a central co-ordinator of information, usually a social worker, who will become the key worker. One task is to contact those with information and check the important facts and opinions, carefully drawing distinctions between the two types of information.

A general practitioner might say

> I've known this family for five years and I'm sure these parents couldn't injure their baby

but may go on to say that the mother has been on anti-depressant medication following the birth of the baby and only last year lost her own mother with cancer. He may say

> I don't see much of the father, he rarely comes in but I was asked for a report for a recent

insurance medical and he was overweight and had recently been drinking rather more heavily than usual.

The health visitor might say

This is the first baby and the pregnancy went reasonably smoothly, although the mother needed a lot of support at the time of delivery and was noted to be withdrawn and tearful whilst she was in hospital. We wondered about a psychiatric opinion, but decided to let the general practitioner know on discharge. The father visited but didn't seem to be a great help. The home is usually very clean and tidy, perhaps a little spartan, but recently mother hasn't been managing with the housework as the baby has been keeping them up a lot at night with crying. There was a brief admission to hospital when we thought he had pyloric stenosis because the mother described projectile vomiting, but he settled very quickly and took his bottles well. I've called two or three times when there has been no one in, or at least no one answered the door, but on one visit there was a tiny mark just by the side of his eye which his mother said she thought could have been caused by a rattle in his cot.

The information must be collated quickly and accurately but will be discussed in more detail at the case conference. The police may or may not know the family, but if a name and date of birth are available they will be able to check if there is a history of violence or assault against children.

Medical examination

Medical examination (Buchanan 1989) is an essential step in the identification of physical abuse. Doctors should be experienced with children, understand growth and development and have forensic skills. They should be able to write clear and concise reports and give evidence in court.

Examination of physically abused children requires a calm, unhurried approach with attention to detail, good note-keeping and an ability to cope with distressed children and parents. The room should be appropriately equipped, including toys and soft furnishings, and be quiet and private.

Important points in medical examination

- Full paediatric history, including careful note of explanations of injury, times, details, etc.
- Developmental history
- Parents' expressed difficulties with child – behaviour, health, development
- Detailed examination of whole child to include:
  - growth – height, weight, arm circumference, head circumference (plotted)
  - nutrition
  - general demeanour and appearance
  - signs of neglect, sexual abuse, emotional disturbance
  - development including language, social skills
- Documentation of injuries

Documentation of injuries

Diagnosis of physical abuse usually involves the assessment of lesions which are visible to the unaided eye. Accurate documentation should be by means of words, drawings and photographs. Each method has its own particular merits which are complementary. Accurate and detailed documentation permits others – including police officers, courts, social workers and other doctors providing additional opinions – the opportunity of assessing the injuries for themselves. Descriptions should be brief but detailed and include:

- probable nature of the lesion and approximate age (colour for bruises)
- site
- shape
- size (in cm)
- any unusual distinguishing features
- where possible, an estimate of likely causation.

Injuries should be listed one by one and related to body drawings which give the best indication of patterns. Drawings should be outline with sizes (e.g. of bruises) marked.

Photography

Taking photographs is now a routine part of the documentation of child abuse cases (Ricci 1991,

Hobbs and Wynne 1995a), and the American Medical Association's diagnostic and treatment guidelines for the abused child recommend that all visible lesions be photographed. It is usual to ask permission of both parent and child where appropriate.

The main functions of photography in child abuse are:

- to document findings, particularly visible injuries
- to provide information for discussion with colleagues, courts, other professionals and those with responsibility for the child, including parents
- for teaching and research purposes.

Photography may be used to record:

- injuries, e.g. bruises, burns
- genital and anal signs (usually injury or infection)
- aspects of growth and development.
- the overall appearance, including demeanour, emotional signs and features associated with neglect.

Procedure for photography

Photographs should be taken as soon as reasonably possible after an injury has been observed. In some cases serial photographs may be required, for example in bite mark recognition, but this is exceptional.

Many hospitals have departments of medical photography with professionally trained photographers who are used to photographing medical subjects. However, the photographer is only able to achieve satisfactory results when he or she is working with clear and detailed instructions of exactly what is to be photographed and how the lesion would be best demonstrated; for example, if it is a torn frenulum it may not be sufficient to write 'mouth injury' on the request card. For best results it is preferable for the examining doctor to be present during the photography to ensure the best views are taken as well as a fully comprehensive set where there are many injuries. With small frightened children, the mother or a skilled nurse to hold and comfort the child will be essential. Again, for similar reasons, it is often best to photograph the child on the ward rather than have the child visit the photographic studio, although in some cases where this is appropriate better results can be achieved.

Incorporation of a measure in the photograph is often recommended. Our policy is to measure lesions and record on diagrams to simplify photography where there are multiple lesions. Facial view will assist in identification. Always keep spare film and batteries with camera.

The doctor as photographer

With modern technology, moderately skilled physicians can obtain excellent results by taking photographs themselves. Many doctors use a single lens reflex camera (SLR) to record injuries in the consulting room. There are a few points to bear in mind:

- Modern fully automatic SLRs incorporating a programme for electronic flash exposure and utilising an interchangeable lens system are appropriate.
- There should preferably be arrangements through a department of medical photography to handle exposed films so as to maintain quality control and support.
- A system of recording patient's name, lesions and date is required using photographed identifier card, standard frame counters and/or data-back information.
- Slides or prints are acceptable. The police prefer and use prints, but 35 mm slides can be used in court with a hand viewer or projector and screen, which gives the doctor the opportunity to demonstrate the injuries to the court, pointing out the important features.

Useful tips for photography

- A macro lens of longer focal length (90–105 mm) allows detailed photographs of individual lesions
- For bruises it is useful to take exposures at different distances to allow both detailed

examination and an appreciation of the pattern and position of bruising in relation to the body as a whole. If the photograph is taken from too far away, small bruises will not be visible

- Use a neutral background. A non-reflective green surgical towel is ideal
- Faint and fading bruises may not show with electronic flash on camera. Studio lighting or reducing the exposure with an exposure compensation setting may be more effective. However, photography must not be used to enhance or exaggerate the trauma that is present

Using photographic evidence in court

Photographs can and should on occasions be used in court to supplement oral evidence. It is necessary to verify legally that the photographs are of the child in question, when they were taken and by whom. Despite anxieties, medical photographers have not in our experience been asked to attend court. In cases where prosecution is likely, the police may arrange to have their photographer take photographs for them, but they may also use 'medical photographs' in evidence.

Classification of injuries

- Superficial (dermatological): bruises, abrasions, lacerations, scratches, bites, stab wounds, pin pricks, pinch marks, ligature marks, broken or avulsed hair or nails, burns or scalds (see Ch. 5), chemical injury
- Deeper lesions: haematoma, cephalhaematoma, mouth injury (tear of lip frenulum), strangulation
- Fractures, dislocations, wrenched limbs, periosteal injury
- Thoracolumbar internal injury – stomach, gut, solid viscera, lung
- Intracranial (including eyes) and spinal injury: whiplash, shaken, subdural haematoma, cerebral haemorrhage, contusion or oedema, spinal cord injury
- Asphyxia, drowning and poisoning
- Fabricated disorders (factitious illness, Munchausen by proxy)

Superficial injury

Bruises

Bruises are present in 90% of physically abused children. Bruises arise when blood is lost from the intravascular space into the skin and subcutaneous tissues. Except in rare cases of severe bleeding disorder, trauma is always implicated in their causation. Bruises do not blanch on pressure and have a characteristic colour. They can be mimicked by paint or pen marks, dye from clothes, birth marks, mongolian blue spots or café au lait spots.

Ageing of bruises

The configuration, delineation and colour in theory provide a guide enabling ageing to be attempted. If there is any doubt that a lesion is a bruise, serial examination will decide the matter.

The apparent discrepancies highlight the caution that doctors should adopt when discussing the ages of bruises in court. Recent reviews (Schwartz & Ricci 1996, Stephenson & Bialas 1996) have emphasised the difficulties of ageing bruises. The time taken for a bruise to develop depends on the depth of injury, deeper bruises taking longer to appear. The colour of the bruise also depends on the depth, yellowish tinges appearing in 3 days in superficial bruises, while in deeper bruises the yellow colour may take 7–10 days to appear. Studies have confirmed that yellow bruises are older than 18 hours (Langlois & Gresham 1991) and that other colours – red, blue, purple or black – can occur in bruises from any time from 1 hour to resolution. Bruises of identical age and cause on the same person may not appear as the same colour and may not change at the same rate. Multiple bruises have often been inflicted on a number of occasions and there will be different ages as well as size and shape. This polymorphic pattern of injury is typical of abuse. After a single accident, bruises will be of the same age and few in number. Falls downstairs are not associated with multiple bruises in many sites and of different ages.

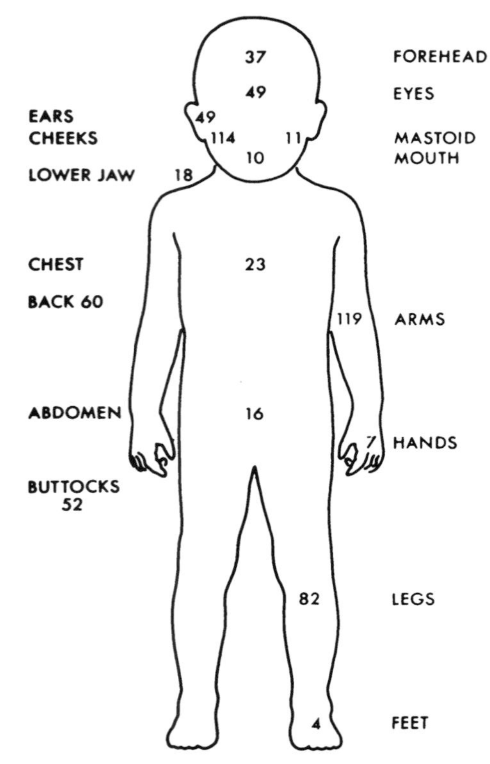

Fig. 4.2 Sites for superficial injury in 251 non-accidental injury cases. Sites, not number of children, are totalled. (Reproduced by courtesy of Dr M F G Buchanan.)

Sites for inflicted bruises

Buchanan (1989) analysed sites for superficial injuries of all kinds in 251 abused children. The figures refer to the number of injuries and the total obviously exceeds the total number of children, denoting that injuries were present in several sites in some children (Fig. 4.2).

- Bruises on the buttocks, lower back and outer thighs are often related to punishment.
- Injuries to the inner thigh and genital area suggest either sexual abuse or punishment for perceived toileting misdemeanours.
- The penis may be pinched or pulled and sometimes tied with string, hairs or rubber bands.
- Injury to the head and neck is common.
  - Slap marks are found on the sides of the face and ears, extending on to the scalp.
  - Bruises on the external ear are unusual following accidents because of the protective effect of the triangle created by the shoulder, skull and base of neck which greatly reduces injury to the ear following a fall.
  - Bruises on the lower jaw and the mastoid are strongly associated with abuse.
  - Other sites are round the neck, suggesting choking, and the eyes and mouth.
  - Black eyes can occur in normal schoolchildren from a direct injury but it takes a very hard blow to the forehead for blood to track down around one or both eyes.
  - Injury to the upper lip and its frenulum may follow forced feeding, and an old tear of frenulum will persist.
- Bruises distal to the elbow and knees generally carry less significance than those on thighs and upper arms.
- Bruises to the trunk (chest and abdomen) are also suspicious of abuse and lower abdominal bruises should suggest sexual abuse.

Patterns of bruising

Inflicted bruises show a number of different patterns:

- hand marks

- marks of implements – e.g. straps, sticks, buckles
- bruises from throwing, swinging or pushing the child on to a hard object
- bites
- bizarre marks (including petechiae)
- kicks.

Hand marks

- grab mark or fingertip bruises, for example on limbs, face, chest wall
- hand print or linear finger mark
- slap mark – often vaguely two or three finger-sized linear marks are seen with stripe effect
- rings may leave a tell-tale mark
- pinch marks – a pair of crescent-shaped bruises, facing one another
- poking marks – fingernail may cut the skin
- fist – diffuse, often severe, bruising to face, penetrating recesses, e.g. eye socket (see Fig. 4.2).

Marks from implements

Newson & Newson (1986) found, amongst a sample of 700 children, that by 7 years of age 26% of boys and 18% of girls had been hit with an implement of some kind. In both use and threat, the order of preference was:

1. strap or belt
2. cane or stick
3. slipper
4. miscellaneous objects.

- Belts or straps leave parallel-sided marks which tend to curve with the contours of the body, whereas stick marks are less clearly defined linear marks over prominent areas, usually thinner than strap marks. Loops of flex show circular closed-end thin lines. Large confluent areas of bruising, commonly on buttocks, arise from slipper beatings.
- Ties or ligatures cause circumferential bands around limbs and gags cause abrasions from the corner of the mouth. Look for petechiae on the upper eyelids and face as well as bruising to the neck in strangulation.

Identification of implements requires cooperation between doctor and police officer who may be able to identify the object during a search at the child's home.

Bite marks

Bites are always non-accidental in origin. They can be animal or human, adult or child (Bernat 1992). Identification of the perpetrator is possible if the mark is recent and clear. Animal bites, e.g. dog or cat, result in puncturing, cutting and tearing of the skin by the carnivorous dentition. Recently, the importance of attacks by animals on children has finally been taken seriously. Dog bites should be preventable.

The human diet is omnivorous and the teeth similar in size, shape and prominence. The resulting bruises are crescent-shaped and individual tooth marks may be identified if the injury is recent. However, bite marks may suffer distortion from the contours of the area bitten, and by movement at the time of biting. Appearances may not be typical in some areas, e.g. fingers or toes. In a very aggressive bite, the skin may be broken. To differentiate between the bite of an adult and a young child (under 8 years) it should be remembered that the intercanine distance (measurement across the mouth between the third tooth on each side) is greater than 3.0 cm in the adult or older child and less than 3.0 cm in a young child with primary teeth.

Arch width differences between a 5-year-old child and an adult are 4.4 mm in the maxilla and 2.5 mm in the mandible, i.e. not great (Moores 1959). In the same study, the cumulative widths of the six upper deciduous teeth were 10 mm smaller in the primary than in the secondary dentition. In the lower arch, the difference was approximately 7 mm.

Suspect identification can be attempted with the help of a forensic dentist or odontologist. A series of photographs, starting as soon as the injury is identified, should be taken at intervals of 24 hours with a millimetre rule incorporated. Suspected perpetrators are asked to provide a dental impression to compare with the photographs.

ABO blood grouping can be determined from saliva washings of the skin surrounding a bite.

Approximately 0.3 ml of saliva are deposited and it can be difficult to obtain sufficient by swabbing.

Is it a bite?

- Human or animal?
- Adult or child?
- Photograph with rule, daily × 7
- Washing for saliva (ABO group)
- Perpetrator identification – forensic odontologist

Bizarre marks

- Unusual bruises may arise when a child is struck through clothes; the pattern of the weave may appear.
- Puncture wounds (e.g. from a nappy pin), cord burns and self-inflicted injuries all produce unusual non-accidental marks.
- Petechial (pinprick) bruises are common and arise when capillaries rupture, producing small haemorrhages around them. They can be seen on an arm if it has been held tightly, around the neck or between the fingers of a handslap. Extensive petechiae involving the upper part of the trunk, upper arms, face and neck have accompanied crushing injuries to the chest. Typically the distribution ends at the waist. Although it is usual to consider platelet abnormalities and viral aetiologies, trauma is the commonest cause for localised petechiae.

Kicks

Usually on the lower half of the body, kicks produce large, irregularly shaped bruises occasionally reflecting the shape of the shoe.

Injuries in a community population

In non-abused children, up to 12 bruises may be seen. In 400 children in the community aged from 2 weeks to 11 years, some injury was found in 37% but with increasing prevalence towards the end of the third year of life (Roberton et al 1982). The commonest sites were the lower leg (21.5%), thigh and buttock (9.25%) and arms (8.5%). In contrast, bruises to the head and face were found in only 6.5% of non-abused compared to 60% of 119 non-accidentally injured children. Accidental injury to the shins, bony prominences (e.g. foreheads) in toddlers and to the hands and feet were prominent, but bruising to the lumbar region showed a marked variation with age, being unusual before the age of 3 but present in 15% of children between the ages of 6 and 11 years. Bruising in young babies (2 weeks–2 months) was found in only 4 out of 60, and in 2 cases there was a clear history of injury. Bruising was uncommon between 3 and 9 months (only one in eight children affected) but increased as the children became more mobile and active, so that 50–65% of children aged between 12 months and 11 years had lesions, usually minor bruising. Injuries to genitalia (two children, both easily explained) and to chest and upper back (maximum 5% in all the age groups) were uncommon, as were burns (three only), and none had fractures.

Non-traumatic causes of bruising, aiding in differential diagnosis, are shown in Table 4.3. Occasionally non-accidental injury is suspected and a bleeding disorder is encountered. Wheeler & Hobbs (1988), over 10 years, found that 23 out of 50 children with lesions suspicious of non-accidental injury were referred with possible bruising. Of these, five had bleeding disorders. Of the other possible causes of confusion, mongolian blue spots, capillary haemangioma, allergic periorbital swelling, and dye, ink or paint were described.

O'Hare & Eden (1984) reported that routine tests of clotting in every child with bruising suspected of being non-accidental in aetiology resulted in abnormal initial investigations in 16%. Although children with spontaneous bleeding or bleeding from trivial trauma were found, many other children had several features supporting a diagnosis of non-accidental injury. The coexistence of a bleeding disorder and physical abuse does occur and the diagnoses are not mutually exclusive. The risks from abuse to a child who has a bleeding disorder may well be greater, so that concern for the

Table 4.2 Differential diagnosis of bruising

Presentation	Differential diagnoses	Features	Investigations
?Bruise	Blue spots, haemangioma, café au lait spots, prominent veins	Static lesions, no evolution with time	Follow up Re-examine
?Bruise	Bleeding disorder, e.g. ITP, haemophilia, haemorrhagic disease of newborn, platelet disorder	Bruising with minimal trauma, sites usual accidental ones Family history, prolonged bleeding	Haematological investigations (see Table 4.3)
?Bruise	Infection, vasculitis: meningococcal septicaemia disseminated intravascular coagulation Henoch–Schoenlein disease	Ill child, rapidly developing purpuric rash Distribution of purpura Joint, abdominal, renal features	Blood culture Lumbar puncture Haematology Urine microscopy Urine dipstick for protein
?Bruise	Allergy – periorbital swelling	History of allergy Contact, appearance, evolution	IgE, eosinophilia
?Bruise	Skin disease: Ehlers–Danlös syndrome Erythema nodosum, other skin disease	Low elasticity, poor wound healing, easy bruisability Painful, warm, erythematous Pretibial joint pain	Seek dermatology opinion Biopsy
?Bruise	Ink, paint, dye, dirt	Removable	Soap and water

child's well-being may increase on discovering an abnormality.

Haematological investigation of bruising, bleeding or purpura

Excessive bruising, bleeding or purpura may be due to explained or unexplained injury, following surgery or spontaneous due to an underlying bleeding disorder. The presence of a bleeding disorder may be coincident with otherwise unexplained injury. The following investigative guidelines were suggested by Dr S Kinsey (pers. comm.).

First line investigations

- history including family history
- full blood count (0.5 ml EDTA anticoagulated blood)
  - white cell count
  - haemoglobin
  - platelet count
  - film to be reviewed by haematologist
- coagulation screen (1.8 ml citrated blood)
  - prothrombin time (PT)
  - activated partial thromboplastin time (APTT)
  - thrombin time
  - fibrinogen.

These tests will not exclude a platelet function defect. If there is any suspicion of a platelet problem then discuss with a haematologist and proceed to second line investigations.

Table 4.3 A child with bruises: is it a haematological disorder? (From Harvey D R, Kovar I Z Child health. 1991 Churchill Livingstone, Edinburgh, with permission.)

Disease	Platelet count	Bleeding time	PTT[a]	Pt[b]	Factor VIII level	Factor IX level
Idiopathic thrombocytopenic purpura	Low	N	N	N	N	N
Haemophilia	N	N	P	N	L	N
Von Willebrand's disease	N[c]	P	N or P	N	L	N
Factor IX deficiency	N	N	P	N	N	L

[a] *Partial thromboplastin time.*
[b] *Prothrombin time.*
[c] *Defective platelet aggregation.*
L, low; N, normal; P, prolonged.

Second line investigations

- Von Willebrand screen
- factor assays
- platelet aggregation studies
- bleeding time

In addition, the drug history is important – for example salicylates can induce a platelet disorder.

Other superficial lesions

Scratches are common in abused children and may result from fingernails, nappy pins, etc. Children have also been stabbed with knives. Fingernails or toenails can be pulled out and traumatic alopecia results if the child is grabbed by the hair. The hair may spiral, following overstretching at the broken end and the scalp may be tender with petechiae at the hair roots. Differentiation from alopecia areata which is common in deprived, poorly nourished children involves the absence of loose hair at the periphery, inflammation or scaling of the scalp. Violent traction forces on the scalp, such as those incurred by lifting the child by the hair, can lead to the diffuse extensive boggy swelling of a subgaleal haematoma between the scalp aponeurosis and the calvarium. These may present without history and then abuse should be implied.

Fractures and bony injury

Abusive fractures usually result from the more extreme forms of violence and represent serious injury. They may coexist with other signs of trauma: external, e.g. bruises, scratches, or internal, e.g. subdural haematoma, retinal haemorrhage or ruptured gut, or may be an isolated injury. However, the hypothesis that absence of bruising around the fracture excludes a non-accidental cause has been effectively rebutted (Taitz 1991). Fractures may occur in any bone, being single or multiple, clinically obvious or occult and then detected only on radiograph. Bony injury in the presence of normal bones provides incontrovertible evidence of substantial trauma. Fractures are an important finding in fatal outcome following abuse.

The recognition of fractures prompted identification of what Caffey (1946) called the *parent–infant stress syndrome*, later renamed the *battered baby syndrome* (Kempe et al 1962). Caffey drew attention to the metaphyseal avulsion at the end of long bones which he thought resulted from indirect traction, stretching and shearing (i.e. acceleration and deceleration stresses on the periosteum and articular capsules rather than direct impact stresses on the bone itself). He linked this to the whiplash shaking syndrome. Since that time the spectrum of injury to the infant and young child's skeleton has widened. Injury to almost every bone has been described in abuse, but certain patterns have emerged and our understanding of the relationship between cause and effect has improved.

Prevalence of fractures in abuse and accident

Fractures of the long bones were found in 4% of 4037 physically abused children; 2% had fractures in other bones (Creighton & Noyes 1989). The majority of abusive fractures occur in infants and pre-school children. One study of physically abused children (Herndon 1983) typically found that 58% were under the age of 3 years and sustained 95% of the fractures. In non-abused children Worlock et al (1986) found that 85% of fractures occur over the age of 5 years.

In the first year of life not only are fractures more likely to follow an assault but, looking at the whole population of infants with fractures, they are more likely to be the result of abuse than at any other time. A high index of suspicion is therefore required.

McClelland & Heiple (1982) studied 34 infants up to 1 year with 55 fractures. They found that 15 patients were injured in accidents and 19 by abuse. Worlock et al (1986) calculated that one in eight infants with fractures had been abused.

Leventhal and colleagues (1993) studied 253 consecutive fractures in 215 children under 3 years who were seen at their hospital over a 5-year period. Of these 24.2% were categorised as abuse, 8.4% unknown and 67.4% uninten-

Table 4.4 Falls in children (modified from Hobbs 1994)

Authors	Number of subjects	Age of subjects	Type of fall	Injuries
Kravitz et al (1969)	255	Birth–1 year	Elevated surfaces at home Clinic in poor area Private practice	Any head injury 105 Bruise scalp 95 Laceration 5 Skull fracture 3 Subdural haem. 1 Extremity fracture 0
Helfer et al (1977)	161 home 85 hospital Total 246	<5 years	Beds, sofas (height <36 in; in 7 cases height >36 in) Beds, cots, Examination tables (height ≤36 in)	Any injury (bumps, lumps, bruises, scratches) 54 Fractured clavicle 3 Skull fracture 3 Humerus fracture 1 Life-threatening injury 0
Lyons & Oates (1993)	207 124 cots 83 beds All hospital cases	<6 years	Cots (height 32 in or 54 in if over sides) Beds (height 25 in or 41 in if over rails)	Superficial injury (all trivial) 29 Fractures: clavicle 1 (21-month-old over cot side) simple skull 1 (10-month-old from cot)
Nimityongskul & Anderson (1987)	76	Birth–16 years	Reported hospital falls (bed, cot, chair) Height: 1–3 ft	Scalp and facial bumps and lumps 14 Lacerations 9 Fractured skull 1 Fractured tibia (osteogenesis) 1 Loose tooth 1 Minor or nil 48
Levene & Bonfield (1991)	328 falls	<16 years	Reported accidents in hospital	Skull fractures: Fall from bed 1 Fall off chair 1 Limb fractures: 3 m fall off climbing frame 1 Non-weight-bearing child with previous fracture 1
Barlow et al (1983)	61 (70% boys, 52% 4 years or less)	1–15 years, peak 1–3 years	Falls from a considerable height on to concreted surfaces/piles of rubbish – 1 or more house stories 77% accidents 23% fell or pushed	3 stories or less – 100% survival 5–6th floor – 50% died Injuries: Concussion 25 Head injury 56 Skull fracture 17 Brain contusion 11 Subdural haematoma 1 Chest 17 Abdominal 44 Other fractures 70
Joffe & Ludwig (1988)	363	1 month–18.7 years, mean 55 months	Stairway falls, 1–24 steps (mean 7)	Abrasion or contusion 200 Laceration 94 Fracture: Skull 6 Extremity 16 Femur 0 Humerus 2 Distal fracture 86% Fractures at separate locations 0 Dental 4 Injury to >1 body part 9

tional. The ratio of abuse to unintentional injury was in inverse relation to age, from 8% abuse in cases older than 23 months to 39% abuse in the age range 0–11 months. There must therefore be a high index of suspicion of abuse in infants with fractures.

Injuries following falls

One of the commonest explanations offered for an injury is that the child fell (Hobbs 1994). A history of a fall from an elevated surface or downstairs is commonly encountered. Various studies have emphasised that fractures are an unusual outcome following such ordinary childhood accidents in hospital and at home (Table 4.4).

Roberton et al (1982) recorded no recent fractures although, as discussed earlier, many had bruises. In infants and toddlers falls from up to about 1 m (3–4 ft) account for most accidents which reach medical attention, but the chance of fracture is low: 1–2% or less. About half of such fractures are uncomplicated single linear fractures of the skull.

Consistent with the findings of these studies, Chadwick and colleagues (1991) found in cases brought to a children's trauma centre that most children who died had allegedly fallen 4 feet (about 1 m) or less. In 100 children who fell less than 4 feet seven deaths occurred, whereas only one child died after falling between 10 and 45 feet. They concluded that when children die in falls of less than 4 feet the history is incorrect. The same authors also found that only one out of 338 young children with head injury sustained at a day care centre was classified as serious, although the child recovered in hours from concussion (Chadwick & Salerno 1993).

There is accumulating evidence from falls from outside buildings in the USA that falls from less than three stories are unlikely to be fatal (Barlow et al 1983, Musemeche et al 1991, Williams 1991).

Falls downstairs have also been studied (Joffe & Ludwig 1988, Chiaviello et al 1994). In the larger study, Joffe and Ludwig described the injuries that resulted, pointing out that life-threatening injuries and those which required intensive care were not seen. Stairway falls consist of a series of short falls and high velocities were not attained. Limb fractures were usually distal and there were no femoral fractures. Injuries in more than one site were encountered in only nine cases. In the other study the higher incidence of intracranial injury including one child with subdural haematoma was claimed to be related to falls with care takers. Such a history, however, must be viewed with caution.

History

When fractures follow genuine accidents, the child is usually presented promptly, there is a clear history of an accident, and the development of immediate pain, loss of function and rapidly developing swelling. In abuse the history may be vague, inconsistent or absent. Medical attention is then more likely to be sought for swelling or loss of function after a period of delay. Sometimes the discovery of the fracture may be unexpected, e.g. rib fracture in a radiograph taken for a medical cause or in a skeletal survey after bruising has been noticed.

Correlation must be attempted between:

- the type of injury observed
- the known mechanisms required for its production
- the proposed mechanism of its production.

If there is a lack of correlation then abuse must be suspected.

Fractures: some common-sense points

- Fractures are sudden, painful and lead to immediate loss of function
- If children are said not to cry or express pain, ask why. Abused children are sometimes too frightened to complain and the frozen and watchful child can be recognised in the Accident and Emergency department (Ounstead 1975)
- Children do not continue to walk or play normally with a fracture, but parents who have abused may ignore the injury

- Pain is at a maximum at the beginning and swelling, bleeding and bruising take a while to develop in full. As these develop, pain may lessen. However, pain continues until the fracture is healed
- Many fractures show no bruising
- As many of the fractures in abused children involve areas of bone dislodged from the main shaft (metaphyseal) or incomplete (greenstick) breaks, all the classic signs of fracture are not always present. Loss of function is the most important sign of a recent fracture. Once healing is under way there may be no clinical signs of fracture detectable, but radiology will reveal the old injury. In abuse, this is especially important because fractures of different ages may be evident on the skeletal survey

Patterns of injury in abuse

The fracture which follows abuse may be single or multiple, recent or old, or a combination and be found in one or more sites. Important patterns include:

- single fracture, e.g. humerus with excessive unexplained bruising
- multiple fractures in various bones, different stages of healing (classic battered baby syndrome)
- metaphyseal–epiphyseal fractures at the end of long bones (these are often multiple after violent shaking and associated with head injury including subdural haematoma)
- rib fractures, single or multiple
- periosteal new bone formation
- skull fracture with intracranial injury.

Although injuries are never interpreted in isolation, some radiological findings carry a higher and some a lower specificity for abuse (Kleinman 1987) (Table 4.5).

Table 4.5 Specificity of radiological findings

High specificity
Metaphyseal lesions
Posterior rib fractures
Scapular and sternal fractures
Spinous process fractures
Moderate specificity
Multiple fractures, especially bilateral
Fractures of different ages
Epiphyseal separations
Vertebral body fractures and subluxations
Digital fractures
Complex skull fracture
Common but low specificity[a]
Linear parietal skull
Shafts of long bones
Clavicle

[a] *Lesions of moderate and low specificity become high specificity when history of trauma is absent or inconsistent with injuries.*

Long bone fractures

Fractures of the long bones are common in children. A variety of different injuries are encountered:

- metaphyseal lesions carry a high specificity for abuse (Silverman 1987): radiologically, corner and bucket-handle fractures are described
- cartilaginous epiphyseal plate injuries (Salter & Harris types I and II) occur in both accident and abuse (Salter & Harris 1963)
- transverse, oblique and spiral shaft fractures
- subperiosteal new bone formation is seen after injury but is also seen with other pathology, including infection and metabolic disease
- other fractures include compound, comminuted, impacted and pathological (underlying bone disease).

Metaphyseal fractures

Disruption through the relatively more fragile growing part of the bone results from indirect trauma. The fracture appears in a corner or bucket-handle configuration depending on the orientation of the X-ray beam. Most often a whole disc-like fragment results from complete separation. These injuries result from pulling or twisting forces and are often multiple. They have a strong association with non-accidental aetiology (Kleinman 1987). These fractures may be associated with soft tissue swelling. With healing, periosteal new bone formation may be seen in the more severe injuries. It is, however, frequently absent in milder injuries (Kleinman 1987).

Epiphyseal plate injuries

Although most injuries to the growing ends of long bones involve the primary spongiosa of the metaphysis, there are some which involve separation of the epiphysis as a result of disruption of the cartilage of the epiphyseal plate. The fracture may involve bone and cartilage or cartilage alone. In the latter case, detection of the fracture will be difficult until healing signs appear, usually at least 7–10 days later.

Transverse, oblique and spiral fractures

Worlock et al (1986) described 35 children with fractures which resulted from abuse and 826 with fractures following accidents. They commented that long bone injuries strongly associated with abuse were subperiosteal new bone formation and spiral or oblique fractures of the shaft resulting from gripping or twisting. In the study, spiral fracture of the humerus was significantly more common in abuse than in the control group. However, they concluded that the fracture alone in most cases would not enable differentiation.

The mechanisms of production of the four basic types of linear fracture (transverse, oblique transverse, spiral and oblique) are discussed by Alms (1961). This may be useful in checking the validity of a history. Alms concluded that the mode of production of the four basic fracture types is deduced on the grounds of simple mechanical theory:

- transverse fractures are the result of angulation: this can occur following a direct blow
- oblique transverse fractures are the result of angulation (or bending) with axial loading (or compression)
- spiral fractures are the result of axial twists with or without axial loading
- oblique fractures are the result of angulation and axial twisting in the presence of axial loading
- axial loading applies to bones, e.g. tibia, which are weight bearing at the time of injury.

Table 4.6 summarises the significance of limb bone fractures in abuse and accident.

CASE HISTORY 4.2

A 14-month-old girl was brought to the Accident and Emergency department with an obvious recent fracture of the forearm. A history was given that she had attempted to climb out of the high chair in which she was being fed and fell. In falling her arm had been caught in the structure of the side of the chair.

In fact, one or two unusual bruises to the thigh, a pattern of failure to thrive and the child's frozen appearance raised concerns. Later it was admitted that during a frustrated feeding session the mother's boyfriend, who had been left to feed the reluctant child, swung her by the arm. In both instances angulation without axial loading could have produced the transverse fracture which resulted.

Periosteal new bone formation

The periosteum comprises inner osteogenic and outer fibrous layers. Subperiosteal haemorrhage causes elevation of the periosteum and separation of the osteogenic layer from the cortex of the bone. Radiographs are initially normal (there may be soft tissue swelling) but after about 7–10 days a thin layer of subperiosteal new bone is formed. Earlier detection of these changes can be achieved by radionuclide bone scanning. The new bone formation may be localised or generalised. Although this is an important finding in abused children, being thought to occur when limbs are grabbed, pulled or twisted, it is itself a non-specific finding encountered in a range of other conditions. These include osteomyelitis, congenital syphilis, rickets, scurvy and vitamin A intoxication, Caffey's disease and leukaemia. In most instances differentiation will be straightforward leaving trauma as the probable cause which, if unexplained, will strongly suggest abuse. Caffey's disease is nowadays little heard

Table 4.6 Significance of limb bone fractures

Bone	Fracture type	Accident	Abuse
Humerus	Spiral/oblique	+	++
	Supracondylar	+	+
	Metaphysis	±	+++
Forearm	Shaft	Common	Direct/indirect injury
	Metaphysis	Rare	Uncommon
Hand (small bones)	Shaft	Uncommon	Occasionally described
Femur	Shaft	Older child uncommon	<2 years, high risk
	Metaphysis		+++ (lower end)
Tibia	Shaft-periosteal	–	+
	Spiral	+	+
	Metaphysis	Rare	++
Fibula	Shaft	+	Kick +
	Metaphysis	Rare	+
Foot (metatarsal)	Metaphysis	–	Highly specific, uncommon pre-school
Pelvis	Pubic ramus	Only after major trauma	Periosteal reaction
Scapula	Various injuries	Rare	Indirect force, high specificity

–, ±, +, ++ *and* +++ *indicate weighting of likelihood, least to most*

of in clinical practice and careful differentiation from abuse is required.

Fractures in specific bones

Femur

Femoral fractures have a long association with abuse, the age of the child being an important variable. Abuse is the predominant aetiology in infancy (Anderson 1982, Gross & Stranger 1983). Anderson found that out of 117 children with 122 femoral fractures, 18 were under 13 months of age. Of these 15 (83%) were abused. Up to 2 years of age, 79% were abused including two-thirds in whom the fracture was the only injury. In older children abuse as a cause is less common. Gross & Stranger (1983) found that in 74 children up to 6 years of age with femoral fractures, abuse was identified in 34 (46%) but in 65% of infants under 1 year. Thomas et al (1991) found 60% to be abusive under 1 year, although surprisingly they described femoral metaphyseal fractures after falls in infants. In three toddlers, one fell from a fire escape, one was in a motor vehicle collision, and in the third case a jacked-up car slipped and crushed the child's leg. These authors suggested that children who are old enough to run can trip or stumble and fracture a femur. However, it may not always be possible to be certain how such a fracture occurs and with injury to such a large bone substantial force is usually implied. Caution in interpretation is required.

Obviously, making a certain diagnosis of abuse when a fractured femur is the only injury may be difficult, but it is important to remember that trivial injury is unlikely to cause a fracture in an otherwise healthy child. In abuse the fracture usually occurs during violent twisting or swinging of the leg or child by the leg. A spiral fracture of the shaft could occur accidentally but only a major fall (e.g. from a first-floor window) would be likely to generate sufficient force to injure this substantial bone. Several studies have found that no particular type of femoral fracture was associated with abuse.

Metaphyseal fractures occur more often in the distal end of the bone. Fractures of the femur account for around 20% of fractures seen in abused children.

Tibia

Fractures of the tibia are described less frequently than femoral fractures in abuse and are most often metaphyseal injuries or subperiosteal new bone formation. The tibial spiral shaft fracture may follow abuse or occur in toddlers learning to walk. The toddler fracture has been defined as 'an undisplaced oblique fracture of the distal tibial shaft in patients aged from 9 months to 3 years, when weight bearing is just beginning' (Shravat et al 1996). The usual symptom is 'unable to weight bear'. The mechanism of injury is considered to be relatively trivial and there is usually an absence of local swelling and bruising. More severe forces may produce a displaced spiral or oblique fracture (Kleinman 1987).

Humerus

The humerus is one of the most frequently injured bones in abuse. Thomas et al (1991) found 14 humeral fractures in children up to the age of 3, of which 11 were judged to have been abusive. All the abusive fractures were diaphyseal or distal metaphyseal, and the accidental ones supracondylar. In abuse the infant is violently grasped by the arm, pulled, swung or jerked, resulting in a range of fractures to the shaft and to both ends of the bone. In the shaft, oblique or spiral fractures usually result although a direct blow may produce a transverse break. Supracondylar fractures occur more typically in accidents although they can occur in abuse. An apparent dislocation of the distal end may in fact be a displaced epiphysis.

Recently two cases were reported of infants aged 3 months and 5 months with spiral-oblique humeral fractures where videotape evidence of the actual incident in one infant and a reconstruction of the alleged incident in the other sought to convince the author that the injuries had occurred unintentionally. The mechanism involved rolling the infant over from prone to supine, with the fractured limb initially extended out from the body and with the limb unable to adduct when the infant was rolled. The trunk was not lifted during the manoeuvre (Hymel & Jenny 1996).

Hands and feet

Injuries to the digits, metatarsals or metacarpals are occasionally found in abuse. There may be little indication of injury clinically, and direct impact is thought to account for some of these. Fusiform swelling of the digits may mimic juvenile arthritis.

Other bones

The clavicle is one of the most commonly fractured bones in childhood. Injury to the lateral part, less common than the midshaft fracture, may be more suggestive of abuse. Scapular and sternal fractures, which nearly always result from direct impact (blows), are highly suggestive of abuse although very uncommon.

Rib fractures

Rib fractures in infants comprise between 5 and 27% of fractures in abused children (Akbarnia et al 1974, Barrett & Kozlowski 1979, Herndon 1983). They can occur antenatally and a case is described of a woman who had attempted to abort her fetus by banging her abdomen against tables and by falling downstairs. Multiple healing rib fractures in the fetus were discovered radiologically (Gee 1975). Care is needed in determining whether a rib fracture occurred as a result of birth trauma as, for example, when an over-vigorous assistant attempts to extract a breech delivery by grasping the child's thorax too hard. This must be very uncommon.

Cardiopulmonary resuscitation rarely, if ever, causes rib fractures and can be safely disregarded as a factor (Feldman & Brewer 1984).

In a recent study, 91 infants who had undergone cardiopulmonary resuscitation before death showed no rib fractures on radiological or autopsy examinations (Spevak et al 1994). Other non-abuse causes of rib fractures include motor vehicle accidents, rickets, osteoporosis, surgery and osteogenesis imperfecta. If there is no history of specific major trauma and no radiological evidence of intrinsic bone disease, unexplained rib fractures are highly specific for abuse.

Diagnosis

Rib fractures, usually only diagnosed radiologically, are frequently multiple and bilateral and most often situated posteriorly near the costotransverse process articulation. Fractures can also occur further anteriorly and are sometimes multiple in the same rib. Kleinman (1987) suggests that rib fractures occur when a child is violently shaken. Anteroposterior compression occurs when the infant's chest is held with palms situated laterally, thumbs anteriorly and fingers posteriorly. In evidence of this, he quotes an abuser's confession and the findings of periosteal disruption and new bone formation on the ventral aspect of the ribs' surface. The rib cage is viewed as a single functional unit comprising a series of parallel struts, and forces are distributed widely throughout the cage leading to multiple fractures of similar age.

Radiology

Acute changes may be invisible, especially if they are situated posteriorly close to the costovertebral junction. Even with healing in this position, only slight widening of the neck of the rib will be seen.

Lateral and anterior fractures are less commonly seen and special oblique views may be needed to identify them, especially in the acute phase. Bone scans have been found to be useful where radiology has produced negative results. Callus formation enhances identification of the fracture and is usually well developed within 2 weeks. The only remaining evidence after a month may be slight cortical thickening.

Spinal injury

Injury to the spine usually results from forced extension and flexion injuries causing damage to several levels. Defects in the lucency of the anterior superior edges of the vertebral bodies, often in the lower thoracic and upper lumbar region, with narrowed disc spaces are typical. There may be no associated spinal cord injury (Swischuk 1969). Injury to the posterior element of the vertebra is less common and is usually associated with injury to the body; the most usual injury is fracture of the spinous process and posterior ligamentous injury.

Skull fractures

Diagnosis

Diagnosis of a skull fracture is usually only made after radiological examination. Occasionally depressed or wide ('growing') fractures can be palpated and the presence of bleeding or cerebrospinal fluid from an ear or nose may lead to a presumptive diagnosis of fracture. A swelling over the scalp may or may not be associated with a fracture of the skull but it should certainly suggest the possibility that one exists. A large haematoma is very likely to be associated with an underlying fracture even if not immediately obvious on radiology.

Skull fractures cannot readily be aged and, because they heal without callus, the usual timetable of events is not applicable. Because it is not usual practice to follow up skull fractures to check on healing, the rate at which they disappear is imperfectly understood. Except for medico-legal purposes, or occasionally when a fracture begins to 'grow', follow-up radiographs serve little useful clinical purpose.

Difficulties in diagnosis arise in infancy because of the presence of aberrant suture lines. Occasionally experienced radiologists may disagree in a difficult case, but usually consultation between the clinician and radiologist enables an accurate diagnosis to be made.

Significance

Injury to the skull is all too common in the severely battered child. Fracture of the skull implies an impact between a solid object and the head. When a child has been violently shaken there may be serious intracranial injury without skull fracture unless impact against a blunt object has also occurred.

Accidental skull fractures in young children usually follow falls, but it is as well to emphasise that this is an infrequent occurrence in the usual kind of accidents which occur. In two series (Kravitz et al 1969, Helfer et al 1977), with a combined total of 594 young children sustaining falls of up to 90 cm (about 3 feet) from table or worktop height, only 5 (1–2%) sustained a skull fracture – all single and linear. None sustained intracranial injury. The surface on to which the child falls is also relevant (Nimityongskul & Anderson 1987).

Patterns

Fractures should be accurately described and measured, either on the radiograph or at post-mortem. The following classification (Hobbs 1984) depends on these definitions:

- Single (linear). A single fracture consisting of an unbranched line in straight, zigzag or angled configuration. The fracture margins are closely opposed with the maximum width between them usually no more than 1–2 mm and often less than 1 mm.
- Multiple or complex. This term applies where there is more than one fracture or where a single fracture has multiple components including a branching pattern. There may be a stellate configuration with several branching lines converging on a central point.
- Depressed. This is a fracture where the normal curvature of the skull is interrupted by the inward displacement of bone. There may be comminution of the fracture with a fragment displaced inwards.
- Growing fractures (Lende & Erickson 1961). These are enlarged linear fractures, usually 3 mm or more at maximum width. They may continue to enlarge over time, sometimes with the formation of a leptomeningeal cyst.

Reports of skull fractures should include:

- site – which bone(s)
- whether suture lines crossed
- configuration – e.g. linear, crazy paving, stellate, branching
- orientation – horizontal, vertical, oblique
- length (cm) of each component – maximum width (mm)
- other features – e.g. depression, growing
- presence of soft tissue swelling (use bright light source)
- comment should also be made on sutures, whether widened or not, with a measure of width.

Table 4.7 gives figures from a study of 89 children aged 0–2 years with skull fracture, 29 of whom were abused.

Site

The most commonly fractured bone, in either accident or abuse, is the parietal which is large, prominent, relatively thin and vulnerable to injury. Frontal fractures are much less commonly seen, either in abuse or accident, whilst occipital fractures have a special predominance in abused children. A depressed occipital fracture is virtually pathognomonic of abuse.

Fractures of the temporal bone and anterior and middle fossa are also uncommon and usually follow severe trauma.

It is frequently possible to recognise that, in the child accidentally injured with fracture(s) involving more than one bone or non-parietal

Table 4.7 Anatomy of skull fractures in abuse and accident (Hobbs 1984)

	Accident	Abuse
Number of cases	60	29
Single linear	55	6
Multiple complex	3	23
Depressed	3	12
Maximum fracture width (3 mm or more)	4	10 (of 13 measured)
Growing	2	6

Table 4.8 Site and extent of cranial fractures (Hobbs 1984)

	Accident	Abuse
Number of cases	60	29
Parietal	57	27
Occipital	3	16
Frontal	0	4
Temporal	1	5
Anterior or middle cranial fossae	1	4
Number of bones involved		
1	56	7
2	3	11
3 or more	1	11

bones, the history denotes a more severe fall. For example, one child with a fracture extending from the parietal across into the temporal bone sustained his injury when he fell from a first floor window (4 m) on to the ground below. Such an injury would be most unlikely to arise from a fall of 1–2 m. This child suffered from disturbed consciousness for 2–3 days but made a full recovery.

Growing skull fracture

Most fractures which occur innocently following falls of a few feet are narrow, hairline cracks, usually in the parietal bone. The width can be measured on a radiograph with a millimetre rule. Occasionally wider fractures of 3 mm or more are seen and rarely a fracture may exceed 5 mm in width. These latter fractures are considered to be growing (Lende & Erickson 1961) and require special consideration.

Growing fractures are uncommon, although they are reported in small numbers in the neurosurgical literature. The essential features are:

- a skull fracture in infancy or early childhood
- a dural tear at the time or injury
- brain injury beneath the fracture
- subsequent enlargement to form a cranial defect.

Out of 89 cases of skull fractures of all kinds in the children studied in Leeds (Hobbs 1984) aged up to 2 years, there were three growing fractures which required surgical treatment. By the time that this kind of treatment is required, the defect is obvious as a smooth swelling over the defect which is pulsatile. The edges of the skull defect are palpable. Growing fractures are linked to severe injury, and abuse should be suspected if such a fracture is found.

Differentiating abuse from accident

The same question must be asked as with all other injuries, i.e. does the injury fit the explanation? As most histories in young children usually involve relatively minor falls or impacts, every skull fracture will need to be evaluated carefully. Differentiation on the basis of fracture characteristics on radiological findings alone is not possible. Obviously those findings which are associated with greater severity of impact (complex, multiple, large depressed areas, wide, involving ' one bone, basal, occipital, associated with intracranial injury) should be accompanied by a history of appropriate severity. Studies have confirmed that uncomplicated linear parietal fractures are the most frequently encountered fractures following both abuse and accident (Meservy et al 1987, Leventhal et al 1993).

Dating fractures

Fractures in child abuse often present late. Recognition of discrepancy between the claimed age and the age ascertained from radiological assessment is strong presumptive evidence of abuse. The presence of fractures of different ages and at different stages of healing is also strong evidence of abuse. There are many factors which can affect the process of healing: severity of injury, degree of displacement at the fracture site, degree of immobilisation and, in abuse, repeated trauma to the same site may complicate the process of healing (O'Connor & Cohen 1987). See Table 4.9.

Refracture of a healing fracture may lead to 'exuberant callus'.

Stages in the process of healing

- *Induction* is the interval between instant of injury and appearance of new bone. During this phase haemorrhage and swelling occur and pain subsides – sometimes as early as 1–2 days after injury. The process of repair begins with ingrowth of capillaries, removal of non-viable tissue and cellular reorganisation.
- *Soft callus* stage. Osteoblasts proliferate and lay down new bone, often seen first around the periosteum. In older children this takes 10–14 days, less in infants. This stage lasts around 3–4 weeks until the fracture line begins to obliterate.

Table 4.9 Timetable for radiographic changes in children's fractures. Reproduced with permission of the authors and publishers from O'Connor J F, Cohen J 1987 In: Kleinman P K (ed) Diagnostic imaging in child abuse. Williams and Wilkins, Baltimore.

Category	Early (days)	Peak (days)	Late (days)
1. Resolution of soft tissues	2–5	4–10	10–21
2. Periosteal new bone	4–10	10–14	14–21
3. Loss of fracture line definition	10–14	14–21	
4. Soft callus	10–14	14–21	
5. Hard callus	14–21	21–42	42–90
6. Remodelling	3 months	1 year	2 years to epiphyseal closure

Repetitive injuries may prolong categories 1, 2, 5 and 6.

- *Hard callus* stage. The fracture is solidly united and lamellar bone replaces periosteal and endosteal bone. In adults this takes 2–3 months, less in children. Infants' fractures may unite in a quarter of the time of those in older children.
- *Remodelling*. The gradual restoration of the original configuration of cortex and medulla can be complete in a stable fracture in a young infant in 3 months while in an older child with angular deformity or displaced fracture may continue for 1–2 years after the original injury. The potential of this process to achieve extreme degrees is maximal in children.

Metaphyseal injuries

Metaphyseal fractures differ from the growth plate fractures of older children in that the tightly adherent periosteum is not disrupted and periosteal reaction is not initiated. Other more subtle changes with healing are described and experienced radiologists can provide an estimate of age in some cases (Chapman 1992).

When birth injury is considered, the absence of periosteal new bone 11 days after birth should suggest the possibility of abuse (Cumming 1979).

Skeletal survey

It is not always necessary to undertake a full skeletal survey in every child where physical abuse is suspected. A skeletal survey should be considered in the following situations:

- presentation with a fracture which suggests abuse
- physically abused child under 3 years of age
- older child with severe soft tissue injury
- localised pain, limp or reluctance to use a limb
- previous history of recent skeletal injury
- unexplained neurological symptoms or signs
- child dying in suspicious or unusual circumstances.

Carty (1989) suggests that the following radiographs are required when conducting a survey for occult trauma:

- skull anteroposterior and lateral
- chest, spine and pelvis anteroposterior
- anteroposterior view of long bones including the hands.

Frasier and colleagues (1991) recommend the following:

- anteroposterior arms
- anteroposterior forearms
- anteroposterior femur
- anteroposterior lower leg
- anteroposterior and lateral skull
- anteroposterior pelvis
- lateral lumbar spine
- anteroposterior (grid) chest for ribs.

All films should be on separate plates.

It must be emphasised that these are the minimum radiographs and must be supplemented with local views in at least two projections of any suspicious area to establish a firm diagnosis. Repeat skeletal survey where abnormality has been identified or thought likely to be present revealed additional information in 14 of 23 cases

Table 4.10 Differential diagnosis of skeletal disorder

Condition	Features	Radiology	Investigations
Normal variant pseudofracture	Aberrant skull suture Symmetrical periosteal reaction Minor abnormality	Often symmetrical, identical to changes of trauma	Consult specialist, large textbook
Birth trauma	Clavicle, humerus, femur, rib, depressed skull, etc.	Absence of callus after 2 weeks = not birth trauma	Check history at birth
Osteogenesis imperfecta (Taitz 1987, Ablin et al 1990, Carty 1991) heterogeneous rare condition, types I–IV	Fractures with minimal trauma Blue sclerae, deafness, family history, wormian bones, dental changes, easy bruising, growth retardation, scoliosis	Osteopenia, thin cortices, angulation and bowing of fractures	Diagnosis on clinical and radiological features No laboratory test available
Osteoporosis (Hobbs & Wynne 1995)	Heparin, disuse e.g. cerebral palsy, osteogenesis, copper deficiency	Poor mineralisation	History, clinical and radiological diagnosis identified cause
Copper deficiency (Shaw 1988)	Rare, temporary Features: sideroblastic anaemia,neutropenia, hypotonia Occurs in preterm, low birth weight, fed by TPN	Osteoporosis, cup shaped and frayed metaphysis, sickle-shaped spurs, symmetrical fractures	80–90% Hb <10 gm/dL neutropenia $<1.0 \times 10^9$/L plasma copper <40 μg/dL caeruloplasmin <13 mg/dL
Osteomyelitis congenital syphilis	Systemic signs and symptoms variable in early infancy Local signs may predominate	Multifocal metaphyseal lesions, periosteal reaction, no corner fractures, bone destruction	Blood cultures, aspirates positive for *Staph. aureus*, coliforms, group B *Strep. meningococcus* Syphilis serology positive, mother and baby
Caffey's disease	Rare disease of infants – painful periosteal thickening in multiple bones	Any bones, especially mandible, clavicle and ulna No fractures or metaphyseal irregularity	Clinical diagnosis Course of disease
Rickets	Premature infant, TPN, confusion after discharge from neonatal unit Older child – fractures unusual	Cupping, fraying costochondral junctions and metaphyses Decreased bone density, Looser's zones	Low serum calcium, low or normal phosphate, raised alkaline phosphatase Low 25-hydroxyvitamin D
Scurvy, vitamin A intoxication	Rare, related to bizarre feeding practice	Periosteal and metaphyseal changes	Vitamin A or C levels in blood

Other diseases include rare genetic syndromes, e.g. congenital indifference to pain, Menke's syndrome, cleidocranial dysostosis, Hajdu–Cheney syndrome, Hutchinson–Gilford disease, homocystinuria, hypophosphatasia, osteoporosis-pseudoglioma (Zinn 1994).

(61%) in one study (Kleinman et al 1996). Increased radiation dose will need to be considered.

Differential diagnosis

Table 4.10 summarises the differential diagnosis of skeletal abnormality in children.

In a review of 10 years of non-accidental injury in Leeds (Wheeler & Hobbs 1988), out of 2578 referrals there were 1912 children with suspected physical abuse. Of these, 50 children had lesions resembling abuse where another cause was found, excluding accidents, and 8 of them had bony lesions:

- birth injury (clavicle) 1
- calcified cephalhaematoma 1
- osteoporosis secondary to neuromuscular disorder 1
- Caffey's disease 1
- congenital hydrocephalus 1
- normal skull variant 1
- scoliosis 1
- osteomyelitis 1

From a medico-legal point of view, osteogenesis imperfecta and copper deficiency are worth careful consideration. Abuse is common and both these conditions are rare, but they may occasionally cause confusion. Metabolic bone disease in the newborn only rarely causes confusion.

Osteogenesis imperfecta

Osteogenesis imperfecta is an inherited disease of connective tissue characterised by fragile, matrix depleted bones which fracture easily following minor injury (Sillence et al 1979, Ablin et al 1990, Hobbs & Wynne 1996). The disease is uncommon with an incidence of 1 in 20 000 births. It is variable clinically: there are four main varieties which are divided into various subtypes (Table 4.11).

In the differential diagnosis of fractures it is the mild forms (types IA and IVA) which may cause diagnostic difficulty.

Types IB and IVB refer to patients with osteogenesis and dentinogenesis imperfecta characterised by fragile, eroded, discoloured deciduous and permanent dentition. Once the teeth are erupted they provide a good diagnostic marker for the condition.

Other features are as follows (see Table 4.11):

- type I: autosomal dominant associated with blue sclerae
- type II: very severe, multiple fractures at birth and early death
- type III: similar to type II, but less severe. cortical thickening, tendency to fracture: unlikely to cause confusion in terms of accident, abuse or organic disease
- type IV: rare autosomal dominant with occasional mutations, osteoporosis possibly present, sclerae not blue.

Clinical picture of mild osteogenesis imperfecta type IA in infancy

- Family history of collagen disorder and fractures, blue sclera, early onset deafness and joint laxity. Careful confirmation of the appropriate history of repeated fractures with minimal injury is required

Table 4.11 Osteogenesis imperfecta

Sillence type	Type I	Type II	Type III	Type IV
Incidence	1 : 30 000	1 : 30 000	Very rare	Unknown
Usual inheritance	Autosomal dominant	Sporadic dominant	Autosomal dominant	Autosomal dominant
Severity	Mild to moderate	Lethal	Moderate to severe	Mild to moderate
Fractures at birth	IA: 10%, IB: 25%	100%	60%	Unknown
Death	Old age	Stillborn or neonate	20–30 years	Old age
Sclerae	Blue	Blue	Blue early then grey	White
Early onset deafness	40% at 40 years	–	5%	As general population
Teeth	IA: normal, IB: abnormal	–	–	IVA: normal, IVB: abnormal

- Hypotonia can be assessed using the Beighton index
- Infant presents with fracture with minimal trauma but pain and dysfunction present
- First fracture usually delayed until weight bearing/ambulation
- Blue sclera: distinguish from normal blueness of infancy and older infants with glaucoma or hypophosphatasia
- Triangular face, growth failure and skeletal deformity unlikely in mild cases in infancy
- Hernia and endocardial defects
- Skin soft, bruises easily, vessels fragile
- Wormian bones: >10 measuring 6 mm by 4 mm are significant (Cremin et al 1982) but may not be present in neonates or preterm infants in early months. (NB wormian bones also occur in Hajdu–Cheyney syndrome, Mencke's disease, progeria and central nervous system abnormalities (Pryles & Khan 1979).
- Osteopenia may not be apparent and normal healing may take place in mild cases in infancy
- Skull, rib and metaphyseal fractures, retinal haemorrhage and intracranial injury are not part of mild osteogenesis imperfecta
- 10% of cases are sporadic

Clinical picture in mild osteogenesis imperfecta type IVA in infancy

- Rare: accounts for 5% of all cases
- Usually a family history but occasional sporadic cases occur
- Normal teeth and sclera
- History of fracture with minimal trauma
- Diagnosis difficult in absence of family history, normal sclerae, radiology normal (wormian bones are usual) and mild disease

Types I and IV enter into the differential diagnosis of child abuse. Easy bruisability is also a feature. However, fractures of ribs, skull, metaphyses, intracranial injury and multiple bruises are not part of the disorder. Fractures which no longer occur in protective care also point to abuse.

A diagnosis of osteogenesis imperfecta is encouraged by the presence of blue sclerae, osteopenia, thin cortices, a tendency to bowing and angulation of healed fractures, a family history, dentinogenesis imperfecta, deafness, presence of wormian skull bones. Although most children would have at least one or more of these associated findings, the possibility of encountering a sporadic type IV case with none does exist, but it has been estimated at between one in 1 million and one in 3 million births. The probability of encountering such a child in comparison to meeting one who has been abused is very small and, as Taitz (1987) points out, medical witnesses need to formulate their opinion in the light of such odds. Provided care is taken, osteogenesis imperfecta does not provide a satisfactory reason for unexplained fractures in otherwise healthy babies. Recent suggestions that there is a 'temporary brittle bone disease', a variant of osteogenesis imperfecta, have been dismissed on the grounds that there is no evidence for this condition. Most authors believe that this is really child abuse by another name.(Ablin & Shashikant 1997, Chapman & Hall 1997).

Copper deficiency

Copper deficiency has also been raised as a possible cause of unexplained skeletal abnormalities, including fractures (Shaw 1988).

Skeletal manifestations of copper deficiency

- Retardation of bone age
- Osteoporosis
- Metaphyseal cupping
- Increased density of the zone of provisional calcification
- Metaphyseal sickle-shaped spurs.
- No skull or metaphyseal fractures

The changes occur late and are distributed symmetrically throughout the skeleton. Copper deficiency is rare (100 reported cases) with fractures in 16 (5 term infants). Fractures usually occur in abnormal long bones, ribs in preterm infants only and never in skull.

Other features of copper deficiency include:

- preterm infants (40% of cases of copper deficiency are in preterm infants)
- abnormal feeding pattern (not in breast-fed or formula-fed infants)
- psychomotor retardation, hypotonia, pallor, hypopigmentation of skin and hair, prominent scalp veins, sideroblastic anaemia resistant to iron therapy, neutropenia.
- low serum copper: all cases have levels below 43 μg/dl term, 33 μg/dl preterm.
- response to copper supplements.

An experienced radiologist should be able to differentiate between child abuse and the abnormal bones of copper deficiency, but it is wise to check the presence or absence of other features.

Metabolic bone disease (Ryan 1996)

- Occurs in ill preterm infants with prolonged nutritional compromise
- Fractures occur in ribs or long bones in the neonatal unit or soon after discharge
- Metaphyseal and skull fractures have not been described
- Rickets and osteoporosis are associated with raised blood alkaline phosphatase level and hypophosphataemia
- Is preventable and readily reversible with improved nutrition.

Intracranial injury

The prognosis of a head injury relates to the intracranial component. Injury to the brain is the commonest cause of death from physical abuse. In the first year of life 95% of serious head injuries result from abuse and serious head injury following an alleged minor fall in a baby should alert the clinician to the possibility of abuse (Billmire & Myers 1985, Hobbs 1993).

There are two major categories of head injury:

- *Impact injury* when the child is thrown violently against a wall, floor or other object or struck. This results in trauma to the brain as well as its coverings including scalp, skull and meninges and vasculature.
- Violent *acceleration/deceleration injury* from shaking. In this situation the child is held, often with both hands by the chest and violently and repeatedly shaken back and forth. The relatively large and unsupported head undergoes wide amplitude whiplash type flexion and extension movements frequently with associated rotation. In this pattern of trauma there may be no superficial injury or fracture either to head or other parts of the skeleton. In other cases, however, metaphyseal and rib fractures may be found and bruises where the infant was held. Cervical spine injuries are infrequent.

These two mechanisms of injury frequently coexist and overlap in effects.

The pathology of head injury includes:

- scalp injury: bruises, traumatic subgaleal haematoma
- skull fracture
- subdural, subarachnoid and intraventricular haemorrhage
- cerebral contusion, haemorrhage and oedema
- eye and other associated injury.

Subarachnoid haemorrhage

Subarachnoid haemorrhage rarely occurs spontaneously in childhood (Newton 1989) and then follows rupture of an arteriovenous malformation or aneurysm in two-thirds of cases. No cases in children under 1 year old have been reported. Subarachnoid haemorrhage, detected by the finding of bloodstained cerebrospinal fluid, may occur as part of a wider pattern of injury following trauma. Misdiagnosis has resulted when bloodstained fluid has been dismissed as traumatic tap (Apolo 1987). This can be avoided if the infant's retinae are carefully evaluated (preferably by an ophthalmologist) and if bloodstained cerebrospinal fluid is inspected after centrifuging and cytology undertaken. Association with subdural haemorrhage is common.

Subdural haemorrhage

Subdural haemorrhage is likely to give rise to concern over the possibility of non-accidental injury when it arises in infants and young children (Caffey 1946, Newton 1989).

A number of rare conditions have been reported to be associated with subdural haemorrhage in childhood. It is not always possible to say from the reports that these cases had not also suffered abuse. They include *Haemophilus influenzae* and pneumococcal meningitis, haemophilia, malignancy, arteriovenous malformation/aneurysm, post-cardiopulmonary bypass, glutaric acidaemia, Algelle's syndrome, disseminated intravascular coagulation and Mencke's disease.

It is now considered to be extremely unlikely that the condition of benign subdural collection of infancy exists, and that infants who were previously given this diagnosis had been shaken.

As is noted above, in an otherwise healthy infant, subdural haemorrhage is invariably traumatic in origin. Although theoretically a clotting disorder may present with subdural haemorrhage, in practice this is rarely seen. Appropriate investigation should be considered on clinical grounds.

Over half the cases of subdural haemorrhage present without evidence of skull fracture or other sign of injury to the head. This gave rise to the notion of 'spontaneous origin' or arising from 'minimal trauma' until the mechanism by which these children had been injured was appreciated. It is now accepted that these children have been violently shaken. The infant's anatomy – with a large, heavy, relatively poorly supported head – predisposes to violent acceleration and deceleration forces in the 'whiplash shaken syndrome' (Guthkelch 1971, Caffey 1972). The soft, pliable skull and brain lead to stress on the bridging veins as they attach to the sagittal sinus, causing disruption and bleeding into the subdural space, often over a wide area bilaterally. The expanding intracranial mass produces symptoms which depend on its rate of growth and may be acute or chronic. In the chronic slowly accumulating case, failure to thrive, poor feeding, sporadic vomiting, unexplained anaemia and fever with late onset of fits and accelerated head growth may occur. In the acute case, irritability, vomiting, fits, decreased responsiveness, coma, stupor, irregular breathing and apnoea may suggest the diagnosis in the presence of a tense fontanelle. The infant appears shocked and distressed.

It is increasingly recognised with more sophisticated radiological techniques and detailed neuropathological examination that there is a spectrum of non-accidental head injury in infancy which correlates with eye injury.

The scheme in Table 4.12 is based on the work of Green et al (1996). The authors suggest that the same shaking forces which produce the subdural haemorrhage also apply to the vitreous producing the subhyaloid and intraretinal haemorrhages and in many instances retinal detachment.

Diagnosis of subdural haemorrhage is confirmed readily by computed tomography (CT) scan. Prior to the introduction of this technique, diagnosis in life was made by subdural taps through the anterior fontanelle which were both diagnostic and therapeutic. Post-haemorrhagic anaemia is a usual finding if the bleeding has been extensive.

On CT scans, subdural collections have a high attenuation when fresh. They most often lie over the convexity of the hemispheres although less commonly lie in the inter-hemispheric fissure or posterior fossa. The high attenuation value of fresh blood falls with age thus allowing the opportunity to age the collection(s). CT may not always detect very fresh blood (<2 hours). Magnetic resonance imaging (MRI) supplements CT by demonstrating:

- small subdural collections
- subdural haematomas of different ages
- shaking injuries that are not visible on CT (Sato et al 1989).

Table 4.12 Fatal non-accidental head injury

Grade of injury	Head injury	Eye injury
Less severe	Subdural haemorrhage	Subhyaloid and intraretinal haemorrhage
More severe	Intracerebral subarachnoid haemorrhage	Perineural (subdural) optic nerve haemorrhage
Most severe	Cerebral laceration	Retinal detachment Choroidal and vitreous haemorrhage

Table 4.13 summarises the diagnosis of intracranial injury.

Retinal haemorrhage

Many studies have documented the association of retinal haemorrhages with child abuse (e.g. Harcourt & Hopkins 1971). The presence of retinal haemorrhages may be the first clue to the diagnosis of an intracranial injury in an infant with no external signs of trauma. Retinal haemorrhages can occur in other conditions but confusion with abuse is unlikely.

Non-abusive causes of retinal haemorrhage

- Birth trauma: 2.6–50% of newborn babies have retinal haemorrhages depending on when examined. More common after vaginal delivery than Caesarean section. They disappear from 24 h to 6 weeks
- Acute leukaemia
- Other haematological disorders – thrombocytopenia, hyperviscosity
- Meningitis (<5% of cases)
- Other rare causes (Kaur & Taylor 1990)

In abuse, the haemorrhages persist much longer and occur in association with brain trauma. Sudden elevation of the intracranial pressure causing compression of the central retinal vein and increased pressure at the choroidal anastomosis at the optic disc may be responsible.

Table 4.13 Diagnosis of intracranial injury (Zimmerman et al 1979, Alexander et al 1986, Wissow 1990)

History	No injury or minor household accident ('rolled off settee')
Presentation	May suggest illness: fits, unconsciousness, lethargy, apnoea, delay in presentation
Examination	May be no external findings of injury
Child's condition suggests	Meningitis, encephalitis, toxic state, metabolic disease and others
Useful physical signs	Full or bulging fontanelle Low haematocrit (earlier injury) Separation of sutures Increased head circumference Retinal haemorrhages
Investigations	Skull radiograph Skeletal survey Lumbar puncture (may be bloody) CT scanning: diffuse cerebral oedema, subarachnoid haemorrhage, subdural haemorrhage MRI: posterior fossa and intraparenchymal lesions

This blockage of circulation leads to rupture of intraretinal capillaries which leak blood into the retinal tissues. Various patterns are described – flame, dot, etc.

Retinal haemorrhages are present in between 75% and 90% of shaken babies (AAP 1993) but even in those infants with no haemorrhages detectable on clinical examination, intracranial and optic nerve sheath abnormalities are demonstrable on histopathology (Budenz et al 1994). Table 4.14 summarises abusive ophthalmic injuries found in children.

Cerebral contusion, haemorrhage and oedema

Areas of cerebral injury may be scattered throughout the brain leading to fits, raised intracranial pressure and long-term handicap. Between 3% and 11% (Buchanan & Oliver 1972) of children in hospitals for those with severe learning difficulties were handicapped as a result of physical abuse in one study. Epilepsy, post-traumatic hydrocephalus and changes to visual pathways and cerebral infarction leading to atrophy and microcephaly result.

Children presenting without a history of trauma who have unexplained hydrocephalus, raised intracranial pressure or fits may have been

Table 4.14 Ophthalmic injuries in abuse (Allen Gammon 1981)

Structure	Result	Lesion	Effects
Eyelids, periorbital tissue	Blunt trauma, e.g. fist	Bruising – 'black eye'	Recovers
Cornea, conjunctiva	Blunt or penetrating trauma, burns, chemicals	Haemorrhage, laceration, abrasion, ulceration, scarring	Variable, depending on severity in visual axis
Lens, anterior structures	Blunt or penetrating trauma	Iris sphincter rupture Dislocated lens	Vossius ring glaucoma Intraocular scar formation Cataract
Posterior structures, vitreous, retina	Anterior injury transmitted to back of eye Whiplash, shaking Fractures of orbit	Vitreous haemorrhage Retinal haemorrhage Retinal detachment Optic nerve injuries	Retinal scarring Papilloedema Optic atrophy Resolution and visual loss variable
Visual cortex	Head injury Contrecoup	Cerebral contusion Haemorrhage	Cortical blindness

abused. The fundi should be carefully examined for retinal haemorrhages and skeletal survey considered. Differential diagnosis of 'non-traumatic' presentation includes herpes simplex encephalitis, meningitis and tumour as well as the administration of drugs and poisons. Other useful investigations include a lumbar puncture and computed tomography.

Shaken impact syndrome

A study by Duhaime and colleagues (1987) has suggested that the original hypothesis for the mechanism of injury in the 'shaken baby syndrome' may be inadequate to explain the severity of the injuries often encountered.

The classic description has the assailant holding the infant around the chest wall between his or her hands. As the infant is violently shaken the head and limbs flail, so producing the subdural and retinal haemorrhages and the long bone fractures. Duhaime's team found difficulty in reconciling the injuries in 48 infants thought to have been shaken with the histories and clinical findings. In addition, when infant-sized dolls were shaken by adult volunteers, the forces measured by transducers were thought to be insufficient to account for the severity of injury expected in the clinical situation. In contrast, accelerations caused by impact exceeded shake accelerations by a factor of almost 50. Out of this work has grown the concept of the shaken impact syndrome.

A further aspect of this syndrome is its repetitive nature. Alexander et al (1990) described 24 children who had been shaken, 12 of whom had external head trauma in addition to being shaken. There was evidence of prior abuse, neglect or both in 71%, and 33% were known to have been previously shaken. It is important, therefore, to recognise the complex factors responsible for head injuries in child abuse.

Radiological investigation of suspected intracranial injury

The detection of intracranial injury following child abuse depends on the threshold for investigation as well as the method of examination used. Prior to the introduction of CT, recognition of intracranial injury relied on clinical, surgical or post-mortem findings. Many cases of intracranial injury are undoubtedly missed because the clinical signs appear insufficient to warrant CT scanning. It is also believed that some intracranial injury is not detectable on CT. CT findings include:

- diffuse or focal cerebral oedema
- subarachnoid haemorrhage
- subdural haemorrhage (interhemispheric, convexity – acute or chronic)
- intraventricular haemorrhage
- contusional haemorrhage
- post-traumatic hydrocephalus and cerebral atrophy.

The reversal sign of anoxic/ischaemic encephalopathy is a finding which carries a poor prognosis indicating irreversible brain damage.

MRI is a valuable adjunct to CT in the evaluation of brain injuries in infants. Detection of subdural collections, particularly those orientated transversely or in difficult areas proximal to bone e.g. posterior fossa is enhanced (Frasier et al 1991) and intraparenchymal lesions including non-haemorrhagic white matter contusions and shearing injuries is significantly improved (Sato et al 1989). Ageing of injuries is also facilitated. Rebleeding into an existing collection can be detected.

Outcome of inflicted intracranial injury

The outcome depends on the severity of the shaking episode or episodes. Anoxia during the event may also contribute to brain injury. Morbidity and mortality are high when the infant at presentation is unconscious, with 60% dying or profound learning and/or motor disabled in one study (Sinal & Ball 1987).

Long-term follow-up studies of whiplash shaken infants suggest that few escape unscathed. In one recent study from Belgium (Bonnier et al 1995), of 13 infants fulfilling the criteria for whiplash/shaking injury, there were six with a sign free interval and seven without. These seven remained severely and permanently abnormal from the time of injury with one death. Of the six, five (sign free) who appeared to recover well on later follow-up at between 6 months to 5 years were found to have done badly. Problems included hemiparesis (2), severe learning difficulties (5) and severe behaviour disorder (3).

There is a risk of re-injury if returned home, and only 10–20% of victims of the shaken baby syndrome turn out reasonably normal (Fischer & Allasio 1994).

Inflicted submersion injury

Holding a child's head under water was described as a physical control strategy in a recent study (Smith 1995). Clinical cases, including fatal ones, may present difficulty in diagnosis. In one study (Gillenwater et al 1996) 8% of 205 submersions were judged to be inflicted from other signs of abuse or incompatibilities in the history. Victims were young (mean age 2 years) and immersions in baths were more often inflicted. Kemp et al (1994) looking at bathtub immersions found that 20% were suggestive of abuse. They found that most bathtub submersions they considered to be accidental occurred to children aged 8–15 months. In epilepsy-related drownings, a child with epilepsy aged over 24 months was left alone in the bath.

Non-accidental drownings were usually outside the 8–15 months age group and histories were inconsistent with late referral to hospital. Victims were less likely to be revived by bystanders and more likely to die. Accounts of events collected by multiple professionals around the time of the incident proved crucial in the diagnosis of abuse. They often changed and were inconsistent with the child's stage of development or extent of the injury. Deliberately leaving a young infant alone in a bath of water would constitute at best highly inappropriate parenting, neglect or passive abuse, in the latter instance the adult being conscious that a serious outcome would probably result. Table 4.15 summarises the finding, in accident and abuse.

Abdominal injury

Abdominal injuries are less commonly recognised in physical abuse than limb fractures or craniocerebral injuries (McCort & Vaudagna 1964,

Table 4.15 Submersion/drowning: features in accident and abuse (Kemp et al 1994)

Feature	Accident	Abuse
Age	8–15 months	Older or younger than accidental range
History	Left briefly alone	Inconsistent, late presentation, different versions of history
Other signs	No signs of abuse	Other signs of abuse
Carer	With sibling, mother preoccupied with other children	Maternal mental illness, inappropriate carer

CASE HISTORY 4.3

The mother of a 6-year-old boy returned home to find him ill in bed. His stepfather was in the house with the boy's three siblings and no explanation was given for the injury initially. It was later stated that he had been playing on a nearby building site and that something may have fallen on him. Even later the stepfather said that the child had returned from the building site, got himself in and out of the bath and then gone to bed.

On arrival at hospital it was immediately obvious that the child had an acute abdominal catastrophe. A plain radiograph showed free gas in the peritoneum. Recent abrasions over the right lower chest wall and overlying the lumbar spinous processes were noted. At operation free blood, bile and pancreatic juice were found in the peritoneum. There was a laceration in the liver, and traumatic transection of the pylorus with complete transection of the head of the pancreas. The duodenum was devitalised, the common bile duct and pancreatic duct were transected. There was bleeding from the middle colic vein.

Touloukain 1968, Cooper et al 1988). Their importance lies in the threat to life, particularly if there is a delay in diagnosis. Intra-abdominal trauma usually results from a kick or punch, and injury to gastrointestinal as well as solid organs may result.

Diagnostic points

- There may be no signs of external injury, e.g. bruising
- Delay in presentation and denial of a history of trauma make diagnosis difficult and mortality high
- Doctor's attention is attracted to other injuries, e.g. head and limbs
- Free gas is found in a minority of cases
- A high index of suspicion is required, especially if the general condition of the child is poor or shock is present.

Types of injuries

- *Perforation of gut*: stomach, duodenum and duodeno-jejunal flexure, jejunum, ileum
- *Haemorrhage*: major vessel
- *Laceration, contusion, haematoma*: liver, spleen, duodenum, pancreas, mesentery, kidney.

Mechanics of injury

- *Compression*. A punch or kick to the abdomen will squeeze the intestinal tract, especially the stomach or colon. Susceptibility to injury is greatest when the organs are distended by food or gas. The result is likely to be rupture if the organ is unable to withstand the increased pressure
- *Crushing injury*. If an organ is compressed against the spine or rib cage, crushing or shaking forces result which lead to damage. An example is in blunt abdominal trauma, certainly to the upper abdomen, where the relatively fixed duodeno-jejunal flexure is crushed against the spine producing shearing forces which result in rupture or bleeding into the wall. Other susceptible organs include the pancreas, liver, spleen and kidney
- *Sudden acceleration/deceleration injuries*, as where the child is swung or thrown into a solid object. This is likely to interrupt the vascular supply to the bowel, with or without perforation

Investigation

Urgent laparotomy is the most appropriate way to confirm the presence and site of a perforation and other abdominal injury. Other investigations are as listed below (see Hobbs 1994a)

Clinical abdominal examination

- Is there distension?
- Insert nasogastric tube, empty stomach. Is blood, food or bile obtained? Does distension remain?
- Is rectal examination required? Are there signs of injury (sexual abuse can perforate the rectum in infancy), blood, anterior tenderness?

Laboratory investigations

- Serial haematocrit for blood loss
- Serum amylase (raised in pancreatic and in some cases of splenic injury because the spleen lies close to the pancreas)
- Serum aspartate aminotransferase, alanine aminotransferase, lactate dehydrogenase (raised in liver laceration)
- Urine: gross or microscopic haematuria (>20 red blood cells per high-power field suggests damage to the kidney or urinary tract)

Radiology

- *Chest radiograph*: rib fracture, pneumothorax, pleural fluid/haemothorax
- *Posteroanterior abdominal and chest radiographs*, taken in supine and erect positions, allows visualisation of free air and fluid levels following perforation of a hollow viscus
- *Plain radiographs of abdomen* may reveal ground-glass appearance of intraperitoneal haemorrhage(or fluid from other cause)
- *CT scanning* is the most sensitive method of identifying injuries of the lungs, pleura and solid abdominal organs, including pancreatic injury and duodenal haematoma.

Specific injuries

Stomach

Rupture of the stomach is rare following both accidental and non-accidental injury, with the majority of cases in children, predominantly boys (Schechner & Ehrlich 1974, Case & Nanduri 1983).

Gastric injuries may follow motor vehicle accidents, but a few cases have reputedly followed vigorous cardiopulmonary resuscitation. The injury was then assumed to be the result of the ventilatory dilatation of the stomach with air. The few cases in the literature relating to abuse are in children presumed to have received a blow to the upper abdomen. Cases of spontaneous rupture of the stomach are found almost exclusively in infants during the first 2 weeks of life and are related to birth trauma, congenital defects, peptic ulcer, septicaemia, hypoxia or oxygen therapy. However, the study relating to this predates our current knowledge of abuse, and cases of abuse would not have been recognised (McCormick 1959).

The usual site of laceration is along the anterior wall and greater curvature; the lesser curvature is less commonly involved. Other abdominal injuries – including to the liver, bowel, spleen and pancreas – often coexist. Severe shock may follow release of gastric contents and hydrochloric acid into the peritoneum; mortality varies from 10 to 66%. Delay in presentation, diagnosis and surgery increases morbidity and mortality.

CASE HISTORY 4.4

A 5-month-old baby was found dead by his grandmother around dawn, after his mother had left him and his 2-year-old sister alone and unattended overnight in her flat. At post-mortem examination, he showed signs which suggested severe anoxia before death (petechial haemorrhage to thymus, brain and lungs) and greater curvature rupture of the stomach which contained milk solids. There was bruising to the liver and diaphragmatic tissues, but not to the skin of the abdomen. Thirty-six hours earlier he had appeared to be a well, thriving, uninjured infant when presented to a paediatrician because his mother had claimed previous sexual abuse by the infant's father of her 2-year-old daughter. The grandmother stated that she had found the baby and could not wake him. She had pressed his abdomen and called an ambulance. No prosecution followed.

Duodenum and small bowel

Injury to the duodenum and duodeno-jejunal flexure is well recognised in blunt abdominal trauma (Woolley et al 1978, Hamilton & Humphreys 1985). As with abdominal injuries in general, the majority of children are under 4 years of age and, in a review of 21 small intestinal perforations in 17 abused children, the average age was 2 years. In the same series, 60% involved the jejunum, 30% duodenum and 10% ileum.

Perforation may be intraperitoneal, leading to different clinical pictures. Intraperitoneal perforation results in abdominal pain, distension, fever, shock, leukocytosis and signs of peritonitis. There may be free gas in the peritoneal cavity. It may be visible radiologically, although sometimes with difficulty. Supine and erect films should be taken where there is any suspicion of abdominal injury.

Retroperitoneal perforation from duodenal injury may not produce typical signs of peritonitis and the signs are more insidious. Radiology is often unhelpful. Intramural haematomas of the duodenum and jejunum have been recognised in abuse only recently. If a bleeding disorder is excluded, the aetiology is presumed to be trauma. The haematoma may be localised or diffuse, and present with vomiting and abdominal pain, sometimes delayed for hours or days after the injury. There may be significant blood loss and elevated white cell count.

Radiological examination may reveal signs of upper intestinal obstruction and a filling defect may be visualised in the lumen of the gut on barium examination. The mass encroaches on the lumen, is smooth and rounded and produces varying degrees of obstruction. Specialist radiological assessment is essential for accurate diagnosis. Providing there is no perforation, conservative treatment is indicated. When a duodenal haematoma is recognised in a child, child abuse should always be considered and appropriate search for other injuries and an appraisal of the child's and family's history undertaken. One author found clear evidence of abuse in 50% of cases of duodenal haematoma.

Pancreas

Acute pancreatitis is a rare condition in childhood. It may be due to drugs, viral infection, systemic disease or – most commonly – blunt abdominal trauma (Hartley 1967, Slovis et al 1975, 1980). Drugs associated with pancreatitis include high-dosage corticosteroid therapy, valproic acid, sulfasalazine and thiazine.

Pancreatitis may occur in cystic fibrosis, systemic lupus erythematosus, antitrypsin deficiency, diabetes mellitus, Crohn's disease, glycogen storage disease type 1, hyperlipidaemia types I and V and familial (hereditary) cases, hyperparathyroidism, Henoch–Schonlein purpura, Reye's syndrome, and malnutrition. Alcohol-induced pancreatitis should be considered in older children. Obstruction to the pancreatic ducts by stones, tumours or choledochal cysts is a rare cause.

Trauma may be accidental or non-accidental. Car accidents (as passenger or pedestrian), bicycle handlebar injuries and falls against objects are typical examples. The injuries are not always considered serious at the time and some children have been sent away from Accident and Emergency departments only to return later. The onset of pancreatitis may be rapid, or gradual and insidious. The commonest injury pattern seen is the pancreatic pseudocyst; contusion, laceration, disruption and complete transection are less common. Some 60% of pseudocysts are due to trauma and the origins of around 30% are unknown but almost certainly include some cases of unrecognised trauma. Increasing evidence linking pancreatitis and pseudocysts with blunt abdominal trauma indicates that, if there is no satisfactory history, abuse must be a strong possibility and should be investigated as such.

Lying across the spine, the pancreas is vulnerable to blunt trauma by crushing against the vertebral bodies. Pancreatitis develops when damage occurs to the glandular acini or ducts, leading to seepage of enzymes into tissue spaces and consequent autodigestion. Clinical features are persistent abdominal pain, bilious vomiting, fever, leukocytosis and elevated serum amylase. An epigastric mass is frequently palpable in patients with pseudocysts. Radiology, including CT and ultrasonography, is useful in diagnosis, especially in defining the presence of a pseudocyst. Where there is peritonitis, high levels of amylase may be found in the fluid obtained by paracentesis. Pleural effusions may be present and bony lesions from fat necrosis consist of intramedullary necrosis and new bone formation, difficult to distinguish from leukaemia, sickle cell infarction or bony metastases. Involvement of a paediatric surgeon in consultation in management is valuable, although conservative management is successful in many children with acute pancreatitis.

Liver

Injury to the liver usually arises from direct injury from blows or following sudden deceleration (Cooper et al 1988). Major injuries are uncommonly seen and are identified at laparoscopy or post-mortem examination. Smaller contusions and lacerations may go unnoticed and undiagnosed. Only if the newer imaging techniques are routinely used (ultrasonography, radionuclide or CT) are these injuries detected.

The most common injuries are laceration, capsular tear and haematoma. More serious injury can lead to vascular damage (e.g. to hepatic veins and vena cava) with massive haemorrhage. There will frequently be other evidence of injury elsewhere, but the mortality from liver trauma is high.

Spleen

The spleen is a commonly injured abdominal organ in childhood trauma. There is, however, little in the literature relating splenic injury to child abuse. It must be considered as a possible injury in the abused child with abdominal pain, especially in the left upper quadrant. Increased uptake of ^{99m}Tc methylene diphosphorate by the spleen in a 5-year-old child scanned to detect skeletal injury was related to a subcapsular haematoma outlined by ^{99m}Tc sulphur colloid scan.

Kidney

As with the other solid abdominal organs, injury to the kidney is very uncommon in child abuse (Morse 1975). Injury can be classified as contusion, laceration or rupture. The most serious injury may involve damage to the renal vessels. Posterior rib fractures may be noted, together with bruising to the back and loin regions. There may be haematuria, loin pain and usually evidence of injury elsewhere. A tender mass in the flank may be palpable. In suspected renal trauma urine must be obtained for examination, by catheter if necessary, and imaging techniques including intravenous urography and radionuclide scintigraphy used to visualise the kidneys.

Recently it has been recognised that acute renal failure following major soft tissue injury in abuse may relate to myoglobinuria secondary to rhabdomyolysis.

Chest injuries

Bruising to the chest wall and rib fractures are common in abused children. Underlying injuries to the pleura, lungs, heart and mediastinal organs are rarely recognised.

CASE HISTORY 4.5

An abused infant of 3 months presented acutely ill. An empyema necessitatis was thought to be related to an inflicted puncture wound of the overlying chest wall. Other injuries included an avulsed toe nail and multiple bruises.

The flexibility of the rib cage in a young child appears to protect the intrathoracic organs from injury from compression or blows. Underlying pulmonary contusion is seldom clinically significant. Injury to bronchi has not been reported in child abuse and tension pneumothorax must be extremely rare. Injury to the heart is limited to single case reports, but the possibility of penetration injury should always be considered. One child with sewing needles lodged in the heart has been described.

Management of child and family

The aims of management are to secure a safe environment for the child, to provide for his future needs and prevent further abuse. After a period of assessment, the small number of children for whom substitute or alternative care is required should be identified. The majority of children will return or remain at home with a plan of management to protect the child.

Strategies include:

- addressing the source(s) of stress within the family
- alleviating material difficulties – housing, debt
- empowering parents to improve their parenting skills
- provision of day care
- improving community support
- use of family aides, home helps
- promoting non-violent ways of coping with stress
- facilitating improved relationships within family and extended family
- information about child development.

The plan should incorporate inputs from a variety of different agencies (e.g. statutory and voluntary) and be coordinated by the key worker. Concerns about the children must be honestly expressed to the parents and the need for change spelled out clearly. Expectations and standards of care must be explicitly stated. If there is a legal order, control is with the statutory authority within the terms of the order. Otherwise cooperation must be achieved voluntarily – often difficult in child abuse work.

In addition to addressing the needs of the child, it is important that the parents' needs are addressed; otherwise they will not be able to provide differently for their child. Sometimes a separate worker is assigned to give special attention, for example to a mother or a father, leaving the key worker to focus on the child's needs.

Part of successful management is the periodic assessment of the child's well-being and development. It is useful for the family and closely involved 'face workers' to receive an assessment by a paediatrician who can comment on the child's progress, highlighting improvements as well as areas of development which need to be addressed. Encouraging the parents to make their own observations and assessments is also part of such programmes as the Child Development Project being used by health visitors in some areas.

When satisfactory progress has been made, and the family appears to be functioning at an acceptable level, the child's name may be removed from the register and the intensity of work reduced, although contact will usually be maintained after this time.

Summary

1. Accidental injury is extremely common in childhood.
2. Differing patterns of injury allow distinction of accidental injury from abuse, in the majority of cases.
3. 1–2% of children are recognised as being physically abused at some time during their childhood. However, recent research confirms that most violence to children goes unreported.
4. There is a strong relationship in reported cases with adverse social circumstances.
5. Mothers are more often implicated as perpetrators than men, because they are the principal carers.
6. Bruises are the most commonly encountered injury followed by fractures and brain injury.
7. Subdural haemorrhage and retinal haemorrhage are almost always the result of abuse.
8. Rib, certain patterns of skull and long bone metaphyseal fractures are all strongly suggestive of abuse.
9. Abdominal injury is the second most common cause of death and is frequently missed in diagnosis. Injuries to the stomach, duodenum and pancreas are most often seen.
10. Differential diagnosis includes bleeding and clotting disorder, bone disease, congenital abnormalities and skin conditions.
11. Physical abuse commonly coexists with other abuses, e.g. one in six are also sexually abused.
12. Acute injury is often a crisis in a childhood of violence.

13. The importance of minor injury in babies cannot be overstated.
14. Interventions aimed to protect children and support families must be mindful that children may be permanently damaged or die.
15. When giving evidence in court, build up the diagnosis to explain the final opinion.

REFERENCES

AAP 1993 American Academy of Pediatrics. Shaken baby syndrome: inflicted cerebral trauma. Pediatrics 92:872–875

Ablin S A, Shashikant M S 1997 Non-accidental injury: confusion with temporary brittle bone disease and mild osteogensis imperfecta. Pediatric Radiology 27:111–113

Ablin S A, Greenspan A, Reinhart M, Grix A 1990 Differentiation of child abuse from osteogenesis imperfecta. American Journal of Radiology 154:1035–1046

Akbarnia B, Torg J S, Kirkpatrick J, Sussman S 1974 Manifestations of the battered child syndrome. Journal of Bone and Joint Surgery 56A: 1159–1166

Alexander R C, Schor D P, Smith W L 1986 Magnetic resonance imaging of intracranial injuries from child abuse. Journal of Pediatrics 109:975–979

Alexander R, Crabbe L, Sato Y, Smith W, Bennett T 1990 Serial abuse in children who are shaken. American Journal of Disease in Childhood 144:58–60

Allen Gammon J 1981 Ophthalmic manifestations of child abuse and neglect. In: Ellerstein N S (ed) Child abuse and neglect. A medical reference. J Wiley, New York, pp 121–139

Alms M 1961 Fracture mechanics. Journal of Bone and Joint Surgery 43:162–166

Anderson W A 1982 Significance of femoral fractures in children. Annals of Emergency Medicine 11:174–177

Apolo J O 1987 Bloody cerebrospinal fluid: Traumatic tap or child abuse? Pediatric Emergency Care 3:93–95

Barlow B, Neiminska M, Gandhi R P et al 1983 Ten years experience with falls from a height in children. Journal of Paediatric Surgery 18:509–511

Barrett I K, Kozlowski K 1979 The battered child syndrome. Australian Radiology 23:72–82

Bernat J E 1992 Dental trauma and bite mark evaluation. In: Ludwig S, Kornberg A E (ed) Child abuse: a medical reference. Churchill Livingstone, New York, Chapter 14

Billmire M E, Myers P A 1985 Serious head injury in infants: accident or abuse? Pediatrics 75:340–342

Bonnier C, Nassogne M, Evrard P 1995 Outcome and prognosis of whiplash shaken infant: Late consequences after a symptom free interval. Developmental Medicine and Child Neurology 37:943–956

British Psychological Society 1992 Submission to Scottish Law Commission Report on Family Law, Scottish Law Commission. HMSO, Edinburgh

Buchanan A, Oliver J E 1972 Abuse and neglect as a cause of mental retardation: A study of 140 children admitted to subnormality hospitals in Wiltshire. British Journal of Psychiatry 131:458

Buchanan M F G 1989 Physical abuse of children (videotapes and accompanying booklet). University of Leeds Audio-Visual Service

Budenz D L, Farber M G, Mirchandani H G, Park H, Rorke L B 1994 Ocular and optic nerve hemorrhages in abused infants with intracranial injuries. Opthalmology 101:559–565

Caffey F 1946 Multiple fractures in the long bones of infants suffering from chronic subdural haematoma. American Journal of Roentgenology 56:163–173

Caffey J 1972 On the theory and practice of shaking infants. American Journal of Disease in Childhood 124:161–169

Carty H 1989 Skeletal manifestations of child abuse. Bone 6:3–7

Carty H 1991 Differentiation of child abuse from osteogenesis imperfecta. American Journal of Radiology 156:635

Case M E S, Nanduri R 1983 Laceration of the stomach by blunt trauma in a child: a case of child abuse. Journal of Forensic Sciences 28:496–501

Chadwick D L, Salerno C 1993 The rarity of serious head injury in day care centers. Letter to editor. Journal of Trauma 35:968

Chadwick D L, Chin S, Salerno C, Landsverk J, Kitchen L 1991 Deaths from falls in children: How far is fatal? Journal of Trauma 31:1353–1355

Chapman S, 1992 The radiological dating of injuries. Archives of Disease in Childhood 67:1063–1065

Chapman S, Hall C M 1997 Non-accidental injury or brittle bones. Pediatric Radiology 27:106–110

Chiaviello C T, Christoph R A, Randall Bond G 1994 Stairway-related injuries in children. Pediatrics 94:679–681

Childhood Matters 1996 Report of the National Commission of Inquiry into the Prevention of Child Abuse. Stationery Office, London

Children and Violence 1995 Report of the Gulbenkian Foundation Commission. Calouste Gulbenkian Foundation, London

Cooper A et al 1988 Major blunt abdominal trauma due to child abuse. Journal of Trauma 28(10):1483–1487

Creighton S J, Noyes P 1989 Child abuse trends in England and Wales 1983–87. NSPCC, London

Creighton S J, Russell N 1995 Voices from childhood: A survey of childhood experiences and attitudes to child rearing among adults in the United Kingdom. NSPCC, London

Cremin B, Goodman H, Spranger J, Beighton P, 1982 Wormian bones in osteogenesis imperfecta and other disorders. Skeletal Radiology 8:35–38

Cumming W A 1979 Neonatal skeletal fractures. Birth trauma or child abuse? Journal of the Canadian Association of Radiologists 30:30–33

Dawkins J L 1995 Bullying in schools: doctor's responsibilities. BMJ 310:274–275

Dawkins J L, Hill P 1995 Bullying: another form of abuse? In: David T J (ed) Recent advances in paediatrics 13. Churchill Livingstone, Edinburgh
DES 1994 Bullying – don't suffer in silence; an anti-bullying pack for schools. Department of Education. HMSO, London
Duhaime A-C, Gennarelli T A, Thibault L E, Bruce D A, Margulies S S, Wiser R 1987 The shaken baby syndrome: a clinical, pathological and biomechanical study. Journal of Neurosurgery 66:409–415
Elliott M 1991 Stop bullying. Booklet for parents and children. Kidscape, 152, Buckingham Palace Road, London SW1W 9TR
Feldman K W, Brewer D K 1984 Child abuse, cardiopulmonary resuscitation and rib fractures. Paediatrics 73:339–342
Fischer H, Allasio D 1994 Permanently damaged: Long-term follow-up of shaken babies. Clinical Pediatrics 33(11):696–698
Frasier L D, Smith W L, Alexander R C 1991 Clinical presentation and imaging studies in child abuse. Hospimedica May 1991:28–35
Gee D J 1975 Radiology in forensic pathology. Radiology 41:109–144
Gillenwater J M, Quan L, Feldman K W 1996 Inflicted submersion in childhood. Archives of Pediatric and Adolescent Medicine 150:298–303
Green M A, Lieberman G, Milroy C M, Parsons M A 1996 Ocular and cerebral trauma in non-accidental injury in infancy: Underlying mechanisms and implications for paediatric practise. British Journal of Opthalmology 80:282–287
Gross R H, Stranger M 1983 Causative factor responsible for femoral fractures in infants and young children. Journal of Pediatric Orthopedics 3:341–343
Guthkelch A N 1971 Infantile subdural haematoma and its relationship to whiplash injuries. British Medical Journal 11:430–431
Hamilton A, Humphreys W G 1985 Duodenal rupture complicating childhood non-accidental injury. Ulster Medical Journal 54:221–223
Harcourt B, Hopkins D 1971 Ophthalmic manifestations of the battered baby syndrome. British Medical Journal 3:398
Hartley R C 1967 Pancreatitis under the age of five years: a report of three cases. Journal of Pediatric Surgery 2:419
Helfer R E, Slovis T L, Black M 1977 Injuries resulting when small children fall out of bed. Paediatrics 60:533–535
Herndon W A 1983 Child abuse in a military population. Journal of Paediatrics and Orthopaedics 3:73–76
HMSO 1989 An introduction to the Children Act 1989. HMSO, London
Hobbs C J 1984 Skull fracture and the diagnosis of abuse. Archives of Disease in Childhood 59:246–252
Hobbs C J 1993 Head injuries. In: Meadow S R (ed) ABC of child abuse. BMJ Publications, London, pp 14–16
Hobbs C J 1994a Child abuse. In: Addy D P (ed) Investigations in paediatrics. W B Saunders, London, Chapter 11, pp 157–171
Hobbs C J 1994b Could it have happened when he fell, doctor? Child Abuse Review 3:148–150
Hobbs C J, Wynne J M 1990 The sexually abused battered child. Archives of Disease in Childhood 65:423–427
Hobbs C J, Wynne J M 1995a Physical signs of child abuse – a colour atlas. W B Saunders, London
Hobbs C J, Wynne J M 1995b Spontaneous fractures in cerebral palsy. BMJ 310:873–874
Hobbs C J, Wynne J M 1996 Fractures in infancy: are the bones brittle? Current Paediatrics 6:183–188
Hymel K P, Jenny C 1996 Abusive spiral fractures of the humerus: a videotaped exception. Archives of Paediatric and Adolescent Medicine 150:226–227
Joffe M, Ludwig S 1988 Stairway injuries in children. Pediatrics 82:457–461
Kaur B, Taylor D 1990 Retinal haemorrhages. Archives of Disease in Childhood 65:1369–1372
Kemp A M, Mott A M, Sibert J R 1994 Accidents and child abuse in bathtub submersions. Archives of Disease in Childhood 70:435–438
Kempe C H, Silverman F N, Steele B F, Droegmueller W, Silver H K 1962 The battered child syndrome. JAMA 181:17–24
Kennedy H 1995 Banged up, beaten up, cutting up. Report of the Howard League Commission of Inquiry into penal institutions for young people. Howard League for Penal Reform, London
Kleinman P K 1987 Diagnostic imaging of child abuse. Williams & Wilkins, Baltimore
Kleinman P K, Nimkin K, Spevak M R, Rayder S M, Madansky D L, Shelton Y A, Patterson M M 1996 Follow-up skeletal survey in suspected child abuse. American Journal of Roentgenology 167:893–896
Kravitz H, Driessen G, Gomberg R, Korach A 1969 Accidental falls from elevated surfaces in infants from birth to one year of age. Paediatrics (suppl) 44:869–876
Langlois N E I, Gresham G A 1991 The ageing of bruises: a review and study of the colour changes with time. Forensic Science International 50:227–238
Lende R A, Erickson T C 1961 Growing skull fractures of childhood. Journal of Neurosurgery 18:479–489
Levene S, Bonfield G 1991 Accidents on hospital wards. Archives of Disease in Childhood 66:1047–1049
Leventhal J M, Thomas S A, Rosenfield N S, Markowitz R I 1993 Fractures in young children – distinguishing child abuse from unintentional injuries. American Journal of Disease in Childhood 147:87–92
Lyons T J Oates R K 1993 Falling out of bed: a relatively benign occurrence. Paediatrics 92:125–127
McClelland C Q, Heiple K G 1982 Fractures in the first year of life. A diagnostic dilemma? American Journal of Disease in Childhood 136:26–29
McCormick W F 1959 Rupture of the stomach in children. Archives of Pathology 67:416–426
McCort J, Vaudagna J 1964 Visceral injuries in battered children. Radiology 82:424–428
McMurray J 1989 Case conferences. In: Meadow S R (ed) ABC of child abuse. BMJ, London, pp 42–44
Meservy C J, Towbin R, McLaurin R L, Myers P A, Ball W 1987 Radiographic characteristics of skull fractures resulting from child abuse. American Journal of Roentgenology 149:173–175
Messages from Research 1995 Child protection: messages from research. HMSO, London
Moores C F A 1959 The dentition of the growing child. Harvard University Press, Cambridge, MA, pp 79–110
Morse T S 1975 Renal injuries. Pediatric Clinics of North America 22:379
Musemeche C A, Barthel M, Cosentino C et al 1991 Pediatric falls from heights. Journal of Trauma 31:1347–1349
Newell P 1989 Children are people too. The case against physical punishment. Bedford Square Press, London
Newson J, Newson E 1986 Findings on use of physical punishment on 1, 4, 7 and 11 year old children, together with some sequelae in later life. Child

Development Research Unit, University of Nottingham
Newton R W 1989 Intracranial haemorrhage and non-accidental injury. Archives of Disease in Childhood 64:188–190
Nimityongskul P, Anderson L D 1987 The likelihood of injuries when children fall out of bed. Journal of Paediatric Orthopaedics 7:184–186
O'Connor J F, Cohen J 1987 Dating fractures. In: Kleinman P K (ed) Diagnostic imaging in child abuse. Williams & Wilkins, Baltimore, pp 103–113
O'Hare A E, Eden O B 1984 Bleeding disorders and non-accidental injury. Archives of Disease in Childhood 59:860–864
Ounstead C 1975 Gaze aversion and child abuse. World Medicine 12(17):27
Pryles C V, Khan A J 1979 Wormian bones – a marker of CNS abnormality. American Journal of Disease in Childhood 133:380–382
Rao V 1995 Bullying in schools – a more aggressive preventive strategy is required (letter). BMJ 310:1065
Ricci L R 1991 Photographing the physically abused child: principles and practice. American Journal of Disease in Childhood 145:275–281
Roberton D M, Barbor P, Hull D 1982 Unusual injury? Recent injury in normal children and children with suspected non-accidental injury. British Medical Journal 285:1399–1401
Ryan S 1996 Nutritional aspects of metabolic bone disease in the newborn. Archives of Disease in Childhood 74:F145–F148
Salter R B, Harris W R 1963 Injuries involving the epiphyseal plate. Journal of Joint Surgery 45A:587–622
Sato Y, Yuh W T C, Smith W, Alexander R C, Kao S C S, Ellerbroek C J 1989 Head injury in child abuse: evaluation of MR imaging. Radiology 173:653–657
Schechner S A, Ehrlich F E 1974 Gastric perforation and child abuse. Journal of Trauma 14:723–725
Schmitt B D 1987 The child with nonaccidental trauma. In: Helfer R E, Kempe R S (eds) The battered child, 4th edn. University of Chicago Press, Chicago
Schwartz A J, Ricci L. 1996 How accurately can bruises be aged in abused children? Literature review and synthesis. Pediatrics 97:254–256
Shaw J C L 1988 Copper deficiency and non-accidental injury. Archives of Disease in Childhood 63:448–455
Shravat B P, Harrop S N, Kane T P 1996. Toddler's fracture. Journal of Accident and Emergency Medicine 13:59–61
Sillence D O, Senn A, Danks D M 1979 Genetic heterogeneity in osteogenesis imperfecta. American Journal of Medical Genetics 16:101–116
Silverman F N 1987 Radiology and other imaging procedures. In: Helfer R E, Kempe R S (eds) The battered child. University of Chicago Press, Chicago, pp 214–246
Sinal S H, Ball M R 1987 Head trauma due to child abuse: serial computerised tomography in diagnosis and management. Southern Medical Journal 80:1505–1512
Slovis T L, VonBerg V J, Mikelic V 1980 Sonography in the diagnosis and management of pancreatic pseudocysts and effusions in childhood. Radiology 135:153–155
Slovis T L, Berdon W E, Haller J O et al 1975 Pancreatitis and the battered child syndrome. Report of two cases with skeletal involvement. American Journal of Roentgenology 125:456
Smith M 1995 A community study of physical violence to children in the home, and associated variables. Poster presented at ISPCAN Vth European Conference on Child Abuse and Neglect, Oslo, Norway 1995
Smith M, Bee P, Heverin A, Nobes G 1995 Parental control within the family: the nature and extent of parental violence to children. Quoted in Child protection: messages from research. HMSO, London
Smith S M, Hanson R 1974 134 Battered children: a medical and psychological study. British Medical Journal 4:666–670
Spevak M R, Kleinman P K, Belanger P L, Primack C, Richmond J M 1994 Cardiopulmonary resuscitation and rib fractures in infants. JAMA 272:617–618
Stephenson T, Bialas Y 1996 Estimation of the age of bruising. Archives of Disease in Childhood 74:53–55
Swischuk L E 1969 Spine and spinal cord trauma in the battered child syndrome. Radiology 92:733
Taitz L S 1987 Child abuse and osteogenesis imperfecta. British Medical Journal 295:1082–1083
Taitz L S 1991 Child abuse: some myths and shibboleths. Hospital Update 5:400–404
Tattum D P, Lane D A 1988 Bullying in schools. Trentham, Stoke on Trent.
Thomas S A, Rosenfield N S, Leventhal J M, Markowitz R I 1991 Long bone fractures in young children: distinguishing accidental injuries from child abuse. Pediatrics 88:471–476
Touloukain R J 1968 Abdominal visceral injuries in battered children. Paediatrics 42:642–646
Waterhouse L, Pitcairn T, McGhee J, Secker J, Sullivan C 1993 Evaluating parenting in child physical abuse. In: Child abuse and child abusers. Jessica Kingsley
Wheeler D M, Hobbs C J 1988 Mistakes in diagnosing non-accidental injury, 10 years' experience. British Medical Journal 296:1233–1236
Whitney I, Smith P K 1993 A survey of the nature and extent of bullying in junior/middle and secondary schools. Educational Research 35:3–25
Williams R A 1991 Injuries in infants and small children resulting from witnessed and corroborated free falls. Journal of Trauma 31:1350–1352
Wissow L S 1990 Head and internal injuries. In: Child advocacy for the clinician, an approach to child abuse and neglect. Williams & Wilkins, Baltimore
Woolley M M, Mahour G H, Sloan T 1978 Duodenal haematoma in infancy and childhood. Changing aetiology and changing treatment. American Journal of Surgery 136:8–14
Working Together 1988 Working together: a guide to arrangements for inter-agency co-operation for the protection of children from abuse. HMSO, London
Working Together 1991 Working together under the Children Act 1989. A guide to arrangements for inter-agency co-operation for the protection of children from abuse. HMSO, London
Worlock P, Stower M, Barbor P 1986 Patterns of fractures in accidental and non-accidental injury in children: a comparative study. British Medical Journal 293:100–102
Zimmerman R A, Bilaniuk L T, Bruce D, Schut L, Uzzell B, Goldberg H I 1979 Computed tomography of craniocerebral injury in the abused child. Radiology 130:687–690
Zinn A B 1994 Genetic disorders that may mimic child abuse or sudden infant death syndrome. In: Reece R M (ed.) Child abuse – medical diagnosis and management. Lee and Febiger, Philadelphia, ch 17, p 414

5

Burns and scalds

Burns and scald injuries to children are common. The majority result from accidents which involve varying degrees of parental inattention, including cases of neglect. A small number involve deliberate abuse and their detection poses an important challenge to doctors who see large numbers of children. Doctors in the front line of accident and emergency work see the more severe injuries at the all-important time of presentation and their records and observations are vital to assessment. They work closely with paediatricians as well as surgeons who are responsible for treatment. Less severe injuries may never be seen in hospital; general practitioners, health visitors and school nurses may be the first to see them and question how they have been caused.

The parent who abuses may wish to hide the consequences, which are then only discovered by the vigilance of others, for example nursery nurses or schoolteachers. It is interesting to note how often concealment is partial or imperfect and this seems to reflect the ambivalence of the parents.

Statistics

The causes of 11.1% of all accidental deaths (Jackson 1985) are classified as burns or scald injuries, although this figure include children who die in house fires where the inhalation of smoke may play an important part. Children in house fires may have been left alone, unattended or unsupervised, and have played with fires or matches. In one well-publicised case in which a child died and the sibling was severely burned, the parents deliberately set fire to the house and then made it look as though they had been the victims of an arson attack. There had been previous fires over a period of a few years including one which had lead to the family being rehoused. Repeated and inappropriate fire-setting (e.g. in the bedroom) in children is a good marker of abuse. Some learn that it is a sure way of raising concerns which can lead to removal into safety.

In England and Wales each year there are over 5000 discharges and deaths from hospital of children with burns and scalds; four-fifths of these are in children aged 0–4. Accidental injuries of this type are very much a problem in younger children, who have to be taught of the risks and dangers of heat and fire. Attendance without admission to hospital is even more common – one estimate from a Home Office Surveillance system run by the Department of Trade and Industry puts the number of attendances at all Accident and Emergency departments offering 24-hour cover in 1983 at 13 900 for burns and 21 900 for scalds, with a similar age distribution as for children admitted (see Table 5.1).

A downward trend has been recorded in burn and scald injuries in children over the past 20 years (Chapman et al 1994). The number of flame burns has declined with proportionately more scalds. As in virtually all childhood accidents (horse-riding excepted), boys outnumber girls in the cases of burns and scalds by 3 : 2.

The majority of these injuries occur in the home, which for young children is understandably the most dangerous environment. It is against this background – in which burns and scalds are common injuries, particularly in the younger child – that one faces the task of identifying abuse. The proportion of children with burns and scalds resulting from abuse is not accurately known, with estimates from 4% to 39% (Stone et al 1970, Phillips et al 1974, Hight et al 1979, Showers & Garrison 1988). The few British studies (Raine & Azmy 1983) suggest 1–2% of admitted children, but a typical study from America in one hospital found 8% of suspected inflicted injury with 4.2% later substantiated (Phillips et al 1974). In Melbourne the figure of 6% was found, whereas in Michigan – in one of the largest studies over 6 years and involving 872 children admitted to a burn centre in the children's hospital – 16% were thought to have been inflicted (Hight et al 1979). It is suspected that underdiagnosis is the rule, as with abuse in general.

Table 5.1 Common accidents resulting in admission to a children's surgical ward (adapted from Hobbs 1986)

Scalds	134
Drinks, food, pans, kettles	112
Baths, sinks, domestic hot water	22
Contact burns	12
Room heaters	9
Tools, appliances	3
Other	17
Fat, caustic, flame, electrical	

Burns and scalds occur in around 10% (Martin 1970) of physically abused children, occasionally in association with other injuries such as bruises or fractures. The highest proportion of physically abused children with burns or scalds is the early UK study of Smith & Hanson (1974) in Birmingham, where 20% had burns and scalds. These figures of course reflect hospital experience and serious abuse. Bruising is still far commoner than burns or other injuries.

Accidental burns and scalds

A great deal could be done further to reduce accidental burns and scalds, which occur principally to young children (Jackson 1985). Kitchens, and to a lesser extent bathrooms, remain the focus of danger; the living room fire is much less a danger in these days of central heating and gas and electric fires with improved safety features, but it must still be viewed as negligent for there to be an unguarded fire with young children in the house.

The peak age for these accidents is between the first and second birthdays, when children acquire mobility without the means to protect themselves. Exploratory behaviour is at a peak and cups of tea, kettle flexes or pan handles all pose dangers. Washing machine hoses can be pulled out of sinks and an older toddler may be able to climb into a bath into which scalding hot water has been run. Even a spilled cup of tea contains a considerable amount of heat if freshly poured and the presence of clothes will keep the liquid in contact with the skin for longer and with larger volume and hence heat.

Some of the most serious accidents ensue when a flex from an electric kettle or jug is pulled, dragging the kettle and contents off a table or work surface above a child. As the water cascades down, the child's head, shoulders and upper trunk bear the brunt of injury with possible secondary injury to arms and feet. The use of coiled kettle flex is being introduced as a means of reducing this kind of accident.

Tap water scalds

Although the pour scald injury still accounts for the majority of scalds, accidents involving domestic hot water from taps or showers in baths and sinks are also important (Hobbs 1996). It is often in these circumstances that the possibility of abuse is raised. Adults do understand the burning dangers of tap water, and non-impaired adults do not sustain bath scalds. This implies that when children sustain such injuries, a very careful examination of the circumstances is required and some kind of abuse or neglect assumed until proved otherwise.

Causation of burns and scalds

Explanations for accidental tap water scalds

- Fall into an excessively hot bath (running of bath by sibling or inadequately supervised by adult)
- Tap turned on by child or sibling when child in the bath
- Child put hand into hot water in sink or bath (e.g. to retrieve toy or to prevent self from falling in)
- Child accidentally placed in a bath of too hot water by a carer
- Plastic/portable bath fell over on to child
- Water from hosepipe (draining washing machine) spilled on to child

The relationship of time and surface temperature in the causation of burns was explored by Moritz & Henriques (1947). The relationship expresses the time taken at a particular temperature to produce a full thickness burn. For example, above 70°C burning may be almost instantaneous. The relationship is logarithmic and holds until 44°C when injury becomes less predictable (Fig 5.1).

Department of Health and Social Security engineering data (DHSS 1977) based on more recent research, and experimental work at the now defunct Industrial Injuries and Burns Unit of the MRC gave the results shown in Table 5.2. These results differentiate between partial and full thickness burns. The results were obtained with the use of heated metal sources, commonly a copper container heated internally with circulating water at the appropriate temperature. They represent animal experiments and the use of the (relatively thin) skin of the human forearm in adults. The information which is provided in the form of guidance on safe temperatures for heated surfaces and hot water supplies in health–care buildings recommends that a safe average temperature is 42–43°C for a heating surface for patients at risk (elderly, handicapped, children). The maximum tolerable temperature for handwashing is 49°C and 44°C is comfortably hot for a bath.

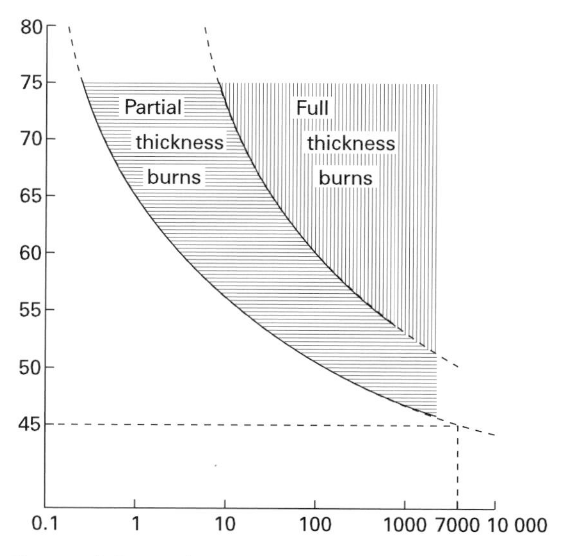

Fig. 5.1 Relation of time and temperature (contact with heated metal) to produce injury or discomfort.

Table 5.2 Temperature and duration of exposure sufficient to cause burns in thin areas of skin (DHSS 1977)

Temperature (°C)	Partial thickness burn (seconds)	Full thickness burn (seconds)
65	1	20
60	5	80–100
54	35	700–800
50	60	

The importance of this information will become apparent when careful forensic assessment of bath-scald injuries is undertaken, and it also enables us to estimate the potential dangerousness of a domestic hot water system for a child (Fig. 5.2).

Accidents from tap water are serious because they are frequently extensive and severe, requiring the care of a special burns unit. Over one-third in one study involved a quarter or more of the body surface area. The major factor causing these injuries is the high temperature of domestic hot water in many homes. Studies in North America have confirmed that many homes have water temperatures higher than 54°C, which will produce a partial thickness scald in around 30 seconds, sometime shorter in a child. Obviously, if thermostats are not working properly, the temperature may be even higher than 65°C. A safe temperature of 49°C has been proposed for domestic baths and showers to avoid accidents, but this is unlikely to be widely adopted and a maximum of 54°C seems to be a more realistic figure adopted by bodies concerned with safety in the home.

A change in the law in Washington State, USA to limit the temperature of water heaters to a maximum of 49°C resulted in a reduction in frequency, morbidity, and mortality of tap water burn injuries in children. Lower water heater settings proved acceptable to the consumer (Erdmann et al 1991). There appears to be no study of hot water system temperatures in homes in Britain.

Table 5.3 Published series including tap water scalds in children

Authors	Date	Location	Findings
Feldman et al	1978	Seattle, USA	28% of hospitalised tap water scalds were abusive
Raine & Azmy	1983	Glasgow, UK	472 children <3 years, 387 scalds – 48% tap water. 10 children referred for NAI investigation
Hobbs	1986	Leeds, UK	5 of 8 abusive scalds from tap water. 25% of all abusive thermal injuries were scalds
Purdue et al	1988	Dallas, USA	Scalds were most frequent cause of inflicted thermal injury (83% from tap water)
Tennant & Davidson	1991	Edinburgh, UK	758 children including 91 with bath scalds. No cases of NAI, social services involved with 5 families
Renz & Sherman	1992	Georgia, USA	26% of paediatric burn admissions were the result of abuse – scalds were the commonest injury
Yeoh et al	1994	South Wales, UK	6% of bath-related scald injuries were the result of forced immersion (abuse)

Contact burns

One major group of accidental thermal injuries, contact burns, has shown a reduction in recent years. Room heaters are important as causes of burns in accidents, neglect and non-accidental injury. Properly designed and fitted fireguards protect children, but loose or poorly fitted guards may be circumvented by exploring hands, resulting in serious burns, especially from the electric bar fire. Contractures caused by deep palmar burns may occur if the hand adheres to the element.

Other sources of contact burns, both accidental and non-accidental, include irons: the flex is grasped by the young child who pulls the iron off the ironing board, the iron landing on the lap of the child sitting in a buggy, for example. A

CASE NO: ______________________ POSSIBLE PERPETRATOR'S NAME: ______________________

PRESENT DATE: ______________________ CHILD'S NAME: ______________________

PLACE WHERE INJURY OCCURRED ________

BATH OR SINK MEASUREMENTS:

Width: ______________________ Inches

Top length ______________________ Inches

Bottom length: ______________________ Inches

Inside depth: ______________________ Inches

Construction ______________________ (porcelain, fibreglass, metal, plastic etc.)

RUNNING WATER TEMPERATURE - HOT:

Seconds	Degrees
0	______
5	______
10	______
20	______
______	______ Peak Temp.

RUNNING WATER TEMPERATURE - COLD:

Seconds	Degrees
______	______

RUNNING WATER TEMPERATURE (FULL HOT AND COLD):

Seconds	Degrees
______	______ Peak Temp.

FULL HOT WATER STANDING 5 INCHES DEEP (TEMPERATURE MEASURED IN MIDDLE OF BATH/SINK AT MID-DEPTH):

	Fill Time			
Inches	Minutes	Seconds	Minutes	Degrees
			0	______
1	______	______	______	______
2	______	______	______	______
3	______	______	______	______
4	______	______	______	______
5	______	______	______	______

PARENT RAN A TUB OF WATER ON MY REQUEST. RESULTS: DEPTH 5 INCHES — 1 MINUTE AFTER WATER OFF — TEMPERATURE __________ DEGREES. MEASUREMENT WAS MID-BATH/MID-DEPTH.

INVESTIGATOR #1: ______________________ I. D. # __________ DIVISION: ______________

INVESTIGATOR #2: ______________________ I. D. # __________ DIVISION: ______________

Fig 5.2 Pro forma for immersion scalds (modified from an evidence worksheet provided by P J Peltier, Office of District Attorney, San Diego, California).

variety of small household appliances including soldering irons, hair crimpers and heated rollers are potentially dangerous. The external surfaces of cookers and cooker doors may be hot enough to produce a burn.

Other accidents causing burns

Conflagrations and flame burns

Flame burns occur most commonly in young school-age children, with flammable liquids, cigarettes or lighters, outdoor fires and house fires responsible in that order (Mercier & Blond 1996).

Smokers' materials – matches, cigarettes, lighters – can all be responsible for fires which result in injury or death. Paraffin heaters and liquid petroleum gas cylinders are other potential sources of hazard to families. Deaths from clothes and nightdresses catching fire from open fires have fallen dramatically with improved safety regulations, and recently introduced safety regulations regarding furniture construction should assist further. Smoke alarms can reduce the risk of serious injury but battery powered ones may suffer from poor use and maintenance.

Faulty wiring, bare wires and faulty appliances may be responsible for fires or electrocution; children are at high risk if these problems are left unattended or go unnoticed. Older children may be burned making fires in the open or playing with fireworks.

Non-accidental burns

It is disturbing to think of an adult deliberately inflicting a burn on a child. Because of this, it is less likely that the possibility will be considered and the inflicted injury may be overlooked.

Burning a child may be an impulsive immediate response – to a child playing with a fire, for example. one parent held her child's hand against the fire to demonstrate to the child that it was hot when she found the child playing with the fire's controls: a superficial burn resulted.

In other instances there may be deliberate premeditation, as when the child who has wet or soiled is plunged into a bath of hot water. It takes time to run the water and undress the child. Where burns are linked to sexual abuse (Hobbs & Wynne 1990) it seems likely that there is a wish to inflict pain, sometimes as a way of threatening the child into silence. Here the adult may obtain gratification from sexual aggression and the power of control over the child. Children who have been abused in this way are often terrified and find difficulty in relating what has happened to them. Inflicted burns are sadistic and may be part of ritual abuse.

Diagnosis

Presentation is either as:

- acute injury
- neglected or old injury
- healed burn or scar.

Figure 5.3 summarises the pathway of referral for non-accidental burns.

General features of non-accidental burns (Scalzo 1994)

- Delay in presenting the child for treatment – in one study a delay of over 2 hours correlated with abusive causation (Feldman 1988)
- Presentation after a delay if a complication develops (Purdue et al 1988)
- Presence of other injuries, old and new
- Pattern of repeated burns/scalds to children in the family
- Evidence of neglect including non-organic failure to thrive
- Responsible adults allege that there were no witnesses to the 'accident' and that the child was merely discovered to be burned, thus hoping to discourage any further inquiry
- Scald attributed to action of sibling or other child (this is often a false explanation for abusive scalds but if found to be true, then the wider implications require careful consideration)
- Child reported to cry little/experience little pain at the time of injury or to show unusual response to the injury/ treatment

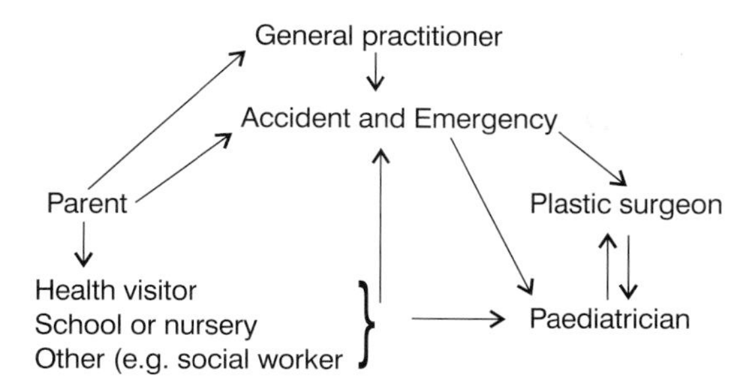

Fig. 5.3 Pathway of referral for non-accidental burns.

As with all non-accidental injuries, the cardinal point is a history which does not match the injury. It has to be said that the more carefully taken the history, the clearer the picture will be of how the injury supposedly happened. Until there is a completely clear picture further questions should be asked and information sought. Sometimes only a visit to the scene or an examination of the fire or bathroom enables an understanding of the incident and if there are doubts after the usual history taking it is better to wait, admitting the child to hospital until it is clear.

Delay or avoidance of treatment is common and the reasons must be explored. One family said the doctor's surgery was closed so they did nothing. This might be just about acceptable in a minor burn, but most families know that Accident and Emergency departments at hospital stay open 24 hours a day. If the burn looks older than the history claims, then the views of an experienced nurse are sought. Nurses dress burns often, and soon get an idea of how old a burn is. Their experience is vital in recognising the abused burned child.

Many parents say they did not witness the incident, perhaps being in another room or attending to another child. This was the case in two out of every three abused children seen in Leeds, but in only about 10% of true accidents in another study (Martin 1970). It should be borne in mind that most of the children burned are under 5 years of age, and the commonest age for burns from abuse is less than 3 years. These children are normally close to their parents and there is usually little doubt about what has happened when an accident occurs. In abuse the parent may describe the cause of the injury accurately but obviously not the way it happened. Where parents say they do not have any idea how the injury occurred, they should be encouraged to speculate, to list all the sources of heat in the house and to suggest possibilities. In this way the source of injury will often be mentioned. Persistent inability to explain the injury may sometimes indicate that the parent has left the child alone or poorly supervised: in families who abuse their children this is not uncommon.

In abuse, parents rarely take responsibility. They usually feel that the child deserved it and may even blame the child for the injury. He or she may have tripped over, been pushed by the dog or a sibling or be playing with the taps yet again despite being told repeatedly not to do so.

Sometimes of course these stories are true, but concern should always be aroused if the parent is hostile towards the child. Even though the child obviously contributes to many of the accidents we see, parents usually feel guilty and blame themselves. Parents of children with accidental injuries naturally feel uncomfortable about being questioned and their feelings of guilt should not be misinterpreted.

Denial of the injury is another important clue. This can be manifested by non-presentation or trivialisation of the injury or the child's response. 'It wasn't bad, he didn't even cry' is not uncommon. Sometimes the denial is complete. One mother swore that the deep circular ulcer on one buttock of her child was a nappy rash when her health visitor, general practitioner, a paediatrician and paediatric nurse all said it could not be nappy rash and had to be a burn (Plate 64). She steadfastly refused to accept their diagnosis. In the case of another child, the mother stated firmly that the child had scraped his back playing in the garden when the lesion was obviously a burn. The finding of an old, healing, unpresented burn across his younger sister's bottom provided further evidence with which to confront the family. Of course there are some lesions which look like burns but about which it is impossible to be certain. This is particularly true of small, poorly defined, healing lesions which could have a number of causes.

Confessions are not common but are sometimes made to doctors who gently confront parents' concerns about injuries which don't add up.

Checklist of points in diagnosis of abuse

- History – does it explain features of injury:
  - extent
  - depth
  - pattern
  - type
  - age
- Is there a more likely explanation if history does not fit?
- Is burn compatible with child's ability and development?
- Are there other injuries which might suggest abuse?
- Are there signs of sexual abuse, or failure to thrive, or neglect?
- Has the child given a history:
  - in parents' presence?
  - elsewhere?
- Have the parents responded reasonably to the injury and are they cooperating with treatment?
- Who is taking responsibility? Are the parents detached or lacking concern for the child?
- How is the child behaving? May need to wait for initial panic and shock to subside before child's more normal behaviour becomes apparent. Is he withdrawn, frozen, or hyperactive, anxious, aggressive?
- Has anyone visited the home, seen the fire, bath, etc?
- Is there information from other professionals, e.g. at a case conference?

Perpetrators

There are few reports of the identity of perpetrators from the literature. Showers & Garrison (1988) found that 70% of the alleged perpetrators of burn and scald abuse in their series of 139 children were females, with mothers the majority of abusers (52%). This perhaps reflects the young age of many of these children, the time spent with their mothers and the events reported as precipitating the abuse (e.g. anger over dirty nappies, soiling events).

CASE HISTORY 5.1

One mother talked for an hour about the burn on her baby's hand, finally saying, 'You don't believe it was an accident do you? Well, I'm having some difficulty but if someone did that on purpose I think they must need help. Would they go to prison if they did that?'

The response was 'It's not possible to predict that and the police would have to know but it's not automatic and where someone has taken responsibility and accepted help, there is more likely to be a sympathetic response.'

'Well, I did it and I deserve what's coming. I can't cope with my children any more.'

This mother took responsibility, accepted a period with her two children away from her and then, with their return home, accepted help and support and continues to care for them. She herself was sexually abused as a child between the ages of 6 and 8 but never told her mother, whose father had been the abuser.

Other parents are unable to admit what has happened but make sure they are found out.

CASE HISTORY 5.2

One mother who had been struggling for some time with two children brought her 3-year-old daughter with glove scalds to both hands. The history that the child had fallen full length and fully clothed into a bath of hot water without sustaining scalds elsewhere was clearly so inconsistent with the injury that abuse had to be suspected. Despite having had the inconsistencies pointed out to her, the mother stuck rigidly to her story but did not deny very vigorously the suggestion that the child had been abused.

These case histories are important because they demonstrate the help-seeking behaviour shown by parents who are abusing their children. Failure to recognise and intervene leaves the children at further risk.

Child's history

Unprompted statements made by the child in hospital undergoing treatment are common.

'Mummy did it' may not imply abuse as such but 'Mummy did it because I was bad' is more significant.

CASE HISTORY 5.3

One mother who had five boys, two of whom in the past had had worrying burns (one on his bottom and the other on his abdomen), came to the hospital because a third, 3-year-old, child had been noticed in nursery school to have an oblong-shaped burn at the top of his thigh. His mother agreed it was a burn but steadfastly refused to offer an explanation, although after some time she said it could have been the iron but would say no more. Judging that little progress was being made, it was decided to address a question to the boys, who were all in various parts of the room playing with toys. 'Do any of you know how this burn happened?' One by one the children slowly shook their heads, quietly and avoiding eye contact. However, a voice from one corner of the room from beneath a chair said 'Mummy did it'. The hostility with which she turned on this child left all concerned about his safety. Although it could not be ascertained what had happened, it was a worrying exchange.

Child's developmental ability

In assessing the feasibility of the history it is important to consider the developmental capabilities of the child and whether the child could have been burned in the way suggested. Here visits to the scene of injury are important.

This can be a crucial part of the history when, for example, it is alleged that the child took an active part in producing the injury. In one case (Plates 65, 66) three closely opposed burn marks on the upper thigh from a heated ring at the end of an expandable curtain wire were very unlikely to have been caused by the 2-year-old child concerned. Clearly the necessary fine motor skills had not yet developed. In another case, where it was alleged that a child had climbed over the edge of a bath, it was shown that the child did not have the necessary skills to do this.

A general understanding of child development is essential to making clear decisions about what it is possible for a child to do, but an alternative is to observe the child in this situation and gauge what can be achieved.

A 9-month-old baby allegedly crawled backwards into a central heating radiator, sustaining burns to the soles of both feet (Plate 67). Although the radiator was not particularly hot, it was envisaged that had the feet maintained contact for several seconds a burn could have ensued. The question raised was whether a baby of this age would try to push away from the radiator, thus maintaining contact for longer. In practice, it was found that a rapid withdrawal response from his feet was observed when placed in contact with an aversive stimulus, thus indicating the unlikelihood of the proposed theory.

It is important in bathtub incidents to take careful note of the height and depth of the bath, the taps, position and style of the control part of the tap. Turning a round faucet is considered possible after 24 months of age (Johnson 1996). Small children entering a bathtub are unlikely to enter feet first and cannot 'step' into the water. They would be expected to slide in sideways or head first and to move and splash as they attempt to get away from the hot water (Johnson 1996).

Types of thermal injury

Characteristics of different thermal injuries are shown in Table 5.4. Depending on the age, it is often possible to make a reasonable assessment of the likely type of burn present. In abuse, several patterns have been recognised.

Dip scald or forced immersion injury

Dip scald or forced immersion is a relatively common non-accidental-injury (Lenoski & Hunter 1977, Feldman et al 1978) affecting hands, feet, buttocks or sometimes the whole child. As the child is held in the hot water, unable to struggle, clear demarcation lines are found between scalded and spared skin. This gives the glove and stocking distribution (Plates

Table 5.4 Characteristics of various types of thermal injury

Type of injury	Appearances
Scalds	Variable thickness between and within different lesions Contouring of depth, tendency to be deepest in the middle Dip, splash or pour patterns. Smooth circular edges Peeling and sloughing Skin loss in sheets Moist, macerated, soggy lesions spread into flexures, depressions, e.g. natal cleft Blisters pronounced
Contact burns	Delineated margins Square and straight edges Depth variable but generally uniform Dry, scabbing
Cigarette burns	Circular, 0.5–1.0 cm diameter In abuse: often full thickness cratered, leaving circular, depressed, paper thin scars In accident: superficial, eccentric with tail from brushed contact
Flame burns	Tissue charred Hair singed
Chemical burns (e.g. from caustic liquid)	Scald-like distribution ± staining May be deep with underlying tissue destruction
Friction	Occurs over body points, e.g. nose, point of shoulder Usually superficial Intact blisters not seen
Electrical burns	Deep, small, localised Exit and entry points Hands and fingers common sites Tissue charring and deeper necrosis Nuclear streaming on microscopy
Microwave burns	Unusual, sharply demarcated, full thickness burns widely distributed on body (opposite microwave emitting devices) Deeper burns to muscle described

68, 69), modified if the fist is clenched or if the sole of the foot presses against the cooler base of the bath. With the child's buttocks, the central area may be spared if pressed to the cool bath base, leaving the 'hole in the doughnut effect' (Plate 70). Such children will not have the splash marks expected of children who accidentally fall into the bath. Water will find its way into hollows in the child's body but, where surfaces are opposed, the skin will be spared. If, therefore, the legs are flexed and the child dunked, confluent areas of non-scalded skin in opposition will be seen.

Splashed, thrown or pour scald injury

Unusual sites for these injuries, for example genitalia, or a pattern of separated areas, as when fluid is thrown, may suggest abuse, although examination will be less conclusive than with the forced immersion scald. The backs of the hands are uncommonly scalded in accidents but are affected when the hand is held under a flow of hot water.

Mechanisms in abusive scalds

- Child (extremity, limb, buttocks) immersed forcibly in bath/sink, etc.
- Child (extremity, limb, buttocks) held under flowing hot water from tap
- Wet cloth/ flannel held on to skin
- Hot water splashed, poured or thrown on to the child

Specific features of inflicted scalds

- Glove or stocking distribution of scald to one or both hands/feet
- Absence of splash marks implies restraint of the child
- Clear 'tide mark' may be present
- Soles may be spared if feet pressed on to cooler base of bath – presence of shoes and clothes may modify pattern of injury
- Scalds to the buttocks, either isolated or associated with immersion scalds to feet. Central sparing implies buttocks pressed against the cooler base of bath ('hole in doughnut' effect)
- Pour or thrown pattern which may involve unusual sites, e.g. back of hand, genitalia, face
- Age of scald inconsistent with history given
- Child unable to create the situation where injury alleged because of developmental level (e.g. 12-month-old unable to climb into sink)
- Pattern of injury is not consistent with the history, e.g. there could not be flexural sparing at the knee if the child was said to be standing in the

bath. Investigators should use models/dolls to work out body position from photographs/drawings of the pattern of injury

- Bath water temperatures from 'scene of crime investigation' inconsistent with account by carer

Food burns

If a child is accidentally given hot food with a high moisture content, the lips and mouth are the likely sites to be burned. If a beaker or dish of food is pushed into a reluctant child's face, the burns are centred around the mouth but are also present on the face, including the cheeks. Sticky foods such as hot porridge can concentrate heat and produce unpleasant scalds.

Scalds in the groin have been seen, when a bowl was tipped into a child's lap and a scalded foot when a child put his foot in his bowl of porridge on the floor. Although unusual, these were accepted as accidents.

Contact burns

Holding a hot object against a child's skin is possibly the commonest way of abusing a child. The child may also be pressed against a hot object, such as a fire or hotplate. If there are multiple burns, particularly if they are on different 'sides' of the child such that contact must have occurred on several occasions, abuse is more likely. Children soon learn to avoid hot objects and the intense pain which accompanies a burn.

Common objects used to inflict burns include fire grills, irons and curling tongs; the heated top of a cigarette lighter was mentioned in one study (Keen et al 1975). An object such as a poker may be heated in the fire and applied like a brand. The distinct configurations allow one to compare the object with the injury, giving positive identification (see Plates 65, 66). The depth of burn depends on the temperature and factors preventing the child from escaping the heat. The commonest sites are the backs of hands, outside of legs, buttocks and feet.

One of the commonest contact burns encountered is that caused by a clothes iron (Batchelor et al 1994). Most of these are on the upper extremity. Burns to the dorsum of the hand are particularly worrying. The history is usually that the mother was not present when the injury occurred and had switched the iron off leaving it somewhere she thought the child could not reach (work surface, ironing board) but also sometimes on the floor. The child is usually aged about 1–3 years and is mobile. Although the incident is rarely said to have been witnessed, it is suggested that the child picked the iron up, or the iron may have fallen on to the child's hand and is frequently found on the floor, table, etc. When the child is discovered, he or she is no longer in contact with the iron. The burn may be of full thickness and in some cases require skin grafting. A clear-cut outline of the edge of the iron is visible (Plate 71).

Differentiating abuse from accident in this situation requires a carefully taken history and a full assessment of the circumstances. The position on the back of the hand decreases the likelihood of accident (Johnson 1996). Associated injuries, burns to unexposed area, time and developmental inconsistencies would assist a diagnosis of abuse.

Cigarette burns

Cigarette burns are increasingly seen as a manifestation of child abuse. A proportion of children referred with suspected cigarette burns turn out to have other skin pathology, frequently impetigo (Wheeler & Hobbs 1988).

It is not known how long it takes to produce a deep, cratered, circular, full-thickness burn, but it is suspected that it is a second or two, or possibly more. This is far longer than the milliseconds which will elapse in a brushed contact which leaves an area of reddening, often with a tail or elliptical shape. Sites include the hand, foot, limbs, forehead, neck, breast or back (Plate 72).

Cigarette burns may be single or multiple; a look-out should be kept for scars which may appear as shallow craters (Plate 73). Cigarette burns carry a particularly high emotive significance; it is wise to be clear of the certainty that the lesion is a cigarette burn before giving evidence in court.

Other burns

Flame, caustic, radiant, electrical and friction burns are all seen in abuse. Their features are described in Table 5.4, but none is particularly common. Children have been forced to stand in front of a fire until their legs were burned from radiation; they are dragged across a carpet on their face producing friction burns, or burns occur where ropes have been used to restrain a child. If a caustic substance is placed on the skin, destruction of the tissue may continue for some time and lead to deep injuries with considerable scarring. Certain caustic substances, e.g. hydrofluoric acid, have been used in criminal assaults, but this is rarely described in child abuse.

Severe and extensive sunburn in a young child is not uncommon and could be viewed as indicating poor care. Erythema and blistering result. Recently microwave ovens were reported to produce full thickness burns in children placed inside them (Alexander et al 1987).

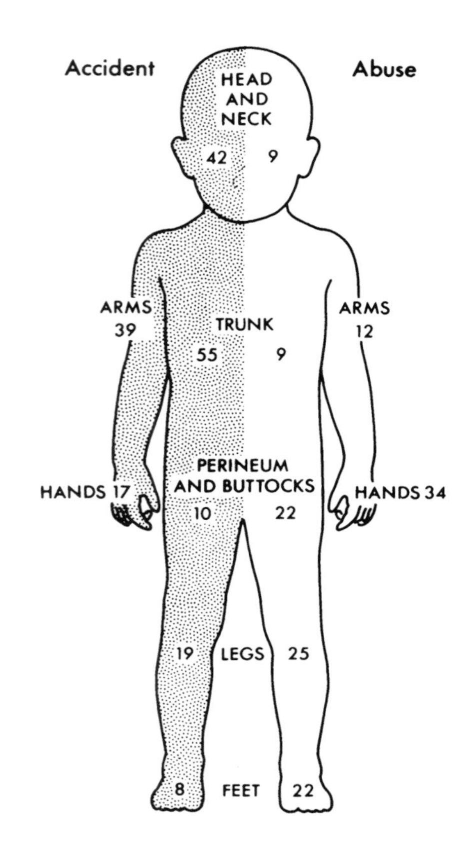

Fig. 5.4 Percentage frequency of sites involved in burn and scald injuries in accident and abuse. Data from 195 children (165 accidents, 30 abused) with burns and scalds. (Reproduced with permission from Hobbs C J 1986 When are burns not accidental? Archives of Disease in Childhood 61:357–361.)

Sites in abuse

It is always essential to consider the part of the child's body affected. There are no sites which are specific to abuse, but the hands (Johnson 1990), buttocks, genitalia and feet are especially important (Fig. 5.4). Isolated burns on the buttocks commonly arise from abuse. The backs of hands are not usually burned accidentally. As the child explores it is usually the fingers that are burned, not so much the flat of the dorsum or the back of the wrist.

Burns on the soles of the feet should also cause concern, unless of course there is a sensible history. Any site can be the target and nowhere is spared. In one seriously abused infant, the cornea was burned, probably by a cigarette. The child was presented to the family doctor and treated for an eye infection but only later when the child had been seriously bruised around the face and sustained a skull fracture was the corneal ulcer demonstrated with fluorescent staining.

Self-inflicted burns are rarely encountered and then only in very disturbed children who have usually also been abused. As with scratches and bruises, the arms and hands are the predominant sites.

Often, further evidence later clarifies the picture. Where suspicion is high, a full investigation is warranted and requires coordination of a team response for the child. Caution is required in some cases to be certain that a lesion is in fact a burn. Table 5.5 illustrates conditions where there has been confusion with burns.

Table 5.5 Differential diagnoses of burns

Presentation	Differential diagnoses	Features	Investigations
?Scald or cigarette burn	Infection – impetigo	Irregular, golden crusts, tend to spread, prompt response to antibiotics	Skin/nasal swab: *Staphylococcus aureus* or β-haemolytic streptococcus
?Scald or burn	Staphylococcal scalded skin syndrome	Erythematous, painful lesions, +ve Nikolsky's sign	*Staphylococcus aureus* phage group II, types 70 or 71 from skin/nasal swabs
?Scald or burn	Nappy rash, with or without infection	Distribution, pattern, blisters	History
?Scald or burn	Photodermatitis	Sensitisation by contact with certain plant/fruit substances Burn produced by light	History. Sensitivity testing of small areas
?Scald or burn	Folk medicine practice: cupping, coin rubbing or rolling	Red lesions, erythema, bruises. Middle East, Latin America, SE Asia, E Europe	History
?Scald or burn	Fixed drug eruption	Purple/red plaque clearly demarcated border in same site repeatedly follows drug ingestion	History: usually salicylate, tetracycline, sulphonamide

Exotic and unusual burn accidents

There are situations in which the history sounds unlikely or there is no satisfactory explanation. One child had lesions which resembled scalds around both ankles. The explanation that this was a vinegar burn was doubted until the vinegar was found to be glacial acetic acid (pH 1.5) which required dilution at 1 in 10 before use. Another case was described where a baby placed in a car seat in a car that had stood in the sun sustained a burn on his abdomen, for which at first no explanation was forthcoming. The belt buckle had been hot enough to burn him and, as he had often cried before on being placed in the seat, his distress had not been heeded. Black vinyl plastic seats have been implicated in similar circumstances.

The most common differential diagnosis remains between accident and abuse.

Management

The primary consideration in treatment of most burn or scald injuries is the medical or surgical treatment of the injury and child. In small healing or healed burns, the issues of child protection may be the prime and sole concern. Medical and surgical management of burn injury is not discussed in this text and the reader is referred to other sources for details.

Approach to investigation

When concerns arise that a burn may be non-accidental it is important that there is a procedure for investigation.

Procedure for investigation of burns

- Take full detailed history of the injury, including time and place, witnesses, precise detail of the events surrounding the injury, action taken following the injury and child and parent's responses
- Take full paediatric history including family and social history, history of siblings, previous injury including other burns, child's behaviour
- Examine the child fully for any injury
- Make a detailed drawing of the burn including measurements, site, pattern (consider position child was in at the time of injury), depth of injury (in conjunction with surgical team). Is there sparing, e.g. soles/palms in immersion injury? Consider effects of clothes
- Obtain consent for genital and anal inspection (links with sexual abuse)
- Assess child's development and ability to act in the way stated, e.g. can this child turn on a tap or climb into a bath?

- Attend strategy meetings, work closely with police, social services, surgical team and family. Information must be freely shared and discussed. A series of meetings at different stages of the investigation may be helpful in some cases
- Visit the home to view the scene of injury. Re-enact the scene according to the description of the carer present at the time of injury. This can be a very revealing exercise, as well as a distressing time for the carer, and needs to be handled with care and sensitivity. Exact details of temperature and time should be obtained as well as heights, depths of water, nature of materials. Scientific advice, manufacturer's data, etc. may be required
- Ask to see appliance/heater alleged to have injured. Does it fit? What was the likely temperature at time of alleged injury? May ask to see clothing*
- Assess likely time of contact from temperature (if known) time graph*
- Arrange photographs of injury, appliance, environment, etc.*

* Usually carried out jointly with the police

CASE HISTORY 5.4

An 18-month-old boy was brought to hospital with symmetrical partial thickness immersion scalds to both hands and forearms to a distance of 10 cm from the wrist to just below the elbow, with palmar sparing. There was a clear line of demarcation at 90° to the axis of the arm and no splash marks or scalds elsewhere and no other injury. The mother described how she filled the bath using only the hot tap and briefly left the room for a few seconds only. On return the child had climbed into the bath and was discovered on all fours in the kneeling position screaming. He wore a vest, T-shirt, wool jumper and nappy but no trousers.

A visit to the home re-enacted the events as described by the mother. It was confirmed that the water heater had been switched on as before and that no one had just used significant amounts of water from the hot water system. At the same time of day, the temperature of hot water leaving the tap was measured using a mercury glass thermometer to be 61°C, and the temperature in the bath was 58°C. It took 5 minutes to obtain a depth of 3 inches and 6–7 minutes to obtain a depth of 4 inches (10 cm), i.e. the depth of immersion from the injury measurement. The temperature of 58°C was maintained up to 9 minutes when the hot water began to run colder. It was judged difficult if not impossible for the child to have climbed into the bath, although this was not tested in practice.

It was concluded that:

- it would have taken longer than suggested by the mother to fill the bath to the depth described by her and even longer to fill the bath to the depth calculated to have been present to scald the child.
- at the temperature of water found, it would have taken between 5 and 100 seconds to produce a partial thickness scald to an adult, somewhat less for a child. Given the depth of scald it is likely that the time of contact was probably in excess of the lower limit, i.e. certainly several seconds.
- the description of the child kneeling in the bath is inconsistent with the pattern of vertically immersed upper limbs only.
- the pattern of no splash marks and clear demarcation of scalded from non-scalded skin indicates forced immersion, i.e. the child's limbs were held in such a way that he could not move despite feeling obvious severe pain.
- sparing of the palms of the hands may indicate that the palms were pressed on to the cooler base of the bath or that the fists were clenched.

This case was referred for full joint investigation by police and social services.

Close cooperation of paediatricians with surgical teams undertaking the management of the injury is vital if the future safety of the child is to be ensured. Where abuse is suspected, early assessment by the paediatrician experienced in physical abuse in conjunction with the surgical and nursing staff treating the injury should allow discussion of the likely mode of injury to take place. Examination as soon as possible after arrival of the child at hospital, coupled with further examinations as the boundaries of the injury become clearer, is valuable and can be coordinated with dressing changes if required. Photography, both close-up and whole body to show overall pattern, is invaluable for later reference and study and to assist with the presentation of evidence in court. Drawings are also helpful. The usual assessments of developmental level, growth and behaviour of the child are made.

Clinical histories of examples of abusive burn and scald injuries

- 5-year-old boy whose father had heated a dining fork and applied it to his ear while laughing.
- 5-year-old with superficial linear burn on buttock said to have been caused when child deliberately stood against radiator. Signs of sexual abuse in child and sibling. Previous unexplained bruising in child.
- Cup of coffee thrown at girl of 3 years by drunken father. Scalds to chest, upper arm and face.
- Full thickness contact burn from iron on dorsum of hand in 12-month-old boy who had played with an iron turned off for 'at least 5 minutes'. Untreated longstanding genital warts were found in both 4-year-old sister and the father who had recently left home.
- Triangular shaped scald on forehead wrapping around front and side of head in 15-month-old girl said to have fallen against gas fire. Further scald on arm and unexplained bruises on thigh. Family had just finished a meal of pizza.
- Deep burn on back of neck in 11-year-old girl in school for children with moderate learning difficulties. Stepmother admitted to burning child with spatula while frying eggs.
- Ulcerated burn on glans penis only visible with foreskin retracted. After repeated questioning parents eventually suggested that child may have stood too close to a central heating radiator whilst passing urine. Family fled the area before investigation could proceed but further concerns regarding abuse identified in another city.
- 13-month-old girl said to have climbed on to the worktop and sat on the cooker. Two sets of concentric circular radiant ring burns, one on buttocks and one on thighs.
- 14-month-old girl with full thickness burn on instep and sole of one foot. Parents said they saw smoke and heard the sound of frying bacon when she stood on a cool fire surround. They suggested electrocution for which there was no evidence. Both parents were intravenous drug abusers. The child was also failing to thrive.
- 3-year-old boy said by father to have fallen into a bath of hot water with shoes and socks on. Bilateral, severe, symmetrical, scalds in stocking distribution present to both feet with sparing of dorsum of feet. No splash marks were present and upper limit clearly demarcated. Appearances those of forced immersion scalds while wearing shoes.

Presentation of evidence in court

Where a child has bruises or other typical non-accidental injuries, the burns should be included in the evidence, although the exact aetiology may remain open in terms of medical opinion unless it is clear exactly how the injury was inflicted. It would be unusual for the doctor to be able to be dogmatic about the exact nature of many of the burns in this situation. Where the injury is exclusively a burn, which may be extensive or serious, and where the history permits a clearer opinion to be formed, it is often the best policy to present to the court the reasoning behind the diagnosis.

CASE HISTORY 5.5

The mother's story was that a 4-year-old child with stocking distribution scald had been left alone and happy for a few minutes in the bath in warm water which could not have scalded him. On his mother's return he had got out of the bath, was dripping wet and his feet were badly scalded in a symmetrical stocking distribution.

It is reasonable to examine the various possible scenarios one by one for the court, starting with the accidental version (e.g. he turned the tap on, the water got hot and he got out) followed by what it is thought really happened. The pros and cons of each argument are weighed up with a final statement of which one – on the balance of probabilities – seems most likely.

In this way the court is able to follow the reasoning and explore the possibilities, hopefully coming to an agreement as to what is likely to have happened. Using this method, it is possible to avoid making a direct statement of an opinion that the child has been abused at too early a stage in the evidence. The phrase 'I found it difficult to see how it could have happened in the way stated' is useful. Another useful phrase is 'one is left with few other reasonable alternatives than that this burn was deliberately inflicted on the child'. Caution is required but cases can be brought for child protection on the 'balance of probability' rule if there is general agreement that the history is not adequate.

Follow-up

Follow-up is often undertaken with a paediatrician or plastic surgeon with an interest in burns. Behaviour problems are common in this group of children. Foster-parents may come to recognise the signs and symptoms of other forms of abuse, notably sexual. Psychological help may be necessary for the most disturbed children.

Psychological effects of injury

The psychological and emotional consequences of inflicted burns are likely in general to be more severe than the physical effects. They may have a devastating effect on the psychological health of the child, who may show persistent behavioural difficulties extending into adult life.

Sequelae

Burns and scalds in children are associated with acute and chronic physical and psychological sequelae. The child with physical scars will have a constant reminder of his abuse, which may reinforce the emotional difficulties and interfere with psychological healing. Adults have sometimes revealed scars which they acquired in childhood burns, expressing confusion and anxiety when attempting to remember how they might have been caused.

Repetition of burns in childhood

Burns cause extreme pain, and repetition of accidental injury is uncommon. In contrast, repeated incidents are not uncommon in abuse and should arouse suspicion. Children with several separate burns which could not have arisen at the same time are likely to have been abused.

Summary

1. Most burn and scald injuries in childhood occur in pre-school children and should be prevented.
2. Accidents follow brief lapses in protection, neglect as part of a pattern of inadequate parenting and abuse when injury is deliberately inflicted.
3. Burns and scalds following abuse are under-reported.
4. Evaluation is difficult requiring a careful and detailed history. A visit to the home may be necessary.
5. Non-accidental thermal injuries include forced immersion and pour scald, contact, friction and chemical burns.
6. Sites in abuse particularly include backs of hands, buttocks, genitalia and feet. No site is exempt.
7. Significant points in the history are unwitnessed incidents, delayed presentation, minimisation of severity of injury, surprising lack of pain, repeated burns.
8. Differential diagnosis includes other skin pathology, especially infections.
9. There is a particular association between sexual abuse and burns.
10. Repeated burns are a dangerous form of neglect.
11. Burns may be associated with any form of abuse.

12. Medical assessment is often complex and requires the opinion of plastic surgeons, A & E surgeons and nurses experienced in treating burns.
13. When giving evidence in court, build up the diagnosis to explain the final opinion.
14. Emotional sequelae are expected to be severe and long-lasting.

REFERENCES

Alexander R C, Surrell J A, Cohle S 1987 Microwave oven burns to children: an unusual manifestation of child abuse. Pediatrics 79:255–259

Batchelor J S, Vanjari S, Budny P, Roberts A H 1994 Domestic iron burns in children: a cause for concern? Burns 20(1):74–75

Chapman J C, Sarhadi N S, Watson A C 1994 Declining incidence of paediatric burns in Scotland: a review of 1114 children with burns treated as inpatients and outpatients in regional centre. Burns 20(2):106–110

DHSS 1977 Safe temperatures for heated surfaces and hot water. Reference DN3.3, DHSS Engineering Data

Erdmann T C, Feldman K W, Rivara F P, Heimbach D M, Wall H A 1991 Tap water burn prevention: the effect of legislation. Pediatrics 88(3):572–577

Feldman K W, Schaller R T, Feldman J A, McMillan M 1978 Tap water scalds in children. Pediatrics 62:1–7

Hight D W, Bakalar H R, Lloyd J R 1979 Inflicted burns in children. Recognition and treatment. JAMA 242:517–520

Hobbs C J 1986 When are burns not accidental? Archives of Disease in Childhood 61:357–361

Hobbs C J 1996 Tap water scalds. Child Abuse Review 5:214–217

Hobbs C J, Wynne J M 1990 The sexually abused battered child. Archives of Disease in Childhood 65:423–427

Hollyoak M A, Muller M J, Pegg S P 1994 Electric iron contact burns in an Australian paediatric population. Paediatric & Perinatal Epidemiology 8(3):314–324

Jackson R H (Chairman) 1985 Report of a working party on burn and scald accidents to children. Child Accident Prevention Trust. Bedford Square Press, London

Johnson C F 1990 The hand as a target organ in child abuse. Clinicial Pediatrics (Philadelphia) 29(2):66–72

Johnson C F 1996 Physical abuse. Accidental versus intentional trauma in children. In: Briere J, Berliner L, Bulkley J A, Jenny C, Reid T (eds.) The APSAC handbook on child maltreatment. Sage, London, Chapter 12

Keen J H, Lendrum J, Wolman B 1975 Inflicted burns and scalds in children. British Medical Journal iv:268–269

Lenoski E F, Hunter K A 1977 Specific patterns of inflicted burn injuries. Journal of Trauma 17:842–846

Martin H L 1970 Antecedents of burns and scalds in children. British Journal of Medical Psychology 43:39–47

Mercier C, Blond M H 1996 Epidemiological survey of childhood burn injuries in France. Burns 22:29–34

Moritz A R, Henriques F C 1947 Studies of thermal injury: the relative importance of time and temperature in the causation of cutaneous burns. American Journal of Pathology 23:695–720

Phillips P S, Pickrell E, Morse T S 1974 Intentional burning. A severe form of child abuse. Journal of the American College of Emergency Physicians 3:388–390

Purdue G F, Hunt J L, Prescott P R 1988 Child abuse by burning – an index of suspicion. Journal of Trauma 28:221–224

Raine P A M, Azmy A 1983 A review of thermal injuries in young children. Journal of Pediatric Surgery 18:21–26

Renz B M, Sherman R, 1992. Child abuse by scalding. Journal of Medical Association of Georgia. 81(10):574–578

Scalzo A J 1994 Burns and child maltreatment. In Monteleone J A, Brodeur A E (eds.) Child maltreatment. A clinical guide and reference. G W Medical, St Louis, MO

Showers J, Garrison K M 1988 Burn abuse: a four year study. Journal of Trauma 28:1581–1583

Smith S M, Hanson R 1974 Battered children – a medical and psychological study. British Medical Journal iii:666– 670

Stone N D, Rinaldo L, Humphrey C R, Brown R H 1970 Child abuse by burning. Surgical Clinics of North America 50:1419–1424

Tennant W G, Davidson P M 1991 Bath scalds in children in the south-east of Scotland. Journal of the Royal College of Surgeons of Edinburgh 36:319–322

Wheeler D, Hobbs C J 1988 Mistakes in diagnosing non-accidental injury, 10 years experience. British Medical Journal 296:1233–1236

Yeoh C, Nixon J W, Dickson W, Kemp A, Sibert J R 1994 Patterns of scald injuries. Archives of Disease in Childhood 71:156–158

6

Neglect

Expectations and definitions

Child rearing in modern society is complex and the responsibility for enabling children to reach their full potential is shared between carers and the state.

Cantwell & Rosenberg (1990) wrote that

> The child has a right to expect, and the adult care-taker has a duty to provide: food, clothing, shelter, safekeeping, nurturance and teaching. Failure to provide these constitutes neglect.

The Inquiry into Child Abuse Prevention (1996) used a wide definition of child abuse as the basis for an effective prevention strategy (not to increase numbers on child protection registers): Child abuse consists of anything which individuals, institutions, or processes do or fail to do, which directly or indirectly harms children or damages their prospects of safe and healthy development into adulthood.

This is in tune with the Children Act 1989 (England and Wales) which clearly states that the welfare of children is paramount and the carers have a responsibility to meet the child's needs but that local social service departments must take the lead and collaborate with key agencies to establish effective services for children who have unmet needs (children at risk of abuse or neglect are 'in need').

Working Together (1991) has a narrow definition of neglect:

> The persistent or severe neglect of a child, or the failure to protect a child from exposure to any kind of danger, including cold or starvation or, extreme failure to carry out important aspects of care, resulting in the significant impairment of the child's health or development, including non-organic failure to thrive.

This raises the threshold for recognition for practitioners and so restricts or rations resources so only the most needy or neglected children and families are assisted. From March 1997 in England Children's Services Plans have to be agreed and in place for children in need as defined by the Children Act, but '. . . within available resources'. Kempe & Goldbloom (1987) wrote 'neglect can be a very insidious form of maltreatment. It implies failure of the parent to act properly in safeguarding the health, safety and well being of the child'.

The National Child Abuse and Neglect Data System (NCANDS 1995) in the US defines neglect as 'a type of maltreatment that refers to failure to . . . provide needed, age appropriate care'. NCANDS continues with the important notation that neglect is typified by an *ongoing* pattern of inadequate care, and is, in contrast to physical or sexual abuse, observed (and accommodated) by individuals in close contact with the child. Helfer (1987) widened the definition to beyond an individual's (parent's) responsibility to that of society, when he described the 'litany of smouldering neglect' whereby many children in the USA are brought up in poverty, do not have access to health care, do not finish their education, cannot read, and drift into drugs, crime and jails. The long-term adverse consequences are well recognised in the US (Rosenberg & Cantwell 1993) and the UK (Messages from Research 1995).

In 1991 the UK government became a signatory to the United Nations Convention on the Rights of the Child (1989). The first General Declaration on the Rights of the Child was in 1924 – but Declarations are not binding, Conventions are. Thus broad statements such as Article 24 'the right of the child to the enjoyment of the highest attainable standard of health and the facility for the treatment of illness and rehabilitation of health' are agreed. Countries should take measures to diminish infant and child mortality, promote health education and prevent accidents. It is also stated in Article 19 that legislative, administrative, social and educational measures should be taken to protect children from all forms of physical and mental violence, injury and abuse (including sexual abuse) and negligent treatment.

Unfortunately UK governments have continued to ignore the rights of children, despite having ratified the Convention (UK Agenda for Children 1994). This is seen against the background of increasing childhood poverty, not listening to children's views and the detention of children. The UN committee which looked at the implementation of the Convention in the UK in 1995 noted progress in the reduction of the incidence of sudden infant death syndrome, the attention paid to bullying in schools and the interdisciplinary approach to child abuse. Concern was raised as to how the rights of children (as agreed in the Convention) were being implemented, and this included economic, social and cultural rights. It was noted that children were begging and sleeping on the streets. The concern about the low age of criminal responsibility and juvenile justice with emphasis on imprisonment and punishment was clear. The lack of access of gypsy and traveller children to basic services was noted.

The UN Committee made over 20 suggestions and recommendations as to how the state could improve children's' rights, but these have not been heeded (Children's Rights Office 1995).

Effects of unemployment, poverty and homelessness

In the UK the National Children's Bureau (NCB 1987) had already written of the social measures necessary to have a real impact on the welfare of children and in particular to affect

- perinatal and infant mortality
- immunisation rates
- child health
- levels of child abuse
- cigarette smoking
- drug and substance abuse.

The improvements in social conditions required attention to

- unemployment
- homelessness
- poverty.

Although unemployment overall has decreased in the UK in the 1990s the proportion of children with unemployed parents rose from 6% to 17% between 1981 and 1991 (Roberts & Power 1996) and the proportion of children growing up in poverty has risen from one-tenth to one-third between 1979 and 1993 (CPAG 1996). (Fig. 6.1). In other words, 4.3 million children in England and Wales are poor (Oppenheim & Harker 1996). The extent of income inequality has increased faster in the UK than any comparable country except New Zealand. From 1979 to 1993 the poorest tenth of the population have experienced an 18% fall in real income, and the next tenth no increase, whereas the whole of society has had a 37% rise (DSS 1995). In 1995 there were 3.1 million children in the UK living in families living on income support compared with less than a million in 1979.

Poverty is related to unemployment, low pay (especially if large families), lone parent families (Judge & Benzeval 1993) and black and ethnic minority groups. Consequences of poverty include poor diet, economies in the use of heating and water, and debt which may lead to disconnection, eviction, fines and even imprisonment (Kempson 1996). Use of addictive drugs and alcohol leads to further social disadvantage and crime.

Income inequality and the association with inequality in health is well described from infant mortality to life expectancy at birth to morbidity and especially accident rates (pedestrian accidents, drowning, house fires), all of which was well described in the Black Report (DHSS 1980, Townsend et al 1992), and is found in rural as well as urban areas (Reading et al 1993), and has not improved despite improvements in the UK economy (HMSO 1995, Mackenbach 1995, Black 1996, Davey Smith 1996).

Poverty is highly correlated with neglect. Many carers given appropriate resources are able to provide better for their children but others do not care or understand, or refuse to work to improve the care of their children.

Homelessness has more than doubled in the last 15 years (Kumar 1993) There were 134 000 homeless households in England in 1993; 54 000 were placed in temporary accommodation such as bed and breakfast hotels and hostels. Studies of the health of people living in temporary housing shows that mental health problems are common in the adults and children have a higher level of emotional and behavioural problems (delayed development, aggression, poor sleep patterns, enuresis). Homeless women are more likely to have small, premature babies (Arblaster 1995). Although homeless people use the health service twice as much as local residents they may have difficulty registering with a local practitioner and this too may lead to an inappropriate

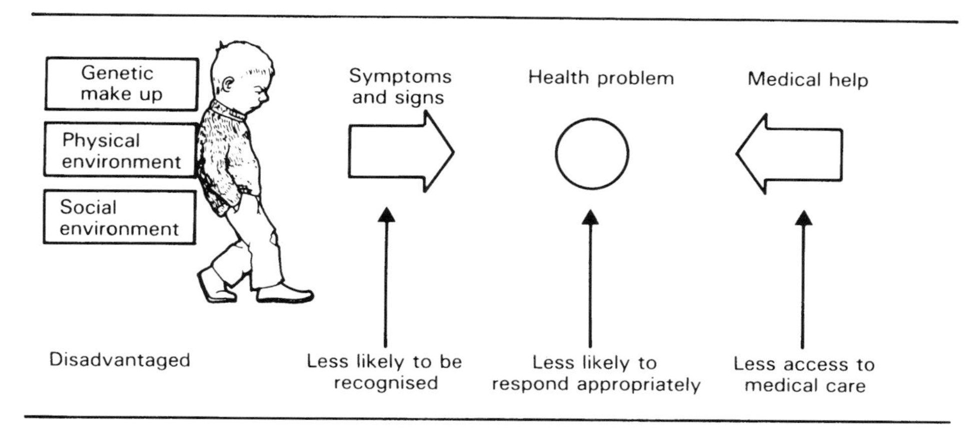

Fig. 6.1 The disadvantaged family. The members of a family at disadvantage are more likely to fall ill, they have fewer personal and material resources to cope with illness, and there are fewer medical resources available to them. (Reproduced from Polnay L, Hull D 1985 Families and homes. In: Community paediatrician. Churchill Livingstone, London.)

use of 'emergency doctors', Accident and Emergency departments and a greater likelihood of hospital admission (Spencer et al 1993). Adverse life events such as loss of job, bereavement, assault on mother, house move are more frequent in those in temporary accommodation (Lissauer 1993). All these factors make child raising more difficult as disadvantage is piled on disadvantage and the child's needs are not met.

Clearly issues of social policy require attention if the adverse effects of childhood poverty are to be addressed. Helfer (1990) wrote of the increasing 'de-emphasis' on the neglect of the children whereby even those professionals mandated to report neglect may not, feeling nothing will be done (or can be done) by overwhelmed, under-resourced child protective service agencies.

As Helfer continues, the needs of children are known and understood and the consequences of a neglected childhood predictable. Childhood is a vulnerable time and needs not met during the child's period of growth may have irreversible consequences, especially in terms of intellectual development and social adjustment (Rosenberg & Cantwell 1993, Gibbons et al 1995).

The emphasis of the Children Act 1989 (in England and Wales) on 'children in need' and the requirement that there are 'Children's services plans' to meet those needs may mean that disadvantage will be addressed and alleviated. What appears more likely is that thresholds of need will be raised and the expectation that preventative work is possible will recede as resources remain limited.

Incidence of neglect

It is difficult to know how many children are neglected in the UK (Table 6.1). Certainly those who are registered (on child protection registers) represent only the tip of the iceberg. In a survey of child protection registers (DoH 1988) 13% of registrations were because of neglect, 2% because of neglect and physical abuse, less than 1% were because of neglect, physical abuse and sexual abuse, and less than 1% due to neglect and sexual abuse. The NSPCC statistics 1983–87 (Creighton & Noyes 1989) record only 6% of children on registers because of neglect in their sample of 10 areas. This figure was static over the 5-year period, which clearly needs explanation. Were all the workers engulfed in the rise of recognition of child sexual abuse? Conditions for children had not improved during those years. In 1988, 6% of registrations again were because of neglect, rising to 8% in 1990. If neglect in association with physical or sexual abuse or both is included, the percentages are 7.5% in 1989 and 10% in 1990. An additional 2% and 3% were registered because of emotional abuse (Creighton & Noyes 1990). The average age of children registered because of neglect was 4 years 9 months.

Table 6.1 Children on child protection registers (% in category). Figures in brackets from Leeds; others from NSPCC (Creighton and Noyes 1990, Leeds ACPC 1996)

Year	Neglect	Neglect and abuse[a]	Emotional abuse
1983–87	6.0	—	—
1988	6.0	7.5	2.0
1990	8.0 (10.0)	10.0 (1.6)	3.0 (3.3)
1993	(15.0)	(15.0)	(7.0)
1996	(23.0)	(27.0)	(9.0)

[a] *sexual, physical and emotional abuse.*

The Leeds Area Child Protection Committee statistics show that in 1990 4% of registrations were due to neglect and 4% to emotional abuse. A radical change in registrations has taken place and in 1996 23% of all registrations were due to neglect and 9% to emotional abuse. The total numbers on the child protection registers were 1013 in 1990 and 1012 in 1996 but the category 'Grave concern' ceased in 1992/3 as did 'child of the family'. The numbers of sexually and physically abused children remain of the same order but 'combined abuse' accounts for 27% (see Table 6.1). The child protection registers in England and Wales (1996) recorded a total of 32 000 children (a 7% decrease from 1995). There were about 40% of children registered because of risk of physical abuse, 32% of neglect and 22% at risk of sexual abuse.

Worldwide, child labour is the commonest form of abuse and neglect (Reddy 1995, Sharp 1996, Silvers 1996).

The serious consequences of neglect should not be dismissed in the short or the long term.

Although this chapter emphasises the insidious long-term damage caused by neglect, the importance of neglect is not always recognised in mortality figures (Browne & Lynch 1995, Hobbs et al 1995).

In the US child neglect is the most common form of child maltreatment reported to the public child protective services representing 49% of substantiated cases of abuse. Neglect is responsible for 42% of the deaths from abuse; children under 5 years are the most vulnerable, 46% being under the age of 1 year. It is estimated that 2000 children die annually from neglect. Parental substance abuse was involved in 29% of fatalities, a pattern which is now seen increasingly in the UK. 'Neglect' deaths are further discussed in Chapter 16.

It is estimated that 8 of every 1000 children in the US experience physical neglect, 4.5 of every 1000 educational neglect, 3 of every 1000 emotional neglect and fewer children experience medical neglect (NCANDS 1995). As with physical abuse, neglect continues throughout childhood but is not usually acknowledged in older children. Neglect and emotional abuse are commonly cited by young runaways as the reason why home life became intolerable for them.

Recent research has shown that young people who are poor have a higher risk of death or disease (Dennehy et al 1997):

- four times the risk of dying by age 20 years (injury and poisoning)
- respiratory problems
- mental health problems (three times the risk of suicide)
- more pregnancies, with additional risk of dietary deficiencies
- greater misuse of tobacco, alcohol and drugs
- disabled teenagers are at greater risk of poverty
- children leaving care (10 000/year) are often poor because of inadequate welfare benefits, unemployment (low achievement educationally), poor housing.

The researchers conclude that '. . . improvement to young people's health will only be made if the underlying problem of poverty is addressed'.

CASE HISTORY 6.1

A 2-year-old boy was found dead in bed. He had had measles and autopsy showed he had died of bronchopneumonia. The family were well known to professional agencies. The boy had 'failed to thrive', and was not immunised. The family had recently moved into temporary housing known to be cold, with a leaking roof. They were not registered with a general practitioner and when the emergency call service (emergency doctor service) arrived it was too late. It was Christmas Day.

CASE HISTORY 6.2

A lone mother and her children aged 3 and 1 years lived in sheltered housing. The mother was very independent and known to be 'difficult'. She had a past history of drug abuse but was not currently abusing drugs or alcohol. Her three older children were in the care of their father. When the younger child became ill his mother said that the doctor was not needed. Three days later his mother rushed screaming to the warden's office that her son was dead. He died in the ambulance. Autopsy showed that the 14-month-old child had died of septicaemia secondary to otitis media.

CASE HISTORY 6.3

Twins 4 years old were playing on the railway line. Their mother had left them for the afternoon with their father and his partner, neither of whom wished to share the care of the boys. One boy was hit by the footplate of a passing express train and killed. The coroner commented on the need for British Rail to keep their fences in better repair.

In the first case death was recorded as due to 'natural causes', that is measles. There are 15 deaths each year in the UK due to measles. Some may be inevitable but others are preventable. In the second case proper medical care was denied to the child, and the twins were not protected from danger. These three deaths were due to neglect; many like these go unrecorded and unrecognised as part of Helfer's (1990) neglected neglect.

In disorganised, stressed, poor families preventable accidents are more common whether seen as ingestions of medicines, home accidents, road traffic accidents and house fires (Kemp & Sibert 1995, Squires & Busuttil 1995, Spencer 1996). The number of house fires increased in the period 1983–92 at a time when the number of families in temporary accommodation increased by a factor of 5 and lone parent families from 12% to 21%. It is known that the risk of house fires is greatest in the poorest council homes, temporary accommodation, lone parents and families who live in poverty. The use of fire alarms is lowest in these circumstances.

The Health of the Nation Strategy (DoH 1992) established the reduction of child injury death rates as a priority: the mortality is falling but there are steep social class gradients (Roberts & Power 1996). From 1981 to 1991 the decline in deaths in social classes I and II was 32% and 37% respectively, but in social classes IV and V the figures were 21% and 2% respectively.

Family factors in cases of neglect

The NSPCC statistics (Creighton & Noyes 1990) record only 15% of mothers and 39% of fathers in paid employment, mostly semi-skilled and unskilled manual jobs. 'Debt' was a significant stress in 22% of families, 'marital problems' were the commonest recorded stress factor noted in 30% of families. Of the children registered because of neglect, 38% were living with their mother alone. The professional assessment in neglect cases was most likely to be that the primary stress factor was 'inability to respond to the maturational needs of the child'.

Substance and alcohol abuse are increasingly factors in the neglect by carers and it is essential that professionals working with the adults, for example workers based in addiction units, also work closely with childcare professionals (Coleman & Cassell 1995, Jaudes et al 1995, Chaffin et al 1996, Wolock & Magura 1996).

CASE HISTORY 6.4

Mother was a heroin abuser but went on to methadone during her latest (third) pregnancy. Baby born 3 weeks pre-term, birth weight 2.1 kg, admitted to 'transitional care' and treated over the next 4 weeks for withdrawal symptoms. Discharged home to mother with support from the addiction unit and social services. The baby failed to thrive, he was not taken for his immunisations or health surveillance. When the baby was 6 months old the 2-year-old brother was admitted to intensive care with a near-fatal ingestion of methadone. The 5-year-old sister was rarely at school; her behaviour was very immature, demanding and aggressive towards her siblings. Money was very short, the family moved house repeatedly and there were frequent break-ins (looking for drugs) and police searches. The mother worked as a prostitute when she began to take heroin – a £60/day habit. The children were physically and emotionally neglected, they were at risk from all the adults who visited, there was no structure to their lives, they were not learning and were frightened of the noise, the fights, the police, and their mother when she was intoxicated.

Carers with mental health problems and/or learning problems may also neglect their children and, again, joint working by professionals is essential (McGaw & Sturmey 1993, Cassell & Coleman 1995, Gath 1995).

Family life and child rearing in a changing society

Child rearing is difficult in a complex, rapidly changing society. The effects of these changes will be evident in the well-being of children. Disadvantage in one aspect of life begets disadvantage in other fields. The UN Convention (1989) in the preamble states

> that the child, for the full and harmonious development of his or her personality, should grow up in a family environment, in an atmosphere of love and understanding.

The composition of families has changed radically in the last 50 years in the UK. Statistics (OPCS 1990, HMSO 1991a) show that:

- almost one-third of births were outside marriage in 1991 compared with 12.5% in 1981, although the parents may be in a stable

relationship and half of these babies are registered in the name of both parents
- marriage rates and remarriage rates are falling as cohabitation rates rise. In 1991 71% of children lived with both parents, compared with 83% in 1979 (Smith 1996), and cohabitation rose from 1 to 3%
- divorce rates are rising; an estimated 164 834 children under 16 years were affected in England and Wales in 1994 (HMSO 1995) and by the year 2000 it is estimated that around one-third of children under 16 years will have experienced at least one parental divorce (NCB 1996)
- in 1994 in the UK 19% of all families are lone parents (over 90% lone mother) and one-third of children will experience lone parenthood in childhood. 60% of lone families experience relative poverty, compared with 25% two-parent families.
- in 1992 there were 1.4 million lone parent families in the UK containing 2.3 million children – twice the number there were in 1971
- around half of lone parents marry, or re-marry within 5 years (Ermisch 1986)
- cohabitation, reconciliation and the non-dependence of teenagers contribute to 'outflow' from lone parenthood (Edwards 1991)
- in 1994 15% of fathers and 3% of mothers had biological children not living with them (1994 British Household Panel Study)
- 1 in 4 children are brought up in families where there is no breadwinner, hence the increase in poverty from 1 in 8 in 1979 to 1 in 3 in 1993
- there is a growing division between no-income families and dual-income families. The factors associated with low income are well known but what may be the social and emotional consequences of dual-income families, especially given the recognised shortage of good, affordable child care in the UK (Bradshaw 1996)
- 100 000 14–16-year-old children disappeared from home in 1989 (24 000 more than in 1987)
- increased social mobility means that many 'nuclear families' receive little support from their extended families.

The Children Act 1989 emphasises that children need families. A main principle of the Act is that 'wherever possible, children should be brought up and cared for within their own families' and parents are to be supported to help bring up their children (in need). The Act also ensures that the wishes and feelings of the child should be considered in the context of the child's age, understanding and circumstances.

Research shows that, in general, children do better when cared for by their birth parents and that children are hurt when this relationship breaks down. The divorce rate in the UK is currently one-third of all marriages and is rising. Remarriage fails to repair the damage caused by divorce; 'grief and disruption' is long lasting (Phillips 1991).

It is evident that social policy must take account of these new patterns of family life. Children need stability and security but adults need assistance to provide for the needs of children. Phillips (1991) suggests that, to improve support, family relationship measures would include:

- improving the economic position of families
- educating all children about relationships and parenthood
- a network of counselling services to help family relationships in trouble.

Poverty is a major stress in many families, particularly lone parent families, and improving their economic status will alleviate some of the sequelae of separation. It will not, however, resolve the rejection many children feel following divorce. The consequences of a lower income and changed lifestyle combined with the breakdown of emotional relationships within families lead some children to leave home early, to premature cohabitation, marriage, parenthood and divorce. Education and ultimate career prospects for some children are jeopardised by the divorce of their parents and the consequent social disruption.

There are clear links between ill health and social deprivation. Adversities tend to be multiple and further adversity compounds disadvantage. Wedge & Essex (1982), Kumar (1993) and Spencer (1996) have demonstrated the overlap between:

- lone parent or large family
- low income
- poor housing
- impaired health in children and adults
- increased mortality in children and adults
- poor diet
- poor growth in childhood
- school failure
- history of accidents
- families from ethnic minorities and travelling families are over represented in terms of childhood poverty and disadvantage (Spencer 1996, Cemlyn 1995).

The term *childhood deprivation* is used to describe the condition of children whose needs are not met – whether emotionally, socially or in terms of learning opportunity. Patterns of disadvantage tend to continue from one generation to the next as children from impoverished families become inadequate parents themselves. However, children are resilient and many, in spite of difficult childhoods, do survive and become successful adults. The more vulnerable do not (Crittenden 1988).

Childhood poverty, defined as living below 50% average income after housing costs, is increasing in the UK (Kumar 1993).

- 1 in 4 or 1 in 5 children were living below the poverty line in 1987 (Delamothe 1991) rising to 1 in 3 by 1992–93 (DSS 1995).
- Over 65% of lone parent families depend entirely on income support (HMSO 1991b).
- Except for Ireland and Portugal the UK has the highest proportion of children in the EC living below 50% of average expenditure level (Smith 1991).
- 10% of families do not have money for out-of-school activities and 14% lack an outing for children once a week (Smith 1991).

Childhood poverty and health are closely associated (Smith 1991, Spencer 1996). Table 6.2 summarises some of the statistics relating child mortality to occupational class.

Tudor Hart (1971) wrote 'the availability of good medical care tends to vary intensely with the need for it in the population served'. Webb (1998) has added that the inverse care law also operates in the use of the provided services. The least disadvantaged, who require the least care, make the best use of available facilities.

Table 6.2a UK vital statistics for children under 1 year (OPCS 1987, Kumar 1993)

	IMR[a]	PNMR[b]	NMR[c]	PMR[d]	SBR[e]
1971	17.9	NA[f]	12.0	22.6	12.6
1981	11.2	4.3	6.7	12.0	6.6
1990	7.8	3.2	4.5	8.1	4.6
SC[g] I	7.0	3.0	3.9	6.6	3.4
SC[g] V	11.8	5.9	5.9	9.6	6.8
Illegitimate	14.3	9.0	6.1	9.1	4.9
NCWP[h]	14.2	6.5	6.8	18.0	

[a] *Infant mortality rate per 1000 live births.*
[b] *Post-neonatal mortality rate per 1000 live births.*
[c] *Neonatal mortality rate per 1000 live births.*
[d] *Perinatal mortality per 1000 live and stillbirths.*
[e] *Stillbirth rate per 1000 live births.*
[f] *NA, not available.*
[g] *SC Social class.*
[h] *NCWP New Commonwealth and Pakistan.*

Neonatal and perinatal deaths

Neonatal deaths are related to maternal age, poverty, social class, place of birth and region, birth weight, and legal status of the infant (Madeley 1991). Although the levels of neonatal mortality reflect the effectiveness of maternity services, a closer relationship, particularly worldwide, is with income. Even in the UK there are marked regional differences (Table 6.3).

The perinatal mortality rate, stillbirths and infant deaths are high in disadvantaged Asian communities (Table 6.4).

Although consanguineous marriage, high maternal age and parity have an influence on these figures, poverty, poor nutrition and housing are likely to be more important (Black 1991). Access to appropriate medical care is difficult for those not educated in the UK and made worse where there are language difficulties.

Post-neonatal deaths have a marked seasonal variation in the UK, not mirrored in Scandinavian countries which are colder but have better, warmer housing. The potential for prevention is in good childcare, especially during cold weather, improved nutrition, and housing. Sir Donald Acheson (then the Chief Medical Officer) in launching 'The Health of the Nation' said 'Health inequalities will be eradicated only

Table 6.2b Relative risk of child mortality by social class and age (Kumar 1993)

Social class	1–4 years	5–9 years	10–15 years
I and II	1.00 (0.83, 1.21)	1.00 (0.80, 1.25)	1.00 (0.84, 1.20)
IV and V	2.08 (1.75, 2.49)	1.71 (1.39, 2.12)	1.37 (1.14, 1.64)
Unoccupied[a]	2.21 (1.88, 2.61)	2.56 (1.98, 3.30)	4.14 (3.43, 4.99)

[a] *90 % are economically inactive lone parent families. Numbers in brackets are confidence intervals.*

Table 6.2c Childhood morbidity (parentally reported), ages 0–15 in the UK 1985–89 (Kumar 1993). Figures are percentages

Social class	Males			Females		
	Chronic	Limiting[a]	Acute	Chronic	Limiting[a]	Acute
I	14.7	5.5	10.9	11.8	3.4	14.4
V	21.4	9.5	13.3	13.8	6.3	12.4
All	17.2	7.4	12.2	13.4	5.2	12.2

[a] *Chronic illness which limits the child's activities.*

Table 6.3 Infant mortality 1986–88 by geographical situation

Location	Perinatal deaths[a]	Infant deaths[b]
Bradford	13.5	14.3
Gateshead	12.1	10.2
Powys	12.3	7.3
Huntingdon	5.1	5.1
England and Wales	9.1	9.3

[a] *Rate per 1000 stillbirths and deaths in first week of life.*
[b] *Rate per 1000 live births.*

Table 6.4 Standardised mortality rates, stillbirths and deaths up to 1 year: SMR ratios by mother's country of birth (Balarajan et al 1989)

Country of origin	UK	India	Bangladesh	Pakistan
SMR ratio	96	134	118	23

by government measures to tackle poverty and improve conditions in which people live' (Smith 1991). It has been assessed that if all children in the UK enjoyed the same survival chances as the children of professionals and managers, over 3000 deaths a year might be prevented (Whitehead & Dahlgren 1991).

Sudden infant death syndrome

Infant deaths, and particularly deaths from sudden infant death syndrome (SIDS), are related to social disadvantage. Over-represented are families with young, single mothers, living in socially disadvantaged areas. The baby is more likely to have been born preterm, of low birth weight, twin pregnancy and been bottle fed, and live in a household with smokers. The incidence of SIDS in families where there has been previous child maltreatment is higher than might be expected.

The recent campaign in the UK to nurse infants of less than 6 months supine, to encourage breast-feeding and discourage smoking appears to have decreased the incidence of SIDS in the UK, but a significant proportion of 'SIDS' deaths are of concern in terms of aetiology.

CASE HISTORY 6.5

Mr and Mrs A had three children living at home; the youngest was a baby of 3 months. Mrs A's first child was neglected and made the subject of a care order and adopted aged 4 years.

The parents had a fierce argument about Mr A's excessive drinking. Mrs A stormed out and disappeared (as she had done many times before). Mr A went to collect the two older children from day nursery. He told the staff he needed help with the baby. Social Services arranged for the baby to go to foster-parents.

The baby arrived at the foster-parents' home at 7:30 p.m., brought by the social worker. When the baby failed to take his feed this was put down to a change of routine. The baby was put in his cot by the foster-mother who noticed he was hot and had a 'funny cry'. Half an hour later the baby was found dead in his cot. Autopsy revealed the baby had an upper respiratory tract infection but nothing more. Did the foster-parents, without prior knowledge of the baby or his behaviour, fail to recognise the symptoms of an ill baby? (Stanton et al 1978).

CASE HISTORY 6.6

A baby aged 6 months was found dead in his cot. He was very thin, had numerous bruises on his chest and back and scratches on his face, and he was dirty with severe nappy rash. Two children were subsequently born to this family. They were severely neglected and care orders were made at the age of 2 and 1 years.

Following the death of the first child an autopsy report commented on the poor growth and superficial injuries of the baby. No cause of death was found. The parents were reassured and told 'they had nothing to reproach themselves for' by the coroner.

Why did he die? Cot death, neglect or filicide?

The difficult task of the differentiation between SIDS and smothering is reviewed in more detail in Chapter 12 (Emery & Taylor 1986, Meadow 1990, Newlands & Emery 1991, Hobbs & Wynne 1995) The rate of SIDS in the UK is approximately 2 per 1000 live births. A small proportion of these are thought to be due to filicide (Emery 1985). The features which may assist in the recognition of smothering have been suggested by Meadow (1989):

- previous episode of unexplained apnoea, seizures or 'near-miss cot death'
- an infant over 6 months of age
- previous unexplained disorders affecting the child
- other unexplained deaths of children in the same family.

Oliver (1983) explored these unexplained deaths in childhood by studying the deaths of children from families known to social services because of abuse or neglect, over a 20-year follow-up period. Of a total 560 children in 147 families, 41 children died. This is about 7% of the children, all before they were 8 years old and the majority under 1 year, and 29 of the deaths were thought to be due to abuse or neglect.

Excess mortality in vulnerable families

It is difficult to tease out the various strands which contribute to the excess mortality of babies and children in socially disadvantaged families. Important factors include:

- low birth weight
- poor nutrition
- lack of immunisation
- damp, cold housing
- cigarette-smoking carers
- increased rate of respiratory disorders
- poverty (causing stress, poor diet, bad housing, etc.).

Access to medical care is often less than ideal in socially disadvantaged families and this adds to the difficulty in providing optimum care (Hart 1971, Webb 1996). As many as 1 in 7 families in inner-city areas are not registered with a general practitioner. This is partly due to frequent house moves, which are themselves disruptive to family life. Medical care is thus limited to 'emergencies' and health visitors have the difficult task of contacting these highly mobile families where statistics show there is an increased incidence of medical and developmental disorders in the children. It is estimated that 'preventable' causes of infant death are three times as common in social class V as in social class I (Spencer 1991).

Child–adult morbidity and poverty

Whitehead & Dahlgren (1991) wrote '. . . social inequalities in health are evident for most diseases and from birth to old age. . .'. Barker (1990) also saw the continuum of poor socio-economic circumstances in childhood leading into disease developing in later life. Smith (1990) described adults in social class V with a life expectancy 8 years shorter than social class I, three times as much mental illness, more coronary heart disease, lower self-esteem and lower immunisation rates. The origins of these disparities in health were in:

- perinatal and infant morbidity
- low birth weight
- infectious disease, respiratory disease
- accidents
- height (an indicator of nutrition in childhood)
- dental health.

Low birth weight is a major cause of morbidity and has a strong social class gradient. Additional evidence is accumulating that social disadvantage may effect the development of diseases in later life (Smith 1991). The standardised mortality ratio for men in social class V is twice that for men in social class I, much the same picture as for children in social class V compared with those in social class I (OPCS 1988). The effect of social disadvantage is shown particularly in respiratory, circulatory, musculoskeletal disorders, stroke and stomach cancer (Davey-Smith 1998). Thus not only do the poorest have shorter lives but their health is worse from childhood onwards (Davey Smith et al 1990).

Medical neglect

The failure by carers to provide appropriate health care to their children (assuming that this care is available) constitutes medical neglect. It may include failure to have the child immunised, attend hospital clinics, ensure the child follows a course of treatment, wears hearing-aids and so on.

Neglected children often have indifferent health with repeated chest, skin and gastrointesinal infections, and infestations (scabies, lice). Medical neglect may make it very difficult to treat children with common disorders such as asthma and more demanding regimes; for example for a child with acute leukaemia may prove almost impossible to clinically manage. Chronic conditions which require careful management such as diabetes mellitus or phenylketonuria may be haphazardly controlled, compounding the risk of both short- and longer-term adverse sequelae.

Children with disability are at greater risk of neglect (see Chapter 10) and this may have an equally compounding effect on the child's prognosis.

Occasionally a carer has a belief that certain treatments are 'wrong' and deny the child care. This may be very serious and children have died because of lack of insulin or a blood transfusion. In this situation an urgent legal opinion is needed.

CASE HISTORY 6.7

A boy of 6 years was admitted to a children's ward very ill due to pneumonia. He was wasted, stunted and anaemic. A tracheo-oesophageal fistula had been repaired at birth. Early surgical follow-up showed good progress. At 3 years he was referred to a paediatrician because of 'asthma'. He was lost to follow-up at 4 years. The family were known to various agencies as a 'problem'. On admission aged 6 years his mother said he had been unwell for more than a year. He weighed less at 6 years than at 4 years. The pneumonia proved untreatable and lobectomy was performed. Was this neglect? Could the family, GP, school health service have recognised this earlier? Did the hospital fail to pass on to primary care the need for follow-up?

CASE HISTORY 6.8

A boy of 7 years was admitted to a children's ward 'acutely' ill with empyema and septicaemia. He nearly died. He has been left with impaired respiratory function. At review various other medical problems were identified in the boy and his 9-year-old brother:

- severe dental caries requiring extractions and dentures
- failure to thrive
- untreated hypospadias and undescended testes.

As in Case 6.7, a 'difficult' family, and an inadequate health surveillance system conspired to impair the health of these boys.

Nutrition

Nutrition is related to growth and health (see Chapter 3). Low income families have not only to spend a high percentage of their money on food (30%), calorie for calorie 'unhealthy' foods are cheaper (Spencer 1991).

Poor housing

Housing is clearly related to health and social disadvantages. Nearly 100 000 households involving children were registered homeless in 1988 (Lowry 1991). Over half the bed and breakfast, bedsit and hostel accommodation fails to meet health and safety standards (Gillen 1991). Thus not only are children living in cramped, unsuitable housing – it is also damp, cold, unhygienic and unsafe. High-rise flats are unsuitable for children, young and older, who need safe, supervised playing areas. Mothers too become depressed and isolated when separated from friends and family.

Accidents

Accidents are a major child health problem in the UK and many more children from socially disadvantaged homes are killed or maimed, adding disability to disadvantage. Half of the deaths in children aged 1–15 years are due to 'accidents' and over half of these are caused by road traffic accidents. Much of the serious morbidity due to accidents follows traffic accidents.

Deaths from road traffic accidents (where the child is usually a pedestrian), drowning in canals or deaths on railway tracks show a 5–10-fold variation with social class. This reflects not only lack of supervision of children but also the inadequacy of play areas in many inner-city areas, and a failure by road planners to protect children from traffic. Mortality from childhood injury is falling but the fall is differential in that the decline is much slower for social classes IV and V than social classes I and II (21%, 2%, 32% and 37%, respectively) in the period 1979–92 (Roberts & Power 1996).

Accidents within the home are related to lapses in supervision, for example another child is ill and the mother is distracted. Antecedents of accidents are that the family have just moved, the parents split up or the mother is depressed. Accidents also happen to more boys, especially those described as over-active, distractable or 'accident-prone', often in socially disadvantaged families.

Accidents in children

- More than 50% of deaths in childhood are due to accidents, poisoning, violence
- 20% of children have a significant injury each year
- More than 60% of pedestrian deaths are on minor roads (near home)
- Peak age for pedestrian deaths is 4–6 years (majority under 10 years)
- Peak time for pedestrian deaths is late afternoon
- Twice as many deaths due to road traffic accident in boys as compared to girls
- Death rates from injury and poisoning are falling in all social classes but in social class V are five times the rate in social class I

Repeated accidents

- More boys
- More inner city, no garden
- Children described as restless, fidgety, disobedient, enuretic, nail biters, destructive, aggressive
- Families known to social services
- Frequent house moves
- Young, depressed, stressed mothers

CASE HISTORY 6.9

A boy of 10 years was admitted to the intensive care unit unconscious having been involved in a road traffic accident. His sister, aged 8 years, and he had been chased home by a gang of boys from the same school. In their escape they had run across a busy road and into a car. The boy had learning problems and was supported in mainstream school, having an educational statement of special needs. He was tall, clumsy and poorly cared for, being dirty and smelly. His lone parent mother was out at work when the children came home from school. The family were constantly harassed in the neighbourhood; the eldest boy was in prison.

The injured boy recovered but has suffered permanent brain damage.

The overall death rate from injury has decreased in the UK in the last 20 years. Deaths from road traffic accidents have fallen, but the morbidity from head injury remains high.

Disagreement continues as to who is responsible but the Child Accident Prevention Trust (Jackson et al 1988) advocates the need for education and a multidisciplinary approach to the problem of accidents in children. A suggested model is given in Figure 6.2.

Neglect and education

Educational neglect occurs when a child of school age does not attend school, has many unexplained absences or is regularly late for school. For older children it may be condoned truancy. The consequences for the child are many and include a failure to learn basic skills of literacy and numeracy, failure to develop social skills including peer relationships and ultimately reduced career opportunities (Kendall-Tiackett & Eckenrode 1996).

Even 4–5-year-old children may have very disruptive behaviours, and older pupils may opt out of school completely. Such children, from the age of 10 years upwards are at risk of developing increasingly antisocial behaviours as they are bored and want money and excitement.

The number of children expelled from schools is increasing. These children may have difficulty gaining acceptance in alternative schools and the local authority may only offer part-time education at a special centre. Urgent research and resources are needed if this disaffected and alienated troubled and troublesome group of children are to be helped. Almost 13 500 children were permanently excluded from school in England in 1995–96, an 8% increase on the previous year. In 1991–92 the figure was below 4000 (Bright 1998). There is also an apparent increase in the numbers of children 'looked after' by the local authority and it may be that the trigger has been the increase in exclusions leading to children loitering on the streets, turning to crime and inevitably, increased family problems.

CASE HISTORY 6.10

A boy was born 12 weeks pre-term to a 16-year-old girl with moderate learning problems (it was learned later that she had been sexually abused from the age of 12 years by her uncle) and a 20-year-old casual acquaintance who had been in care because of neglect and his sexual abuse of his younger sisters. The baby did well after a brief period of ventilation and treatment including gentamycin for septicaemia. Discharge was delayed because of concern as to the couples' parenting skills.

The child was repeatedly admitted to hospital in the first two years because of colds, chest infections and failure to thrive. The general practitioner

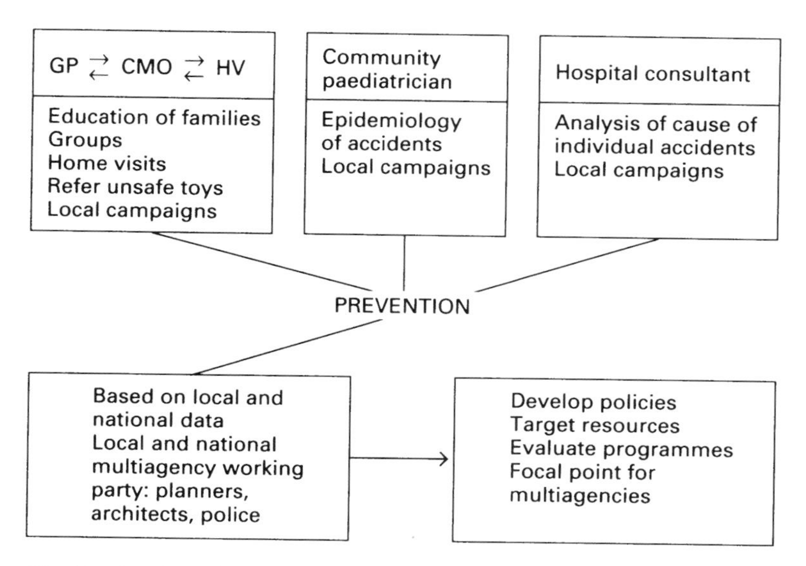

Fig. 6.2 Coordinated accident prevention within a health district. GP, general practitioner; CMO, clinical medical officer; HV, health visitor.

immunised him at home. When he became mobile he had many minor accidents and was frequently seen at the local Accident and Emergency department.

His development was delayed in his attention, play, language and social skills, and a bilateral hearing loss of 80 dB was discovered. At around the age of 2 years the social services began 'care proceedings by notice'. The family worked much more constructively with their health visitor and social worker and the child began to thrive better, the parents went to classes to learn British sign language. The social services department finally sought a Supervision order and the child's name remained on the child protection register in the category of neglect.

By the age of 5 years the boy had eating, sleeping and behavioural difficulties. He was not toilet trained. He had grown better, from the third to the 50th centile for height but was under weight being on the third centile. He had poor attention, knew few words or signs but clearly had better understanding than his expressive language. His hearing aids were rarely worn unless at school: they were either lost, eaten by the alsatian, in the fish tank or away for repair. His mother did not think he needed any more language – 'he understands me' and his father went rarely to a local signing class. The family was often in bed when the school transport arrived. On the occasions he went to school he 'loved the attention, enjoyed play, appeared to have untapped potential and ate very well . . .'. At 6 years in a foster-home with a signing foster-mother and deaf older girl he made rapid progress socially and in his use of language. His parents were reassessed and were increasingly clear that the needs of their son were too demanding for them to meet. His mother 'never wanted him' and she wanted help for herself. His father put his energies into a local group (in charge of the lighting) and although he did not want his son 'in care' he was not prepared to work to meet his son's, by now, increasingly complex needs.

Consequently the boy showed in foster care he had much more potential in all fields of development than had been apparent but his long-term outlook is uncertain, especially socially.

This boy was neglected physically and emotionally and denied appropriate learning opportunities. Professionals worked very hard to support the family but – in retrospect – perhaps for too long?

Responsibility and rights

In 1991 the UK government became a signatory to most of the UN Conventions on the Rights of the Child. Under Article 27 the Convention is clear on the need for family and state responsibility:

- the parents have the primary responsibility to secure the conditions of living necessary for the child's development
- the state shall assist parents, and in cases of need provide material assistance, particularly with regard to nutrition, clothing and housing.

Society therefore has a view as to child-rearing practice but is the responsibility for children to be shared, with parents enabled and empowered, or is the current trend in the UK to prevail, with an increasing devolution on the individual? Helfer (1987) has written of the consequences of a society which neglects its children, at the family and societal level.

Poverty makes child-rearing difficult; the least able in society are the poorest and thus they have to function particularly efficiently to overcome the effects of social disadvantage and be successful parents. Money is a buffer which is taken for granted by those with adequate means, whereas poverty increases stresses on the often impoverished emotional resources of the family, which further impairs coping skills.

Child health clinics and paediatric outpatient clinics are populated with parents of all social classes who are experiencing difficulty in child-rearing. Although neglect in the terms outlined in this chapter is associated with poor physical care and often poverty, emotional abuse and deprivation occur at all income levels and also lead to unhappy, disturbed, underachieving children (Ch. 7).

Parents who neglect their children fail to care for their children physically or to supervise them and do not engage the developmental needs of the child in terms of cognitive stimulation (Skuse 1993). As the child grows the parents do not respond to him or provide for his complex and changing needs.

Childhood – which should be joyful, exciting and full of promise – becomes an existence, the child being cold, hungry, tired, uncomfortable, unloved and consequently showing a lack of interest in people and his surroundings. Neglected children are emotionally deprived children and may also suffer other abuses, such as physical or sexual abuse.

- In infancy, neglected children will be recognised by their poor physical state and their failure to thrive and achieve age-appropriate developmental skills.
- The pre-school child may not only be small, thin, poorly cared for and developmentally delayed, but may also have difficulty in forming relationships and show behavioural problems.
- At school the neglected child will have learning problems (especially in language and attention), as well as increasingly evident emotional difficulties.

Emotionally abused children may be physically well cared for but suffer the same consequences in terms of learning and emotional development. Neglected children are physically neglected and emotionally deprived. The progress neglected and emotionally deprived children make when moved into well-functioning alternative families may be dramatic. The longer a child is neglected, the worse the outcome in terms of emotional competence and the acquisition of educational and social skills needed in adult life.

What are a child's needs?

Children have differing needs at different ages, but all children need adequate nutrition, warmth, housing, love, understanding, security, education and health services. Children need protection from illness, accident, cruelty, neglect, exploitation (child labour) and discrimination (colour, race, gender). In the UK this is best provided by two caring adults who care for each other as well as the children.

Needs of children

- Food
- Warmth
- Clothing
- Shelter/protection
- Grooming
- Fresh air/sunlight
- Activity/rest
- Prevention of illness and accident
- Affection
- Continuity of care
- Security of belonging
- Personal identity
- Opportunity to learn/have career opportunities
- Opportunity to achieve success
- Opportunity to become self-disciplined
- Opportunity to achieve independence

What does a newborn baby need?

Food, warmth, comfort, company, sleep, grooming and movement are the essentials for a baby. How the parents will meet the newborn baby's needs depends on their knowledge and understanding of child-rearing, social and cultural influences and whether they themselves were warmly nurtured as children. Parents who have been neglected themselves may have great difficulty in parenting, but this is not inevitable. Education in schools is essential to supplement deficits in knowledge provided at home.

Practical needs of the baby

- Milk – breast/bottle (sterilisation equipment)
- Warm room
- Access to hot water
- Access to feeding 3–4 hourly

Emotional demands

Rearing a baby is a 24-hour commitment, 7 days a week.

- Was the child planned?
- Was the baby wanted in order to be a provider of love?
- Is the baby difficult, a slow feeder needing small (3–4 hourly) feeds, irritable and so relentlessly testing the mother's skills?
- Is the mother depressed, tired, young, educationally slow, inexperienced, alone?
- Is the house adequate or is it difficult to keep warm or clean, or obtain hot water?
- Does the mother get help, both physically and emotionally?
- If she gets tired or becomes depressed, can she respond to the needs of the baby?
- Does the baby become cross and more irritable or apathetic and disinterested?
- Is this baby just one stress too many in the household?

It is easy to see how babies become too much for parents without support or with inadequate support systems, and care deteriorates as the parents struggle with their own unmet needs and difficulties, as well as the increasing demands of the baby.

What do older babies and toddlers need?

As babies grow it is no longer appropriate that they sleep so much; they sit up, want to move and explore, use their hands and begin to talk. Feeding is more difficult as the baby needs solids, a variety of foods and to be spoon-fed. All these needs require more planning, time and patience on the part of the parents. As the baby becomes mobile the home needs modifying to enable the baby freedom to explore, but it also needs 'child-proofing'. Stairgates, fireguards, cooker guards are simple protective devices which are often not used, yet may allow the child space in safety.

By eye contact, smiles, laughs and coos the child communicates pleasure. Waving and clapping are early signs in communication.

It is expected that the child is taken to the well-baby clinic to be weighed, to be immunised, to have development screened and hearing checked and any problems discussed. Babies are seen in clinic most frequently in the first 12 months of life, on average six times, but social classes I and V mothers attend least frequently.

As children grow older they are dependent on carers to continue to provide materially, but also to talk, play and show interest.

Needs of the pre-school child

A child who is not spoken to, or hears only occasional commands, does not learn to listen and pay attention. Visual and auditory attention are essential if the child is to benefit from the learning opportunities in the environment. Sitting on mother's knee from 12 to 15 months, looking at pictures in a book, pointing, listening, experimenting with sounds, the child will learn to look, hear, pay attention and communicate. Delay in language development is universal in neglected children.

At mealtimes children have to learn to sit at the table, not to wander and to use implements rather than finger-feed. They have to be toilet-trained and shown how to dress. If they have not learned these basic skills by school entry they will already be severely disadvantaged.

Needs of the schoolchild

At school children are required to sit, listen to a story or follow complex instructions, hold a pencil, cope with dinner and playtime, change for PE and use the toilets appropriately. Their language should be at the level of 'reading readiness'. They need to be able to separate from their mother, and also needs to be able to form relationships with his peer group and previously unknown adults.

Children need to belong and be the 'same'. At school children need to be clean and tidily dressed and not to smell. They do not want to look or feel different from their peers. They do not want their parents to dress or behave differently, especially in school, from other parents.

Children need home to be organised with a routine for getting up, having meals, baths, clean clothes, going to bed. To succeed at school a child needs to be on time and to attend regularly. Poor school attendance, whether due to intercurrent illness or family disorganisation, leads to a discontinuity which slows academic progress.

Neglected visual or auditory impairments disadvantage the child who is trying to learn to read.

Children of all ages need encouragement and success to allow them to develop confidence and self-esteem. Parental support and their appreciation of the value of education is essential to help motivate the child.

Children need to start to take responsibility to help in the home, care for pets and may visit relatives. They need increasing experience and activities outside the home to develop greater independence as they learn more of their world.

The child's emotional development, and the acquisition of social skills, is largely determined by his relationship with the main care-givers, usually the mother. Clearly, relationships with the other parent, siblings and grandparents are also important, as is the relationship between the parents. It is essential for emotional development that in the longer term the child forms at least one close, positive and secure relationship. This does not have to be with the mother, but the relationship with the caring adult should be long-term and close. The lack of such a relationship does not mean that the child will inevitably become stunted emotionally but it makes it more difficult for him or her to form good secure attachments in the long term.

It also appears that some children are less vulnerable than others in that they are more able to form other relationships and develop social networks outside the emotionally neglecting home. This gives children the opportunity to have alternative social experience and aids their emotional growth. Thus, although many emotionally neglected children have problems initially with peer relationships which continue to affect adult relationships, this is not inevitable.

Needs of the teenager

Teenagers need much the same as children, and more in many ways than younger children. They continue to need family organisation and routine but also boundaries to test, to discover the tolerable limits of their behaviour. They need constant love and emotional support to help them cope with the demands of peers, school and their own aspirations. They need adults who can cope with the excesses of their behaviour and do not reject them.

Teenagers need adults to help with school work and to provide an environment in which it can be done. They also need adults outside the home in whom they may confide. Teenagers worry about health, sex, sexuality, drugs, acne, careers, everything, and need informed caring adults, not always parents, to advise.

Clinical aspects of neglect

Neglected children present in many ways to the doctor (Table 6.5): the baby with severe cradle-cap who is failing to thrive, the toddler of 2 years who has ingested his mother's iron tablets, the 5-year-old suffering the complications of measles or the 8-year-old child who is failing at school. Essentially, neglect and its consequences are preventable and so present a challenge to all who work with children and their families, especially in primary care.

The clinician's task is primarily that of assessment of the child's growth, development and physical health (Table 6.6). This is put in the context of a family assessment in collaboration with the health visitor. It is always necessary to have a clear idea of normal development and not to accept 'his language is the norm for the area' when told of a neglected child with language delay. Usually children are seen over a period of time and by undertaking careful assessments it is possible to monitor the child: is he or she progressing at an adequate rate or is slipping even further behind? Good records are essential to allow review and if the extra nursery time, health visitor and social work support are not effecting a change for the child, is it time to discuss alternative care? (Table 6.7).

Some doctors will wish to join the parents and other professionals in looking at any feeding problems, behavioural and learning difficulties and work together to plan a strategy to help the child within his family. Others will offer to monitor (objectively) the effects of the intervention.

Table 6.5 Physical manifestations and consequences of neglect

Deprivation	Result	Long-term effect
Supervision or safe environment	Accidents: falls, scalds, ingestions, RTA, drowning, house fires[a]	Morbidity from accidents, e.g. brain damage
• lack of car seat belt or cycling helmet	Accidents/death	As above
Medical care		
• failure to immunise	Measles, rubella, mumps, whooping cough, etc.	Deafness, brain damage, death, lung damage fetal damage
• failure to seek advice for ill child	Illness recognised when child seriously ill or dying	Persisting morbidity, e.g. empyema, suppurative otitis media, brain damage
• failure to attend for developmental surveillance	Squint, deafness, other disorders not recognised	Amblyopia Poor speech Learning difficulties
• refusal of medical care	Prolonged illness, avoidable complication, death	Avoidable death and morbidity
Hygiene in home	Repeated episodes of gastroenteritis, skin infections, head lice, zoonoses	Fail to thrive Poor self-esteem Ostracised at school
• clean (smoke- and mould-free) air	Dirty child Infection: especially respiratory, asthma	Chronic respiratory disease
• clean water	Increased lead burden	Behavioural and learning disorder
Warmth	Cold injury – red, swollen hands and feet Hypothermia, hypostatic pneumonia Infection, especially chest	Frostbite – loss of part of toes rarely
Food	Malnourished – small, thin, protuberant abdomen	Impaired physical well-being
• inadequate calories	May be stunted 'emotional dwarf' with apparent adequate nutrition	Apathy
• inadequate feeding	Impaired brain growth (especially <2 yrs), vitamin deficiencies	Learning difficulties
• innapropriate diet (including fads)		Stunted as adult (adapt to smallness)
Drink	Inappropriate patterns of drinking – e.g. from WC, drains – causing GI infections	
Physical care		
• grooming	Dry, thin, sparse hair, alopecia, cradle-cap, nappy rash, spotty skin, maceration in skin folds Thickened yellow nails Dirty, smelly body with infestations, e.g. nits Vulvovaginitis, especially in young girls Clothing inappropriate, inadequate, dirty	Socially unacceptable at nursery/school Shunned by peers, i.e. additional emotional deprivation

[a] *Other sources of environmental pollution include lead from motor vehicle exhaust or old lead paint; radioactivity from nuclear power plants; toxocara in parks, playing fields; dog bites.*

Pathway to neglect

Why are children neglected and what are the antecedents? There clearly is a 'cycle of deprivation'. Neglected children are at risk of growing up into adults with limited skills in all sorts of areas and becoming inadequate, neglectful parents. In the community there are many families being monitored by health and social work professionals: an example case history is given in Figure 6.3.

Assessing families

Much useful work has been undertaken recently to look at why parents may neglect children and how they may be helped to parent more adequately. The result of assessment may be that the

Table 6.6 Clinical assessment of neglect

Appearance	Note clothing, hair, skin, nails, odour
Growth	Height and weight (serial measurements to check growth rate) Head circumference Mid-upper arm circumference
Physical examination	Signs of disorder e.g. squint, asthma, heart murmur, dental caries, undescended testes, congenital dislocation of hips, signs of physical or sexual abuse
Development	Gross motor skills Fine motor skills Vision and hearing (by age-appropriate technique) Language – receptive and expressive Play Behaviour • observed in clinic • information from third party

Table 6.7 Additional information for assessment

Report from day nursery	Nursery nurse or teacher or school
Assessment of care at home	Health visitor or school nurse or social worker
Physical state of home	As above
Care of other children	As above

Table 6.8 Neglecting families (after Crittenden 1988)

'Neglected' parents	Neglected in own childhood Slow, even mentally handicapped Unemployed, or unskilled work Partner similar Several children when young Extended family large but poor support Few expectations for self or children Live from day to day
'Secondary incompetence' of parents	Become neglectful due to adverse circumstance, e.g. head injury psychiatric illness, drug or alcohol abuse Extreme beliefs, e.g. nutritional, religious, cultural
Environment	Poor, overcrowded housing, unfenced gardens Cold, damp, poor repair Bed and breakfast accommodation Temporary housing, e.g. caravan Unsafe surroundings, e.g. dangerous or no play areas, busy roads, unfenced railways, waterways Poverty: insufficient food, electricity or gas disconnected
Over-reliance on or rejection of professionals	May have large numbers of professionals Professionals' anxiety may be very high Professional help may be totally rejected

particular parent or parents are not able at this point to provide adequate care. A framework for categorising families is given in Table 6.8 (Crittenden 1988).

- Why are the parents failing?
- Are they able or motivated to change?
- What can be done to support the child and parents and improve their environment?
- Is the extended family helpful or destructive?

Before statutory proceedings are considered, a thorough assessment and programme of support should be implemented to see if the family can change in time for this child. Parents do mature, do learn new skills and, if their material position improves, they may feel success is possible. Mild to moderate depression is endemic in mothers in inner cities. Their feelings of hopelessness – coupled with the enormity of the task of rearing children well, often alone, usually in poverty, in an impoverished environment – are real. In some circumstances it is too dangerous to leave a baby at home and statutory proceedings have to be initiated early in the assessment. Rehabilitation to home is always an option after a full review.

Which families are resistant to change?

Some families have overwhelming problems which are multiple; given that resources are limited the overall outcome may be dependent upon the presence of:

- mental retardation of the adults
- adults who have severe difficulty with interpersonal relationships
- limits of resources; neglecting families may consume vast amounts of professional time and other resources.

The parents may have little awareness of their inadequacies in child-rearing and the longer the neglect continues, the more difficult it is to help the children effectively. Parents may also feel unable to change and are overwhelmed by their day-to-day poverty and struggle to survive. If the adults have mere survival as their goal, their

Professional input	*Family*
Family known to SSD Housing Probation	Parents unemployed 7 children, 3 attend special school, 2 left home.
	3rd child, a girl, now aged 15 yrs
Paediatrician →	*PMH* FTT infancy
Health visitor/GP continue	Minor physical abuse 2 yrs
Paediatrician →	Special school 7 yrs (moderate learning difficulty)
Social worker →	? CSA by brothers 12 yrs
Teacher special school →	*PH* Pregnant, no antenatal care
recognised pregnancy School nurse supports	Smokes 10–15 cigs/day
Leaves school 15 years — education complete	
Community Midwife (MW) →	Pregnancy 28 weeks
Hospital services — → Paediatrician, nurses, HV, MW, SW, Community MW	Pre-term delviery 30 weeks, 1.5 kg Baby ventilated 1 week Discharge delayed to 8 weeks
CASE DISCUSSION HELD HOSPITAL/COMMUNITY STAFF ⇄	because of comments about handling and home conditions ↓
GP, MW, SW, Parents } Attended case discussion at hospital too	*Discharged* home to mother and 20-y-old unemployed partner — council maisonette, 12 steps to front door, no garden, all electricitiy heating
Family aide appointed	
Follow-up at home HV/SCBU (special care baby unit) midwife/ SW/Family aide GP	*Home* baby 8 weeks, poor weight gain, slow feeder ↓
Attends CHC (child health clinic) weekly HV GP/CMO (clinical medical officer)	9/52, 10/52, 11/52, 12/52. *13/52* Failing to thrive (FTT) *14/52* FTT, nappy rash
Hospital paediatrician Ward nurses Liaison HV/SW } →	*Hospital* — thrives — nappy rash heals ↓
GP/HV/SW/Family aide →	*Home* 15/52 ↓
Infectious disease paediatrician Ward nurses Liaison HV/SW } →	*Hospital* 18/52 — gastroenteritis — FTT/nappy rash *Home 20/52* ↓
Attends HV GP/CMO SW/Family aide } →	Poor weight gain unresponsive baby ↓
Hospital paediatrician Ward nurses Liaison HV/SW } →	*Hospital* 6/12 Chest infection FTT/nappy rash 'Slow, floppy' No immunisation
CHILD PROTECTION CONFERENCE HELD ←	

Decide
1. Child Protection Register — neglect
2. SSD — key worker
3. Plan of support
4. Reconvene in 3/12 to see outcome (or sooner)

HV, GP, CMO, SW, Family aide nursery nurse — all anxious — all continue to be involved.	*Baby* now 7/12 at day nursery, attends with mother and father, starts to become more alert. IMMUNISED AT NURSERY
All continue except Family aide withdrawn.	*Baby* slowly puts on weight and development accelerates.
OP appointment missed.	*Squint* diagnosed — fails to attend for first appointment.
2nd OP appointment taken by SW. Nursery nurse takes mother to hospital and learns to do therapy at nursery	*Baby* now 12/12 *Mild cerebral diplegia* — weekly physiotherapy arranged.

Summary 1. Unplanned, unsupervised pregnancy leads to preterm delivery for unprepared young mother.
2. Consequences:
(i) for baby — cerebral palsy, squint, possible learning problems later, poor parenting leading to undernutrition, impaired learning opportunities, ill health (Table 6.8).
(ii) for mother — pregnancy when 15 years, has few coping strategies, becomes dependent on professionals, will she be able to learn in time to meet this child's needs?
(iii) for father — pitched into parenthood with as few skills as mother.
(iv) for professionals — vast use of resources, will change be effected? What are their responsibilities to the child and the parents? When does parenting become 'not good enough'?

Fig. 6.3 Case history to illustrate management: PMH, past medical history; PH, presenting history.

aspirations for their children will be low too. Their extended family and neighbours may feel a similar hopelessness and parents and children are enmeshed in an impoverished family and social system resistant to change.

Neglecting parents often feel bad about themselves, do not laugh much or have fun. They do not know how to play with their children. They often find difficulty in showing and receiving affection from partners and children.

Directions for intervention include:

- enabling the adults to feel change is possible
- reducing the level of family dysfunction and improving parenting skills in a structured but supportive way
- fostering normal emotional development, including skills of communication between the adults as well as the children
- focusing on the family as a whole, rather than the child alone, and improving the quality of life of the adults, which it is hoped will be of lasting benefit to the children
- giving attention to the extended family but with sensitivity so as not to alienate, as without the support of those wider networks any change in the family is liable to be rendered ineffective
- providing support, which will be needed for years.

Specific help for neglected children

- An interesting environment where children can learn to focus attention and to talk; for example, a good day nursery
- Enabling them to feel competent, responsive to others, be individuals in their own right and able to have an effect on their future
- This involves individual work, as in good day care
- Ideally the child's carer is not only involved in these improvements but also in work at home with coordinated home visits by social worker, nursery nurse, teacher, family aid, Home Start, Newpin, NSPCC, Family Service Unit and other voluntary agencies

Conclusion

Neglect is a prevalent form of maltreatment in the UK. It is insidious and adversely affects children in many ways including retardation of growth and development, as well as poor general health. Neglected children may also be abused in other ways. A summary is given in Table 6.9 (Skuse 1993).

Neglecting families have a poor prognosis for change. The earlier intervention takes place, the

Table 6.9 Key features of neglect and emotional deprivation (after Skuse 1989)

	Infant	Pre-school	School child	Teenager
Physical	FTT Recurrent infection Repeated admissions Severe nappy rash	Short ± underweight Unkempt, dirty Microcephalic Thin, pulled hair (Verbov 1993)	Short ± underweight Unkempt, dirty Thin, pulled hair	Short + underweight + obese Poor general health, unkempt, dirty, delayed puberty
Development	General delay	Language delay Poor attention Emotional immaturity	Learning difficulties Poor attention Lacks confidence Immature	School failure
Behaviour	Attachment disorder: anxious, avoidant Socially unresponsive	Over-active Aggressive, impulsive Indiscriminate friendliness Physical comfort from stranger	Over-active Aggressive Withdrawn Lacks confidence Poor relationships Poor school progress Wetting, soiling Destructive	School non-attendance Smoking, drinking, substance abuse Run away Sexual promiscuity Stealing Lying Destructive (self, others, property)

greater the chance for progress. The whole family, including the mother's partner, should be involved. Separation, even in day care, should be careful and involve the mother as, with weak bonds in the family, dissolution can occur. Support should be structured and supportive, but not unduly coercive as this often provokes anger and withdrawal from services. Professional help will be needed in the long term.

Assessments

Ongoing assessment of the growth, development and health of the children in neglecting families is needed. If, despite support, the children continue to fail, alternative care (foster-care) may be needed, with early planning towards permanency if the prospects for change at home remain poor.

The paediatric assessment in neglect (Table 6.6) must include:

- physical state – skin, hair, nails, clothes
- growth – growth rate, nutrition
- development – gross motor, fine motor, speech, hearing, vision
- emotional well-being
- information from other professionals (Table 6.7).

A paediatrician may review the child's progress. Detail is important.

- Notes of failed hospital appointments, failure to immunise, poor attendance for speech therapy or nursery should be included.
- Is this child failing to grow because of a lack of calories?
- Why doesn't the child get enough food?
- Has anyone observed a mealtime?

It is necessary to compile a logical detailed report which demonstrates that this child is failing to grow and develop in the absence of a medical disorder. In the first instance the aim of paediatric intervention is to help the parents care for their child, to assess the child's needs (by a thorough physical and developmental check) and then suggest how these needs might be met. Referrals for audiometry, the dentist, support of a nursery place and advice on sleep problems are positive ways in which the child and parents may be helped.

If the child still fails to grow and develop the doctor must say so and be prepared to tell the parents and other professionals. Finally it may be necessary to give evidence in court. This is difficult, especially when parents are clearly disadvantaged by their own past. However, protection of the child is paramount; children have rights too, and failure to grow and develop is a denial of every child's inheritance.

Table 6.10 Summary: Neglect, parenting and social exclusion

'Parenting is probably the most important public health issue facing our society' (Hoghughi 1998) Neglect occurs when parenting is not 'good-enough' (Cooper 1985)	'Children and the inverse care law' (Webb 1998) 'social exclusion is associated with poor health and very poor access to health services'
Parenting is a buffer against adversity, poverty and delinquent influences. It protects children from harm, promotes physical and emotional health and develops a child's potential	> 30% of children are brought up in conditions of socio-economic deprivation 8% of children are brought up in conditions of *profound* socio-economic deprivation
Parenting is the single largest variable in: illness of children, accidents, teenage pregnancy, substance abuse, truancy, unemployability, child abuse, crime, mental illness, conduct disorder	Profoundly marginalised groups include: homeless children, children in care, travellers (30 000 children in the UK), refuges (Women's Aid: 35 000 children pass through each year), minority ethnic communities, runaways, refugees, children in custody
Parenting may be a mediator of damage e.g. child abuse, parental depression, substance/alcohol may damage children	
Preventive measures to assist parents, rather than later intervention Early recognition of 'risk' Integration of services	Strategies are needed to prevent poor health and long-term sequelae: e.g. adequate income, access to services (especially primary care housing), education i.e. to reverse inverse care law

Summary

1. Neglect is insidious, pervasive and damaging; recently there has been an increased professional acknowledgement of this form of maltreatment as shown by increased registrations in the category of neglect on child protection registers (Leeds ACPC 1996).
2. Neglect, as defined in the Children Act (1989), will be considered as to whether it involves actual or likely 'significant harm', and whether it involves 'ill treatment' or 'impairment of health or development' (in each case as defined by the Act).
3. Most of the children reported are under 5 years of age but neglect extends throughout childhood and adolescence.
4. There is a strong relationship in reported cases with adverse social circumstances. Poverty makes parenting more difficult (Tregeagle & Voigt 1993) and poverty is strongly correlated with neglect (Pelton 1993).
5. Neglect may be recognised in socially advantaged families but is less well recognised as parents may buy solutions on the private market (King & Trowell 1992).
6. Although neglect reflects wider social issues, it is in the microcosm of the family in which it achieves expression (in western society). Families are changing and by the year 2000 only 50% of children will have been brought up in traditional nuclear families (Walker 1996).
7. Children have emotional, physical, educational, health and social needs; neglected children have these needs inadequately met.
8. Patterns of neglect are recognisable to extended families, neighbours, professionals and may be tolerated over long periods of time. Neglect should be named, described clinically in an objective way and then addressed.
9. The hallmark of neglecting behaviour is the failure of carers to recognise and/or meet their children's needs, and to comply with professionals' advice.
10. Preventable accidents are a major cause of morbidity and mortality in neglectful families. The significance of repeated accidents should be recognised in the Accident and Emergency department. Reduction of child injury death rates

is a priority in the Health of the Nation strategy (DoH 1992).

11. The cycle of deprivation is well demonstrated in neglecting families.
12. Interventions in neglecting families must be goal directed, time limited, and always involve the parents. Progress is often slow.
13. Prevention of neglect must be broad-based, involving social policy as well as education and development of parenting skills.
14. Presentation of evidence in court demands a comprehensive assessment over time with reference to attempted interventions.
15. Unless government rhetoric on social class gradients in health is matched with appropriate action, the Health of the Nation's (DoH 1992) targets for accidents will be met for in the non-manual social classes but not for those in the manual classes' (Roberts & Power 1996)
16. 'Child health inequalities can be tackled by social, economic and health policies which are aimed at reducing income disparities and improving the access of the poor to essential services, including primary health care, food, water and education' (Spencer 1996). Health workers can work to reduce health inequality and promote equity in health, but health services alone cannot address the fundamental problem of poverty.
17. 1999 will mark the fortieth anniversary of the Declaration of the Rights of the Child. The aims of this basic statement of human rights have not been achieved in practice.

REFERENCES

Arblaster L 1995 Housing and health. Yorkshire Medicine, Spring: 8–9

Balarajan R, Raleigh V S, Botting B 1989 Mortality from congenital malformations in England and Wales; variations by mother's country of birth. Archives of Disease in Childhood 64:1457–1462

Barker D J P 1990 The fetal and infant origins of adult disease. British Medical Journal 301:1111

Black D 1996 Deprivation and health. Journal of the Royal College of Physicians of London 30(5):466–471

Black J A 1991 The medical needs of ethnic minority children in Britain. Current Paediatrics 1:53–58

Bradshaw J 1996 Working together 10 years on – the Sieff Conference, London

Bright M 1998 Teachers now allowed to hold, push and pull unruly pupils *Guardian* July 1998

Browne K, Lynch M 1995 Editorial in special edition. Fatal child abuse: the nature and extent of child homicide and fatal abuse. Child Abuse Review 4:309-315

Cantwell H B, Rosenberg D A 1990 Child neglect. National Council of Juvenile and Family Court Judges, University of Nevada, Reno, Nevada

Cassell D, Coleman R 1995 Parents with psychiatric problems. in: Reder P, Lucey C (eds) Assessment of parenting. Routledge, London, Ch 11

Cemlyn S 1995 Traveller children and the state: welfare or neglect. Child Abuse and Neglect 4(4):278–290

Chaffin M, Kelleher K, Hollenberg J 1996 Onset of physical abuse and neglect: psychiatric, substance abuse, and social risk factors from prospectve community data. Child Abuse and Neglect 20(3):191–204

Children's Rights Office 1995 Making the Convention work for children. Expression Printers, London

Coleman R, Cassell D 1995 Parents who misuse drugs and alcohol. In Reder P, Lucey C (eds) Assessment of parenting, Routledge, London, Ch 12

CPAG 1996 Poverty: the facts. Child Poverty Action Group, 1–5 Bath Street, London EC1V 9PY

Cooper C 1985 Good-enough parenting, a framework for assessment. London, British Agency for adoption and fostering, Practice series 12:58–80

Creighton S J, Noyes P 1989 Child abuse trends in England and Wales 1983–87. NSPCC, London

Creighton S J, Noyes P 1990 Child abuse in 1989. Research briefing No 11. NSPCC, London

Crittenden P 1988 Family and dyadic patterns. In: Browne K, Davies C, Stratton P (eds) Prediction and prevention of child abuse. J Wiley, Chichester

Davey Smith G 1996 Income inequality and mortality: why are they related? British Medical Journal 312:987–988

Davey Smith G, Bartley M, Blane D 1990 The Black Report on socio-economic inequalities in health 10 years on. British Medical Journal 301:373–377

Davey-Smith G, Hart C, Blane D, Hole D 1998 Adverse socioeconomic conditions in childhood causes specific adult mortality British Medical Journal 316:1631–1634

Delamothe T 1991 Social inequalities in health. British Medical Journal 303:1046–1050

Dennehy A, Smith L, Harker P 1997 Not to be ignored – young people, poverty and health. Child Poverty Action Group, 1–5 Bath Street, London EC1V 9PY

DHSS 1980 Inequalities in health: report of a research working group (the Black Report). DHSS, London

Ditch J, Bradshaw J, Eardley 1996 Developments in national family policies in 1994. Social Policy Research Unit, University of York

DoH 1989a An introduction to the Children Act 1989. Department of Health. HMSO, London.

DoH 1989b Children and young persons on child protection registers. Year ending 31 March 1988. Government Statistical Service. HMSO, London
DoH 1992 Health of the nation. HMSO, London
DSS 1992 Households below average income, a statistical analysis 1979–88–89 (revised edition 1995). HMSO, London
Edwards R 1991 Lone parent families poverty and employment highlight, No 102. National Children's Bureau, London
Emery J L 1985 Infanticide, filicide and cot death. Archives of Disease in Childhood 60:505–507
Emery J L, Taylor E M 1986 Investigation of SIDS. New England Journal of Medicine 315:1676
Ermisch J 1986 The economics of the family: applications to divorce and remarriage. Discussion Paper No 140, Centre for Economic Policy Research
Gath A 1995 Parents with learning disability. In: Reder P, Lucey C (eds) Assessment of parenting. Routlege, London, Ch 13
Gibbons J, Gallagher B, Bell C, Gorden D 1995 Development after physical abuse in early childhood: a follow-up study of children on protection registers. HMSO, London
Gillen D 1991 Poor housing, vulnerable people. Leading article, British Medical Journal 303:667
Graham P J 1995 Chair of Working Party – Report. Summary of alcohol and the young. Journal of the Royal College of Physicians of London 29(6):470–474
Hall D, Lynch M A 1998 Violence begins at home. British Medical Journal 316:1551
Helfer R E 1987 The litany of the smoldering neglect of children. In: Helfer R E, Kempe C H (eds) The battered child, 4th edn. University of Chicago Press, Chicago
Helfer R E 1990 The neglect of our children. In: Child abuse. Pediatric Clinics of North America 37(4) 923–942
HMSO 1991a Population trends 66. HMSO, London
HMSO 1991b House of Commons Security Committee. Low income statistics: households below average income tables 1988
HMSO 1995 The health of our children. HMSO, London
Hobbs C J, Wynne J M, Gelletie R 1995 Leeds Inquiry into Infant Deaths: The importance of abuse and neglect in sudden infant death. Child Abuse Review 4:329–339
Hoghughi M 1998 The importance of parenting in child health. British Medical Journal 316:1545
Hoghughi M, Speight A N P 1998 Good enough parenting for all children – a strategy for a healthier society. Arch Dis Childhood 78:293–300
Jackson R H 1988 The doctor's role in the prevention of accident. Archives of Disease in Childhood 63:235–237
Jackson R H, Cooper S, Hayes H R M 1988 The work of the Child Accident Prevention Trust. Archives of Disease in Childhood 63:318–320
Jaudes P K, Ekwo E, Voorhis J V 1995 Association of drug abuse and child abuse. Child Abuse and Neglect 19(9):1065–1076
Judge K, Benzeval M 1993 Health inequalities: new concerns about children of single mothers. BMJ 306:677–680
Kemp A, Sibert J 1995 Preventing scalds to children. BMJ 311:643
Kempe R S, Goldbloom R B 1987 Malnutrition and growth retardation in the context of child abuse and neglect. In: Helfer R E, Kempe C H (eds) The battered child, 4th edn. University of Chicago Press, Chicago
Kempson E 1996 Life on a low income. Joseph Rowntree Foundation
Kendall-Tackett K A, Eckenrode J 1996 The effects of neglect on academic achievement and disciplinary problems: a developmental perspective. Child Abuse and Neglect 20(3):161–170
King M, Trowell J 1992 Children's welfare and the law: the limits of legal intervention. Sage, London.
Kumar V 1993 Poverty, deprivation and children's health. In: Poverty and Inequality in the UK. National Children's Bureau, London
Leeds ACPC 1996 Report. Leeds Area Child Protection Committee, Merrion House, Leeds
Lissauer T, Richman S, Tempra M, Jenkins S, Taylor B 1993 Influence of homelessness on acute admissions to hospital. Archives of Diseases of Childhood 69:423–429
Lowry S 1991 Housing and health. BMJ Publications, London
McGaw S, Sturmey P 1993 Identifying the needs of parents with learning disabilities. Child Abuse Review 2(2):101–118
Mackenbach J P 1995 Tackling inequalities in health. Editorial. British Medical Journal 310:1152–1153
Madeley R J 1991 Recent trends in infant, neonatal and post-neonatal mortality rates. Current Paediatrics 1:49–52
Meadow S R 1989 Suffocation. In: Meadow S R (ed) ABC of child abuse. BMJ Publications, London
Meadow R 1990 Suffocation, recurrent apnoea and sudden infant death. Journal of Pediatrics 3:351–357
Messages from Research 1995 Child protection: messages from research. HMSO, London
NCANDS 1995 Child neglect and childhood fatalities due to child abuse and neglect. National Resource Center on Child Abuse and Neglect information sheets 6/95 & 7/95
NCB 1987 Policy and Practice Review Group. Investing in the future: child health 10 years after the Court Report. National Children's Bureau, London
Newlands M, Emery J S 1991 Child abuse and cot death. Child Abuse and Neglect 15:275–278
Oliver J E 1983 Dead children from problem families in NE Wiltshire. British Medical Journal 286:115–117
OPCS 1987 Occupational class and mortality. Office of Population, Censuses and Surveys. HMSO, London
OPCS 1988 Occupational mortality 1979–1980 and 1982–1983 (Childhood Supplement Series B5 No 8). Office of Population, Censuses and Surveys. HMSO, London
OPCS 1990 Mortality statistics, perinatal and infant: social and biological factors. Series DH3, No 21. Office of Population, Censuses and Surveys. HMSO, London
Oppenheim C, Harker L 1996 Poverty: the facts. Child Poverty Action Group Community Care 24.8.1996
Pelton L H 1993 Is poverty a key contributor to child maltreatment? Yes. In: Gambrill E, Stein T J (eds)

Controversial issues in child welfare. Allyn and Bacon, Boston, pp 16–28
Phillips M 1991 Divorce and its burden of pain. *Guardian* 6 December 1991
Reading R, Jarvis S, Openshaw S 1993 Measurement of social inequalities in health and use of the health services among children in Northumberland. Archives of Disease in Childhood 68(5):626
Reddy N 1995 Child labour: a hidden form of child abuse. Child Abuse Review 4(3):207–214
Roberts I 1995 Deaths of children in house fires. BMJ 311:1381–1382
Robert I, Power C 1996 Does the decline in child injury mortality vary by social class? A comparison of class specific mortality in 1981 and 1991. BMJ 313:784–786
Rosenberg D, Cantwell H 1993 The consequences of neglect: individual and societal. In: Hobbs CV Wynne UM (eds) Child abuse. Balliére Tindall, London, Ch 10
Sharp D 1996 Child labour versus child work. Report given to IPSCAN Conference, Dublin 1996, reported in Lancet 348:539
Silvers J 1996 When they were very young. *Independent on Sunday* 28 April 1996
Skuse D 1993 Emotional abuse and neglect. In: Meadow R (ed) ABC of child abuse. BMJ Publications, London
Smith F B 1990 The BMJ and poverty. British Medical Journal 301:734
Smith P 1991 Child poverty – who says? Concern 78:4–5
Smith K 1996 Parents and families. Parenting Forum Newsletter 5. Winter
Spencer N J 1991 Child poverty and deprivation in the UK. Archives of Disease in Childhood 66:1255–1257
Spencer N J 1996 Measuring child health. In: Poverty and child health. Radcliffe Medical, Oxford, Ch 3
Spencer N 1996 'Race', ethnicity, poverty and child health. In: Poverty and child health. Radcliffe Medical, Oxford, Ch 7
Spencer N J, Lewis M A, Logan S 1993 Multiple admissions and deprivation. Archives of Diseases in Childhood 68:760–762
Squires T, Busuttil A 1995 Child fatalities in Scottish house fires 1980–1990 – a case of child neglect? Child Abuse and Neglect 19(7):865–873
Stanton A N, Downham M A P S, Oakley J R, Emery J L, Knowledon J 1978 Terminal symptoms in children dying suddenly and unexpectedly at home. British Medical Journal 2:1249–1251
Townsend P, Davidson N, Whitehead N 1992 Inequalities in health (incorporating the Black Report and The health divide). Penguin, London
Tregeagle S, Voigt S 1993 Empowerment of families through family support. In: Mason J (ed) Child welfare policy: Critical Australian perspectives. Hale and Iremonger, Sydney, pp 197–209
Tudor Hart J 1971 The inverse care law. Lancet (I) 405–412
UK Agenda for Children 1994 Children's Rights Development Unit, 235 Shaftesbury Avenue, London WC2H 8EL
United Nations 1989 Convention on the Rights of the Child. HMSO, London
United Nations 1995 Concluding observations of the Committee on the Rights of the Child: United Kingdom of Great Britain and Northern Ireland. CRC/C/15/ADD.34
Verbov J 1993 Hair loss in children. Arch Dis Child 68:702–706
Walker J 1996 Continuity and change in families. Parenting Forum Briefing Sheet No.4
Webb E 1998 Children and the inverse care law. British Medical Journal 316:588–590
Wedge P, Essex J 1982 Children in adversity. Pan, London
Whitehead M, Dahlgren G 1991 What can be done about inequalities in health. Lancet 338:1059–1063
Winter 1996 Relate Centre for Family Studies, University of Newcastle upon Tyne
Wolock I, Magura S 1996 Parental substance abuse as a predictor of child maltreatment reports. Child Abuse and Neglect 20(12):1183–1194
Working Together 1988 Working together: a guide to arrangements for inter-agency co-operation for the protection of children from abuse. HMSO, London
Working Together 1991 Working together under the Children Act 1989. A guide to arrangements for inter-agency co-operation for the protection of children from abuse. HMSO, London

RECOMMENDED READING

Brown K D and Lynch M A (eds) 1998 Editorial and review articles. Child Abuse Review 7(2):73–115
Iwaniec D 1996 The emotionally abused and neglected child. Wiley, Chichester
Reder P, Lucey C (eds) 1995 Assessment of parenting. Routledge, London

7

Emotional maltreatment

Though emotional abuse is becoming a more accepted category in the registration of children who have been abused, it is probably the most complex form of abuse in terms of definition, recognition, management and registration. It is rarely absent when a child has been abused physically or sexually, is failing to thrive non-organically, or has been neglected, and yet the statistics point to a very low incidence rate both in the USA and Britain (Creighton & Noyes 1989). The Department of Health 1995 figures show that there is now a considerable increase. In 1992 registrations of emotional abuse reached 2800 but by 1994 the figure had risen to 4400, a dramatic increase of 57%. Studies of prevalence and incidence are still few and far between, and in terms of registration it is still the smallest category – a worrying factor. According to Glaser & Prior (1997), 'there is a delay in arriving at the point of registration for emotional abuse'. Though there may be many reasons for the non- or late registration of children who have been emotionally abused, the short- and long-term consequences are not acceptable for the child and a rethinking is needed: something Glaser & Prior have started to address.

The long-term effects for children are described by Egeland & Erikson (1986, p. 667):

> The sharp decline in the intellectual functioning of these children, their attachment disturbances and subsequent lack of social/emotional competence in a variety of situations is cause for great concern. The consequences of this form of maltreatment are particularly disturbing when considered in the light of a

careful re-examination of our society's definition of child abuse and a consideration of means for early identification and intervention to help prevent the cumulative malignant effects of this form of maltreatment.

As Garbarino et al (1988, p. 7) so aptly stated

> rather than casting psychological maltreatment as an ancillary issue, subordinate to other forms of abuse and neglect, we should place it as the centerpiece of efforts to understand family functioning and to protect children.

CASE HISTORY 7.1

Martin, aged 6, woke up every morning with a bucket in the corner of his sparsely furnished room. '. . . and I went to do my pee in the bucket, then my dad would come and unlock the door'. Martin was not allowed to touch his father because his father had told him that he, Martin, had the devil living in him. Father also told him that anyone who touched Martin could catch 'it'. Martin was often referred to as 'devil' by all members of his family and his father had told Martin that he was the son of the devil. Martin was not allowed to sit at the table with the rest of his family but had to sit on the floor. He had his own cup and plate and had to wash them up separately, so as not to 'contaminate' the others. Martin was often beaten by his parents as part of drumming the devil out of him. He was criticised continually and often had to sit with the large dogs in the garden. Martin was terrified of the dogs, because his father had told him that the dogs would 'get him'. Martin ran away from home only once and hid but his father and the dogs found him and Martin was threatened that they would tear him to pieces if he ran away again. When the school became very concerned about Martin the parents took him to a social services office and said that the child was out of control and that they would not take him back home with them. Martin, looking dirty, clad in ill-fitting clothes, thin and unable to speak, was taken into care. It took considerable time before this story emerged.

History of childcare

Ill-treatment, punishment and even child killings are recorded in the history of many societies and civilisations; for the child the years of infancy were the most dangerous ones, not only because the infant's life was not a very valued one. The period of childhood was always poorly defined – the infant would be seen as a nonentity with no feelings and treated with little understanding. The most important thing a child had to do was to grow up and become an adult. Adult values pertained on this path of growth and the fact that children might have age-appropriate needs did not occur to most people. Plato advocated that children would learn through play, but for the most part it was believed that the only way children would grow up was by repressing their spirits, the foolishness of the child, by beating them severely with the aim of driving this spirit/devil out of them. Scott (1977) showed that in medieval times childcare practices fell back into benightedness:

> If babyhood was survived, all but the most favoured children became little adults and a convenient source of labour. Instances of barbarous treatment of children, infanticide, exploitation, starvation, flogging and mutilation abound; and until comparatively recently these seemed to have caused little public reaction.

Even in the nineteenth century the attitude towards children was one of stern materialism. Infants were killed in order to limit the size of the family and 'baby farming' was a well-known practice whereby children would be handed over to such baby farms if the parent(s) could not care for them. Many children born illegitimately received this treatment.

In England the Education Act and the Children and Young Person's Act were formulated during the 1930s and 1960s, growing out of a wish to grant children rights. However, in general, people remained firm in their beliefs that children had no rights and that they remained the property of their parents to do with as they pleased, or rather as they were best able. With the advent of a more child-centred society parents began to speak of their own often appalling childhoods. It was then that professionals working in the field of child care began to realise that many of the parents of abused children had themselves been maltreated as children. It was also quickly realised that it did not seem to matter in which social class a child grew up. Kempe & Kempe (1978) wrote

> In each generation we find, in one form or another, a distortion of the relationship between parents and children that deprives the children of the consistent nurturing of body and mind that would enable them to develop fully.

Slowly, children's needs have been realised and in some parts of the world a more child-centred attitude has been accepted. However translating this knowledge into practice is still a difficult task for most societies.

Definition of emotional maltreatment

Emotional abuse can be defined as:

> actual or likely severe adverse effects on the emotional and behavioural development of the child caused by persistent or severe emotional ill treatment or rejection. All abuse involves some emotional abuse. (Working Together 1991, p. 49)

This is important, and yet there seems to be considerable hesitation among professionals to register children under this category. This is despite findings (Doyle 1997) that professionals as well as the public at large have no difficulties identifying emotionally abusive events and agreeing.

Lourie & Stefano (1978) defined emotional maltreatment as

> an injury to the intellectual or psychological capacity of the child, as evidenced by an observable and substantial impairment in his or her ability to function within his or her normal range of performance and behaviour with due regard to his or her culture.

Some authorities find emotional abuse too difficult to define (Helfer & Kempe 1980) preferring to choose verbal abuse as a specific category and otherwise pointing to the fact that all maltreated children are victims of emotional harm.

Garbarino et al (1988) discuss 'What psychological maltreatment?' at length and provide definitions from a number of professional angles, including clinical and legal. On page 2 they quote Whiting (1976) as making a useful distinction between emotional abuse and emotional neglect. She indicates that

> emotional neglect is a result of subtle or blatant omission or commission experienced by the child, which causes handicapping stress on the child

and when

> meaningful adults are unable to provide necessary nurturance, stimulation, encouragement, and protection to the child at various stages of their development, which inhibits his optimal functioning.

She also points out that it applies

> when parents resist or refuse co-operative intervention for a child diagnosed as disturbed.

Of course not only children who are already disturbed come into this category, but also those who, for instance, are not sent to school or referred for medical attention when they are not well. Whiting feels that emotional abuse relates to, and is distinguished from, neglect by the 'deliberate parental action' against a child which causes emotional disturbance.

Glaser & Prior (1997) have extended the debate on definitions and helpfully proposed that 'emotional abuse refers to a relationship rather an event' and put the parent–child relationship at the centre of this event. The fact that acts of omission and commission are involved and actual and potential harm can be present it is not difficult to work out the consequences for the child. Iwaniec (1995) identified emotional abuse as

> hostile or indifferent parental behaviour which (if severe and persistent) damages the child's self-esteem, degrades a sense of achievement . . ., belonging, and prevents healthy and vigorous development.

Barnett et al (1991) discussing issues of emotional abuse, speak of parental acts that thwart children's basic emotional needs. They emphasise that children have a right to 'psychological safety' and need to be protected from levels of hostility and violence. Consistent care-giving and encouragement to foster self-esteem in children are high on their list. When children are verbally harassed, ridiculed, shamed and threatened their emotional well-being is at stake.

Incidence of emotional abuse

The American Humane Association reported in 1984 that their statistics collected between 1976 and 1982 showed emotional abuse as occurring in 17% of children registered. In England the NSPCC register of cases between 1983 and 1986 showed 1.5% of all abused children to have been registered under the category of emotional abuse; by 1987 the figure had fallen to 1%. More recent studies and figures have highlighted the fact that registration of children suffering from emotional abuse is increasing despite the fact that professionals are still hesitant and/or delaying in registering under this rubric. From clinical practice it is known that these figures reflect gross under-reporting in this area. It is difficult to interpret such data. It probably highlights the difficulties professionals have in registering this form of maltreatment. Why this should be so is not clear, but the current climate of criticising (emotionally abusing or scapegoating?) professionals may be influential. Overlooking this form of abuse and even denying it are also part of the scenario.

In most cases emotional abuse is not the central reason for the registration of children and other more visible signs of maltreatment have to be present, despite the increasing evidence that emotional maltreatment has considerable effects in the long term on cognitive and emotional development as well as on the capacity to form relationships and other social effects.

Normal emotional development of children

In some sense there is no such thing as 'normal' emotional development; individual differences exist and for the ordinary child, depending on what care he receives, his emotional growth will proceed. However, good emotional development is crucial not only for the individual but also for intergenerational patterns and society as a whole.

It is important to stress that a classification can only be achieved if the age of the child is taken into consideration. What does need to be stated clearly, even though we now have a far better understanding of the child's emotional development, is that the internal (emotional) world of the child is structured by his or her surrounding environment and particularly the parents and care-givers. This process occurs from the earliest days of development and structures the individual's personality through attachments, love and care as well as anxiety and trauma (Bowlby 1969, Winnicott 1988).

Different forms of emotional maltreatment will affect children differently at various ages. It is possible to draw an analogy from fetal development, in which an infection like rubella causes most damage to those organs that are developing rapidly at the time of the infection. Similarly, emotional abuse will affect those psychological functions that are developing at the time. Erikson's (1963) well-known classification of developmental tasks can be used as a way of structuring what is known about age-related effects of emotional maltreatment.

Erikson's theory of psychosocial development centres on the developmental lifespan of human beings. He proposed eight stages through which all human beings need to develop. These eight stages, five of which cover 'childhood', occur at specific age ranges, during which certain tasks will have to be achieved (Table 7.1).

Erikson (1963) also believed that children actively explore all aspects of life and that they have a considerable capacity to adapt to people and situations. Children are not just passive beings who are shaped by their parents, they actively seek to control their environment.

The developmental stages of childhood are briefly set out below.

First year of life

During the first year of life the infant has the 'task' of achieving basic trust or mistrust. Clearly this 'task' is highly influenced and shaped by the adults surrounding the child. It involves learning to trust others to supply basic needs such as food, warmth, love, consistency, etc. If, during this phase, the parents are incapable of providing reasonable care or are rejecting the baby, including giving inconsistent care, the infant is likely to grow in experiencing the world as a dangerous place with untrustworthy or unreliable people in it.

Age 1–3 years

The child grapples with the issues relating to autonomy versus shame and doubt. Children need to learn to be autonomous, to begin to do things for themselves and have a sense of adequacy (putting their clothes on, feeding themselves, etc.). Failing to achieve a certain amount of age-appropriate independence will lead the child to doubt his or her abilities and so feel shame as well as doubt. At this stage the parents are still the main figures in the child's life.

Table 7.1 Child development, related to Erikson's (1963) stages

Age	What the child learns
0–1	To trust
1–3	To be autonomous: age-appropriate independence
3–6	'Initiative v. guilt': the child starts to explore, test boundaries, learns that breaking the rules creates conflicts and guilt, begins to recognise that others have rights
6–12	'Industry v. inferiority': establishing him/herself as competent and achieving; most importantly acquiring social and academic skills
12–20	'Identity v. role confusion': transition from childhood into adulthood, seeking for an identity, coming to terms with being male or female, confusion about sexual and social position. Peers are most important during this stage

Age 3–6 years

The child is in the stage of initiative versus guilt, beginning to explore beyond what he or she is sometimes capable of and trying to take on responsibilities the child often cannot handle. It is the time when children want to be grown up and to do things, or set themselves goals, that they know their parents will not approve of or think are unsafe or even dangerous. Through such excursions the child will come into conflict with parents and siblings, and this is likely to lead to feelings of guilt. In order to leave this stage successfully a balance has to be achieved whereby the child cannot only stay in this exploratory mood and take initiatives but also learn not to interfere with the rights and goals of others. The positive outcome is a child who is purposeful and able to initiate his or her own activities.

Age 6–12 years

Here industry versus inferiority is the issue. The peer group becomes an important factor in the child's life. Competition, particularly in the academic and social sphere, is central during this stage in development. The child needs to establish him- or herself as a competent, self-assured person. Failure to succeed will induce inferiority.

Age 12–16 years

This stage can extend up to the age of 20. The youngster learns about growing up, becoming an adult and about identity and sexuality. Making relationships, particularly with the opposite sex, is essential. The peer group is most influential in shaping the young person's social and occupational path, though the parents remain crucial models.

The importance of attachment throughout childhood

Discussion of emotional maltreatment without taking into account what we now know about attachment theory and attachment behaviours (specific individuals providing a secure base for the infant) would be incomplete. The issues are discussed throughout the book, with a more lengthy discussion in Chapter 3.

Secure, anxious, and avoidant attachments as described by Bowlby (1969) and Ainsworth et al (1978) grow out of the need of the child to be in close proximity to a responsible and responsive adult during development. Bowlby (1969) pointed out that the survival of human beings, in particular of the very small baby, is optimally secured when the infant and child can maintain proximity to one attachment figure or several. As in Erikson's first stage, the baby learns to trust an adult who reacts appropriately to the baby's needs. If all goes well in a family then the baby's cries will elicit the proximity of the mother or care-giver. Since the baby usually cries only because of some form of need (e.g. hunger) or distress, the mother's presence, behaviour and consequent action are essential to help the baby develop a feeling of security. One of Bowlby's (1988) perceptions of what is needed may also throw light on the consequences when attachment is not available for the child. He said

> attachment behaviour is any form of behaviour that results in a person attaining or maintaining proximity to some other clearly identified individual who is conceived as better able to cope with the world. (p. 26)

The child will have a sense of security when an attachment figure is available and responds to the child's needs. Attachment is most in evidence when a child (or adult) is frightened, tired or ill and comfort and care-giving will make things better. As the child grows older this intense need for attachment behaviour becomes less and is only activated strongly at times of need.

The views of Crittenden & Ainsworth (1989) have been influenced and shaped by psychoanalytic theory as well as ethology and evolutionary theory which in turn influenced that aspect of attachment theory which deals with the adaptation of the infant through interactions with the parental system and environment. Further discussion of this concept can also be found in Chapter 15. How trauma influences these patterns is described by Bentovim (1992) and Crittenden (1997).

For the mother/parents to behave in a consistent, loving and nurturing way it is essential that they themselves have experienced something approaching this pattern in their own childhood. When Ainsworth et al (1978) researched attachment patterns in a standardised 'strange situation' they found that children react differently not only at different ages but also depending on their experience of mothering. The major patterns (now further sub-divided by Crittenden) established from this now very well-known research are:

- a secure attachment to specific adults
- an anxious/avoidant pattern of attachment
- an anxious/ambivalent or anxious/resistant attachment.

The baby of about 7–8 months will have formed the earliest attachments, usually to the mother, but also to other people who have been close up to that time. As already indicated, if all goes well the baby will have experienced consistent, loving care and will be securely attached, able to explore in the presence of the attachment figure(s) even in a strange situation and with a stranger present. Children who have been maltreated often show the anxious/avoidant or anxious/ambivalent pattern, or an unusual combination of this pattern.

A securely attached infant who has experienced a responsive mother and/or carer will usually react positively towards her and cry relatively little. When the baby has been distressed because the attachment behaviour has been activated (by separation for instance), he or she is easily comforted and reassured when the attachment figure is close, and goes and attends to his usual activities.

An anxious attachment can be observed most often when a child has to take responsibility for maintaining proximity to the attachment figure (most often the mother). It is here that one might find a child clinging to the mother, and this is interpreted by the onlooker as closeness when in fact it is anxiety that makes the child cling on. Crittenden (1997) also indicated that

> anxiously attached children minimise or exaggerate reality to create an appearance that will motivate the attachment figure to behave as they desire.

Insecure attachment most often occurs and is visible when a child experiences the attachment figure as rejecting.

If the ordinary baby comes to the hospital or is observed at home he or she will be somewhat hesitant at first in exploring the surroundings in the presence of a stranger but this will ease with the mother/attachment figure close by. These children may become distressed and cry, but are comforted by their mother and can be reassured. Children who have been abused show different patterns.

- They may cling to their parents, they may cry and whine and they may become distressed out of all proportion. These children may cause irritation to the parental figures and receive little of the understanding and care which might help them to feel more secure.
- At the other end of the continuum the child may become agitated, charge around, get into every corner, cupboard or drawer, touch everything in sight without any real interest and seem restless and aimless.
- In a third pattern of behaviour the child tiptoes away and watches what goes on from a safe distance; these children often show what is well described as 'frozen watchfulness'. Crittenden & Ainsworth (1989) describe their research in this area where they examined the attachment patterns in families where child maltreatment occurred.

Human beings have difficulties existing without attachment relationships, and this is so particularly for infants and young children because attachment provides them with a base from which they can explore the world and have their needs met. This exploration is vital for the infant's development and reaches optimal levels when a care-giver is there to provide a secure base. The attachment figure, when close to the child, reduces the child's anxiety even in stressful situations and gives him or her the confidence to explore the new and unknown. It is also influential in providing a base from which to form new and lasting relationships in the present and future.

These early attachment patterns lay the foundation for future development. Attachment patterns are dynamic and not static; they can change over time and are dependent on the child's experiences. This is a powerful process which has an influence on the developing self. It achieves this through the development of internal representational models of the attachment figure(s), and of the relationships within which the child is functioning. In turn these internalised attachment figures are later used as models for parenting when the children become parents themselves.

Failure of attachment consequent on early maltreatment

Many children who are being maltreated experience emotional abuse from an early age, quite often as a precursor of other forms of abuse. One way which this interaction between mother and child can develop is recognised in the attachment literature (Bowlby 1969, 1975, 1981, Belsky & Nezworski 1988) and in the writings by Kempe & Kempe (1978). Specific groups of parents may be more likely to abuse their children generally, but emotional abuse can occur in all social strata. Children of very young, inexperienced mothers who come from a deprived background themselves and who may have children in the hope and belief that at last there will be a human being who will love them are at high risk. The bitter disappointment and resentful feelings that arise as it becomes clear that the baby does not provide the longed-for care and love surface in the parent's frustration against the child. The fact that the mother has to provide for the needs of the baby and give affection rather than receive it can lead to considerable confusion in the mother. The recognition of the necessity of providing care and love rather than receiving it from the baby may be a very early beginning to a poor relationship. As a consequence the baby becomes the object of the mother's disappointment and her consequent resentment can lead to physical abuse, neglect, failure to thrive and sexual abuse. Egeland (1988) indicated that one-third of parents who were abused as children are at risk of abusing their own children.

Crittenden (1988) discussed the issues related to parents who have been abused in childhood and found that they often have distorted interpersonal relationships in the past (including their childhood) and the present. The abuse in their childhood has distorted both the attachment figures they have come in contact with, and they also have a distorted sense of themselves. She found that abusing adults often approach others in a distrusting or withdrawn manner and so hope to protect themselves from the pain of unreliable, angry or unfulfilled relationships.

The child's symptoms and adaptation

Understanding the expressions of emotional abuse in a child is a difficult process. In families, children and parents will have to work out between each of them how they respond and behave to each other and those outside the family. These responses and behaviours have been called the 'transactions' between people; this model was described by Sameroff & Chandler (1975) and further developed by Stratton (1977, 1982a) highlighting the complexity of interactions as they occur between the care-giver and child.

An infant experiencing feeding difficulties may not only be tense and anxious but also have a tense and anxious mother. The infant may adapt to the anxious mother by attempting to avoid the traumatic feeding situation and become passive and resistant to taking in food. In turn the mother may become even more tense and anxious and also avoid all aspects of the feeding situation. Once this pattern has been established the result can be that the child loses weight and becomes difficult to handle, possibly even leading to physical abuse as well as rejection and failure to thrive. The transactional process is easy to describe in this kind of example, and it is a common sequence in cases of non-organic failure to thrive. What is so striking is that, even with a clear example like this, at the time it demands a considerable effort of imagination to recognise the pattern of behaviour as an attempt at adaptation within a transactional relationship. Often an outsider has more chance than the mother of observing this pattern and recognising it as being a result of the baby's adaptation. They can then intervene in such a way that the interaction between mother and infant is changed.

The term 'adaptation' acknowledges the fact that the child is not a passive recipient of influence. Under the pressure of maltreatment, the child will take whatever route seems to offer the best chance of minimising risk and pain. Children do not have a long-term perspective on the effects of their behaviour, particularly when they are under the stress of abuse. A tragic consequence is that the attempts of the child to adapt to the abusive situation may actually increase the probability of further abuse. Stratton (1982b) in his section on 'transactional adaptation' unravels some of the complexities in which an infant's adaptations can be understood and how the baby responds to his or her care-giving environment. Bringing the two concepts of transaction and adaptation together gives an insight into how any care-giving situation can elicit responses from the child. These responses then will set up the conditions which will influence the parent's behaviour towards the child.

The underfed child will adapt to the need to conserve energy, and to the anxiety or even antagonism shown by the parents during feeding. Observation of behaviour may suggest that the baby is uninterested in food and feeding. This behaviour (turning away, screaming, keeping the mouth firmly shut, spitting food out, etc.) adaptive in the short term, will make it more likely that the parents can attribute the low food intake to the child being a 'poor feeder'. Parents of children with the label 'poor feeder' are more likely to have little investment in thinking of what the child might like to eat, they may be impatient and give up after only a short time of trying to feed the child or they may become despondent and depressed at their lack of success. All of this or any one of these responses may reinforce the parent's avoidance of the feeding situation. The process of transactional adaptation, which normally works to keep healthy patterns self-sustaining, can also be responsible for the continuation of maltreating behaviours.

In children who have been sexually abused the pattern applies equally, leading to confusion and emotional distress which hinder the child's development and can impair health. Summit (1983) describes the adaptations made by many of the children who have been sexually abused in terms of accommodating the abuse. Their sexualised behaviour towards others (children and adults alike) and themselves is one such example. As these children move through the different developmental stages and grow older, specific aspects of their abusive experiences may become clearer to them. As this happens they may have to adapt once more to the anxieties which are produced by the understanding they have gained. The adaptation may again be in terms of relieving their anxiety and, for instance, lead children to behave aggressively towards anyone who tries to befriend them or come close. The effort of 'accommodation' itself leads to short-term as well as long-term emotional difficulties which are quite unacceptable in terms of adequate childcare.

What professionals need to achieve is a recognition of the patterns of disturbed or disturbing behaviours by children encountered in families, clinics, children's homes, foster-families, schools, etc., and that these disturbing behaviours can be adaptations which first developed in the child's original environment or home. Professionals need to work back and discover the circumstances in which these adaptations originated. To practise and become fluent in such reconstructions it is essential that the signs of a history of emotional or sexual abuse, for instance, are recognised in the behaviour of the child – not just one form of behaviour but the way a child reacts in many situations. As Stratton (1977) pointed out, 'main effect' models are simply unproductive in terms of understanding the negative influences during development. In child sexual abuse the 'main effect' model takes the form of viewing the abuse as a damaging event inflicted on a passive child from outside and that this 'damage', in all its manifestations, should be directly observable. Without in any way diminishing the responsibility of the adult, it is still totally misleading to view the child as a passive recipient of influence, whether good or bad. Moment by moment the child adapts to what is happening, and if there is any sense in which the relationship is transactional, the adult will be influenced by the child's adaptation. The longer-term strategies which the child adopts in order to minimise trauma and immediate threat are the 'characteristics of sexually abused children', described elsewhere in this book (see Chapter 9), and are known to expose the child to further risk. The importance for treatment of the psychological and emotional consequences in such abusive situations is that the maltreating adult and the maltreated child need interventions to break the cycle of their behaviour with each other. Children transfer the behaviours learnt in one setting to another setting. If they are taken into care or are fostered the adaptations will continue and the carers in these situations may also need early and active support to care for these children and avoid being inducted into patterns that reinstate the previous abuse.

Crittenden (1988, 1996, 1997), observing parenting behaviours in maltreating families, described physically abusing parents as interfering and hostile, including becoming verbally hostile and in this way abusing their children both in a physical and emotional way. Neglecting parents seemed to behave differently towards their children. Rather than being active and interfering they did not respond to their children's attempts for attention and were withdrawn. The consequences for the children of neglecting parents were vividly described and are only too easily recognised in clinics. The children under 1 year of age coming from neglecting parents presented as passive and cognitively delayed. It was easy to ignore these children; they were almost 'invisible' to both parents and professionals. However, once they were a little older and able to move about the pattern changed and these children became 'uncontrolled seekers of novel experiences'. They are into everything, quite out of control, and can often be found in dangerous situations (e.g. in the road, exploring dangerous objects, exposing themselves to heights, etc.). At times it can appear as if they are making up for lost (passive) time. The families and, sometimes, professionals may label the child 'hyperactive' and so make the child responsible for the behaviours without considering the interactions and possibly adaptation which will have taken place and which have been described above. Crittenden's research confirms the work undertaken by Dix (1991) quoted below.

'Resilient children'

In recent years there has been increasing interest in the fact that some children raised in adversity progress to a good level of functioning and maturity in adulthood. Rutter (1985) showed that risk factors operate multiplicatively rather than additively. That is, one or two risk factors may have no observable effect, but above three the consequences escalate very rapidly. As would be expected from the account of transactional adaptation (above), the full story involves the fit between the temperament of the child, the forms of parenting failure and the capacity of parents and other carers to cope with the adaptations the child adopts. Werner, in a 40-year longitudinal study of vulnerable children on the Hawaiian island of Kauai, found that 34% of the sample of 210 did considerably better than predicted (Werner & Smith 1982). The phenomenon is not well understood but it does seem that many of the factors identified in research (Rhodes & Brown 1991) are to do with characteristics of the children that elicit positive responses from adults in infancy and later. Anything from an attractive physical appearance to cheerfulness, vitality and an ability to find people who will provide support, helps these children. In detail these findings do not indicate a special capacity to cope with insult so much as an ability to recruit help in overcoming the consequences of adversity.

As Butler (1997) points out, the idea of resilience, let alone Werner's earlier label of 'invulnerability' can easily be misused to blame those children who 'fail' to be sufficiently resilient. The fact that some children survive terrible abuse apparently intact has been used to claim that abuse (usually sexual in this argument) is not in itself damaging. Butler describes how resilience has been used as a justification for reducing support services for abused children, but she also points out that the research findings on resilience do not always point to increased involvement by therapists and statutory services. Joining a religious group, or even a football team, may fit the need more accurately.

As the research on resilience unfolds, and if it can be interpreted within a framework of transactional adaptation, it will undoubtedly show us how to learn from these children what we need to do to help prevent and remediate the damage that emotional and other forms of abuse do to the majority of victims.

Patterns of emotional abuse

Much child abuse includes the verbal degrading of the child as well as the fact that children understand from their poor treatment by their carers that they are not valued members of their family or environment. Their self-esteem is often pitifully low and these children develop ways of expressing their emotional disturbances which can range from daydreaming and withdrawing, to becoming aggressive and antisocial; aggression and anger may be directed against themselves and others (Hanks & Hobbs 1992) and some of the children may become mute and depressed. It is not surprising that the behaviours children show when they have been maltreated overlap and do not always appear to be specifically related to the form of maltreatment. Behavioural problems such as wetting, soiling, poor educational attainment, poor concentration, stealing, lying, depression, etc. may all be expressions of a child's distress caused by being maltreated. In children who have been sexually abused a specific form of emotional distress may show. These children often behave in sexualised ways towards peers, siblings and adults alike, showing and repeating not only what has happened to them but also their confusion and emotional distress.

The child's sexualised behaviour towards others can be interpreted as part of an expression of their feelings, their confusion, guilt and emotional distress. The feelings and behaviours follow one another and accumulate; one moment the behaviour might be followed by feelings, the next moment the feelings may cause behaviours – whichever way round, further disturbance will be the outcome. This relentless cycle will have further damaging effects as the child grows up. The guilt often develops out of a mistaken belief by the child that he alone has initiated the abuse and is to blame.

How the different components of emotional abuse can be defined and separated is not clear at present. Let us take verbal abuse as an example. How can this be defined? How often and to what degree does the child have to be subjected to verbal abuse by parent figures before this becomes damaging? Are there critical ages at which some forms of emotional maltreatment are much more damaging than at other developmental stages? As already indicated, Garbarino et al (1988) made an important contribution to assessing emotional maltreatment in that they identified components of emotional abuse in terms of rejecting, terrorising, isolating, corrupting and ignoring (Table 7.2). This classification has proved a valuable tool in understanding psychological maltreatment in a developmental context. It also helps in viewing the behaviours that many children show as the consequences of abuse in a more meaningful way.

- *Rejecting*: the adult refuses to acknowledge the child's worth and the legitimacy of the child's needs
- *Isolating*: the adult cuts the child off from normal social experiences and contacts and prevents the child from forming friendships, and makes the child believe that he is alone in the world
- *Terrorising*: the adult verbally assaults the child, creates a climate of fear, bullies and frightens the child, and makes the child believe that the world is capricious and hostile
- *Ignoring*: the adult deprives the child of essential stimulation and responsiveness, stifling emotional growth and intellectual development
- *Corrupting*: the adult 'mis-socialises' the child, stimulates the child to engage in destructive antisocial behaviour, reinforces that deviance, and makes the child unfit for normal social experiences (Garbarino et al 1988).

Table 7.2 Components of emotional abuse (Garbarino et al 1988)

Rejecting	Child's needs not acknowledged
Isolating	Child cut off from normal social interaction
Terrorising	Verbal assault on child
Ignoring	Child deprived of essential stimulation
Corrupting	Child involved in inappropriate behaviour

Dix (1991) has provided an up-to-date and comprehensive study 'about the emotions parents commonly experience, about when and why they occur', and importantly, what the consequences for parenting are once specific emotions have been aroused. He concludes that parents'

> positive and empathic emotions motivate attunement to children, facilitate responsiveness to the child's wants and needs, and enables parents and children to coordinate their interactions to the benefit of both. In contrast, distressed parents perceive that they are doing poorly. For complex reasons their concerns are continually undermined. They are unable to select and manage interaction plans so that their concerns are promoted, and, as a result, they experience aversive events and negative emotions at high rates. . . . Because the negative emotions of distressed parents are chronic and intense, they can promote inattention, negative perceptions of children and poor problem solving. Negative emotions can lead to parenting that

is hypersensitive, avoidant, punitive, overly controlling and focused on self- rather than child concerns. (pp. 19–20)

When Claussen & Crittenden (1991) investigated children who had been physically maltreated they found that emotional maltreatment was invariably present in these children. They concluded that the emotional component of their maltreatment was much more likely to cause long-term effects.

Clinical assessment

At the stage of the professional assessment Garbarino et al's (1988) five forms of psychological maltreatment (see above) are particularly helpful. By using these stages one can begin to recognise how the parents behave towards the child and what the parents' interactions with the child are like. The interactions reported or observed can be recorded under the five headings. The next step is to register any visible and observable signs. These may be physical signs: the child may have swollen, red hands and feet, physical delay in growth may be noted, motor movements and/or language may be impaired. There may be bruises or injuries, and alongside these the child may show a number of emotional signs and behaviours which indicate that he or she is unhappy, disturbed, unable to concentrate and learn, unable to interact with others, unable to play and has poor attachment behaviours toward parents or care-givers (Ainsworth 1985, Crittenden & Ainsworth 1989). These observations should be noted and the parents should be asked what their observations are about the child and what they perceive as being the difficulties (Table 7.3).

Once the interactions between parent and child, the child's presentation, the possible delays and the physical state of the child have been established, the psychological and behavioural signs can be mapped and so provide a picture of the child's difficulties and possible delays at any given age. The next stage is to indicate, age-appropriately, what the short- and long-term consequences are most likely to be for the child.

Table 7.3 Child's symptoms or maladaptations

Age	Guidelines
0–1	Sleep/feeding problems, irritability, apathetic, dull, anxious attachments
1–3	As above; also overactive, apathetic, aggressive, attention deficit, language delay, indiscriminate affection, fearful and anxious, inability to play, irritable, anxious and ambivalent attachments
3–6	As above; also peer relationship difficulties, attention seeking, clingy, school failure begins, poor social skills
6–12	As above, though sleep and feeding problems may resolve, inappropriate attachment to carers, rejected by peers, school failure, developing delinquent behaviours, running away, truanting, wetting, soiling, stealing, bullying
12+	As above; also depressions, escalated aggression, anxiety, overdosing self-harm, poor self-image, may continue or begin to wet and/or soil, psychosomatic illness, drug and substance abuse, criminal activities

Psychological assessment of emotional maltreatment

- Behavioural signs shown by the child (positive, negative, delays, etc.)
- Emotional signs observed in the child
- Physical signs noted about the child
- Parental behaviour towards the child
- Likely consequences of the above on the child

These broad categories may be further examined by recording the child's learning difficulties, age-appropriately:

- Can the child read, count, tell the colours; does he know the days of the week, know his address, etc.?
- The level of the child's concentration. Do the parents report that it is good or poor? Does the examiner observe good or poor concentration?
- Can the child play age-appropriately? Can the child use fantasy in play (e.g. pretend to speak through a toy telephone, become engrossed with dolls, cars or trains, etc. and construct a situation), play a game with another (adult or child)?
- Can the child carry out instructions (age-appropriate)?

This list can be developed by the individual clinician and used to comment on the child's state of well-being. Garbarino et al's assessment instruments (1988, p. 234) may be used, however a universal checklist has not been developed as yet and comparisons are difficult to make.

Assessment of child and family

- Provide a child-centred room with toys and drawing materials
- Take the history – develop a family tree (genogram) and map the child's development, milestones and problems from birth
- Observe and make notes on the mother's affect, the child's affect and any interaction between the two, also interactions between siblings and other people present
- Continue with a further detailed history including description of the current difficulties and previous interventions by family and professionals
- Talk with the child, either with parent(s) or alone, recognising the problem for the child, and at least some of the consequences; emotional, behavioural, cognitive disturbances and the child's description of his family
- Collect further information, before or after the interview, from the GP, or school nurse, health visitor, teacher, social worker
- Collate the information and:
  - assess what the problems are
  - assess the motivation for change in the family and professional system
  - plan for intervention including therapy.

Dimensions of emotional abuse (Glaser 1991)

- Persistent negative attitudes expressed verbally and non-verbally
  - negative attributions and attitudes
  - harsh discipline and over-control
- Promoting insecure attachment
  conditional parenting
  inconsistency and unpredictability
- Inappropriate developmental expectation and considerations
  - premature impositions
  - failure of protection or containment
  - overprotection
  - failure to explain
- Emotional unavailability
- Failure to recognise the child's individuality and psychological boundaries
- Cognitive distortions (double binds) exist in the child

Glaser and Prior's (1997) paper discusses issues of protection for these children. Besides these observations, developmental tests such as the Denver Developmental Scale and intelligence tests such as the Wechsler Intelligence Test of Children or the British Intelligence Scale, reading tests, or specific tests for those children with learning difficulties will help to assess the cognitive stage the child has reached.

The recognition of attachment patterns described earlier in the chapter may also be of assistance here.

Consequences of emotional maltreatment

Different forms of emotional maltreatment will produce different short- and long-term effects on children, but it is also important to consider what the effects of such maltreatment are at the different ages and stages of development for the child. Spitz (1948) showed clearly how important the emotional care of the very young child is and that infants need an emotionally rich environment to function and grow appropriately. Infants and children who grow up lacking physical care and nurturance at every level, including lack of consistency in the love they are given, will not only suffer at the time but will also carry the long-term consequences of such lack with them into the future. This can manifest itself in many ways, from total withdrawal at one end of the continuum to more active disturbances like hostility and aggression at other end. It will continue to have an influence on their lives and often express itself in the poor relationships these children make as adults, and intergenerationally in the poor relationships they often make with their own children.

Psychological consequences for emotionally maltreated children

- Often:
  - perform below average on IQ tests
  - are aggressive and lack impulse control
  - are frustrated, anxious and non-compliant
- Have:
  - low self-esteem and confidence
  - problems in social relationships with peers and adults
  - anxious attachments
  - difficulties in accepting and giving affection
  - poor relationships within the family and at school
- Show:
  - a high degree of avoidance
  - non-compliance
- Fail to make transition into adulthood

Presentation in court

Cases of emotional maltreatment rarely result in early statutory intervention. This is not because the consequences are not severe but mainly because they are much more difficult to establish in a legal setting than, for instance, physical abuse. Before taking legal steps to protect the child there is usually a need for a long period of assessment and attempt at intervention by multidisciplinary groups. If evidence is to be presented it must be done logically and as objectively as possible. The application of the 'jigsaw puzzle of abuse' described in Chapter 9 is as valid in this form of abuse as in any other.

The court will often wish to know from the social worker, psychologist or psychiatrist what is likely to be the outcome for the child if he or she stays at home. The court is also likely to want to know what the child's needs might be in the family or in alternative care.

In terms of significant harm the impairment will show particularly in the areas of emotional development, growth and behaviour. These areas need to be clearly described. Comparing the child's ability to learn and his or her achievements may show a realistic gap between what the child would be capable of achieving if the emotional pressure and consequent impairment was reduced or stopped altogether.

Summary

1. Emotional maltreatment is a part of every form of child abuse and should be placed at the centre of our efforts to understand families and protect children.
2. The recognition that emotional maltreatment is as serious as any other form of abuse is vital for the future of these children.
3. The introduction of 'significant harm' has been helpful in the recognition that emotional or psychological maltreatment is a powerful aspect in a child's lack of developmental milestones.
4. It is important to respond as early as possible in cases of emotional maltreatment so as to minimise the effects of the abuse and also to try and avoid formal child protection procedures.
5. Many children are registered and deregistered without effective interventions having been achieved. This is damaging to children.
6. 'The most common form of ill-treatment was found to be developmentally inappropriate interaction', Glaser & Prior (1997).
7. Both omission and commission by carers interacting with children play a part in every child's emotional development.
8. Emotional maltreatment is possible in all families and institutions, social strata and religious adherence not withstanding.

9. The isssues of the 'right of the child' and how to respect the child are central in society as well as families.
10. Resilience in children should in no way be misunderstood or used as a justification for reducing support services for emotionally maltreated children.

REFERENCES

Adcock M, White R, Hollows A 1991 Significant harm. Significant Publications, Croydon

Ainsworth M D 1985 Patterns of infant-mother attachment: antecedents and effects of development and, II Attachments across the life-span. Bulletin of New York Academy of Medicine 61:771–791

Ainsworth M D, Blehar M C, Waters E, Wall S 1978 Patterns of attachment: assessed in the strange situation and at home. Lawrence Erlbaum, Hillsdale, NJ

Belsky J, Nezworski T 1988 Clinical implications of attachment. Lawrence Erlbaum, Hillsdale, NJ

Bentovim A 1992 Trauma Organised Systems. Karnac Books, London

Bowlby J 1969 Attachment and loss. Hogarth Press and Institute of Psycho-Analysis, London

Bowlby J 1975 Separation: anxiety and anger. Penguin, Harmondsworth

Bowlby J 1981 Loss: sadness and depression. Penguin, Harmondsworth

Bowlby J 1988 A secure base. Tavistock, London

Claussen AH, Crittenden PM 1991 Physical and psychological maltreatment: relations among types of maltreatment. International Journal of Child Abuse & Neglect 15:5–18

Creighton S J, Noyes P 1989 Child abuse trends in England and Wales 1983–87. NSPCC, London

Crittenden P 1988 Family and dyadic patterns of functioning in maltreating families. In: Browne K, Davies C, Stratton P (eds) Early prediction and prevention of child abuse. J Wiley, Chichester

Crittenden P, Ainsworth M D S 1989 Child maltreatment and attachment theory. In: Cicchetti D, Carlson V (eds) Child maltreatment. Cambridge University Press, Cambridge

Crittenden PM 1996 Research on maltreating families: implications for interventions. In: Briere J, Berliner L, Reid T (eds) ASPAC Handbook on Child Maltreatment. Sage, California

Crittenden PM 1997 Toward an integrative theory of trauma: a dynamic-maturational approach. In: Cicchetti D & Toth S (eds) The Rochester Symposium on Developmental Psychopathology. Vol 10. Rochester University Press, Rochester

Dix T 1991 The affective organisation of parenting: adaptive and maladaptive processes. Psychological Bulletin 110:3–25

Doyle C, 1997 Emotional abuse of children: issues for intervention. Child Abuse Review 6:330–342

Egeland B 1988 Breaking the cycle of abuse: implications for prediction and intervention. In: Browne K, Davies C, Stratton P (eds) Early prediction and prevention of child abuse. J Wiley, Chichester

Egeland B, Erikson M 1986 Deprivation of attachment. In: Bassard M, Germain R, Hart S (eds) The psychological maltreatment of children and youth. Pergamon, Elmsford, NY

Erikson E H 1963 Childhood and society, 2nd edn. Norton, New York

Garbarino J, Guttman E, Seeley J W 1988 The psychologically battered child. Jossey-Bass, San Francisco

Glaser D 1991 Emotional abuse – identification and treatment. Paper presented at BASPCAN First National Congress on the Prevention of Child Abuse and Neglect, University of Leicester

Glaser D, Prior V 1997 Is the term protection applicable to emotional abuse? Child Abuse Review 6:315–329

Hanks H, Hobbs C 1992 Self abuse and suicide. Current Paediatries 2(1):57–59

Helfer R E, Kempe C H 1980 The battered child, 3rd edn. University of Chicago Press, Chicago

Iwaniec D 1995 The emotionally abused and neglected child: identification, assessment and intervention. J Wiley, Chichester

Iwaniec D 1997 An overview of emotional maltreatment and failure to thrive. Child Abuse Review 6:370–388

Kempe R S, Kempe C H 1978 Child abuse. Fontana Books, London

Kempe R S, Kempe C H 1984 The common secret; sexual abuse of children and adolescents. W H Freeman, New York

Lourie I, Stefano L 1978 On defining emotional abuse. In: Proceedings of the Second Annual National Conference on Child Abuse and Neglect. US Government Printing Office, Washington DC

Rhodes W A, Brown 1991 Why some children succeed despite the odds. Praeger, New York

Rutter M 1985 Resilience in the face of adversity: Protective factors and resistance to psychiatric disorder. British Journal of Psychiatry 147:598–611

Sameroff A J, Chandler M 1975 Reproductive risk and the continuum of caretaking casualty. In: Horowitz F D, Hetherington M, Scarr-Salapatek S, Siegel G (eds) Review of child development research, Vol 4. University of Chicago Press, Chicago

Spitz R A 1948 The importance of mother–child relationships during the first year of life. Mental Health Today 13

Stratton P M 1977 Criteria of assessing the influence of obstetric circumstances on later development. In: Chard T, Richards M (eds) Benefits and hazards of the new obstetrics. SIMP, London

Stratton P M 1982a Significance of the psychobiology of the human newborn. In: Psychobiology of the human newborn. J Wiley, Chichester, pp 17–52

Stratton P M 1982b Emerging themes of neonatal psychobiology. In: Psychobiology of the human newborn. J Wiley, Chichester, pp 391–414

Summit R C 1983 The child sexual abuse accommodation syndrome. Journal of Child Abuse and Neglect 7:177–193

Werner E, Smith R 1982 Vulnerable but invincible: a study of resilient children. McGraw-Hill, New York

Whiting L 1976 Defining emotional neglect. Children Today 5:2–5

Winnicott D W 1988 Babies and their mothers. Free Association Books, London

Working Together 1991 Working together under the Children Act 1989. A guide to arrangements for inter-agency co-operation for the protection of children from abuse. HMSO, London

8

Sexual abuse: the scope of the problem

In the 1980s, child sexual abuse exploded on to the public agenda in England with events in Cleveland. Similar events in Orkney shortly afterwards brought the focus to Scotland. Other countries have experienced similar crises in child care precipitated by confrontation of the issue of child sexual abuse.

The Report of the Inquiry into Child Abuse in Cleveland 1987 (Butler-Sloss 1988) noted that

> We have learned during the Inquiry that sexual abuse occurs in children of all ages, including the very young, to boys as well as girls, in all classes of society and frequently within the privacy of the family.

In the USA professional concern about child abuse is entering its fourth decade (Finkelhor 1996). Finkelhor describes the social movement around child protection which has been a feature of this century and 'is rooted in two profound social changes':

- The growth of a new large class of professional workers who specialise in dealing with children and families (paediatricians, school nurses, health visitors, child and family mental health workers, social service workers and a range of personnel in education, schools and nurseries as well as various therapists and a specialised legal system developed to handle these complex problems).
- The movement of women from the home and into the work force and professions. It was necessary for women to start to discuss sexual abuse they had experienced both as women and children before child sexual

abuse could be addressed. Increasing adult disclosure provided the first glimpses of what Roland Summit (1988) has termed 'society's blind spot'. If one was allowed only a single epithet to describe child sexual abuse, it might be 'hidden'. In a society increasingly willing to examine itself in all aspects, good and bad, it was inevitable that sooner or later child sexual abuse would be discussed.

Historically there is no doubt that child sexual abuse is not new. In the DHSS advice Guidance to Doctors – Diagnosis of Child Sexual Abuse (1988) it is acknowledged that although recognition of child sexual abuse has occurred only recently, Paul Bernard in 1886 reported its existence as a major hazard to child health in France. The laws on incest in this country were enacted from the 1890s onwards but this kind of abuse has in all probability been present in our society for centuries.

A historical perspective on the way children have been treated and maltreated is given in Chapter 2. Just as Freud (1954), Tardieu (1860) and others struggled to grasp the facts of the sexual abuse of children in the context of a prevailing social attitude of disbelief, so others, more recently, have begun to understand the wider psychological resistances which have kept this problem hidden for so long. Sgroi (1978) says that

> those who try to assist sexually abused children must be prepared to battle against incredulity, hostility, innuendo and outright harassment. Worst of all, the advocate for the sexually abused child runs the risk of being smothered by indifference and a conspiracy of silence. The pressure from one's peer group as well as the community to ignore, minimise or cover up the situation may be extreme.

These words may seem to have more than a faint ring of paranoia, but are written from an experience which is repeatedly described by people who work in this field. Anyone who has not shared these experiences is unlikely to have entered into close dialogue with this area of abuse and certainly has not identified with the child's position in this situation. The professionals who were involved in the Cleveland crisis wrote:

> Child sexual abuse is a problem which depends on silence and secrecy. We have experienced something of what happens to abused children when they attempt to speak: we have been disbelieved, rejected and silenced. (Richardson & Bacon 1991)

Definition of child sexual abuse

Issues:

- what is sexual?
- when does what has occurred become abuse?
- how important is age?
- how relevant is consent?

Essential characteristics of child sexual abuse

- Children in general do not like it
- Sexual gratification of the abuser is the usual aim of the abuse
- There is a power/age differential which effectively removes meaningful consent
- The activity is usually secretive, collusive and perpetuated by the more powerful person
- However, sometimes the strong needs of the child for physical affection, attention and dependency lead to the child's apparent complicity or willingness to initiate and maintain the abuse

Sexual abuse is interactive although the responsibility rests entirely with the adult. 'Sexual' relates to any activity which leads to sexual arousal in the adult. It includes a wide range of acts.

There are many definitions (see Glaser & Frosh 1988), for example:

> The sexual exploitation of children is referred to as the involvement of dependent, developmentally immature children and adolescents in sexual activities that they do not fully comprehend, are unable to give informed consent

to and that violate the social taboos of family roles (Schechter & Roberge 1976).

A child (anyone under 16 years) is sexually abused when another person who is sexually mature involves the child in any activity which the other person expects to lead to their sexual arousal (Baker & Duncan 1985)

or, even simpler,

Sexual abuse is the exploitation of a child for the sexual gratification of an adult (Fraser 1981).

No single definition is entirely satisfactory, but the essential aspects are to be found in the ones quoted. Obviously a 10-year-old boy who is attempting to have anal intercourse with a 3-year-old cousin is sexually abusing her. A 10-year-old is not sexually mature, but is sexually capable although still developmentally immature. The issue should be seen from the child victim's viewpoint.

The issue of force or coercion is also important. A child may express power differentials through size in drawings (Fig. 8.1). Although some abuse is clearly the result of violent or forcible acts producing physical injury and best described as rape, molestation refers to a more cautious if equally determined approach to the child who is abused by the use of threats, bribes, trickery and emotional manipulation. In both situations there are powerful emotions at play which overcome any resistance the child may have. Violence is an appropriate description for this abuse of power. The issue of coercion is related to the age difference consideration, although it is almost impossible to define this precisely. Clearly, mutual sexual exploratory play between children of similar ages is not abuse, but where coercion is involved the situation is perceived differently.

CASE HISTORY 8.1

A 10-year-old boy hero-worshipped his 13-year-old cousin with whom he spent time at holidays and weekends. However, his cousin taught him how to masturbate and later involved him in oral sex and

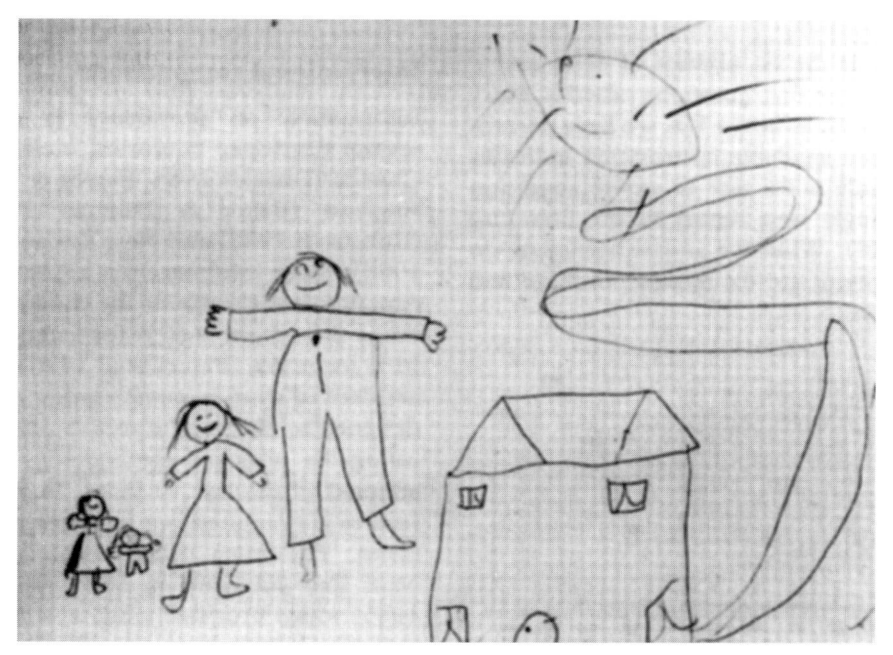

Fig. 8.1 Drawing by a 7-year-old sexually abused girl of her family. The girl is far left with her younger brother, mother and mother's boyfriend in that order on her right. Do the sizes of the figures reflect the child's perceptions of personal power?

attempted buggery. When the younger boy resisted, he threatened to beat him up. The 10-year-old repeatedly asked his mother whether he had AIDS and eventually she elicited the story of what had happened with his cousin. Along with the boy's disclosure, his 12-year-old sister admitted that she had repelled the cousin's attempts to fondle her breasts, although he had masturbated and smeared semen on her, to her disgust.

This case, despite the narrow age difference of the children, clearly indicates that the behaviour is abusive and, from a detailed family assessment, a generational family history of child sexual abuse was elicited from the adults.

Clinical aspects of definitions

It is unusual in clinical practice for long discussions to take place on what does or does not constitute sexual abuse. It is as though the boundary is so clearly defined that serious difficulties do not arise. Of course, there must be encounters between adults and children which might appear worrying and somewhere between normal physical contact and sexual abuse. For example, french kissing seems more prevalent amongst families involved in sexual abuse, but in itself might not be described as sexual abuse. If the activity is leading to sexual arousal of the adult, then this is more likely to have significance. If the activity is perceived as unpleasant or to be avoided by the child, then we should take note. As Glaser & Frosh (1988) have noted,

> the general rule that equates 'sexual contact' with some form of genital involvement is a useful one where questions of the appropriateness of physical encounters are raised.

The 'bathing costume' areas are well understood and although the sensitivity about other parts of the body, for example breasts and thighs, varies from culture to culture, genital awareness is universal.

Normal family sexuality and sexual knowledge in children

Surprisingly little information is available to help define what is normal and abnormal in terms of sexual behaviour in families. It is expected that 40–85% of children engage in some sexual behaviour before the age of 13. Natural and healthy sexual exploration provides information to children by means of exploring each others' bodies, looking and touching (e.g. playing doctor) as well as gender roles and behaviours (e.g. playing house). Children involved are of similar age, size and developmental status, and participate on a voluntary basis (Johnson 1996). Most sex play takes place between children who have an ongoing friendship. The sexual interest is balanced by interest in other aspects of the child's life. Although the child may feel embarrassment, this kind of exploration does not leave the child with feelings of anger, shame, fear or anxiety (Johnson 1996).

Other research reported that coming into the parental bed, touching mother's breasts, being seen masturbating and observing sexual intimacy were all common.

Less common were witnessing sexual intercourse, touching parent's genitalia, seeing violent or horror movies or pornographic magazines (Smith & Grocke 1995). With increasing age, bathing with parents and seeing parents naked decreased. Girls had more detailed knowledge than boys about their sexuality but lack of sexual knowledge remains a problem for children and adolescents.

Incidence and prevalence of child sexual abuse

Definitions

Incidence: the number of new cases occurring in a given time period, usually 1 year (expressed as numbers of cases per year or as a rate per 1000 children). Figure 8.2 shows the numbers of children diagnosed by paediatricians in Leeds over the period 1978–88.

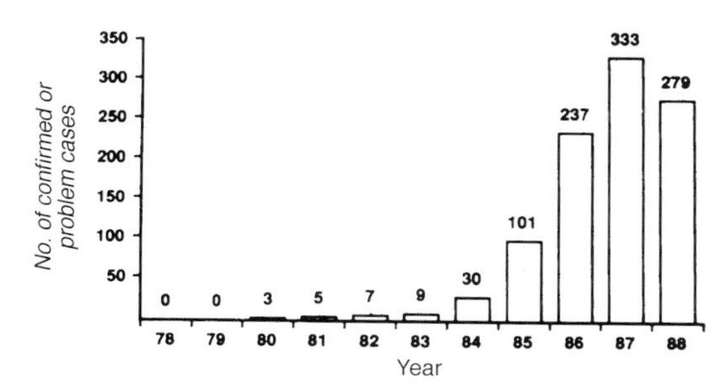

Fig. 8.2 Annual total number of cases of sexual abuse seen by Leeds paediatricians in the years 1978–88.

- *Prevalence*: the proportion of the population that has been sexually abused at some time during the course of childhood (usually expressed as a percentage).

'How common is the occurrence of child sexual abuse?' is one of the first questions raised in every discussion. At present in the UK there are no reliable answers. What we as paediatricians do not know at present are the answers to these and similar questions:

- Is child sexual abuse as common a childhood problem as asthma or febrile convulsions?
- What proportion of paediatricians' time is spent treating and advising on the immediate symptoms and disorders of childhood which arise from this kind of abuse (for example behaviour disorders, psychosomatic problems, recurrent abdominal pains, disorders of elimination, recurrent vaginal and anal conditions)?
- What proportion of bed-wetting children who fail to respond adequately to our tried and tested therapies are wetting as a consequence of child sexual abuse?
- How many children with recessive genetic or unexplained congenital disorders have been born as a result of an incestuous relationship?
- Why are so many mothers vague and evasive about the identity of their child's father?
- How many of the intractable and difficult behavioural problems of handicapped children, both home-based and institutionalised, are related to sexual abuse?

Incidence figures from the USA provide the opportunity to compare sexual abuse with other important problems of childhood (Table 8.1). More recently, in a US telephone survey of 1000 parents concerning disciplinary practices and violence toward their children aged 0–17, 1.9% (2.0% boys, 1.7% girls) reported that their child had been sexually abused in the past year, and 5.7% (6.1% boys and 5.3% girls) ever (Finkelhor et al 1997).

Table 8.1 Incidence of childhood problems in the US (Giardino et al 1992)

Diagnosis	Incidence	Age group
Leukaemia	2000 cases/year	<15 years
Drowning	3200 deaths/year	<4 years
Acute diarrhoea	100 000 hospital admissions/year	All ages
Head injury	250 000 hospital admissions/year	<15 years
Sexual abuse	300 000 cases/year	<18 years

Incidence in the UK

The only large-scale incidence study on child sexual abuse in the UK is that undertaken by the research team of Queen's University, Belfast in 1987 (North Ireland Research Team 1990). In this study 598 cases were analysed; half experienced penetrative abuse, a third non-penetrative sexual abuse. With established cases the incidence rate was 0.9 per 1000 children. For boys and girls the incidence rates were 0.34/1000 and 1.39/1000 respectively. Age-specific rates were 0.28/1000 (0–4 years) and 1.91/1000 (age 15–16 years). These rates are higher than for other regional areas in the UK but lower than US figures at the corresponding times. The figures are also higher than the earlier reported figures of Mrazek et al (1983).

International comparisons

Information on prevalence of sexual abuse is derived from research studies of adult victims designed to elicit retrospective disclosure. Information is available from several developed countries, including the USA, Canada (Badgley et al 1984), England (Baker & Duncan 1985), Sweden (Ronstrom 1985) and New Zealand (Mullen et al 1988). More information is available from North America than elsewhere: the child prevalence rates range there from 6 to 62% for females and from 3 to 31% for males (Peters et al 1986).

Prevalence studies in the UK

- *Mori poll* (Baker & Duncan 1985): 10% of subjects reported having been sexually abused before the age of 16 years (12% females, 8% males)
- *Female only sample of general practitioner's surgery and university students* (Nash & West 1985): 42% of general practitioner and 54% of student sample reported contact and non-contact abuse before the age of 16 years
- *Student sample, University of North London* (Kelly et al 1991): 59% of women and 27% of men reported at least one experience of sexual abuse (defined as unwanted sexual event or interaction) before age 18. 1 in 20 women and 1 in 50 men reported forced sex, rape or coerced masturbation
- *NSPCC survey* (Creighton & Russell 1995): 11% of adult respondents reported sexual abuse involving physical contact during their childhood, one-third perpetrated by relatives, one-third before age 11 years. Girls three times more likely than boys to have been abused.
- *British Crime Survey* (Aye Maving 1995): 1 in 10 girls and 1 in 50 boys aged 12–15 had been sexually harassed in the past 6–8 months by adult men. Half the victims had been very frightened

Data from other countries shows similar results, although the variations between individual studies are large and probably relate to differences of methodology, definition and sample. Some of the major differences in the studies relate to the way in which the information was obtained, with higher rates reported in face-to-face interviews with selected sensitive interviewers (Russell 1983) than in self-administered questionnaires or telephone interviews. Another important observation which was made (Peters et al 1986) in reviewing the various prevalence studies was that the number of screen questions within the protocol aimed at uncovering sexually abusive experience was related to the prevalence rate. Questions such as 'Were you ever sexually abused as a child?' or 'Did anyone ever touch your private sexual parts when you didn't want this'? seem more likely to elicit a positive response if there are more of them in the questionnaire.

In one sense it is surprising not just how many people have been sexually abused but how many are willing to reveal this in the context of a research study. It is in the private and anonymous situation where there are no further consequences that the individual may feel able to disclose. In fact there is good evidence that people use this opportunity to disclose information which they may have been unable to discuss previously.

In reviewing the reasons for success in these studies it is clear that if the respondents are questioned with multiple screen questions which avoid labels like 'sexual abuse' and which give respondents more time and opportunity to remember forgotten experiences or gather courage to reveal embarrassing ones, then responses will be more complete. Recall is also aided by including relationship-specific questions, such as 'Did your brother ever touch you on your genital area when you didn't want it?'

The Mori poll (Baker & Duncan 1985)

The MORI poll, conducted by female interviewers of a nationally representative sample of 2019 men and women, used as its definition:

> A child (anyone under 16 years) is sexually abused when another person who is sexually mature involves the child in any activity which the other person expects to lead to their sexual arousal. This might involve intercourse, touching, exposure of sexual organs,

showing pornographic material or talking about sexual things in an erotic way.

As with most studies, abuse both within and without the family were measured separately, as well as the number of episodes to indicate whether this was a one-off or a repetitious pattern of encounter.

MORI poll: detailed findings

- 10% of subjects reported being sexually abused before the age of 16 years (12% of females, 8% of males)
- no special risks in specific social class categories
- 63% of respondents reported only a single experience
- 23% were repeatedly abused by the same person
- 14% subjected to multiple abuse by a number of people
- 49% of abusers known to the victims
- 14% of all abuse took place within the family
- 51% of the experiences reported as abusive involved no physical contact
- 44% involved physical contact but not sexual intercourse
- 5% involved full sexual intercourse

The University of North London student sample (Kelly et al 1991)

The University of North London study was part of the Department of Health Studies commissioned after Cleveland. The sample was taken from the broad-based intake of a college of further education (as it then was). A total of 1244 young people aged between 16 and 21 completed the questionnaire (62% female).

These findings are not atypical of the kind of results obtained in this area of research. Females tend to report abuse more often than males, but it is very likely that men under-report. The highest prevalence rates are to be found in studies using the most searching and sensitive methods of questioning, suggesting that lower rates in some studies are underestimates of the problem.

Detailed findings of the student sample

- 59% of women and 27% of men reported at least one experience of sexual abuse (defined as unwanted sexual event or interaction) before age 18
- commonest experiences flashing – 27% of experiences, touching 23%
- 1 in 20 women and 1 in 50 men reported forced sex, rape or coerced masturbation
- women 2–3 times more likely to experience sexual abuse than men
- prevalence rate for black and white men and women are the same
- over 25% of assaults committed by peers, with largest group individuals known to child
- 2% reported incestuous abuse, i.e. parent or sibling
- female abusers 15% peer group, 5% by adult
- one-fifth of experiences were attempts which were repelled or escaped
- a half told someone, 90% were believed. Only 5% told an agency

The figures include a wide range of abuses and relationships of abuser to child. Figures for specific patterns of abuse, e.g. father/son, will be correspondingly lower. Important factors which appear not to influence the rates include education and socio-economic status or class, ethnicity or age. Within the USA, where there are sufficient numbers of studies to draw some conclusions, geographical region appears not to be a significant factor. The claims 'Well, the problem is more common in place A than place B', or 'We don't have incest in this town' seem unlikely to withstand close scrutiny.

Possible factors accounting for differences in prevalence rates in research studies include (Peters et al 1986):

- definitions:
  - type of abuse – contact, non-contact, exposure to pornography, verbal acts
  - upper age limit of childhood
  - criteria to define encounter as abusive
  - difference in age between perpetrator and victim
  - experiences with peers included
- sampling differences:
  - age (differences may reflect fluctuating real prevalence rates or changing attitudes towards disclosure
  - social class, ethnicity, education, geographical region, inner v. outer city v. rural
- methodology:
  - sampling techniques
  - response rates (usually many non-responders)
- method of administration of questionnaires/interviews – face-to-face, self-administered, telephone:
  - type and number of questions
  - skill and experience of questioner
  - opportunity for follow-up and support of interviewers.

Conclusions from prevalence studies

Gorey and Leslie (1997) analysed the findings from 16 cross-sectional studies from North America. They found that the two single most important variables were response rate and the operational definition of child abuse, and these together accounted for half the observed variability in the abuse prevalence estimates. People who have been sexually abused are more likely to agree to take part than those who were not, so low response rates favour higher prevalence rates. Adjusted for response rates the aggregated prevalence rates for sexual abuse for girls and boys were 16.8% and 7.9% and, adjusted for operational definitions, 14.5% and 7.2%. Given that the average response rate of the better surveys was still only 69%, a more accurate estimate was suggested: females 12–17%, males 5–8%.

Patterns of abuse

Child sexual abuse occurs in a variety of situations and social settings.

- *Intrafamilial abuse* (Bentovim et al 1988): includes abuse within the nuclear and extended family and may incorporate family friends, lodgers or close acquaintances with the knowledge of the family. Abuse within adoptive or foster-families is also included here.
- *Extrafamilial abuse*: includes abuse with adults frequently known to the child from a variety of sources including neighbours, family friends, schoolfriend's parents, as well as abuse within sex rings.
- *Ritualistic abuse*: can be intrafamilial or extrafamilial and is discussed in Chapter 13.
- *Institutional abuse*: includes abuse occurring within schools, residential children's establishments, day nurseries, holiday camps – e.g. Cubs, Brownies, Boy Scouts and other organisations both secular and religious.
- *Street or stranger abuse*: assaults on children in public places, child abduction.

Intrafamilial abuse

As sexual abuse is a secretive activity where the risks of detection are minimised by the offender; the family offers the safest option. The opportunity to control and manipulate the child into silence, the avoidance of discovery and the taboos which prevent society from believing that parents could sexually abuse their own children provide insurance against discovery.

In the author's experience (Hobbs & Wynne 1987) two-thirds of children are abused by a family member (Fig. 8.3): this includes not only natural parents but also step-parents, unrelated boyfriends and cohabiting friends as well as grandparents, uncles, aunts, cousins, brothers and sisters. Relations who do not live under the same roof as the child will use the collusive secrecy of the family and easy access to the chil-

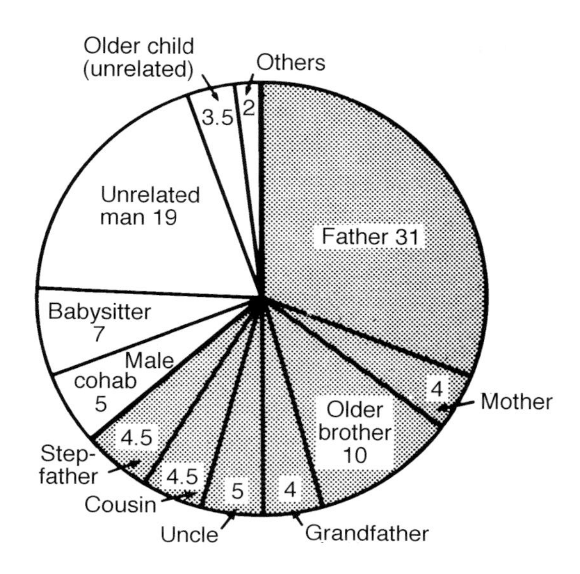

Fig. 8.3 Relationship of perpetrators to children (all ages) in 337 cases of sexual abuse. Shaded area represents relatives of child. Percentages are shown. (Reproduced with permission from Hobbs C J, Wynne J M 1987 Child sexual abuse – an increasing rate of diagnosis. Lancet ii: 837–841)

dren, often in preference to abusing children outside the family. However, evidence from in-depth amnesty studies (Abel et al 1981) in the USA of committed sexual offenders indicate that as many as half of them have abused children both within and without their families.

Abuse occurs when an abuser has access to an available and vulnerable child. In a family setting it is more likely that all the children will be involved, but in institutional settings individual vulnerability may have more influence on the choice of the child.

Intrafamilial abuse is likely to be chronic, to begin in many cases soon after the birth of the child and to extend throughout childhood (Bentovim et al 1988). For some children the abusing relationships continue into adult life; women may bear their father's children and continue to live within their family, participating in the ongoing abuse of the next generation. Intrafamilial abuse, therefore, is more easily perceived as a pattern of relationships in which all the family participates and in which the normal boundaries within and between generations do not exist. The paediatrician who is working in this area should be aware of these generational cycles of abuse (Kaufman & Zigler 1989). When an angry grandmother writes or calls to proclaim her son or daughter innocent, she may be trying to protect them, but it is also likely that she is thinking of the whole family including herself and her husband and all the uncles, aunts, nieces and nephews who will feel threatened and exposed by the uncovering of abuse in a single child. For this reason, it has been the author's experience that arrangements to foster sexually abused children within the wider family have often met with difficulty, including further abuse by other family members. It is common when investigating sexual abuse in a family to make links with other related families where abuse has been recognised. The work of Oliver (1983) in Wiltshire has shown how abusing and neglecting families are connected through extensive kinships and how so much childhood morbidity and mortality is found in these families.

Extrafamilial abuse

There has been less focus on extrafamilial abuse in the literature. Many of the community surveys of sexual abuse report that body contact extrafamilial sexual abuse is more common than abuse in the family. Extrafamilial abuse is the most common form of abuse recognised among boys.

The boundaries between intrafamilial and extrafamilial abuse are often blurred and the recognition of one must lead to a consideration of the other. A boy who has been abused at home by his father may unconsciously allow himself to be in dangerous situations with other men, who may take the opportunity to abuse him away from his family.

Many of the children in sex rings (Burgess et al 1981, Burgess 1984, Wild & Wynne 1986) were found to have been abused at home, but some had not. Often it was the ringleaders who had been victims of parental abuse and had recruited other children into the situation. Although some of these children had been deprived of attention at home and were vulnerable to the rewards of 'prostitution', they had not been sexually abused within their homes as far as one could tell (Wild & Wynne 1986).

In extrafamilial abuse a wide variety of adults, usually known to the child, establish relationships and lure the child into situations where he or she is abused, often in return for something which the child is not receiving at home. The child remains silent because disclosure might evoke parental anger with the child for allowing him or herself to become involved in the relationship. Babysitters and others who claim a genuine interest in helping the family may manoeuvre themselves into positions of trust so that they achieve contact with children in their own or the abuser's home. Some parents are happy that the child is willing to be away for a while to relieve them of the endless responsibility of child care. Others seem less concerned about where or with whom their child spends time. Children who truant from school seem especially vulnerable and this should be viewed in some cases as a warning sign.

Although child protection services may be less interested in extrafamilial sexual abuse, children experience negative effects from the abuse and may suffer emotional and behavioural difficulties at least in the short term (Ligezinska et al 1996). These children therefore are likely to require help after abuse has been detected and stopped.

Characteristics of child sex rings

- One adult (or small group) and several children
- Men and women, boys and girls, usually in separate rings
- Elaborate socialisation process binds and locks children into the ring
- Ringleaders are also often abused within their families
- Children aged 6–16 years including siblings (i.e. school age)
- Adult abusers appear benevolent and encourage children to act out, pitting child members of the ring against one another
- Older children may abuse and manipulate younger ones
- Children are sexually abused individually or as a group with a range of activities from masturbation to intercourse
- Pornography binds children more firmly to the ring and establishes commercial links with other abusers
- Extreme secrecy is maintained by threats, peer group pressure and the fear of discovery
- Discovery depends on dedicated and experienced police officers working closely with other community agencies
- Rings have a life of years, may break and rejoin around another abuser. Children join and leave the rings, maintaining secrecy
- Children are emotionally damaged by the abuse, experiencing subsequent sexual difficulties, acting out behaviour, alcohol or drug abuse. Identification with the abuser is common
- Child sex rings have been discovered in several cities in the UK and in the USA. It is likely that they are a common and widespread form of abuse. Around 300 children were involved in Leeds (Wild & Wynne 1986)
- The term 'child prostitution' has been used because in some cases the abuser will reward the children with cups of coffee, attention and small monetary gifts. For this reason, children from materially or emotionally depriving families may be at greater risk

Families of sexually abused children

Certain characteristics of families who have a child who has been sexually abused are described. The families of both incest and non-incest sexual abuse victims are described as less cohesive, more disorganised, and generally more dysfunctional than those of non-abused children. Areas of difficulty in incest cases include communication, lack of emotional closeness and flexibility, and social isolation (Berliner & Elliott 1996). However, it should be remembered that this information comes from studies of families where abuse has been reported and include an excess of families from poorer socio-economic circumstances. The community surveys supports the view that incest occurs more evenly across the social spectrum.

Family contexts relevant to abuse described by adults who had suffered abuse as children included domestic violence and/or alcohol, parental absence, relationship difficulties between parents, reconstituted family, abuse part of family life for family members, lack of understanding, divorce or separation and substitute care (Childhood Matters 1996). Of these, domestic violence or alcohol abuse was most commonly reported.

Children who are sexually abused

The traditional view of the sexually abused child implied that there was something within the child's make-up which contributed to abuse. These so-called 'child factors' have been much discussed within the context of physical abuse as well as neglect and failure to thrive. It was hypothesised that the child's behaviour, manner or appearance triggered off interest on the part of the adult. In sexual abuse a mythology existed that only certain children at certain ages were abused and that this was related to their 'mini' adult sexuality: hence the view that a teenage girl blossoming into puberty provided a stimulus which to a stepfather, not bound by incest taboos, could be irresistible. Recognition that this scenario was little more than a comforting attempt to normalise deviant behaviour has led to a reappraisal.

Children of all ages are abused, including infants less than a year old. Both in clinical samples and in community surveys of adults, girls usually outnumber boys. Hobbs & Wynne (1987) found a ratio of 2 girls to 1 boy whereas an incidence study in Northern Ireland found 4.4 girls to 1 boy (Northern Ireland Research Team 1991). Boys are less likely to be suspected, to report or to be believed (Rogers & Terry 1984). In view of these confounding variables, it has been suggested that boys may be sexually abused to the same extent as girls (Kempe & Kempe 1984, Hanks et al 1988).

Age at diagnosis does not inform us of age of onset of abuse, but the mean age at diagnosis is around 7 years with the peak at 2–7 years according to data on children diagnosed in Leeds (Fig. 8.4). Age at diagnosis depends more on the ease of diagnosis, willingness to disclose and frequency of physical findings which assist diagnosis. There are good reasons for believing that older children learn the consequences of disclosure, are better able to conceal the fact of their abuse and have a greater sense of the perceived harm which they may suffer if they tell. As well as finding abused children of both genders and all ages, it is quite common to find that all the children in the family have suffered abuse (Hobbs & Wynne 1986, Muram et al 1991).

Rather than child factors being important in determining whether or not abuse occurs when they come into contact with the abuser, it is the indiscriminate behaviour of the abuser which appears to be more important. If this is the case, differences between sexually abused children and non-abused children are more likely to be the result of the abuse than its cause. Recently a 5-year-old girl took to having make-up and nail varnish, having her hair done in a grown-up style and wearing earrings. Sexual abuse by her father and brother was discovered and her transformation to a sexual object gave important clues to her foster-mother that all was not well. If she had been 12 or 13, the alternative explanation that she was sexually precocious and inviting inappropriate attention could easily have been preferred.

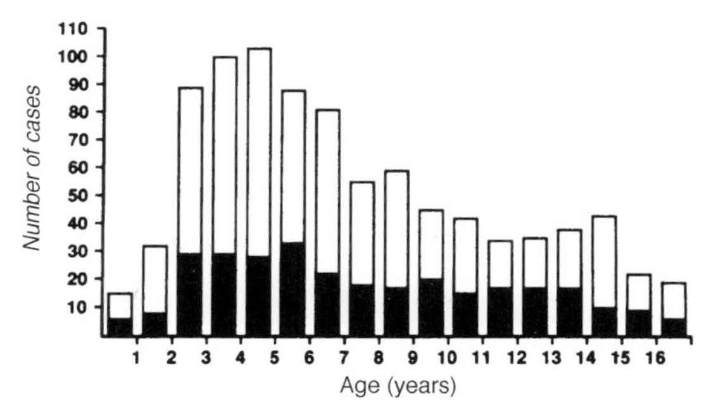

Fig. 8.4 Age/sex distribution of 900 sexually abused children seen by paediatricians in Leeds in the years 1986–88. Black, boys; white, girls.

These children are groomed and trained to respond sexually, the process occurring gradually over a long time. Loss of childhood innocence and the appearance of a child too wise for his or her years are common effects.

The nature of sexual abuse experiences

Multiple abuse episodes are very common in sexual abuse, occurring in half the cases from community research samples and over 75% of clinical cases. Children who have once been sexually abused appear to be at greater risk of further abuse by the same or different perpetrator.

Acts involved in sexual abuse

- Contact:
  - touching, fondling or oral contact with breast or genitals
  - insertion of fingers or objects into vulva or anus
    - masturbation: by adult of him/herself in the presence of the child, including
    - ejaculation on to the child; by adult of child or by child of adult
    - intercourse: vaginal, anal or oral intercourse whether actual or attempted in any degree. (This is usually with adult as the active party but in some cases a child may be encouraged to penetrate the adult)
  - rape is attempted/achieved penile penetration of the vagina (Fig. 8.5)
  - other genital contact; intracrural intercourse where the penis is laid between the legs or genital contact with any part or the child's body, e.g. penis rubbed on thigh
  - prostitution: any of the above abuse which includes the exchange of money, gifts or favours and applies to both boys ('rent boys') or girls. (We have encountered cases where parents have sold their children as young as 3 years for sexual abuse)
- Non-contact:
  - exhibitionism (flashing)
  - pornography of many kinds; photographing sexual acts or anatomy
  - showing pornographic photographs, films, videos
  - erotic talk, telling children titillating or sexually explicit stories
  - other sexual exploitations
  - sadistic activities
  - burning a child's buttocks or genital area

Completed or attempted oral, anal or vaginal penetration occurs in 20–49% of non-clinical subjects and in more than 60% of forensic samples.

At present we have no sure way of assessing or predicting the harm or upset which is caused to a child from these varying activities. The child's responses are individual. Although we all have our own ideas as to which activity is more serious and which likely to be more damaging, it is as well to remember these difficulties. Most people view intercourse as the most serious and exhibitionism the least.

Many children suffer more than one abuse, for example genital fondling, oral and anal intercourse, and it is often considered that the abuses may escalate over time from, say, exposure, involvement in masturbation and intracrural intercourse to vaginal intercourse. However, the high frequency of oral and anal intercourse in pre-school children suggests that this slow seduction is often shortened where children have less ability to resist.

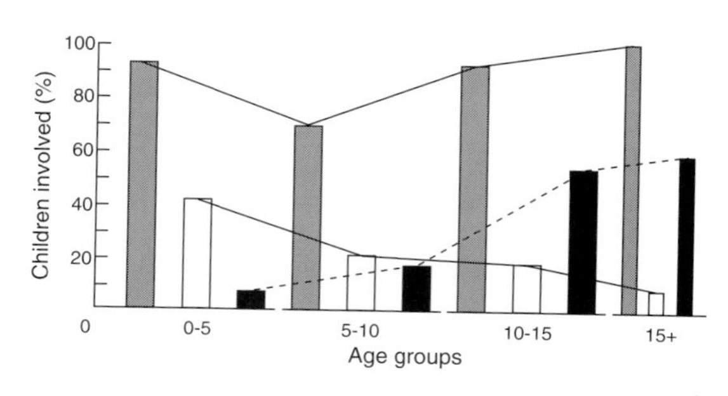

Fig. 8.5 Penetrative sexual abuse. Percentage of children involved in anal and vaginal penetration by age group and gender from a study of 337 sexually abused children. Black, vaginal; grey, anal (boys); white, anal (girls). (Reproduced with permission from Hobbs C J, Wynne J M 1989 Sexual abuse of English boys and girls: the importance of anal examination. Child Abuse and Neglect 13:195–210)

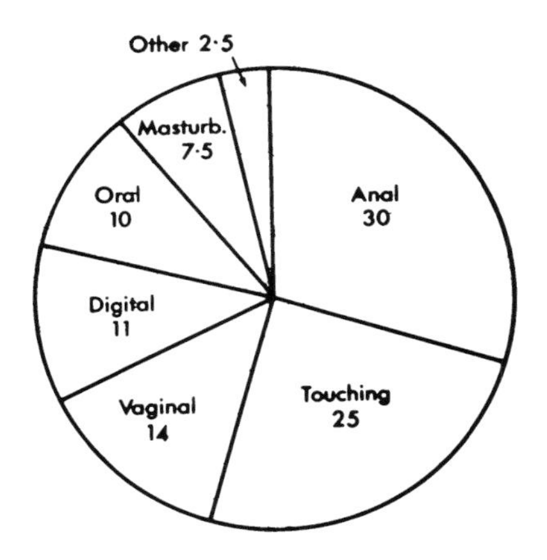

Fig. 8.6 Percentage frequency of different types of sexual abuse in 337 children (Reproduced with permission from Hobbs C J, Wynne J M 1987 Child sexual abuse – an increasing rate of diagnosis. Lancet ii: 837B841)

Figure 8.6 gives the relative proportions of the different abuses seen in our series. Types of abuse will vary depending on the way children are selected; clinical series are likely to have fewer non-contact cases for obvious reasons.

Abusers

Some quotations

> Everyone hates a child molester until it's someone you know. (American police officer)

In response to an article in the *Observer* in August 1989 entitled 'Why do men do it?' we asked 'Why do women do it?', or even 'Why do people do it?' Perhaps the answer is much more simple than it appears – what could be easier than abusing a child?

> Sexual offenders will only tell you the minimum of what they need to say to avoid responsibility for what they have done. The only characteristic that offenders have in common is that they commit deviant sexual acts – and also thought it was okay to do it. (Judith Becker, in a paper presented to a child abuse conference in Glasgow, 1987)

> Child sexual abusers include white-collar workers, priests, doctors, attorneys, judges, blue-collar workers and those who have no job. (S Wolf, at a conference on child protection, Leeds University, 1988)

Facts about abusers

Most abusers or perpetrators are related to or, if unrelated, known to the child. Figure 8.3 demonstrates these relationships in a study of 337 children. Many abusers commit large numbers of offences involving large numbers of children. In one study 232 abusers guaranteed confidentiality admitted that they had attempted 55 250 acts of child abuse and completed 38 727 of them (Abel et al 1985). Recidivism is high after conviction but lower after treatment. Abusers include both men and women. Our expectations and the teaching given to us as children (don't speak to strange men) mean that we underestimate and fail to recognise female abusers. The numbers being recognised are steadily increasing but the true proportion is not known. In clinical and community studies, men heavily predominate. Earlier studies found that 5% of girls and 20% of boys were abused by women. In day care in the US, 40% of abusers were female (Finkelhor et al 1988). In this study, the women were aged 16–77 years, 63% were married, only 21% had no children. The women were more socially respected than the men in the same sample. The women are unlikely to be detected from police checks.

The majority of sexual abusers against children start behaving in this way as adolescents. Many abusers themselves report sexual abuse as children, but not all (Knopp 1984). In almost 20 studies, the reported rate of victimisation among offenders ranged from 0 to 70% but with increased sample size was usually around 20–30% (Hanson and Slater 1988) . Others, however, recall difficult and damaging experiences as children (Becker 1988).

In one study of convicted abusers' childhood experiences (Wolf 1987):

- 17% witnessed sexual abuse

- 23% were victims of emotional abuse
- 27% were victims of sexual abuse
- 30% were victims of violence
- 37% had witnessed violence.

In addition,

- 47% had feelings of isolation
- 100% grew up in dysfunctional families.

In Leeds, 25% of children diagnosed were abused by teenagers (Hobbs & Wynne 1987) and in another study a third of abusers were teenagers (Northern Ireland Research Team 1991). Many of the male abusers have been sexually abused, and other work suggests that female teenage abusers have all been sexually abused (Tranter, personal communication 1991).

Rationalisations and distortions

A common feature of abusers is their distortion of attitude and belief (Beckett 1994). Abusers may say to defend their actions (Donleary & Goodwin 1989):

> The child was sexually provocative, she came and sat on my knee.
>
> If she didn't want to be raped, why did she start developing breasts?
>
> I only did it to teach him about sex.
>
> I just knew she wanted to by the way she was looking at me.

Models for viewing abusive behaviour (Salter 1988)

- *Sexual addiction*: high levels of sexual arousal leading to need for frequent gratification and cycle of addiction. Breaking the habit is extremely difficult. Abusers tell themselves they won't do it again. As with other addictions, the need for increasing 'dosage' leads to escalation of the abuse
- *Paedophile: child sexual fixation* (Groth 1982). 'Children are missing out if they don't have the opportunity to enjoy sexual relations.' Everyone else has got it wrong. The paedophile has no sexual interest in adults. His interest is the world of the child. The paedophile's defences are so unchallengeable that he may never be able to start on the difficult process of treatment. Paedophiles are increasingly organised and may be in touch with others, exchanging information and publications
- *Family models* (Furniss 1984): incestuous families are described as patriarchal and authoritarian but within them the individuals have strong needs and personal weaknesses. Patterns of male or female dominance are often described and the marital relationship is poor. The emotional and sexual difficulties are controlled by the development of inappropriate sexual and emotional bonds with the children. In some families this serves to avoid conflict, in others it seems to regulate the violent and disturbed patterns of family life. It is postulated that these families, however, maintain their fragile and dangerous existence because the terror of abandonment is so much greater. The members of the family collude and keep the secret to maintain the integrity of the family unit. This model helps us to understand that child sexual abuse occurs within the context of emotional deprivation and neglect and never as an isolated finding in an otherwise well-functioning family
- *Sociological models*: within society power is one aspect of relationships between individuals and groups of individuals. Men are typically seen as possessing more power than women and of assuming dominant roles in families. Rich have more than poor and whites more than blacks. Adults have power over children. A misuse of adult power for the achievement of adults' needs, denying the child's own needs, is at the centre of child sexual abuse. Sociologists would say that although these major power differentials exist, the potential for abuse is inherent. Only when society is more fair and just will this be reflected in individual and family relationships

Abusers and denial

Abusers are amongst the best liars and deniers. There is no such person as an abuser who does not deny. Salter (1988b) listed the various components of denial as follows:

- denial of the acts themselves (type and period of time the abuse occurred)
- denial of fantasy and planning
- denial of responsibility for the acts
- denial of the seriousness of the behaviour
- denial of internal guilt for the behaviour
- denial of the difficulty of changing abusive patterns.

There is a continuum from admission with justification to admission with guilt. The more the abuser shifts towards the latter, the less pathological is his behaviour. Treatment of abusers is seen as enabling them to move gradually from the position of denial to acceptance of the responsibility for what they have done, together with a sense of the seriousness of their actions.

Women as abusers

Although the majority of studies traditionally focus on men as sexual abusers of children, more recently there have been studies which show a much higher rate of abuse by female perpetrators (Fritz et al 1981, see also Hanks & Saradjian 1991). Here figures of between 44% and 60% abused by females were recorded. In another recent study (Etherington 1997), 13 out of 25 non-clinical cases of men who responded to advertisements for adult male survivors of child sexual abuse had been abused by females, seven by their mothers.

Of the seven men, six were either single or divorced and related marital difficulties to their abuse. Such abuse is frequently difficult for men to conceptualise, with some preferring to refer to it as 'over-loving'; others unable to see that a woman could ever abuse a male because of socialisation messages. One man was quoted as saying that women were put on earth for cooking, cleaning, and sex for the benefit of men and every man should have several. They were not abusers and were there to be abused upon, so how could he have been abused by one?

Women, like men, abuse both male and female children and we have not detected any gender bias.

There is still a very strong feeling that women, particularly mothers, are closer to their children and just could not commit such acts. Information is emerging, however, that it is just these strong and widely held prejudices that prevent the true extent of female abuse from being recognised.

Women may abuse children on their own, with men or in groups involving both men and women. Hanks & Saradjian (1991) described abuse taking place by women of their own or other women's children in various clinical situations:

- when they live on their own with their children
- in conjunction with men
- as married couples
- as lesbian couples
- when they have a handicapped child (usually a boy).

Clinical features – medical findings:

It is unusual to be able to distinguish the gender of the perpetrator from physical evidence unless semen is detected. The kind of acts perpetrated as well as the degree of violence and force used may be virtually identical.

One useful practical point is that when a case of child sexual abuse is difficult to understand or the intervention is unsuccessful in protecting the child, you should pause to consider whether a woman might be the abuser.

Sexual offender behaviour

Sexual abuse is achieved in various ways. The offender frequently targets a particular child, plans the seduction and manipulates the child into silence.

The process of preparation of the child has been termed 'grooming'. Children may be gradually sexualised, given special favours and involved in what they believe is a special relationship. This process may extend to adults surrounding the child, including the mother and also to unwitting professionals. When confronted, the perpetrator may become victim, attracting sympathy as the 'wrongly accused'. In other cases the abuse occurs unexpectedly and without warning. The perpetrator may use force or coercion or threaten the child. Fear of injury, the child's own death of, or the death of a close relative or loved pet, ensures silence.

Effects of sexual abuse

It is widely believed that sexual abuse is harmful (Finkelhor & Browne 1986, Wyatt & Powell 1988). At best it is unpleasant, at worst extremely frightening and painful, physically and psychologically, for the child. Even older children, physically mature enough to experience pleasurable sexual sensations, are hurt and suffer from its effects. Children tell us that they do not like it, they wish it to stop and usually convey pain and discomfort when attempting to tell us about it. Evidence that child sexual abuse has deleterious effects comes from:

- observation of sexually abused children from around the time of diagnosis
- follow-up of children following recognition of sexual abuse
- studies of the population of adults to assess the frequency of mental health problems in abused and non-abused populations (Mullen et al 1988)
- observations of adult psychiatric patients who have been abused (Whitwell 1990).

Effects may be short-term or long-lasting.

Short-term effects on the child

- *Behavioural disturbances*: e.g. soiling, wetting or self-injury
- *Abnormal emotional states*: e.g. anxiety, depression and withdrawal
- *Educational and learning disturbance*: children may require special educational provision or assistance
- *Distorted social relationships*: they may only be able to relate to adults of one sex and have no class friends, or alienate themselves by involving other children in sexual activities.

Accommodation syndrome

When a child is caught up in a sexually abusive relationship, that child develops an adjustment pattern to the abuse which is known as the accommodation syndrome (Summit 1983). An understanding of this 'normal' behaviour pattern is vital to be able to assist children, including explaining in court why a child is relating in a particular way. The five characteristics of the child sexual abuse accommodation syndrome are:

- secrecy
- helplessness
- accommodation
- delayed disclosure
- retraction.

This pattern is most clearly seen when the abuser is a trusted care-giver, for example a parent or parent figure.

Secrecy

Children are told not to tell. Threats of physical violence, but often promises of withdrawal of love and affection, are all that are needed to secure a dependent child's silence. The child fears disapproval or punishment, and attempts to tell often confirm these worst fears. Retaliation certainly occurs. One 5-year-old child who told her aunt that her stepfather was putting his fingers in her bottom was given a good hiding. Another child, who complained to her mother that her 'tuppence' was sore, told her mother it had happened because daddy took her into the bedroom with him. The mother responded by hitting the child across the face, leaving bruises on her cheek and ear which, when noticed by the grandmother, led to detection.

Older children understand the implications for the family of a police investigation: possible imprisonment of father, loss of income, stigmatisation, shame and the possibility that they may be held responsible for all this. The logical solution for most children is to maintain the conspiracy of secrecy and silence.

Helplessness

Children are unable to stop the abuse in most cases. Although they may resist, at least initially, they find that it is less trouble to lie still, pretend to be asleep and switch off. In this way they attempt to protect themselves. This behaviour is often reflected in the ease with which children are medically examined; during the examination some children even go to sleep. Children will not cry out or struggle to protect themselves and this is often misinterpreted as willing compliance, both by the abuser and society at large. The cost that the child pays for the abandonment of active resistance is insecurity, victimisation and a loss of psychological well-being. The child is helpless, powerless and has no one to turn to.

Entrapment and accommodation

In the position of helplessness and secrecy, the child feels trapped and feels there is no way out of the situation. The only active role the child can play is to hold him- or herself responsible and, in sensing the wrongness and badness of what is happening, attempt to make amends. The victim therefore scapegoats him- or herself, leaving the abuser free of experiencing the child's hostility. Self-blame and guilt are almost universal feelings shared by sexually abused children.

In addition the child faces other pressures:

- the need to protect other children
- the need to protect the other parent
- the need to protect the family home and integrity of the family.

The abuser may tell the child that if he stops abusing her he may have to turn to other, possibly younger children. The child has the power to destroy the family, but the responsibility to keep it together. Parent and child roles have been subtly reversed and in doing so the child has accommodated to the situation at the expense of herself and her needs. The loss of childhood is a useful concept to describe the way in which the child is forced into a pseudo-adult role.

Once in this position, other adults easily view the child as a consenting and willing participant in the situation and come to doubt the child's statements if later the truth is revealed. The child who is able to accommodate effectively to the abuse will cover up the reality in order to protect the parent, but also to allow herself space for survival. It is not unusual for children, for example, to flourish at school where they feel protected and safe, effectively splitting off that part of their life from the threats and insecurity of home. Children's capacity to develop different personalities to cope with their complex feelings leads to psychological disintegration and the multiple personality states seen in some adult survivors (Goodwin 1989a).

Delayed disclosure and retraction

It is likely that many children never disclose their sexual abuse. They may attempt to within the family, but less often outside. Many adult victims disclosing in later life indicate that they never told. Disclosure is favoured by:

- overwhelmingly impossible situation at home
- the presence of a sensitive friend or helper, e.g. schoolteacher
- abuser no longer in contact (e.g. divorce)
- education strategies, telephone helplines
- good luck.

Many disclosures seem to arise almost by chance. Incidents where a chance remark is made by a child when defences are down, picked up by a sensitive listener and carefully expanded upon are not common. However, it is very simple to inhibit a child's attempts at disclosure by not hearing, disapproval or disbelief.

Our experience suggests that disclosure is not particularly favoured at any age (Hobbs & Wynne 1987, Hanks et al 1988). Contrary to the popular view that when the child enters adolescence he or she is more likely to disclose, we find that this is not a particular peak for referrals. At that age children can begin to get out of the situation and that option may be simpler than disclosure and exposure. Disclosure is, however, often delayed (schoolchildren present more often through disclosure than pre-school children – Hanks et al 1988), the abuse will have been going on for some time and the child fears that he or she will not be viewed sympathetically. The disclosure is, therefore, often retracted, may sound unconvincing, often includes details of only one or two incidents and is almost never exaggerated. The types of activity described will often be the less intrusive and upsetting ones for the child. There may be ambiguity which the child does not readily resolve.

CASE HISTORY 8.2

Two sisters aged 10 and 8 years in foster-care visited their alcoholic mother regularly at weekends. She failed to protect them from her violent boyfriends and eventually the older girl said to her social worker that one of the boyfriends had touched her once through her clothes between her legs. Thinking that it was unlikely that there would be any medical evidence and that the abuse did not seem so serious, the social worker delayed a while, but mentioned it to the child's paediatrician when he next routinely saw the children. On questioning the older girl further, she revealed that she had been hurt between her legs and that she was sore for several days. Her younger sister, who up to this point had denied that she had been involved in any way, then reminded her foster-mother that she had on occasions complained of a sore bottom. Both the children readily agreed to medical examination, where signs were found which strongly suggested that the older girl had experienced intercourse. The younger girl also had signs suggesting that vaginal penetration had been attempted.

Even, therefore, when children are being protected and given consistency and security, disclosure can be a slow gradual process, taking months and sometimes years. All these factors, of course, make criminal investigation difficult and often unrewarding; the current conviction rate in Leeds is 5% (Frothingham et al 1991). It is easy to suggest that the child is not being truthful when of course the child will usually conceal more than he or she is willing to reveal. Only an understanding and sensitive interpretation of the psychological processes involved allows the evidence to be properly assessed.

Retraction

Whatever children, adults and even sometimes professional witnesses say about sexual abuse, there is a strong likelihood that they will reverse it under pressure.

For the child, the whole subject is loaded with ambivalence, guilt and self-doubt. A hostile response by family or the outside world soon lets children know that they had better take it all back and say they made it up. The fact that children cannot and do not readily make up stories of explicit sexual activity is quickly forgotten by all concerned as the threat of the child's disclosure recedes. The retraction reassures, encourages disbelief of the original disclosure and may lead to inaction. While it should be viewed as a normal and expected part of the psychological adjustments of sexually abused children. People are happier to believe that children lie than that they are sexually abused (Goodwin 1989b).

Anger and rage

Angry emotions are common in abused children and may find in many ways.

Expressions of anger

- Self-destruction, self-hate, self-mutilation, suicidal behaviour, promiscuity and running away
- Exploitation of others, e.g. as ringleader may manipulate younger children in the ring
- Rejection of non-abusing parent, usually the mother if the father is abusing. There may be good easy-to-hand reasons, for example, 'Why didn't mother stop it, she must have known!'
- Aggressive, antisocial behaviour, wanton destruction, vandalism
- Depression, drug and alcohol abuse
- As the child becomes older, abusing or raping others less powerful

Long-term effects on the adult

The long-term effects of abuse in childhood manifest themselves in many ways (Briere & Runtz 1988):

- *mental health problems*: depression, suicide, self-injury, poor self-esteem, alcohol and/or drug abuse
- *sexual adjustment difficulties*: prostitution, marital difficulties, aversion to sexual contact, fertility control
- *child-rearing difficulties*: repeat cycle of abuse, over-protectiveness, fear of closeness
- *social dysfunction*: delinquency, criminal behaviour/offending, acts of violence, victim role.

Histories of child sexual abuse in women with mental health problems

The extensive literature on the prevalence of childhood sexual abuse among adult female clinical populations has been reviewed (Pilkington & Kremer 1995). High rates of child sexual abuse history were found in various diagnostic groups. These included patients with

- multiple personality disorder
- eating disorders
- chronic pelvic pain
- psychosexual disorders.

Further, it has been found that the risk of developing depression is up to four times greater in adults who were abused sexually as children than those who were not.

Women are more likely to internalise their distress, whereas men may cope by externalising their distress in aggressive and angry behaviour.

A model for looking at the harmful effects has been proposed by Finkelhor & Browne (1986) and includes four separate but inter-related areas of traumagenic dynamics. These different dynamics – traumatic sexualisation, betrayal, stigmatisation and powerlessness – account for the variety of symptoms and effects which we see. For each of the dynamics one can envisage:

- the abusive component
- the shaping effect it has on the child through its impact
- the manifestations which are incorporated into the child's and subsequently adult's behaviour.

Sexual traumatisation

A child may find that he or she receives attention and affection in exchange for sex; for example, many receive gifts for allowing daddy to get his way. The child then confuses sex with love and receiving care and attention. The long-term result will be that as the child grows up he or she may attempt to sexualise all relationships from which affection and attention are expected. The result will be seen as sexual promiscuity, possibly prostitution, and a tendency to sexualisation of relationships with their own children.

At the other end of the spectrum, sexual activity may be perceived as associated with entirely negative emotions and memories, leading to sexual aversion and difficulty in arousal or orgasm, or complete avoidance of sexual intimacy.

Betrayal

Betrayal stems from the loss of trust and disillusionment which a child feels when abused or not protected by a parent. This can produce dependency, clinging in young children, or a search for a trusted person. The impaired ability to judge people may lead to mistrust or misjudgement in relationships, with obvious disastrous implications for marriage or long-term relationships.

Stigmatisation

In child sexual abuse, the wrongfulness of the activity is soon perceived by a child as well as the offender and feelings of being dirty or damaged are common, leading to a sense of worthlessness or poor self-esteem. Such individuals, as they grow up, can become outcasts prone to alcohol or drug abuse, self-injury, criminal activity and isolation (Bagley & Ramsay 1986).

Powerlessness

Sexual abuse is clearly an abuse of the power that all adults have over children. Inability to stop the abuse – through weakness born out of dependency and developmental immaturity – leaves the child feeling powerless, anxious and unable to influence his or her own life. The child, as he or she grows up, may feel anxious, inefficient with impaired coping skills, a tendency to run away from problems, or sometimes despair and depression. Revictimisation is always a possibility but compensatory mechanisms to overcome these feelings include a need to control or dominate and a potentiality for aggression and becoming an abuser (Rogers & Terry 1984).

The Finkelhor & Browne model is useful in understanding some of the basic psychological mechanisms occurring in sexually abused children. It is derived from understanding of a great many facts, for example that prostitutes were very often sexually abused as children (James & Meyerding 1977), that there is a high frequency of a history of abuse in depressed women, and that victims may also become abusers.

What is also clear from the testimony of adults abused as children is that the feelings which accompany thoughts or recollections of these experiences remain hidden for many years and often for a lifetime. Letters from ageing grandparents who disclose abuse for the first time bear witness to the pain and suffering which these individuals have had to deal with all their lives. The process of coming to terms with this may be protracted, slow and incomplete. Repression and denial can be very powerful and the individual unable to confront these feelings except through these defensive mechanisms.

Factors which affect outcome in child sexual abuse

The degree to which a child is emotionally harmed by child sexual abuse in influenced by such factors as the child's prior history, current developmental level and age, as well as the nature of the sexual abuse:

- type of sex act:
  - frequency and duration
  - degree of force/violence and degree of bribery and coercion used
  - relationship with offender
  - age of child when contact first occurred
  - multiple abusers
- other important factors:
  - did the child disclose the abuse?
  - to whom did they reveal it?
  - have family and institutions responded?

Type of sex act

In our culture there is a perceived hierarchy of 'seriousness' of sexual activity ranging from kissing, breast touching and genital touching to intercourse. A similar hierarchy has been suggested for the prediction of trauma in child sexual abuse. Russell (1986) found the following percentage of women traumatised according to the type of act:

- clothed contact, unwanted kissing 22%
- touching of unclothed genitals, breasts 36%
- vaginal, oral or anal intercourse 59%

Penetrative abuse is considered more harmful than non-penetrative (Russell 1986, Briere 1988, Harter et al 1988). In addition to research findings, it is clear that professionals working in this field share this perception. Davenport (1988) interviewed 19 doctors (paediatricians, psychiatrists), social workers and clinical psychologists, all of whom were working actively in this field. She found that penetration was considered the most abusive of all the various acts. This is also reflected in the way in which the law views the seriousness of various offences. The term rape itself implies penetration. The victim's perception (what he or she feels about what has been done to them) and the harm which results are closely and aetiologically related.

Frequency and duration

The balance of evidence favours the view that harmfulness is related to frequency and duration (Tsai et al 1979, Russell 1986). However, chronicity is likely to lead to accommodation which may be associated with fewer symptoms in the short term although it may be associated with greater long-term psychological harm. In chronic abuse, the child is more likely to suffer long-term distortion in development.

Degree of force and violence

Society perceives physical force or violence as abusive, whereas more subtle inducements resulting in the same outcome are often not viewed in the same way. Conversely, although initially force will be immediately traumatising there may be some solace for the victim who is able to perceive later the wrongfulness of the experience and his or her own lack of involvement. Children who are tricked, bribed or seduced to comply may feel complicity and their view of themselves may be distorted in other ways. They often feel more intensely that they are at fault and should have stopped the abuse. The reality – that they would not have been able to do this easily – is lost. However, the degree of violence, according to research studies, remains an important factor although it will certainly interact with other variables (Finkelhor 1979, Bagley & Ramsay 1986, Russell 1986).

Relationship with offender

The relationship with the offender includes family links, quality and closeness, age, gender and maturity of the abuser.

Abuse by close relatives, especially those in a parental or caring role, is generally felt to have the most harmful effects (Finkelhor 1979, Adams-Tucker 1982, Russell 1986). However, no straightforward connection between the closeness of the relationship (nuclear family, versus relative, versus friend, versus stranger) and the effect on the child has been established (Finkelhor 1979). In the long term the quality of other, non-abusing, relationships will also influence the outcome.

Age of child

The child's age is an important and complex factor. With young pre-school children the view that the child does not understand or perceive the wrongfulness of the act is often quoted to indicate that less harm will result. However, many young children exhibit signs of emotional disturbance indicating that, whether or not they have an understanding of right and wrong, the negative effects have been perceived and responses have occurred. In developmental terms the effects are likely to be related to the developmental processes occurring at the time. In the younger child, the development of trust may be harmed and if the abuse continues relationships will become distorted in fundamental ways.

Thus it is our view (Hanks et al 1988) that

> Sexual abuse strikes at the foundation of the child's development as an individual. Abuse occurring in the early stage of a child's life (from birth to 5 years of age) is more likely to lead to major and fundamental changes in normal development and from what we have seen so far to have life-long consequences. These children have been deprived of trust and security within a relationship. What is more, they have come to regard human relationships in a distorted way – a distortion that they are at first not aware of and that cumulatively grows. As they grow older and reach the age of around 9 years they become clearly aware of the taboo which exists about incest and withdraw in shame and guilt, or turn to aggressive or abusive behaviour themselves.

Adolescents have also been considered to be especially vulnerable psychologically to sexual abuse. Adolescence is characterised by a search for identity and an understanding of the meaning of normal and deviant sexual relationships as well as drives towards autonomy and independence. Sexual identity is at the height of its development and will be distorted by sexual abuse. It is often said that guilt is especially common and may be compounded by the pleasurable effects which may at times be felt from the sexual contact. Isolation from peers may also be enforced by the perpetrator. Perpetrators often object to the child having other relationships and prohibitions mount at the possibility of other sexual relationships. Age is therefore an important complex variable, with different effects expressed at different developmental stages.

Multiple abusers

The effect of being abused by multiple perpetrators is to convince the child that the blame for the abuse lies in him- or herself, rather than with the offenders. The harmful effects are therefore compounded and patterns of re-victimisation into adulthood may result.

Effects of disclosure

Children are harmed not only by the abuse, but also by the response of the family and professional system. Disbelief or denial by someone (e.g. mother or father) in a position of responsibility regarding the child is clearly a major source of harm to a child already suffering the effects of sexual abuse. Obviously it will add to the child's sense of betrayal. Even when a disclosure is believed, the immediate effects of disclosure on the family may be extremely traumatising. Disruption of family relationships, suicide, and emotional turmoil and distress are all potentially harmful, certainly in the short term. A positive response and support of disclosure may be therapeutic in assisting the child and may have effects on such outcomes as the 'attitude to men' following abuse (Wyatt & Ray Mickey 1988). Many children still receive little in the way of therapeutic help or positive support, the most usual reaction, even when the abuse is acknowledged and acted upon, being 'to forget about it as quickly as possible' (Frothingham et al 1993).

Iatrogenic harm

It is important to distinguish between the crisis and distress following discovery, which in themselves have not been caused by the professional response, and true components of iatrogenic harm which certainly have (Jones 1991). Jones lists these as follows.

- *Overzealous professional intervention*: the crusader who may end up alienating parents and children alike.
- *Repeated interviewing, multiple interviews.* To this can be added extended, pressured interviews.
- *Repeated physical examinations* (physical examinations conducted against the wishes of the child or insensitively are also included).
- *Social and economic effects on the family.* These cannot in all fairness be called iatrogenic and society needs to confront the needs of families where enforced break-up has led to loss of income, loss of job, etc.
- *Defensive decision making.* Refusal to take any risk leading, for example, to unwarranted removal of the child from the family. It is preferable when possible of course, to remove the perpetrator, leaving the child at home.
- *Attendance in court.* There is evidence that this adds to the harm experienced by a sexually abused child (Flin & Bull 1989, Goodman et al 1989).
- *Withholding of treatment* (often it is simply not available or is withheld to spare the short-term distress often experienced at the beginning of therapy).
- *Overtreatment* for too long where change is impossible. This compounds the situation and the helplessness of the family where earlier use of statutory intervention would have been more helpful.
- *Fostering and residential care.* Further abuse may occur in care and this can be devastating for children placed there for protection. Children who have been sexually abused may be moved around as they are more difficult to care for. Lack of support for foster-parents and drift in placements all have professional components.

Summary

1. Child sexual abuse has recently been recognised as a major cause of morbidity in children of all ages, boys and girls.
2. Prevalence studies of adult survivors suggest substantial under-reporting by children, although reports have been increasing in many countries in recent times.
3. The abuse is an abuse of power and can be perpetrated by male and female adults, and teenagers, as well as older children.
4. Definitions emphasise the developmental immaturity of the child, the lack of consent and the sexual needs of the abuser as well as the deviant and coercive nature of the behaviour.
5. The abuse occurs within and without the family, in institutions, in organised rings, by perpetrators known or unknown to the child. Ritualistic abuse frequently involves sexual abuse.
6. There appear to be few factors which predispose the child to become a victim of sexual abuse, and all children are potentially at risk. The effects of sexual abuse on the child may predispose them to further abuse.
7. Investigators of child sexual abuse need to be aware that children develop complex adjustment behaviours to accommodate to the abuse. Although regular gross abuse is occurring the child may openly present as happy and coping well.
8. The accommodation syndrome includes: secrecy, helplessness, accommodation, delayed disclosure and retraction.
9. Abusers commit large numbers of deviant sexual acts, usually accompanied by denial and justification. The types of abuse include contact and non-contact, penetrative and non-penetrative acts. Prosecution is infrequent.
10. The available evidence indicates the harmful nature of sexual abuse and models for understanding the effects are helpful in helping children's and adults' problems. The harm may be short- or long-term.
11. Many factors influence the harm which children suffer after sexual abuse. The long-term outcome is affected by the child successfully revealing the abuse, being believed and being protected.
12. Professional interventions, while seeking to secure protection and support for the child, must avoid themselves adding to the child's distress.

REFERENCES

Abel G G, Becker J V, Murphy W D, Flanagan B 1981 Identifying dangerous child molesters. In: Stuart R B (ed) Violent behaviour. Brunner/Mayed, New York

Abel G G, Mittelman M S, Becker J V 1985 Sexual offenders: results of assessment and recommedations for treatment. In: Ben-Aron M H, Huckle S J, Webster C D (eds) Clinical criminology: the assessment and treatment of criminal behaviour. MM Graphic, Toronto, pp 191–205

Adams-Tucker C 1982 Proximate effects of sexual abuse in childhood. A report on 28 children. American Journal of Psychiatry 139:1252–1256

Aye Maving N 1995 Young people, victimisation and the police. British Crime Survey findings on experiences and attitudes of 12–15 year olds. Home Office Research and Statistics 140 HMSO, London

Badgley R et al (Committee on sexual offences against children and youth) 1984 Sexual offences against children, Vol 1. Canadian Government Publishing Center, Ottawa

Bagley R 1986 Disrupted childhood and vulnerability to sexual assault. Long-term sequels with implications for counselling. Social Work and Human Sexuality 4:33–48

Baker A, Duncan S 1985 Child sexual abuse: a study of prevalence in Great Britain. Child Abuse and Neglect 9:457–467

Becker J V 1988 The effects of child sexual abuse on adolescent sexual offenders. In: Wyatt G E, Powell G J (eds) Lasting effects of child sexual abuse. Sage, London, pp 193–207

Beckett R 1994 Assessment of sex offenders. In: Morrison T, Erooga M, Beckett R C (eds) Sexual offending against children – assessment and treatment of male abusers. Routledge, London 3:55–79

Bentovim A, Elton A, Hildebrand J, Tranter M, Vizard E 1988 Child sexual abuse within the family: assessment and treatment. Wright, London

Berliner L, Elliott D M 1996 Sexual abuse of children. In: Briere J et al (eds) The APSAC handbook on child maltreatment. Sage, London 3:51–71

Bernard P 1886 Des attentats a la pudeur sur les petites filles. Paris.

Briere J 1988 The long-term clinical correlates of childhood sexual victimization. Annals of the New York Academy of Sciences 528

Briere J, Runtz M 1988 Post sexual abuse trauma. In: Wyatt G P, Powell E J (eds) Lasting effects of child sexual abuse. Sage, London

Burgess A V 1984 Child pornography and sex rings. D C Heath, Lexington MA

Burgess A W, Groth A N, McCausland M P 1981 Child sex initiation rings. American Journal of Orthopsychiatry 51(1):110–119

Butler-Sloss E 1988 Report of the Inquiry into Child Abuse in Cleveland 1987. HMSO, London

Childhood Matters 1996 Report of the National Commission of Inquiry into the Prevention of Child Abuse. Vol 2 Background Papers. Stationery Office, London

Creighton S, Russell N 1995 Voices from childhood: a survey of childhood experiences and attitudes to child rearing among adults in the United Kingdom. NSPCC, London

Davenport C 1988 The traumatizing effects of child sexual abuse. Public and professional opinion. BSc thesis, University of Leicester

DHSS 1988 Guidance to doctors – diagnosis of child sexual abuse. HMSO, London

Donleavy J, Goodwin J 1989 What families say: the dialogue of incest in sexual abuse. In: Goodwin J (ed) Sexual abuse: incest victims and their families. Year Book Medical Publishers, Chicago, pp 65–82

Etherington K 1997 Maternal sexual abuse of males. Child Abuse Review 6:107–117

Finkelhor D 1979 Sexually victimized children. Free Press, New York

Finkelhor D 1996 Introduction. In: The APSAC handbook on child maltreatment. Sage, London

Finkelhor D, Browne A 1986 Initial and long term effects. A conceptual framework. In: A sourcebook on child sexual abuse. Sage, London, Chapter 6, pp 180–198

Finkelhor D, Williams L N, Burns N 1988 Nursery crimes – sexual abuse in day care. Sage, London

Finkelhor D, Moore D, Hamby S L, Strauss M A 1997 Sexually abused children in a national survey of parents: methodological issues. Child Abuse and Neglect 21:1–9

Flin R, Bull R 1989 Child witnesses in Scottish criminal proceedings. In: Spencer J R, Nicholson G, Flin R, Bull R (eds) Children's evidence in legal proceedings. Faculty of Law, University of Cambridge, pp 193–200

Fraser B G 1981 Sexual child abuse: the legislation and the law in the United States. In: Mrazek P B, Kempe C H (eds) Sexually abused children and their families. Pergamon, Oxford, pp 55–73

Freud S 1954 The origins of psychoanalysis: letters to Wilhelm Fliess. Drafts and notes 1887–1902. Bonaparte A, Freud A, Kris E (eds). Basic Books, New York

Fritz G S, Stoll K, Wagner N 1981 A comparison of males and females who were molested as children. Journal of Sex and Marital Therapy 7:54–59

Frothingham T E, Barnett R, Hobbs C J, Wynne J M 1993 Child sexual abuse in Leeds before and after Cleveland. Child Abuse Review 2:23–34

Furniss T 1984 Conflict-avoiding and conflict regulating patterns in incest and child sexual abuse. Acta Paediatrica Scandinavica 50:299–313

Giardino A P, Finkel M A, Giardino E R, Seidl T, Ludwig S 1992 The problem. In: A practical guide to the evaluation of sexual abuse in the prepubertal child. Sage, London

Glaser D, Frosh S 1988 Child sexual abuse. In: Myth and reality: the dimensions of child sexual abuse. Macmillan, London, Chapter 1

Goodman G S, Pyle E A, Jones D P H, England P, Port L K, Rudy L, Prado L 1989 Emotional effects of criminal court testimony on child sexual assault victims. Final report submitted to US National Institute of Justice, Grant number 85-IJ-CX-0020

Goodwin J M 1989a Recognising multiple personality disorder in adult incest victims. In: Goodwin J (ed) Sexual abuse: incest victims and their families, 2nd edn. Year Book Medical Publishers, Chicago

Goodwin J M 1989b Credibility problems in multiple personality disorder patients and abused children. In: Goodwin J (ed) Sexual abuse: incest victims and their families, 2nd edn. Year Book Medical Publishers, Chicago

Gorey K M, Leslie D R 1997 The prevalence of child sexual abuse: integrative review adjustment for potential response and measurement biases. Child Abuse and Neglect. 21:391–398

Groth A N 1982 The incest offender. In: Sgroi S (ed) Handbook of clinical intervention in child sexual abuse. Lexington Books, Lexington MA, pp 215–239

Hanks H, Saradjian G I 1991 Women who abuse children sexually: characteristics of sexual abuse of children by women. Journal of Systemic Consultation and Management 2:247–262

Hanks H G I, Hobbs C J, Wynne J M 1988 Early signs and recognition of sexual abuse in the pre-school child. In: Browne K, Davies C, Stratton P (eds) Early prediction and prevention of child abuse. J Wiley, Chichester

Hanson R K, Slater S 1988 Sexual victimization in the history of sexual abusers: a review. Annals of Sex Research 1:485–499

Harter S, Alexander P C, Neimeyer R A 1988 Long term effects of incestuous child abuse in college women. Social adjustment, social cognition and family characteristics. Journal of Consulting and Clinical Psychology 56(1):5–8

Hobbs C J, Wynne J M 1986 Buggery in childhood – a common syndrome of child abuse. Lancet II:793–796

Hobbs C J, Wynne J M 1987 Child sexual abuse – an increasing rate of diagnosis. Lancet II:837–841

James J, Meyerding J 1977 Early sexual experience and prostitution. American Journal of Psychiatry 134:1381–1385

Johnson T C 1996 Understanding children's sexual behaviors. What's natural and healthy. Available from T C Johnson, 1101 Fremont Ave, suite 101, South Pasadena, CA 91030, USA

Jones D P H 1991 Professional and clinical challenges to protection of children. Child Abuse and Neglect 15 (suppl 1):57–66

Kaufman J, Zigler E 1989 The intergenerational transmission of child abuse. In: Ciccheti D, Carlson V (eds) Child maltreatment. Cambridge University Press, Cambridge

Kelly L ,Regan L ,Burton S 1991 An exploratory study of the prevalence of sexual abuse in a sample of 16–21-year-olds. University of North London

Kempe R, Kempe C H 1984 The common secret: sexual abuse of children and adolescents. W H Freeman, New York

Knopp F H 1984 Retraining adult sex offenders: methods and models. Safer Society, Orwell, VT
Ligezinska M, Firestone P, Manion I, McIntyre J, Ensom R, Wells G 1996 Children's emotional and behavioral reactions following the disclosure of extrafamilial sexual abuse: initial effects. Child Abuse and Neglect 20:111–125
Mrazek P B, Lynch M, Bentovim A 1983 Sexual abuse of children in the United Kingdom. Child Abuse and Neglect 6:263–278
Mullen P E, Romans-Clarkson S E, Walton V A, Herbison G P 1988 Importance of sexual and physical abuse on women's mental health. Lancet ii:841–845
Muram D, Speck P M, Gold S S 1991 Genital abnormalities in female siblings and friends of child victims of sexual abuse. Child Abuse and Neglect 15:105–111
Nash C L, West D J 1985 Sexual molestation of young girls: a retrospective study. In: West D J (ed.) Sexual Victimisation. Gower, Aldershot.
Northern Ireland Research Team 1991 Child sexual abuse in Northern Ireland. Greystone, Belfast
Oliver J E 1983 Dead children from problem families in N E Wiltshire. British Medical Journal 286:115–117
Peters S D, Wyatt G E, Finkelhor D 1986 Prevalence. In: Finkelhor D (ed) A sourcebook on child sexual abuse. Sage, London, Chapter 1
Pilkington B, Kremer J 1995 A review of the epidemiological research on child sexual abuse. clinical samples. Child Abuse Review 4:191–205
Richardson S, Bacon H 1991 Child sexual abuse: whose problem? Reflections from Cleveland. Venture Press, Birmingham
Rogers C M, Terry T 1984 Clinical interventions with boy victims of sexual abuse. In: Stuart I, Greer J (eds) Victims of sexual aggression. Von Nostrand Rheinhold, New York, pp 91–104
Ronstrom A 1985 Sexual abuse of children in Sweden. Perspectives on research, intervention, consequences. Unpublished manuscript. Rodden Barren, Box 27320, Stockholm, Sweden
Russell D E H 1983 The incidence and prevalence of intrafamilial and extrafamilial sexual abuse of female children. Child Abuse and Neglect 7:133–146
Russell D E H 1986 The secret trauma: incest in the lives of girls and women. Basic Books, New York
Salter A C 1988a The role of the offender. In: Treating child sex offenders and victims. A practical guide. Sage, London, Chapter 3, pp 43–53
Salter A C 1988b Offender denial. In: Treating child sex offenders and victims. A practical guide. Sage, London, Chapter 8, pp 91–110
Schechter M, Roberge L 1976 Child sexual abuse. In: Helfer R, Kempe C (eds) Child abuse and neglect: the family and the community. Ballinger, Cambridge, MA
Sgroi S M 1978 Introduction: a national needs assessment for protecting child victims of sexual assault. In: Burgess A W, Groth A N, Holmstrom L L, Sgroi S M (eds) Sexual assault of children and adolescents. Lexington Books, Lexington, MA, pp xx–xxii
Smith M, Grocke M 1995 Normal family sexuality and sexual knowledge in children. Royal College of Psychiatrists/Gorkill Press, London
Summit R 1983 The child sexual abuse accommodation syndrome. Child Abuse and Neglect 1:177–193
Summit R C 1988 Hidden victims, hidden pain, societal avoidance of child sexual abuse. In: Wyatt G E, Powell G L (eds) Lasting effects of child sexual abuse. Sage, Beverley Hills, CA
Tardieu A 1860 Etude medico-legale sur les services et mauvais traitments exerces sur des enfants. Ann Hyg Pub Med Leg 13:361–393
Tsai M, Feldman-Summers J, Edgar M 1979 Childhood molestation: variables related to differential imparts on psychosexual function in adult women. Journal of Abnormal Psychology 88(4):407–417
Whitwell D 1990 The significance of childhood sexual abuse for adult psychiatry. British Journal of Hospital Medicine 43:346–352
Wild N J, Wynne J M 1986 Child sex rings. British Medical Journal 293:183–185
Wyatt G E, Powell G J 1988 Lasting effects of child sexual abuse. Parts II, III and IV. Sage, London
Wyatt G E, Ray Mickey M 1988 The support by parents and others as it mediates the effects of child sexual abuse. In: Wyatt G E, Powell G J (eds) Lasting effects of child sexual abuse. Sage, London

FURTHER READING

Arnold R P et al 1990 Medical problems of adults who were sexually abused in childhood. British Medical Journal 300:705–708
Brown R M et al 1989 Child sexual abuse presenting as organic disease. British Medical Journal 299:614–615
Leventhal J M 1988 Has there been a change in the epidemiology of sexual abuse of children during the 20th century? Pediatrics 82:766–773
Wilkins R 1990 Women who sexually abuse children. British Medical Journal 300:1153–1154

9

Clinical aspects of sexual abuse

PART 1

Presentation, related symptoms, medical examination

Wherever there are children, there will be sexually abused children; an increasing proportion of those children recognised to have been abused have been sexually abused (in 1983, 5% of registered abused children had been sexually abused, in 1995 23% of children on the child protection register had been sexually abused). It has been estimated that up to 100 000 children each year have a potentially harmful sexual experience (Childhood Matters 1996)

The recognition of child sexual abuse depends upon the adult ability to acknowledge that abuse might occur and so be prepared to see and hear. This means not only recognising the warning signs or hearing a disclosure, but also knowing how to handle this concern, or cope with an apparently clear allegation. It is evident that some seriously sexually abused children may not manifest any signs or symptoms; this, however, does not mean that all is well with the child, as is seen for example when one child in a family discloses and it becomes apparent that others in the family have also been abused. When children disclose it is sometimes obvious in retrospect that there were signs which could have been seen. The non-disclosing child may be the more damaged child in a family, and all siblings should be examined (Muram et al 1991).

The emotional distress of a child does of course vary with the child, the abuse, the abuser and the frequency of the abuse, but almost all children subsequently say how much they disliked the abuse (see Ch 8). Children have a right to a childhood free of abuse: that they do not complain, appear clinically distressed or disturbed does not mean that they are not suffering.

There is an increasing debate concerning the role of child sexual abuse in the subsequent physical and mental health of adults; of course most of this abuse was undisclosed in childhood (Peters 1988, Arnold et al 1990, Whitwell 1990). It is probable that boys suffer equally with girls and find disclosure even more difficult. Ideally, children would have the confidence to speak out and expect their parents to protect them; if the abuse is intrafamilial a child's mother may not protect, and then others must listen and act.

Historically it has always been known that some children are victims of child sexual abuse, but the usual notion has been of a teenage girl complaining of sexual abuse by her stepfather. The recognition that sexual abuse may involve the very young, boys as well as girls, and may involve serious assault such as oral, vaginal or anal abuse, is relatively new, although the forensic literature does contain much that is relevant to the current debate (Paul 1984, de la Haye Davies 1987).

Advice and guidance for professionals

- Cleveland Inquiry Report (Butler-Sloss 1988)
- Working Together (1988, 1991) the official guides to arrangements for inter-agency cooperation for the protection of children from abuse.
- Diagnosis of Child Sexual Abuse: Guidance for Doctors (DHSS 1988) gives a framework for doctors to work within clinically
- The American Academy of Pediatrics has published comprehensive guidelines (AAP 1991)
- The Royal College of Physicians of London reported on the physical signs of sexual abuse in children (RCP 1991, 1997)
- Memorandum of Good Practice (HMSO 1992) provides advice on videotaped interviews with child witnesses for criminal proceedings

Referral

Adults are increasingly recognising and listening to children when they speak of abuse. Until professional management improves, children may well feel that it is safer to keep quiet, and abusers have much invested in denial. For the minority of children who are identified, there should be access to a system which is supportive, accepting and helpful in the long term, even if the short term may be emotionally distressing.

All professionals dealing with children should understand local procedures (see Fig. 9.1). A doctor may see a child because of concern voiced by another professional, the child, or the child's family, or another third party. The complaint may be of abuse or one of several presentations for which child sexual abuse may be the underlying cause. The general practitioner will see the child in a health centre, and the paediatrician in a local clinic or hospital. If the parents initially take the child to a police station, the child should not be examined there but referred on, usually to the local district hospital for examination within the child health department. The child is the victim and should not be examined in a police station.

Doctors should not work alone in this field. They should seek advice, cooperate with other agencies and take appropriate responsibilities. If the initial doctor does not feel confident to undertake the physical examination, he or she should refer to an appropriate colleague or arrange a joint examination with an experienced colleague. If the child has presented by disclosing, e.g. to a teacher, a 'planning meeting' should be held (see Fig. 9.1).

A decision whether to refer a particular case of possible child sexual abuse to social services will depend upon the level of concern following the paediatric assessment and discussion with the health visitor or general practitioner, for example. Table 9.1 gives guidelines to help make this decision.

For other children – referred by teachers or nursery nurses to social services, or children referred directly to the police – the decision whether a full child protection investigation is indicated may be made before or after referral to

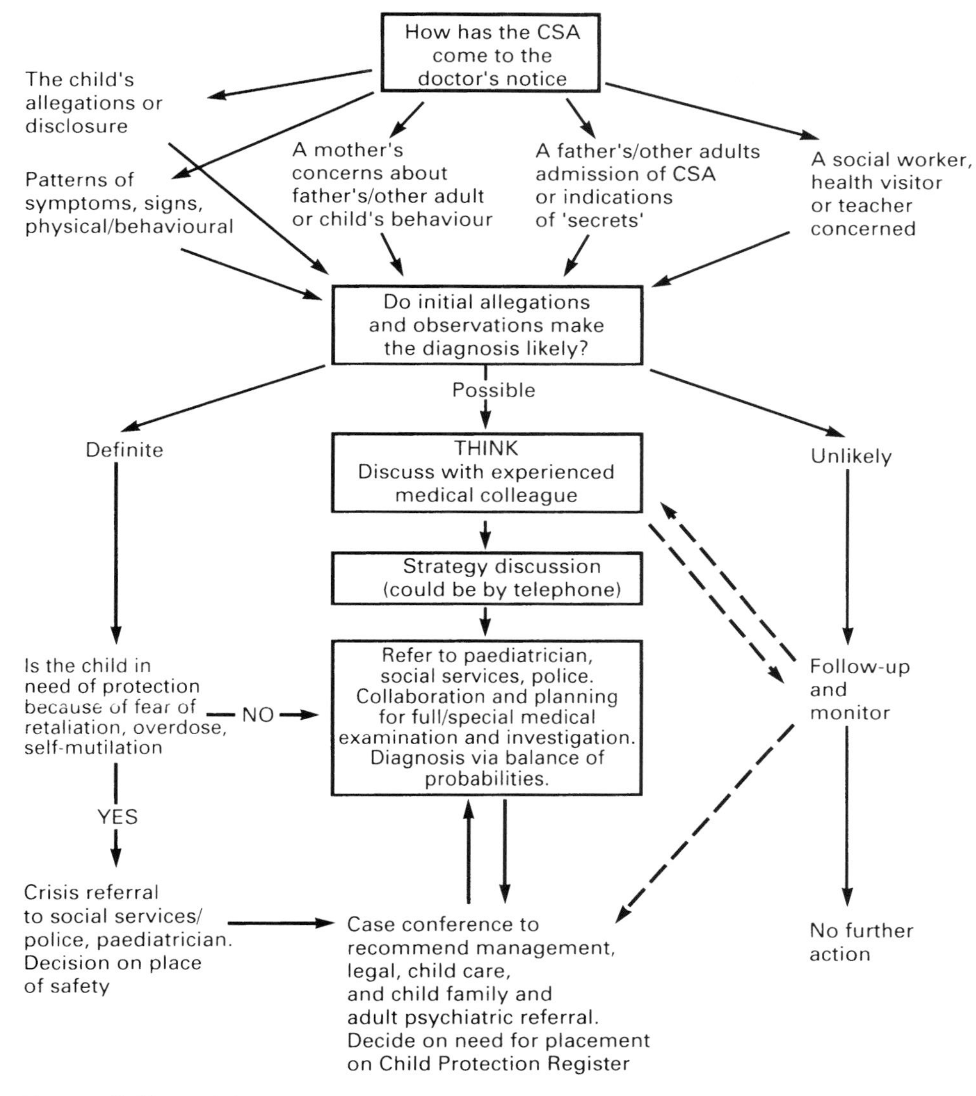

Fig. 9.1 Child sexual abuse. The role of the initial medical contact (i.e. family doctor, A&E, STD, etc.). (Reproduced with permission from Diagnosis of Child Sexual Abuse: Guidance for Doctors (DHSS 1988.)

the paediatrician, depending upon the circumstances. Working Together (1991) gives details of inter-agency working.

Consent to examination should be informed and is equally valid whether given orally or in writing. If a child is capable of understanding the nature and purpose of the examination then he or she is capable of giving consent. The DoH Guidance to the Children Act (DoH 1991) makes it clear that it is the doctor's responsibility to help the child to understand and also to come to a decision as to the child's capability.

The components of informed consent have been described (BAAF 1991) as an understanding of:

- the nature of the examination
- the immediate purpose of the examination

Table 9.1 Guidelines for making the decision to report child sexual abuse to social services (after AAP 1991, RCP 1991, 1997)

History	Examination	Laboratory investigation	Concern	Report
None	Normal	None	None	None
Behavioural changes	Normal	None	Low	±[c]
None	Supportive[a]	None	Possible	±[c] FU[d]
History from parents	Supportive[a]	None	Possible	±[c] FU[d]
None	Diagnostic[b]	None	Probable	Refer[e]
Clear statement	Normal	None	Probable	Refer[e]
Clear statement	Diagnostic[b]	None	Probable	Refer[e]
None	Normal	Gonorrhoea		
Supportive	Semen	Definite	Refer[e]	
Diagnostic	Pregnancy			
Behavioural changes	Supportive	Other STD	Probable	Refer[e]

FU, follow up; STD, sexually transmitted disease.
[a] A supportive physical examination includes signs, e.g. enlarged hymenal opening, scar at posterior fourchette (RCP 1991).
[b] A diagnostic sign includes, e.g., laceration extending beyond the anal mucosa on to the perianal skin (RCP 1991).
[c] Consider reporting on basis of information gathered.
[d] Follow up all cases if there are continuing concerns or unexplained behaviours or physical signs. If in doubt discuss with colleagues and senior social worker.
[e] Suggests that the case should be referred to social services; these children are usually followed up, at least in the short term.

- to whom the resulting information will be given
- the implications for others (this is not the child's responsibility).

From the age of 16 years a child is regarded in law as capable of giving consent. Depending on their level of understanding, younger teenagers or children may give consent. Parental consent must be sought in all situations apart from the above, unless parental responsibilities are invested elsewhere. If in doubt, seek legal advice and remember that if court proceedings are in process the court's permission is needed.

The commonest form of lack of consent is by teenagers, who find physical examination particularly difficult. A follow-up appointment is usually offered in these circumstances.

The more detailed aspects of consent are described in Chapter 14.

Responsibility of examining doctor

- Take a full history
- Physically examine the child if appropriate
- 'Whole child' examination to include growth and development
- Take swabs as indicated:
  - STD screen
  - forensic swabs
- Arrange further investigations as indicated:
  - blood count
  - clotting screen
  - skeletal survey
  - pregnancy test
  - HIV antibody test
  - hepatitis B antibody test
- Talk to child and carers and explain findings
- Check results of swabs and tests
- Talk to other professionals, often before examination has been arranged; include social services and police as indicated
- Write report for GP, Child Health (Community Services) and social services
- Write police statement on request
- Attend case conference
- Attend court
- Arrange follow-up paediatrically
- Refer for treatment of:
  - mental health, e.g. child psychologist or psychiatrist

  - physical complications, e.g. anal warts to paediatric surgeon
- Refer for second (paediatric) opinion)

Joint medical examinations

Joint examinations are examinations undertaken by more than one medical practitioner where the practitioners have separate clinical responsibilities. The police surgeon is employed by the police authority to examine the child and to provide a report for possible criminal proceedings. The paediatrician has a wider responsibility in the short and longer term (see above). However, there are advantages in working with a colleague with complementary skills, although the indications for such examinations are likely to become fewer as paediatricians have more experience of examining sexually abused children.

One example where a paediatrician is likely to request the help of an experienced police surgeon is in a case of stranger rape, when collection of forensic samples, for example fibres, is very important and better done by an experienced practitioner.

Ultimately, as in physical abuse, neglect and all other forms of child abuse, paediatricians will accept responsibility for the examinations, not least because of the long-term sequelae of abuse and consequent need for ongoing care.

It is also necessary to evaluate the efficacy and cost of medicals. Two doctors cost more, there is often considerable waiting time for the child, family and professionals, and the child has two doctors examining him or her (it is a two in one examination, rather than a single one). If there is a conflict of medical opinion, usually over the interpretation of physical signs rather than the signs themselves, it may be very difficult for the social services department to protect and the police to proceed.

Also, if a police surgeon is present the parents must know and this may escalate the investigation in an unhelpful way when it is at a preliminary stage.

Confidentiality

The doctor may be referred to a child where there has been a clear disclosure; alternatively, the suggestion of child sexual abuse may arise during the course of the interview or examination. In the latter case, the doctor may have immediate concerns and feel it necessary to refer to the statutory agencies at once, or in other situations to follow up over weeks or months while collecting further information (Table 9.1).

Once the doctor has reached a point of some concern, he or she should report; confidentiality to child or family is secondary – the General Medical Council states

> 'if you believe a patient to be a victim of neglect or physical or sexual abuse, and unable to give or withold consent to disclosure, you should usually give information to an appropriate responsible person or statutory agency, in order to prevent further harm to the patient'. (GMC 1996)

The diagnostic process in child sexual abuse

The diagnostic process here does not differ from that of any disorder in medicine, except that it is usually complex and sooner or later involves information gathering by other agencies such as social services and the police (Working Together 1988, 1991). As in other disorders, a diagnosis is built up gradually, starting with the history, followed by physical examination and laboratory investigation. Physical, emotional and sexual abuse may all coexist, and the child's growth, development and behaviour should also be considered. Consider the diagnosis as a 'jigsaw' and piece together all the information (Table 9.2).

There are, however, certain points which must be taken into account. The examination of a child who may have been abused is essentially a forensic examination. Although the examining doctor may think he or she is dealing with a child who presents with bed wetting, there may be signs suggesting that the child is a victim of sexual abuse. The doctor may refer the child on for a

Table 9.2 The clinical jigsaw in child sexual abuse

Child's story or disclosure	+	Parents' history	+	Other third party, e.g. nursery nurse observation
Child's past medical history	+	Family history	+	Child's development
Child's physical growth	+	Child's emotional/behavioural state	+	Physical examination
Medical investigations, e.g. STD	=	Initial medical opinion	+	Social work investigations
Police investigation	+	Further opinion	=	Proven abuse (rarely) or probable abuse or possible abuse or abuse unlikely

Medical notes

- Notes should be written at the time of examination (contemporaneously) or immediately afterwards
- Notes should be clear, concise and contain details or questions asked: for example 'no urinary symptoms' is better than nothing, but 'no dysuria, frequency, urgency or haematuria' is better still. Initials such as 'NAD' are not helpful when discussing the physical examination later – what actually was done?
- Any spontaneous remarks made by the child during the examination should be recorded verbatim, as with any answers to questions: e.g. 'What made your tuppence sore?', answered by 'Daddy with his finger like this . . .' and record what the child demonstrates
- Record injuries appropriately: line drawings with annotations are the clearest, suitable charts are available. Describe bruises by position, size, colour (rough age) and think how they may have been caused. Burns, scratches and lacerations are also measured and described (Chs 4 and 5)
- Record abnormalities of the genitalia or anus, again a line drawing is helpful
- In the rare cases of recent assault, usually stranger rape, other factors are important to avoid losing valuable contact evidence. A good description is given in forensic medicine textbooks. A joint medical examination with an experienced police surgeon is useful here (Paul 1984, McLay 1990a, RCP 1991)
- Record which investigations were performed; and ensure results are obtained. Were photographs taken? If used in court proceedings these may need to be sworn by the photographer (Ch 4)
- Record any treatment given
- Indicate if follow-up was arranged

more specialised examination but the initial notes may be required by the court at a later stage.

Presentation of child sexual abuse

Disclosure

The presentation of child sexual abuse is summarised in Table 9.3. Disclosure of abuse by the child is of itself the most important piece of the 'diagnostic jigsaw' (see Table 9.2). When work in child sexual abuse began, the majority of investigations were instigated by an allegation of abuse by the child. But, as professionals have recognised other signs which may be indicative of abuse, the concept of 'disclosure work' began. Jones defined such work as 'the process by which professionals attempt to encourage or hasten the natural process of disclosure by a sexually abused child' (Butler-Sloss 1988, Pt 2 Ch. 11, Jones & McQuiston 1988, Cleveland Report, p. 204).

Some children 'disclose' spontaneously. Disclosure is defined by Jones & McQuiston as

> a clinically useful concept to describe the process by which a child who has been sexually abused (within the family) gradually comes to inform the outside world of his plight.

The young child may speak innocently of behaviour which the adult recognises as abuse. Older children decide to tell, usually in an attempt to stop the abuse and maybe to protect younger siblings. A spontaneous unprompted statement by a child is the most reliable way in which child sexual abuse may be acknowledged.

The question is often asked, how often do children make it up? The answer is that a deliberate fabrication is unusual – largely restricted to older children – and that young children cannot

Table 9.3 Presentation of child sexual abuse (Vizard & Tranter 1988)

Disclosure	By child or third party
Physical indicators	Rectal or vaginal bleeding, pain on defecation
	Sexually transmitted disease (STD)
	Vulvovaginitis/vaginal discharge/'sore'
	Dysuria and frequency? UTI
	Physical abuse, note association of burns, pattern of injury, death
	Pregnancy
Psychosomatic indicators	Recurrent abdominal pain
	Headache, migraine
	Anorexia or other eating disorders
	Encopresis
	Enuresis
	Total refusal syndrome
Behavioural indicators	
Pre-school	Sexually explicit play, 'excessive' masturbation, insertion of foreign bodies (girls), self-mutilation, withdrawn, poor appetite, sleep disturbance, clingy, delayed development, aggression
Middle years	Sexualised play, sexually explicit drawing or sexual precocity, self-mutilation, anxiety, depression, anger, poor school performance, mute
Teenagers	Sexually precocious, prostitution, anxiety, anger, aggression, depression, truancy, running away, solvent/alcohol/drug abuse, self-destructive behaviour, overdoses, self-mutilation, suicide
Learning problems or physical handicap (see Ch 10)	May present with depression, disturbed (including aggressive) behaviour
	Sexualised behaviour
	Attempts at disclosure not understood
	May be physical and psychosomatic indicators as above
Social indicators (see Ch 8)	Concern by parent or third party, sibling, relative or friend of abused child
	Schedule I offender in close contact with child

See also Table 9.9 for specific emotional and behavioural indicators.

fantasise specific sexual acts that they have not experienced.

The incidence of false allegations in various studies ranges from 0.5% to 8% in samples including all kinds of situations. Higher figures have been reported from studies of allegations made during the course of custody and access disputes.

There are a number of ways that false allegations may arise.

- They may arise in the mind of an adult, either a carer or a professional, and be erroneous but sincere or false.
- A parent may misinterpret a child's statement/behaviour, or a physical condition.
- A parent might indoctrinate a child into believing that someone had abused them, an interview may be frankly suggestive, or a parent may suffer from a delusion.
- Another possible explanation may be group contagion – but sexual abuse may also occur to groups of children.
- Finally, a child who makes a false allegation may do so at the request of a parent, or for revenge –the 'true' false allegation.

It is generally recognised that very few children lie about sexual abuse, and the few who do will tend to be emotionally disturbed teenagers. If children complain of re-abuse, they are also to be believed in the first instance, as evidence suggests that they rarely lie. The simple rule is: believe the child initially, and test the statement later.

In disputed custody cases allegations of child sexual abuse should be taken seriously and evaluated rigorously. Many allegations are subsequently validated (MacFarlane 1986).

Children usually tell someone whom they trust, whether this is initially a friend, family member or professional (teacher, school nurse, doctor). After initial 'disclosure' and a strategy discussion between professionals, a formal interview will take place; recently this has usually taken the form of a joint interview conducted by a social worker and police officer from a child abuse unit.

Interviews

Interviewing should be undertaken by staff who have undergone appropriate staff development and training (Working Together 1991). The number of investigative interviews should be kept to a minimum (Butler-Sloss 1988), but although some children who are ready to talk are able to disclose the details of their abuse in one or two interviews, other children 'frozen' by fear or anxiety may only come to talk of their abuse over months to years. This is an unresolved clinical dilemma. There are also children with communication difficulties or who have English as a second language who need interviewers with particular skills.

If an assessment is undertaken in the course of court proceedings the court's agreement is needed as the evidence may not be used in court unless the court agrees.

Recorded interviews

Recording of interviews should be accurate and differentiate between fact, hearsay and opinion.

Video or audio tapes have been made of interviews with the intention of avoiding repeated interviews, and the Pigot Committee (Pigot 1989) had hoped that they would be admissible in criminal court without the need for the child to be present and to be cross-examined. Under the Criminal Justice Act 1991 a video recording may be used as the child's main evidence in certain circumstances, but the child must also be available for cross-examination. The child in court may be helped by the use of screens and contemporaneous video links.

The Memorandum of Good Practice (HMSO 1992) provides assistance to those interviewing children and making a video recording of the interview. It includes the requirements of the Criminal Justice Act 1988 on when, where and how to make a video recording, including the equipment to use and the standards to aim for. There is detailed information about the conduct of the interview, the use of dolls and other props. There is also guidance on the security and storage of tapes.

An important part is the legal constraints and the rules of evidence including the avoidance of leading questions. Hearsay evidence is allowable in family proceeding courts but not in criminal courts.

If videotapes are not made to a very high standard they will not help the child as legal arguments dismiss the evidence. Similarly, minor inconsistencies in evidence given in court when compared with the videotape will imply that the child is unreliable or lying.

Effects on the child

Current research in the UK shows that children who do give evidence have more anxiety symptoms up until the trial than those who do not give evidence, and this manifest anxiety persists for the following 12 months before their levels of anxiety fall to levels of the non-evidence-giving victims.

If the alleged abuser is convicted this may be enabling to the child, but if an abuser is acquitted, for whatever reason, the child may be devastated, feeling that this is a public statement that he or she was lying (Pigot 1989, Spencer & Flin 1990, Smith & Wilson 1991, Spencer 1991).

In a comparative study in Leeds of practices in 1985–86 and 1989 the percentage of cases where the perpetrator was convicted fell from 25% to 5% (Frothingham et al 1992). The reasons for this are speculative.

The current position in the UK remains that children may be better protected in family proceedings court by the use of videotapes of well-conducted interviews, but many parents and professionals caring for children are wary about submitting them to the trauma of an appearance as a prosecution witness in a criminal court. Davies et al have reported on recent practice.

How to interview children

In thinking about interviewing sexually abused children it is important to think of their predicament and to remember that most children do not tell.

- The child has been exploited and misused.
- The person who has exploited them is more powerful than they are.
- Disclosure of sexual abuse is very frequently delayed especially if abuse is by a relative or someone known to the child than by a stranger.

- Victims are frequently disbelieved, subtly or openly admonished or silenced.
- With our increasing knowledge of abuser behaviour, including grooming and manipulation of the child, it is understandable how a child will often have been made to feel responsible for the abuse.
- Children may feel guilt connected to their participation in the abuse, loss of the warmth which the abuser may have provided, and responsible for the fall-out – family break-up, etc.
- Children therefore often disclose in situations of relative safety, e.g. bedtime, to trusted adult, if parents have separated, if in foster home, etc.

Children may be helped to talk using play materials, including anatomically complete dolls, drawing, and plasticine (Table 9.4; Figs 9.2–9.5). However, it must be remembered that in helping the child to tell (Bentovim et al 1988, Glaser & Frosh 1988, Siran et al 1988, Glaser & Collins 1989, Jones & McQuiston 1992) the possibilities are:

- the abuse has occurred and the child is speaking of it
- the abuse has occurred and the child is unable to speak of it or is denying it

Table 9.4 Use of anatomically complete dolls and line drawings

Dolls	Drawings
Sexually explicit play is suggestive of child sexual abuse	May enable child to describe abuse
Non-abused children do not enact adult sexual behaviour	Sexually explicit drawings may be the child's way of disclosing abuse
Abused children may play non-sexually with dolls	The child may find it easier to complete outline figure provided by examiner
Abused children are more likely to treat the male doll roughly	
Helpful to elucidate abuse in young, shy, developmentally slow children	
May cause abused child great distress	
Should be used by skilled professional	

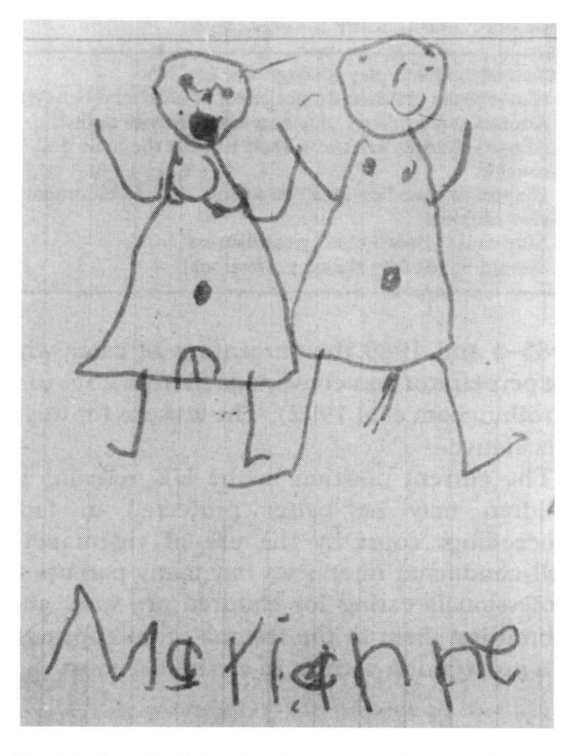

Fig. 9.2 Sexualised drawings by a girl aged 7 years who later disclosed child sexual abuse by her father after reception into care following physical abuse of her brother aged 5 years.

- the abuse has not occurred and the child cannot speak of it.

There are several levels at which this work may be done, and the use of leading, alternative or hypothetical questions should be left to those with special expertise. This may also apply to the use of the anatomically complete dolls.

The following types of interview are described.

- *Screening*, e.g. has anyone touched you down there? This is usually with parent present. Child sexual abuse should be introduced into everyday practice for psychiatrist, paediatrician, social worker, etc.
- *Investigative interview* (usually joint police/social services) to discover whether abuse has happened and as much detail as possible (HMSO 1992).

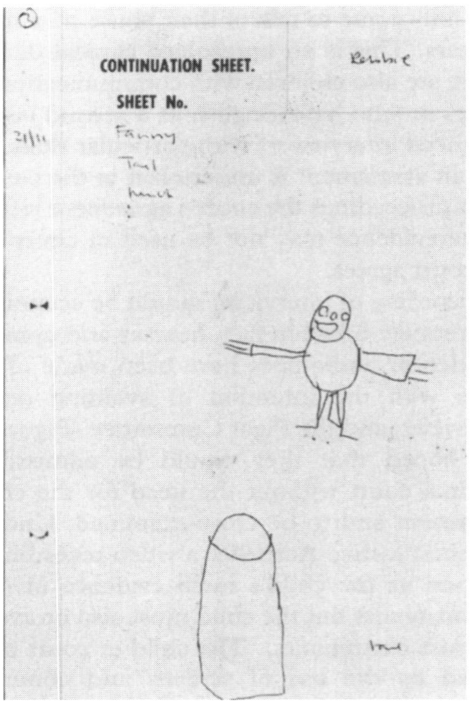

Fig. 9.3 A girl aged 8 years, unable to talk of abuse but in answer to the question 'Why are you sore?' drew a man with a phallus and, by way of further explanation, the enlargement.

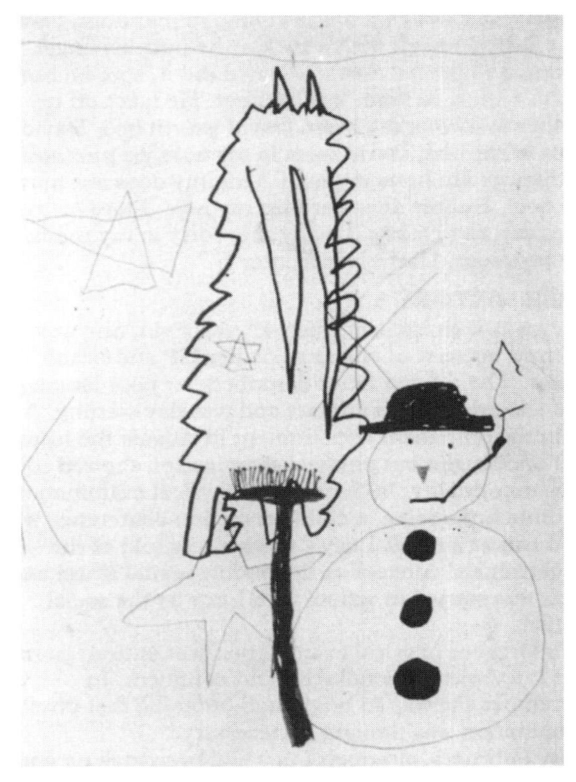

Fig. 9.4 Drawing by a girl aged 6 years with recurrent vaginal discharge and nightmares involving a monster who came to her bed. She later disclosed abuse by her grandfather.

Basic principles of interviewing children

- Interviews for children who 'may' have been sexually abused, i.e open-mindedness
- Don't make promises you can't keep, e.g. 'if you tell me I'll protect you'
- You may need to plan more than one interview
- Go at the child's speed
- Accept that not all children will be able to say when we are sure there is something to say
- Children may tell someone of their choice but not repeat to others in more formal setting, e.g. formal video interview (Glaser 1995)
- Use open, not leading, questions
- Balance need to know against harm of repeated interviewing
- Interviewer must be trained and supported

- *Facilitative interviews* (high levels of suspicion in children with learning difficulties, communication difficulties, psychiatric disorder associated with the abuse, or considerable delays since allegations first made (Bentovim et al 1988). These require special knowledge and skill.

Anatomically correct dolls

The use of anatomically correct dolls has been researched (Glaser & Collins 1989). Possible uses include:

- as an icebreaker – to talk about sexuality
- to assess child's terminology
- as a demonstration – show and tell
- as a memory stimulus to trigger recall

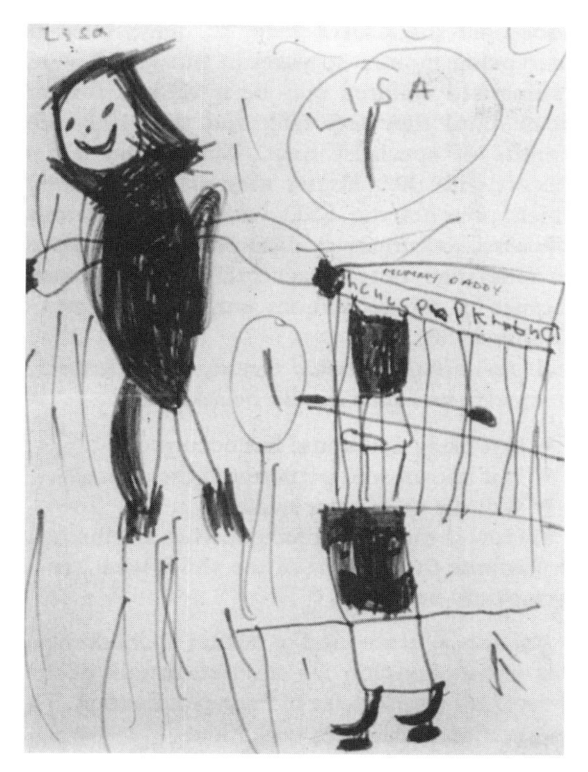

Fig. 9.5 Drawing by a girl aged 7 years explaining that she only felt safe from sexual abuse while her father was in prison.

- as a screening tool – give the dolls to the child and see what happens
- interviewer needs training.

It is important to remember that the dolls are not suggestive or over-stimulating. Their use can help in revealing a child's knowledge. Explicit sexual positioning is normally rare and much more likely to be related to prior experience. The abused chld may demonstrate sexually explicit play. Aggression toward the dolls is another important finding.

Interviewing environment

Interviewing should feel safe and relaxed for the child and be uninterrupted. Children should be interviewed in a suitable and sensitive environment (Butler-Sloss 1988).

Interviews are inevitably part investigation, part assessment and part therapeutic. The dilemma of this situation has not been resolved. The therapeutic needs of the child are not the same as the requirements of the legal system, and the interviewer has to focus on the aim of the interview whilst recognising the need to be sensitive to the child's feelings.

The interviewer should be trained and on occasion have special skills; for example be fluent in sign language for a severely hearing impaired child. The gender of the interviewer is important – most teenage girls would prefer to talk to a woman. If joint interviews are undertaken, one worker leads the interview and the other observes. Children from a young age are interviewed apart from their parents but often one of the interviewers has a relationship with the child, albeit a very recent one.

The interviewer should be well briefed before the session and have a relevant knowledge of the child and his or her family. The interview should have a structure which allows later analysis. Good descriptions of interviewing technique are available (Glaser & Frosh 1988, Vizard & Tranter 1988, Furniss 1991, Jones & McQuiston 1992).

Recording is important and may be by contemporaneous note taking, video or audio taping (see above).

The function of the interview is to:

- investigate the possibility of child sexual abuse
- validate the child's allegations
- assess the child's need for protection
- assess the need for ongoing therapy.

Contents of the interview

As previously described, the interview should be child-centred and child-led. Most sessions start with a rapport building phase and then move on to a free narrative account with the child encouraged to use their own words. Drawing is often helpful in children of 5 years and over. At this stage the use of anatomically complete dolls with younger children (under 7 years) or developmentally delayed or very shy children may be very helpful (see above). The third stage is the questioning phase, starting with the use of open-ended questions and moving on to specific yet non-leading questions. This may include direct enquiry about events, people and places. Whichever method is used, the child must know the context of the interview but care is needed to avoid asking leading questions.

The number of interviews needed to make a proper assessment varies but primarily investigative interviews are usually limited to 1–3. Therapeutic work is described in Chapter 15. Additional disclosures may be made over the intervening months to years in therapy. Severely traumatised children may be unable to communicate until they feel safe, and then only after months of specialist help. While they are in contact with their abuser they may never speak, which presents the social services department with a real dilemma. Likewise, information disclosed in therapeutic sessions may not be acceptable to the courts because of the techniques employed (Vizard & Tranter 1988).

At the end of the initial investigative interview(s) the questions which should be asked are:

- Is it likely that abuse has occurred?
- Is it known who perpetrated the abuse?
- Will the child be protected?
- How is the child affected, what are the plans to continue the support of the child, what are his or her therapeutic needs?

Paediatricians are used to talking to children and it is not uncommon for children to talk of their abuse during the course of their examination. This information needs later validation.

Problems of investigative work

There are major problems inherent in investigative work. Firstly, the child may not be ready to tell. Children formerly have told when they have been ready – unfortunately the need for a 'completed' investigation within a few days (the usual requirement of the police) means children may be under pressure to tell their story and, rather than being encouraged to tell, just clam up or retract. Investigations should be conducted at the pace of the child not the professional.

Research has been conducted into the accuracy of children's statements.

The child's disclosure – is it true?

- The more detail that is recalled the more likely it is to be truthful
- Do the core elements of the story remain consistent?
- Distinguishing details, e.g. taste of semen, smell, 'knife in bum', are not learned from watching sexually explicit material on TV or videos
- Children are known to recall events accurately from pre-verbal stage of development
- Children's memory is no less accurate than adults but children tend to recall less detail. Children relate events within the limits of their language and understanding
- Children can place events in correct temporal order
- Recantations are uncommon, stereotyped, and often use incongruous language
- Children may be silenced by fear, coercion or anxiety
- Children cannot fantasize sexual acts of which they have no experience

Current problems in investigative interviews/children's evidence

The Davies Report was commissioned to report on the workings of the 1991 Criminal Justice Act and the 1992 Memorandum of Good Practice (Davies et al 1995). Concerns raised by professionals included the stress and trauma to the child, particularly of cross-examination, that videos had less impact on juries, and that many of the interviews were legally unacceptable. The report included an analysis of 40 tapes, all of more than 1 hour duration. Although a clear account was given of abuse in 75%, surprisingly 30% were thought to be of no evidential value. The inordinately large number of tapes made in comparison to the very few used in court has pointed to enormous wastage and the need for careful pre-interview assessment and screening.

Despite this there is also evidence of a higher rate of late guilty pleas when application to show the video is made (Glaser 1995).

Criminal prosecution problems included:

- low rate of prosecution
- pre-trial delays
- effects on child witnesses
- low credibility of child.

Current provisions for child witnesses include:

- live TV link
- videotaped interviews at trial in place of child's evidence in chief
- right to cross-examination retained
- Memorandum of Good Practice (HMSO 1992) – guidelines for conduct of interviews.

CASE HISTORY 9.1

Stephen, aged 7 years, was seen at the request of social services as bruising had been noticed by the school nurse. The NSPCC had previously had an anonymous allegation about a 'beating'. Stephen presented as a frightened, underweight, quiet boy with a swollen upper lip and scattered bruises on his back and physical signs compatible with anal abuse.

After examination Stephen was asked 'What makes your bottom sore?' He said, without further questioning but with palpable anxiety, 'Daddy does it . . . lean over bed . . . puts willy in bum, puts willy in mouth . . . willy stands up – goes big . . . sticky stuff comes out . . . it's different from wee, it's got a bad taste – I spit it out. In Daddy's bedroom, lean over bed . . . Mummy knows – seen him do it. Daddy does it.'

CASE HISTORY 9.2

Sarah, aged 4½ years, was seen at the request of social services following referral by her school. She had been playing in the Wendy house when she told the teacher that she went in bed with daddy and he had a stick and hurt her. There was also a history of daytime wetting, occasional soiling and delayed language development. Sarah was a small, sad girl with signs compatible with anal abuse.

She was spoken to alone and would not engage in free play. She repeated 'I want Debbie' (her mother). When asked 'Did anyone hurt you?' she said 'I want Debbie' but went on 'I was crying, in my room, David (her father) hurt it with a stick – he puts his finger . . . (pointed to genital area) – David did it, sore on bum, it was a stick, in bum, lots of times. He takes off my clothes to look at my bum. David gets in bed, David wees in my bed, David wees in my hole, he puts stuff in there. . . . He hurts my hole. Mummy does not hurt my hole. Debbie does not hurt my hole. I love Mummy and Daddy. Daddy says sorry in my room, in my bedroom. David is nice after'.

CASE HISTORY 9.3

Lucy was seen initially when 4½ years old. She was referred because of concerns by her general practitioner and health visitor. The referral letter described her poor language, that she avoided eye contact and was day-wetting. At an initial outpatient appointment in August the history was unchanged but physical examination showed some anal abnormality. In September physical examination was much the same, a child protection conference was held and as a result Lucy's mother was told of the professionals' concern as to possible sexual abuse and work was started in school with Lucy by the social worker.

In October physical examination was entirely normal and Lucy was more talkative and confident. In December she was so bright and outgoing that physical examination was thought unnecessary.

By February, although Lucy had been making good progress generally, there had been two episodes at school when she had been very withdrawn and it was noticed she was becoming aggressive towards her mother. As her behaviour had changed a physical examination was performed and there were minimal genital signs but marked anal signs consistent with abuse. When asked directly what had happened, Lucy said 'A man has hurt my bum and my tuppence. He hurt it with a knife. He didn't say he was sorry. In my bedroom. It's my Daddy'.

CASE HISTORY 9.4

Susan and Elizabeth were aged 4 years and 6 years and seen because of anonymous allegations to the

NSPCC about child sexual abuse. They were very frightened. Neither child would talk and physical examination was normal. When given the anatomically complete dolls, Elizabeth demonstrated oral sex and said the names of her two elder brothers and father. She then put the penis of the man doll between the girl doll's legs and said 'Daddy'. She became very upset and started to cry. The younger sister would not hold the dolls and just looked frightened.

Elizabeth said 'Mummy knows what happens'. The older brothers (aged 8 and 10 years) subsequently made full disclosures of abuse involving both parents and all four children.

Note that currently few paediatricians would use the dolls in an interview like this because of the need for later validation. However, with young or developmentally delayed children paediatricians do have skills which are of use in assessing such children where others are unable to successfully communicate due to lack of experience and expertise.

CASE HISTORY 9.5

Naseem, an Asian girl aged 9 years, was noticed to be unhappy at school. She was thin, and rocked to and fro. She was referred because of her unhappy behaviour, low weight and vaginal discharge. Physical signs were compatible with vaginal interference. Work with the family was unsuccessful and eventually Naseem was taken into care because of emotional abuse and failure to thrive. The question of child sexual abuse was unanswered.

Three days before the final hearing at court, Naseem wrote to the social worker and told of the sexual abuse by her father at home. The fear of returning home following the court hearing was finally greater than the fear of her father.

Physical indicators of child sexual abuse

Physical indicators are important as they may give the first sign that all is not well with the child. They may be the only sign in infants or young children or in other children who, for whatever reason, cannot communicate. They may corroborate the child's story. The significance of a particular indicator is variable, for example vaginal bleeding is a symptom which should always be thoroughly investigated and a sign such as laceration of the hymen is of the highest significance (in the absence of a history of accidental penetration). Caution is needed in the interpretation of signs and symptoms and time is often needed to build up the diagnostic jigsaw (Table 9.2).

It is much easier for a doctor when examining a child who has disclosed abuse to explain that certain physical signs are consistent with abuse; it is much more difficult if similar signs are found incidentally (Table 9.1). Management of such cases needs careful planning and it may be only after weeks to months or even years that the whole picture emerges. In the meantime the child lives in a possibly abusive home, but the limitations of medical examination must be acknowledged (Butler-Sloss 1988, RCP 1991).

Information should be shared (Table 9.1) as appropriate with other professionals at a planning or strategy meeting and responsibility shared (DHSS 1988, Working Together 1988, 1991).

Figures 9.6 and 9.7 show the relative importance of the various signs and the effects of healing or re-abuse on the signs found on examination.

An examination where no abnormality is found cannot exclude child sexual abuse. In a study to evaluate the physical signs associated with child sexual abuse, 382 sexually abused girls, mean age 5.8 years, were examined: 71% had normal findings, including 48% who had been penetrated (interlabially, not vaginally) (Marshall et al 1988). Other authors have emphasised the same point (Muram 1989b, RCP 1991).

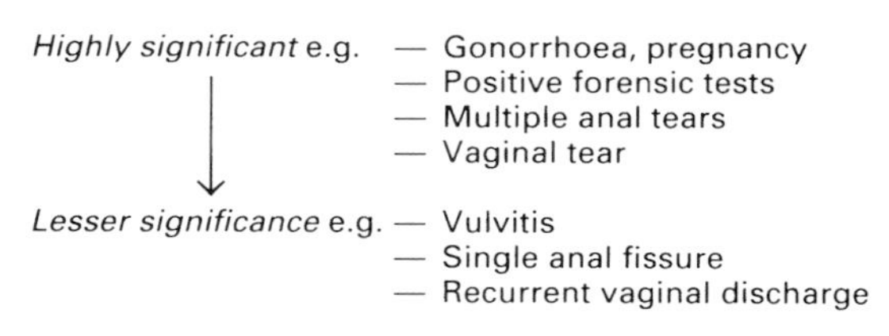

Note: About one-third of the children examined by paediatricians because of possible sexual abuse have *no* abnormality on physical examination

Fig. 9.6 Which signs are significant in child sexual abuse?

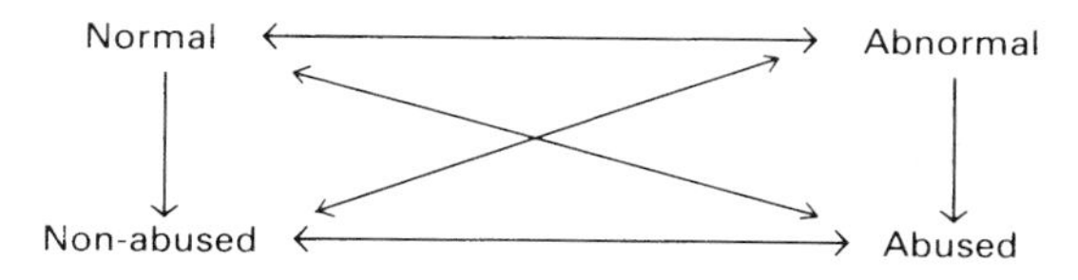

Fig. 9.7 Healing and physical signs: examination.

Healing takes place rapidly and scarring is uncommon (Hobbs & Wynne 1989). Changing physical signs suggest healing, re-abuse, or that a disease process is evolving.

A differential diagnosis of vulvovaginitis, genital and rectal bleeding is given in Table 9.5.

Genital bleeding

Genital bleeding is an important symptom and must always be investigated. Common causes include:

- accident – but there should be a history of a painful fall, most frequently a straddle injury (see later, p. 247)
- early puberty – investigate as precocious puberty
- other regular bleeding, such as each Friday night when the baby-sitter comes
- lichen sclerosus, vulval haemangioma and other rarities.

Rectal bleeding

Rectal bleeding also warrants investigation; organic causes have recently been well reviewed (Raine 1991). In general paediatric practice bleeding is commonly only seen secondary to fissures and infective diarrhoea.

Anal fissures are usually caused by the painful passage of a large hard stool, and faecal masses are palpable in the child's abdomen. A fissure is defined as

> a break in the lining of the anal canal, usually extending from inside the canal to the anal verge, and travelling vertically to the verge.

As is clear from the definition, anal fissures differ from the superficial breaks in the skin which are seen where there is perianal soreness for whatever cause – diarrhoea, threadworms, seborrhoeic dermatitis (McCrae 1985) – where the break in the skin does not cross the anal verge into the anal canal.

Anal fissures are caused by the stretching of the anal margin to a point where splitting occurs, giving a triangular tear with the apex within the anal canal. The aetiology of the fissure – whether it is organic or caused by a foreign body being inserted forcibly – cannot be deduced from its appearance. Fissures are also seen in inflammatory bowel disease, for example Crohn's disease,

Table 9.5 Causes of vulvovaginitis, vaginal and rectal bleeding

Vulvovaginitis	Genital bleeding identical to bloody discharge	Rectal bleeding
Poor hygiene	Onset menses (NB pseudo-menses ≡ trauma)	Fissure
Local irritation – bubblebath, soap, tights	Precocious puberty	Infective diarrhoea, e.g. salmonella, shigella
Candidal infection (after broad-spectrum antibiotics)	Accidental trauma	Inflammatory bowel disorder, e.g. ulcerative colitis
Threadworms	Foreign body – **rare**, ?child sexual abuse	Rectal polyp or other tumour
Part of systemic infection – measles, varicella, streptococcal	Infection, e.g. streptoccal	Child sexual abuse – penetrative, penile or foreign body
STD (see Table 9.10)	STD (see Table 9.10)	Foreign body – ?child sexual abuse
Child sexual abuse causing superficial trauma with secondary infection	Tumour	
Child sexual abuse – self-mutilation	Skin disease	
Associated skin disorder, e.g. eczema, lichen sclerosus		
Foreign body – **rare**, ?child sexual abuse		

but other signs and symptoms will be apparent in the presence of systemic illness.

Anal fissures cause pain on defecation and may be associated with anal spasm. They bleed initially, but usually heal over 1–3 weeks. Healing is impaired if the fissures are being persistently stretched, as in untreated constipation or continuing anal abuse. In these circumstances, a fissure may be seen as a deep, wide cleft, often placed posteriorly. Healing of such a chronic fissure may take months and is more likely to heal with scarring. Large fissures may leave a skin tag as a marker of previous trauma. Such chronic fissures are not painful (RCP 1991) and the skin tag is considered to represent an overgrowth of skin in the healing process.

Anal fissures are seen most commonly in infancy, associated with significant constipation and are usually superficial and may be multiple. They are seen with decreasing frequency after infancy and are uncommon in the school-aged child (Shandling 1987). In older children fissures are usually single and posterior (McCrae 1985).

In one study of 20 children attending a gastroenterology clinic because of severe constipation, 8 children had fissures and they were all in the age group 1–3.5 years (Anderson 1975).

In Clayden's (1981) review of severely constipated children referred to a regional constipation clinic, 1 out of 18 children on presentation had a fissure. Another review by the same author showed that 3 out of 30 children at follow-up had fissures and 16% had a past history of fissure (Clayden 1988). However, Agnarsson et al (1990), in a survey of 136 children with mild to moderate constipation, reported that 35 children had fissures and, most unusually, 10 had two fissures and 8 multiple fissures. That fissures are uncommon even where there is significant constipation has been shown (Benninga 1994), where only one in 111 children had a fissure, 35% had a palpable abdominal mass and 28% had a palpable rectal mass.

In McCann et al's study of children selected for non-abuse, average age 5 years 7 months, none of the 267 children had fissures (1989). By contrast, in a series of children who had been anally abused, 59/69 children aged 0–5 years and 53/143 children of all ages had anal tears or fissures (Hobbs & Wynne 1989).

Fissures following abuse become less likely with increasing age of the child, particularly if lubricant is used. If the child is examined some time after the abuse has occurred fissures may have healed and few leave scars.

Children who have been abused and have fissures often do not complain of as much pain as might have been expected. Some abused children do become constipated.

Fissures are associated with anal abuse (Hobbs & Wynne 1986, AAP 1991, RCP 1991). In the absence of constipation or inflammatory bowel disease, the presence of fissures needs explanation. If a child has two or more fissures (not excoriations) and especially if there are other signs of anal trauma such as bruising, swelling of the anal verge, laxity or dilatation, enquiry into the possibility of abuse should follow.

Bleeding in the absence of fissures may be due to other disorders such as rectal polyp (Raine 1991).

Vulvitis and vaginitis in prepubertal girls

Vulvitis or vaginitis is partially dependent on the oestrogen status of the child. At birth the influence of maternal oestrogen causes the mucosa to be thick and the secretions slightly acidic. The maternal hormonal effect ceases after about 4–6 weeks and the mucosa becomes thin and the pH neutral until puberty.

Pre-pubertal girls are prone to vulvitis and this is said to relate to this relative oestrogen deficiency. Specific infections are also influenced by the child's oestrogen status: trichomonas grows poorly in the absence of oestrogen and the reverse is true for gonorrhoea and chlamydia.

Causes of vulvitis

- poor hygiene
- sensitivity, e.g. to bubblebath, soaps
- threadworms (cause irritation and the child scratches)
- atopic eczema, seborrhoeic dermatitis
- child sexual abuse – causing local trauma and secondary infection
- excessive and inappropriate washing
- sexually transmitted disease

- other specific infections, e.g. streptococcus
- candida – rare except after a course of antibiotics
- not masturbation, unless self-mutilation seen in some sexually abused children (see later).

Symptoms of vulvitis

- soreness
- itchiness
- burning on micturition.

Causes of vulvovaginitis

- non-specific
- group a β-haemolytic streptococcus, *Staphylococcus aureus, Haemophilus influenzae*
- *Gardnerella vaginalis*
- sexually transmitted disease
- rarely, foreign body.

Symptoms of vulvovaginitis

- as vulvitis
- discharge.

Sexual abuse and vulvitis and vulvovaginitis
A high proportion of prepubertal girls who have been sexually abused complain of 'soreness' and have a vulvitis or vulvovaginitis on examination. This is probably due to rough handling leading to abrasions of the mucosa which may become secondarily infected. Hence, when symptoms of the lower genitourinary tract occur – including vulvovaginitis associated with soreness and discharge, or recurrent dysuria in the absence of proven urinary tract infection – child sexual abuse should be considered (DHSS 1988).

Management of vulvitis and vulvovaginitis

- Take a detailed history.
- Include in the history details of usual bathing practices: recent work recognises situations where cleansing becomes excessive and inappropriate causing soreness and even discharge. The child's genitalia may be handled and inspected with resulting physical and psychological harm (Herman-Giddens 1989).
- Enquire into the possibility of child sexual abuse, if not at the first visit then at follow-up – parents increasingly expect this.
- Perform a complete physical examination of the child (remember anus).
- Consider appropriate microbiological investigations: suggest a full screen for sexually transmitted disease (see Fig. 9.8) in older sexually active girls and girls with recurrent symptoms (even if little discharge is present).
- Treat specific infections and threadworms.
- Advise on
  - daily baths – no scrubbing of genitalia, 'sit and soak'
  - avoidance of irritant soaps and bubble-baths
  - no disinfectant in bath
  - cotton pants; avoid tights and closely fitting clothes.

Dysuria

Following child sexual abuse, pain on micturition or even traumatic haematuria may be seen in boys and girls. There may also be frequency of micturition. These symptoms occur when a child has a traumatised urethra which may be evident on examination by bruising, swelling, inflammation or dilatation. Microscopy of the urine and culture should differentiate a urinary tract infection from local inflammation. A history of recurrent dysuria is common in girls who have been sexually abused, particularly young girls aged less than 6 years, when 20% have genitourinary symptoms (Klevan & De Jong 1990). Difficulty in passing urine is also seen in boys and girls, and even retention where there has been more serious trauma.

Proven urinary tract infections are not a good marker for child sexual abuse; in one series of such infections 2/428 children had been sexually abused (Mehl 1990). However, recurrent genitourinary symptoms are an indicator of possible child sexual abuse, which should be considered in the differential diagnosis.

Urethral pathology is uncommon but includes urethral caruncle, haemangioma, prolapse and polyp.

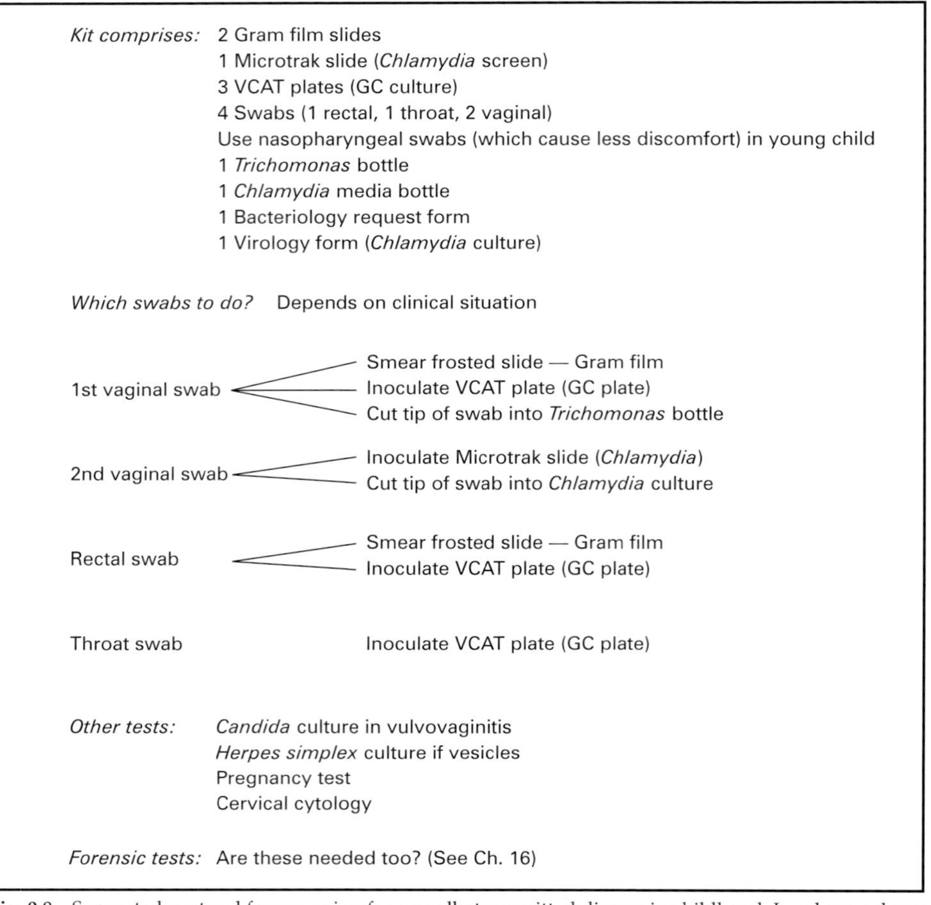

Fig. 9.8 Suggested protocol for screening for sexually transmitted disease in childhood. Local procedures should be worked out with a specialist in genitourinary medicine.

Masturbation

Masturbation does not ordinarily cause any abnormal physical signs. As a pleasurable activity in boys and girls it usually involves rubbing, and is universal in young children. Girls usually rub around the clitoris and so achieve an orgasm. Vaginal penetration, involving stretching and often tearing of the hymen, is painful and not a usual part of masturbation in young girls. Young girls are usually unaware that they have a hymenal orifice.

'Excessive masturbation' is described in some abused children (Corwin 1988). This may be the child's response to the need for sexual arousal, or comfort (Finkelstein 1996), or due to vulval irritation secondary to trauma or infection. If masturbation alone causes a vulvitis this is abnormal and should be thought of as self-mutilation and highly correlated with child sexual abuse. Parents and teachers use the expression 'excessive masturbation' to describe the behaviour of children who are continually rubbing their genitalia in public, both digitally and also by rubbing against furniture, knees or any firm surface. It should be asked 'Why does this child masturbate so much?'

Self-mutilation

Self-mutilation has been long recognised in abused adolescents and is increasingly appreciated, even in young children, where excessive scratching may cause deep lacerations which bleed or become secondarily infected. Children burn, pinch and cut themselves. The mutilation may affect face, neck, arms, abdomen and arms, for example, as well as the genitalia or anus (Hanks & Hobbs 1992).

Foreign bodies

Insertion of foreign bodies into the vagina is unusual in children (Paul 1986). This is because many younger prepubertal girls are unaware they have a vagina and by the time they are more aware of their anatomy they are beyond the age of this kind of behaviour. The classic triad of symptoms produced by a foreign body are bleeding, purulent discharge and odour (Paradise & Willis 1985). If insertion of a foreign body has caused stretching of the hymen it will have caused pain and often bleeding.

Always consider child sexual abuse if a child is seen with a foreign body in the vagina, and particularly if there are repeated episodes (RCP 1991). This is learned behaviour – where did the child learn to put pencils, Lego bricks or other objects inside herself? Herman-Giddens (1994) found that 11/12 prepubertal girls with foreign bodies were either confirmed or suspected victims of sexual abuse. Insertion may be recurrent.

Rectal foreign bodies are only rarely found and are usually associated with sadistic rape of older children.

Threadworm infestation (oxyuriasis)

Threadworms are extremely common during childhood and the incidence is higher in school children aged 5–14 years, with boys and girls equally affected. Incidences as high as 40–50% have been reported in London children (Goldsmid et al 1985).

The gravid female worm emerges from the child's anus at night and usually lays her eggs perianally, but may also migrate to the vulva. The child suffers intense irritation perianally and in the vulval area, and scratches. The perianal skin and vulva become reddened and on occasion excoriated. The eggs may be trapped under the child's nails, the fingers are then sucked and the child re-infects herself or her classmates by touching toys and so on.

Symptoms

- may be no symptoms
- pruritus in perineal area
- vulval irritation leading to scratching, vulvitis and occasionally pyogenic infection of excoriations leading to vulvovaginitis and discharge
- reinfestation rates are high.

Diagnosis

- If a child is heavily infected, worms may be seen perianally.
- A piece of Sellotape is applied perianally in the morning before washing or toileting and then placed adhesive side down on a slide. The adhering eggs are visible under a microscope.
- Stools show eggs in 5–10% of cases.

Treatment

- mebendazole (Vermox) 100 mg stat (over 2 years)
- piperazine (Pripsen) repeat after 14 days
- treat the whole family.

Infantile eczema and seborrhoeic dermatitis

Children with these skin disorders have a tendency to develop vulvitis and perineal soreness.

Lichen sclerosus et atrophicus

Lichen sclerosus et atrophicus (LSA) is an uncommon, chronic skin disorder, but may present with symptoms of vulvitis, the girl complaining of soreness, burning, itching, dysuria, genital bleeding and, if the perianal area is affected, pain on defecation and anal bleeding. It usually affects girls in mid-childhood but boys may be affected and present with phimosis.

The physical signs may be quite dramatic and superficially appear like trauma – hence child sexual abuse may be considered. However, the long history of intense irritation and burning sensations, coupled with the signs of LSA, should make the differentiation from child sexual abuse. There are on examination ivory or white shiny macules and papules that form homogenous hypopigmented atrophic areas on the vulva and perianal skin in a 'figure of eight' pattern if both are affected. There may also be areas of vasculitis or purpura with ecchymoses. Fissures are common perianally. There may be a superadded infection leading to a vulvovaginitis (Handfield-Jones et al 1987). Confusion with sexual abuse has been described (Priestley & Bleehan 1987).

The possibility that trauma including from child sexual abuse is an aetiological factor in some cases has been suggested. Warrington & de San Lazaro (1996) found that in 36% of children with lichen sclerosus, there were concerns regarding sexual abuse, providing some evidence for an association.

Sexually transmitted disease

The increased recognition of sexually transmitted disease in children parallels the recognition of child sexual abuse in general. Non-sexual transmission of sexually transmitted disease is rarely an issue in adults and when these diseases occur in children sexual abuse must be suspected (Foster 1992, RCP 1997). Acquisition or transmission of sexually transmitted disease in childhood is more complicated than in adults, particularly in infancy. The transmission of sexually transmitted organisms is shown in Table 9.6.

Table 9.6 Transmission of sexually transmitted diseases (STD) in children (RCP 1997)

Infective agent	Mode of transmission
Gonorrhoea	Perinatal – but after neonatal period probability is CSA (Emans 1998)
Chlamydia	Perinatal – persistence beyond infancy is controversial
Human papillomavirus	In utero, perinatal, > 2 years probability is CSA
Herpes simplex type I & 2	Perinatal, direct contact, NB clinically similar symptoms
Trichomonas	Perinatal, > 6 weeks probable CSA
Bacteria vaginosis	Direct contact, low probability CSA
HIV	In utero, perinatal
All sexually transmitted diseases	CSA/consensual contact

(Clarke & Lacey 1990).

The presence of a sexually transmitted disease does give corroborative evidence of child sexual abuse and Table 9.7 gives a guide to the probability of abuse (Clarke & Lacey 1990, RCP 1991).

The infections seen commonly in the UK are gonorrhoea, trichomonas, chlamydia, herpes, warts and bacterial vaginosis; rare infections are hepatitis B, syphilis and human innunodeficiency virus (HIV). The incidence of sexually transmitted disease in children depends on the incidence in the adult population including the population of abusers. sexually transmitted disease is diagnosed in 3–13% of sexually abused children, the higher rates being in older children (White et al 1983, Ingram et al 1992). Presenting signs and symptoms are given in Table 9.8.

When to test for sexually transmitted disease

A case could be made to screen all children suspected of being sexually abused for sexually transmitted disease. If history is of non-contact abuse, could we omit? How reliable is the history? Can children have a sexually transmitted disease without symptoms? The answer is probably yes, as in adults. Gonorrhoea may be found asymptomatically in pharnynx or rectum. Also, when should we screen for HIV, hepatitis B or syphilis serologically? This should be done on an individual basis, e.g. where there is a history of contact with an abuser known or suspected to be affected. Our current practice with sexual abuse evaluations is:

- screen symptomatic prepubertal children (soreness plus discharge in genital/anal area)
- screen all pubertal girls
- if one infection is found, e.g. warts, screen for other sexually transmitted disease
- continue to explore new screening methods which are simple to use and acceptable to child, e.g. urine polymerase chain reaction
- have a low threshold for screening for sexually transmitted disease.

Investigation must be carried out meticulously and checked, given the far-reaching con-

Table 9.7 STD and the probability of abuse

STD	Incubation period	Vertical transmission (neonatal disease)	Probability of abuse[a]
Gonorrhoea	3–4 days	Neonatal ophthalmia Neonatal vaginitis (rare)	++ (+++ if child >2 years)
Trichomonas	1–4 weeks	Rare but occasionally seen, usually clears spontaneously	+++ (if child < 6 weeks)
Chlamydia	7–14 days	Neonatal conjunctivitis Neonatal pneumonitis	++ (+++ if child <3 years and organism cultured is child's)
Warts	Several months	Laryngeal papillomata (HPV-II) Genital/perianal?	+
Herpes	2–14 days	Localised or disseminated	++
Bacterial vaginosis	2–14 days		+
HIV	Majority convert in 3 months	If maternal	Sexual assault
Hepatitis B	<3 months	Infection	Recognised
Syphilis	<3 months		+++

[a] *after RCP (1991).*
+, Child sexual abuse possible; ++, child sexual abuse likely; +++, child sexual abuse almost certain.
Full penetrative sexual intercourse (vaginal or anal) is not necessary for infection. Orogenital sex and intercrural contact may transmit pathogens (Branch & Paxton 1965).

sequences of the diagnosis. It is usual to work in close association with a genito-urinary physician. Table 9.9 summarises the tests needed.

Gonorrhoea

Gonorrhoea in childhood is almost always due to abuse. In one series 44/45 1–10-year-olds and 115/116 10–14-year-olds had suffered abuse (Branch & Paxton 1965). Neonatal infection is the only exemption to this rule.

Only just over half the infected children are likely to have symptoms (Table 9.9), and those with pharyngeal infections are likely to be asymptomatic (De Jong 1986). Typing including antibiotic sensitivity profiling may allow comparison of abuser and victim strains of organism. This is of obvious forensic importance.

Trichomonas

Trichomonas is a less common infection in child sexual abuse but is found in older girls in particular (Herman-Giddens et al 1988). Trichomonas vaginalis does not survive long in the prepubertal vagina and so if infection is found the abuse is recent (RCP 1997). Neonatal transmission may occur, the organism persisting for up to 3–6 weeks in the infant's vagina due to maternal oestrogen influence (RCP 1997).

Table 9.8 Presenting signs or symptoms of STD

Signs or symptoms	Possible cause
None	Chlamydia
Discharge (vaginal, penile, rectal)	Gonorrhoea
Itch or soreness (vulval, penile or perianal)	Candida
Pain (vulval or rectal)	Herpes
Ulceration, vesicles, warts (genital, oral, perianal)	Condylomata
Systemic illness	Gonorrhoea

Herpes

Genital herpes is uncommon and is likely to have resulted from child sexual abuse (Kaplan et al 1984). Typing of the virus does not help in identification of child sexual abuse as HSV-1 causes as much genital herpes as HSV-2, and in any event oral sex is common.

Chlamydia

Chlamydia trachomatis was found in 4–17% of sexually abused children who had been routinely screened for sexually transmitted disease (RCP 1991). The diagnosis is ideally made on culture but this is not always available.

Most girls with chlamydia infection are asymptomatic. The usual neonatal presentation is ophthalmia, and persistence of chlamydia infection beyond infancy is controversial, child sexual abuse being strongly suspected beyond the first 1–2 years of life.

Table 9.9 Summary of sexually transmitted diseases

Disease	Organism	Signs and symptoms	Incubation	Transmission	Microbiological investigation **(always repeat)**
Gonorrhoea	*Neisseria gonorrhoeae*	*Newborns:* conjunctivitis	3–4 days	Requires intimate contact with epithelial or mucus-secreting cells, dies in 1 hour	Gram stain: intracellular diplococci, Gram-negative
		Prepubertal: vulvovaginitis ± itchy, discharge, dysuria		Sexual contact	Culture (always repeat)
		Rarely systemic – urethritis is uncommon *Adolescent girls*: asymptomatic, discharge, cervicitis, salpingitis *Adolescent boys:* urethritis, epididymitis, prostatitis *Anorectal:* pruritus, mucopurulent discharge, bleeding		Birth canal (up to 1 month)	Serological typing: types 1–16, specialised lab Investigate trichomonas, chlamydia Diagnosis requires culture of the organism
Trichomoniasis	*Trichomonas vaginalis* (protozoon)	*Newborn*: low risk – 0.5% nasal discharge, vaginitis	4 days–4 weeks	Sexual contact	Microscopy
		Older children: vulvovaginitis, urethritis, cystitis, asymptomatic		Birth canal	Culture Investigate for gonorrhoea, chlamydia
Chlamydia	*Chlamydia trachomatis* subgroup A	Manifestations as for gonorrhoea, may be asymptomatic NB conjunctivitis in newborn	7–14 days	Sexual contact Birth canal (up to1 month)	Culture mandatory for diagnosis Enzyme immunoassay and immunofluorescence not reliable Check for gonorrhoea
Genital herpes	Herpes simplex virus, DNA-containing, types 1 and 2 (HSV-1, HSV-2)	*HSV-1 primary infection*: usually aged 1–5 years, 'cold sores', 10% gingivostomatitis Occasionally other parts – skin, eye, genital tract Rarely encephalitis Tendency to recur Heal 10–14 days	2–14 days	HSV-1 direct contact	Cervical cytology, i.e. pap smear, see multinucleated giant cells and eosinophilic nuclear inclusions
		HSV-2 primary infection: small, painful vesicles develop either singly or in groups, general malaise, lesions usually on penis or vulva, vagina, cervix in women, also perineum, anus, rectum Recurs but attacks tend to come at longer intervals and be less severe		HSV-2 direct contact	Tissue culture, also enables typing of virus
		Newborn: similar spectrum to above, Disseminated disease is often fatal		Neonate by birth canal	Serological methods
				Autoinoculation of genital area with HSV-1	Electron microscopy

Table 9.9 *Continued*

Disease	Organism	Signs and symptoms	Incubation	Transmission	Microbiological investigation **(always repeat)**
				Children with genital herpes, HSV-1, consider child sexual abuse especially in absence of previous cold sores HSV-2, consider child sexual abuse	
Genital and anal warts (*Condylomata acuminata*)	Human papilloma virus (HPV) >50 types, types 6, 11, 18 live on keratinising surfaces, types 16 and 18 only on mucous membranes	Soft verrucous lesions on genital and anorectal area Rarely adjacent thigh or trunk May extend to vagina, cervix, anal canal	Average 2–3 months, to several months, or longer	In utero	Biopsy/histology
		Complications: Invasive carcinoma of cervix Carcinoma of anal canal		Birth canal	Genotyping – genital types HPV-6, 11, 16, 18, 31 Common warts types HPV-1–4
		Children: High index of suspicion of child sexual abuse		Direct contact Sexual abuse	Screen for other STD
		Non-venereal transmission suggested in early infancy, or lesions distant from anogenital area *Differential diagnosis:* Clinically from *Molluscum contagiosum*		Autoinoculation of some types	

Warts

Warts are perhaps the most frequently seen STD in paediatric practice (Gutman 1992, 1994), and management is often difficult. It is reported that 1–2% of abused children have genital warts and 50–75% of cases are due to CSA. Data on the persistence of HPV DNA beyond the neonatal period is inconsistent. Current practice varies, in the UK if the child with warts is two years old or younger a perinatal infection is thought likely, in the US three years is the 'cut off' age. In older children genito-anal warts are indicators of CSA but the relationship is weaker that for gonorrhoea (e.g. Neinstein 1984, Herman-Giddens 1988). Recent work suggests that the more thorough the investigation, the more likely it is that child sexual abuse will be identified (Gutman 1990). Gutman et al (1992) found that 1/3 sexually abused girls had evidence of clinically undetectable herpes virus infection using vaginal wash samples. Tests should be done to exclude other sexually transmitted diseases.

Typing of warts demonstrates only partial site specificity – that is, genital warts are associated with types 6 and 11 and less often types 16, 18 and others. Types 1 and 2 have been found in perianal warts.

Data from children does not yet make the clinical picture clear. Children with anogenital lesions rarely have warts elsewhere but one boy has been reported who had warts on his hands and perianal warts, and type 2 virus was detected in both (Flemming et al 1987).

It is likely that with greater multi-agency experience in investigation of venereal warts in children over the age of 2 years that child sexual abuse will be increasingly recognised in these children.

In order to postulate a non-sexual acquisition of venereal warts there should be (Rock et al 1986):

- a negative social enquiry
- no other signs of abuse
- lesions somewhat distant from the anus or introitus
- child under 9 months when lesions noted.

However, proving that abuse has not taken place may be very difficult (Clarke 1997).

Examination of the child's parents and any siblings for evidence of clinical or sub-clinical herpes virus infection may provide useful information and is helpful (RCP 1997). In addition to a high frequency of warts in the parents (Obalek et al 1990), as many as a half of the mothers may have cervical intraepithelial neoplasia (Handley et al 1993).

Bacterial vaginosis

Bacterial vaginosis is a cause of vulvovaginitis and vaginal discharge. It is a polymicrobial infection including vaginal anaerobes, *Gardnerella vaginalis* and Gram negative organisms. It has been found in association with child sexual abuse, especially if there has been multiple abuse. A review in 1985 of 54 prepubertal girls showed bacterial vaginosis in 8/31 abused girls and 1/23 non-abused girls (Hammerschlag 1988); another review in 1987 showed BV in 14% of abused girls compared with 4% of non-abused (Bartley et al 1987).

Bacterial vaginosis is uncommon in non-abused girls. *Gardnerella vaginalis* is an unusual organism in cultures from virginal women. The probability of abuse on bacterial vaginosis infection alone is not high, but is supportive of the diagnosis.

Hepatitis

Hepatitis A and B may be transmitted by sexual contact, hepatitis A by oral–anal contact and hepatitis B by homosexual and heterosexual intercourse. Hepatitis B has been seen in child sexual abuse in Leeds (1991).

Recovery is the rule after hepatitis A, but hepatitis B may lead to an infective carrier state and chronic hepatitis. This clearly has implications for the child and his or her carers.

Screening for hepatitis B is not routinely done in the assessment of sexually abused children but should be considered in the same circumstances as for HIV testing.

Carers and siblings should be tested if the child is found to have HBsAG and HBeAg in his serum, indicating an infective carrier state. If carers are non-immune they should be offered hepatitis B vaccine.

Concomitant infections with hepatitis B and HIV are common.

HIV

HIV infection has been recognised in child sexual abuse, and the cases due to sexual assault are likely to rise (Gellert 1989). In 1993 over 28 cases of HIV secondary to child sexual abuse had been reported in the USA (Gellert et al 1993). Screening for HIV needs careful consideration and the following protocol is suggested.

Suggested protocol for HIV screening

- A child who is unwell with signs and symptoms suggestive of HIV infection should be tested
- A child who has been involved in high-risk activities, e.g. prostitution or drug abuse, should probably be tested
- If a child (usually a teenager), parent or carer insists on testing this needs careful consideration
- A single act of stranger abuse, a coexistent sexually transmitted disease, previous anal or oral abuse do not currently warrant screening
- HIV antibody testing would be done at the time of the initial examination and after 3 and 6 months
- Counselling for the child and his or her carers is mandatory
- Education of young adolescents about the cause and effects of HIV infection is essential

Molluscum contagiosum

Molluscum contagiosum is an infection caused by a DNA pox-containing virus. Children usually have non-venereal infections with lesions on the face, trunk and limbs, but in a minority there is an association with other sexually transmitted diseases and child sexual abuse.

Investigation of sexually transmitted disease

A protocol for investigation of sexually transmitted disease is given in Figure 9.8. If the child is young the application of swabs may cause distress. The use of small nasopharyngeal swabs dampened with tap water may limit the discomfort. Careful transhymenal insertion using colposcopic visualisation is acceptable to the cooperative child and causes no discomfort. The protocol has been planned to use a minimum of swabs, as indicated clinically. However, if the child cannot cooperate and clinically there is concern, sedation or even a general anaesthetic should be considered. Always consider whether forensic swabs are indicated – usually only if the most recent sexual assault was within the last 72 hours.

An outline of treatment is given in Table 9.10.

Criminal injuries compensation

Criminal injuries compensation is available to victims of child sexual abuse. A consequent sexually transmitted disease may well have serious long-term health implications for the child and should be documented in the report for the Criminal Injuries Compensation Board (see Ch. 14).

Physical abuse

Physical abuse and child sexual abuse are closely related (Reinhardt 1987, Hobbs & Wynne 1990, RCP 1991). Approximately 1/6 of 769 physically abused children and 1/7 of sexually abused children had been physically abused, and deaths occurred (Hobbs & Wynne 1990).

The injuries may be of the kind seen in physical assault, but there are patterns associated with child sexual abuse (Fig. 9.9).

- Grip marks on the inner aspect of the upper arms, the thighs and around the knees are common.
- Signs associated with partial suffocation, such as petechiae around the orbit and linear marks around the neck, are seen – presumably the assailant in an attempt to quieten the child has put a hand over the child's mouth or squeezed the neck.

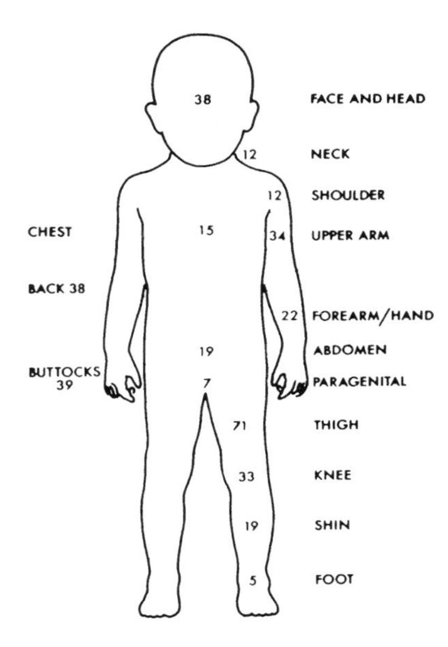

Fig. 9.9 Distribution of bruises by site in 110 physically and sexually abused children. Figures refer to the number of children. (Reproduced with permission from Hobbs C J, Wynne J M 1990 The sexually abused battered child. Archives of Disease in Childhood 65: 423–427.)

- Bruises on the lower abdomen, particularly over the pubis, and also around the hips where the child has been grasped are seen.
- 'Love-bites' are of concern whatever the age of the child and are usually on the neck, or breasts of older girls. Other bites are also relatively commonly seen, often on the back or shoulders.
- Deliberately sadistic acts such as laceration of the dorsum of the penis are also seen or cuts to the labia or perianal area.
- Burns and scalds are one of the least well recognised manifestations of abuse and clinical assessment may be difficult. Sadistic burns are inflicted to the genitalia and other 'abusive' sites such as the back of the hand, buttocks or back of the neck. An important feature in the history is a description of repeated incidents of burning, each burn on its own perhaps having been dismissed as 'minor'.
- Sexually abused children are murdered either in the course of the abuse or in order to silence them.

Table 9.10 Treatment of sexually transmitted diseases

Disease	Treatment[a]	Notes
Ophthalmia neonatorum[b]		Notifiable
Gonococcal	Systemic penicillin, e.g. benzylpenicillin 50 000 units/kg body wt/24 h in divided doses, 2 times/day, 3 days	Rarely generalised infection
	Saline eye baths	May be associated with chlamydia Investigate mother
Chlamydial	Systemic antibiotics, e.g. erythromycin ethylsuccinate 50 mg/kg body wt/24 h in divided doses, 14–21 days	May be associated with pneumonia
	Saline eye baths	Severity of ophthalmia varies Investigate mother
Gonorrhoea	Ampicillin 3 g orally with probenecid 2 g orally	Contacts?
Uncomplicated penicillinase-producing gonococcus or allergy to penicillin	Spectinomycin 2 g i.m. or co-trimoxazole 4 tab orally 2 times/day, 2 days	Other infection?
Trichomonas	Metronidazole 200 mg 8 hourly for 7 days or 2 g as single dose	Do not drink alcohol on drug Contact?
Chlamydia	Oxytetracycline 500 mg 4 times/day, 7–14 days or erythromycin 500 mg 4 times/day, 7–14 days	
Herpes types 1 and 2	Primary attack: Acyclovir 200 mg 5 times/day, 5 days Topically Acyclovir cream Secondary attack: Septrin 2 tabs 2 times/day, 7 days Topically Nystaform-HC cream 3 times/day	Check cervix cytology annually What is appropriate for children?
Genital and anal warts	Adults: podophyllin 10–25% twice a week	May be associated with malignancy, especially types 16 and 18
	Cervical warts: laser treatment Children: refer to paediatric surgeon for excision/diathermy	Follow-up?
Gardnerella or bacterial vaginosis	Metronidazole 400 mg 12 hourly, 5 days	Contact?
Candidiasis	Adults: e.g. clotrimazole as local cream or pessary; systemically, e.g. fluconazole 150 mg Children: local cream, e.g. clotrimazole	Predisposing factors, e.g. diabetes, antibiotics
Molluscum contagiosum	Liquefied phenol or saturated solution of trichloroacetic acid applied to base of lesion with sharp stick	
Viral hepatitis	Prevention in high-risk groups: hepatitis B vaccine Contacts: specific immunoglobulin Infant: active and passive immunisation at birth	Hepatitis A and B may be transmitted sexually
HIV infection	No method of immunisation No specific treatment AZT orally Treat opportunistic infection promptly	

[a] *Adult doses given (except for ophthalmia neonatorum).*
[b] *Defined as conjunctivitis within 21 days of birth).*

CASE HISTORY 9.6

A girl aged 14 years told her mother that her stepfather had been sexually abusing her since she was 6 years old. All the appropriate agencies were involved and the girl left to live with friends, the mother undertaking to protect her. She returned home. The girl was found dead with her mother;

both had been involved in sexual intercourse before they were killed and the stepfather was hanging from the bannister.

CASE HISTORY 9.7

A boy aged 4 years was found unconscious and bruised when his mother returned from shopping. His father said he had been bouncing on his bed and fallen. On examination he had a badly bruised swollen face, retinal haemorrhages and anal signs of recent buggery. He died 5 days later of his head injury.

Pregnancy

Pregnancy in girls should always be questioned and the girl be given time to talk and be counselled apart from her mother. This may be difficult to achieve.

Testing of blood groups, including DNA profiling, may help identify or confirm the alleged father or exclude others.

CASE HISTORY 9.8

A girl aged 12 years was taken to see a paediatrician when a schedule 1 offender moved into the family home. She was too embarrassed to allow a genital examination. The social worker and doctor were very concerned. Six months later she presented 28 weeks pregnant.

Psychosomatic indicators

Psychosomatic indicators are important because this may be the only way in which a child demonstrates distress. The stresses on a child may be very many and range from the weekly spelling test to bullying in the playground or an alcoholic father; added to the list must be 'Is there any child sexual abuse?'

Recurrent abdominal pains

Abdominal pains are particularly common in the 5–10-year age group. The child usually complains of central abdominal pain and nausea, looks pale and may vomit. The pain may last from minutes to hours. The child feels unwell enough to need to lie down but then after a period of rest is completely well and resumes activity. There are no abnormalities on physical examination between attacks. Up to 10% of children complain of such pains at some time and there is often a family history of abdominal pain and also migraine.

Organic causes for the pain should be considered and, although more than 90% of children have no pathology, urinary tract infections and duodenal ulcers occasionally present in this way.

Child sexual abuse is one of the stresses which should be explored, especially in children where the pain persists in spite of reassurance by the doctor.

Headaches

Headaches become more common as children grow into adolescence and on enquiry the majority of teenagers will report recurrent headaches.

A child with severe recurrent headaches may have an underlying disorder such as an intracranial space-occupying lesion; a detailed history and examination are needed. The younger child, with morning headaches not relieved by analgesia and which worsen over weeks to months, clearly needs thorough investigation.

Migraine is the commonest recurrent headache in childhood and is usually associated with nausea or vomiting, visual disturbance, lethargy and unilateral headache. There is often a strong family history. Other 'tension headaches' are described with a heaviness or tight band, or sharp pain, including pain in the neck. Migraine and other headaches are usually a symptom of stress, although there may be an additional association with certain foods such as chocolate, or hunger, or excessive tiredness. Management involves looking into the child's lifestyle for identification of stress factors, one of which may be child sexual abuse. Treatment of headaches involves reassurance about lack of an organic cause (brain tumour) and simple analgesics, but essentially should deal with the stress precipitating the attacks.

CASE HISTORY 9.9

A boy of 11 years presented with migraine which was becoming disabling. He was a keen athlete but had had to withdraw from training because of headache. When examined he was underweight and had scars of self-mutilation on his forearms. Later he disclosed anal abuse by his older brother.

Anorexia and eating disorders

Eating disorders are relatively common in adolescence but anorexia in extreme form has a significant morbidity and mortality. Child sexual abuse is now being recognised as one of the important antecedents to this disorder. Although girls are recognised to have anorexia more often than boys, if affects both sexes.

The age of onset is usually in the early teenage years but children as young as 10 or 11 years are also identified. In a teenage girl it may begin with her being very particular about her diet, the total calories and content, but then eating less and less. She hides food, has tempers about eating food yet remains well and active, while becoming progressively thinner. Many children with anorexia have sessions of bingeing (bulimia); more recently recognised is their physical activity – they may swim, run and exercise in a similarly obsessive way. The girl's periods stop, or may never start.

Management is complex; in serious cases hospital admission is needed and individual family work with a child and family psychiatric team is usual.

Constipation, soiling and encopresis

- *Constipation* involves difficulty or delay in the passage of faeces.
- *Soiling* is the frequent passage of liquid or semi-solid faeces into clothing (Agnarsson & Clayden 1990).
- *Encopresis* is the passage of faeces of normal or near normal consistency into socially inappropriate places (including clothing) (Graham 1991).

Constipation and soiling are commonly seen in paediatric practice but encopresis, which is likely to be associated with considerable emotional trauma (including emotional abuse and child sexual abuse), is more commonly seen in child psychiatric clinics. There are emotional difficulties for any child who is not continent of faeces, and the groups overlap.

Soiling associated with constipation is usually seen in children of 3–6 years. It often follows a febrile illness and the constipation gradually worsens over months with the child painfully, and infrequently, passing large stools and soiling intermittently. Fissures may be caused with consequent pain and further retention of faeces.

Physical examination shows a well child with a distended abdomen and faecal masses easily palpable. Examination of the anus reveals soiling and a large faecal mass above the sphincter. A fissure may be visible but is uncommon, although excoriation and reddening of the perianal skin is a frequent finding.

Organic causes of constipation are uncommon and include:

- anorectal stenosis
- aganglionosis (Hirschsprung's disease)
- spinal cord lesion.

The diagnosis of the above disorders may be made on anal examination, with a tight sphincter and empty rectum in aganglionosis and an abnormally lax sphincter in spinal cord lesions.

Psychological factors in constipation (Graham 1991) include:

- parental factors (training too young, punitive, disorganised household)
- factors in child (delayed development, anxiety, fear)
- association with child sexual abuse (retention of faeces as a response to stress, especially in anal abuse).

Constipation also occurs in severely physically and mentally handicapped children. This may be due to dietary and other factors, but handicapped children may also be abused (Ch. 10).

Management of constipation

- Consider pathology – organic, dietary or functional.

- Empty bowel – laxatives and faecal softeners.
- Enemas are best avoided but occasionally needed.
- Begin a retraining programme – relaxed, positive, gradual.
- Laxatives and softeners may be needed for several months.

Encopresis

At 3 years of age, 16% of children show signs of faecal incontinence once a week or more but at 4 years only 3% (Richman et al 1982), and at 7 years only 1.5% and by 10–11 years 0.8% (Graham 1991).

More boys than girls are affected by encopresis and there are no consistent social class differences. Encopresis usually starts before 5–6 years and may or may not be associated with constipation. The soiling occurs several times a day and may be at school and home or just at home.

Factors in encopresis (Graham 1991) include:

- parental (little significance or aggressive, punitive, conformity, high standards)
- child (developmental delay, fear, part of emotional disorder)
- family factors (tension, disharmony)
- life stress (bullying).

Abused children (child sexual abuse, emotional abuse) may be very angry; encopresis may be an expression of this anger and associated with smearing of faeces and other destructive behaviour. Other children, who may be depressed and fearful, express their distress through soiling. It may also be rationalised by the child 'If I'm smelly and dirty he'll leave me alone'.

Management of encopresis

- Look at probable cause – if the abuse stops, the encopresis may be dramatically cured.
- Look at child–parent relationship.
- Give positive encouragement and reward.
- Behaviour modification
- Psychotherapy.

Enuresis

Enuresis is the involuntary emptying of the bladder at an age when continence is expected. This may be a problem during the day or night. Over 10% of children aged 5 years wet the bed and at least 10% of the bedwetters wet during the day. Around 5% of 10-year-olds wet the bed, diminishing to 1% of adults. Children who have been dry and start to wet have often had an emotional upset, for example parental divorce.

Abused children may only become dry when they feel safe and are protected. Amongst persistent day-wetters there are increasing numbers of recognised victims of child sexual abuse (Bentovim & Boston 1988).

Factors associated with wetting:

- more often boys, and often family history of bedwetting
- more often socially disadvantaged, insecure or unstable family unit
- behavioural problems in child
- other signs of emotional distress in child (particularly in secondary wetting)
- developmental delay
- rigid, intolerant parental attitudes and high expectations
- neglectful parents
- angry child who deliberately wets as a hostile gesture.

Clinically:

- exclude urinary tract infection.
- ensure anatomy is normal, e.g. ectopic ureter.
- check neurologically there are no signs.
- look for signs of child sexual abuse (and other abuse).

Management of of enuresis

Managment measures suggested by (Graham 1991) are:

- enquiry into signs of emotional disturbance, abuse
- depends on age and motivation of child and family
- reassurance of child and parents
- positive rewards
- bladder training
- enuresis alarm
- medication
- psychotherapy.

Total refusal syndrome

Total refusal syndrome is a recent clinical description of the behaviour of a group of seriously psychologically disturbed children, usually adolescents, who take to their beds and in extreme cases will not feed, wash or toilet themselves. Inevitably the differential diagnosis has been with myalgic encephalomyelitis but clinical investigation suggests that a severe traumatic event(s), such as serious emotional and/or sexual abuse, is more important in the aetiology (Tranter, personal communication). Management involves admission to a specialist adolescent psychiatric unit to tackle the practical (i.e. food refusal) as well as the psychological disorder.

Behavioural indicators

Child sexual abuse may present as one of the 'ordinary' emotional and behavioural problems in childhood, such as bedwetting, anxiety symptoms or school failure (Lusk & Waterman 1986, DHSS 1988, Sgroi et al 1988, Brown et al 1989).

The range of behaviours associated with child sexual abuse is wide, as children express their distress in different ways. Occasionally children present with psychotic symptoms apparently precipitated by the stress of coping with sexual abuse in a vulnerable personality.

As with physical signs, some behaviours are relatively specific for child sexual abuse, such as sexually explicit play, whereas others are non-specific, such as nightmares or deterioration in school performance (Table 9.11) (Corwin 1988). An increasing proportion of children seen in child guidance and psychiatry clinics are now recognised victims of child sexual abuse (Lusk & Waterman 1986, Brown et al 1989). Children attending special schools for children with emotional problems are a group of children of whom the question 'why?' should always be put: could it be child sexual abuse (or other maltreatment) that is causing this child's deviant behaviour?

Recently three cases have been described of children demonstrating apparent mental deterioration where the cause was considered, initially, to be a deteriorating organic mental state, but was later shown to be the child's extreme reaction to sexual abuse (Brown et al 1989). The cardinal features of such states have been described as mental deterioration with loss of skills in language and play and general social withdrawal (Corbett et al 1977). The differential diagnosis in these children was considered to be autism, schizophrenia and neurodegenerative conditions such as lipidosis. The three children, all girls aged 5–6 years, improved and disclosed child sexual abuse on admission to a residential psychiatric unit.

Table 9.11 Specific emotional and behavioural indicators of victimisation (Corwin 1988)

Pre-school (0–4 years)	Nightmares triggered by place, person, objects related or including physical movements or vocalisations that are consistent with sexually abusive experience Premature eroticisation • preoccupation with genitals • repetitive seeking to engage others in differentiated sexual behaviour • excessive or indiscriminate masturbation or masturbation with objects • precocious, apparently seductive behaviour • depiction of differentiated sexual acts in doll play Fearfulness • over-determined denial of genital anatomy and exposure to normal nudity • avoidance and anxiety in response to specific questions about differentiated sexual behaviour • unexplained person, gender, place, or object avoidance or fearfulness Child's age-appropriate and circumstantially congruent description of being sexually abused Dissociative phenomena
School age (6–11 years)	As for pre-school, plus: Sexual aggression and coercion towards other children Cross-dressing Prostitution
Adolescents (12–18 years)	As for school age, plus: Extreme sexual inhibition

The medical examination

The mechanics of any medical examination are important in order to minimise trauma for the child and family, but also to ensure that the maximum amount of information is learned from the examination.

The paediatrician may be asked to see a child who has made a clear disclosure. In these circumstances a social worker will usually give details of the disclosure to the doctor, who may need to clarify details of pain felt, or bleeding, but essentially accepts the history presented. A full medical history should still be taken (see below) but the child should not be expected to retell what may have been a distressing story.

On other occasions the child presents 'incidentally' (Table 9.3). In these circumstances some paediatricians will have developed skills in talking to children concerning abuse and feel able to use the anatomically correct dolls, line drawings, and so on. Other doctors prefer to note the physical signs and discuss their findings with colleagues (including a social worker) as described in Figure 9.1. Increasingly social workers and police officers, conduct 'disclosure interviews'. It may well be that the social worker needs to work for weeks or months with a child before the clinical picture does become clear. It has been shown that a too-rapid escalation of investigations may lead the child to refuse to talk, and although the child may be left unprotected in the short term, experienced workers learn to pace the interviews. This may be difficult for police officers if pressurised by senior colleagues to conduct one or two interviews and then make 'yes or no' decision.

Increasingly too, videotapes are made of interviews with children. Again these require skilled interviewers as a poorly conducted interview may be used 'against' the child by lawyers. Few paediatricians have facilities to video their conversations with children, which is unfortunate as the spontaneous disclosures made by children during physical examinations are often not only clear but of good evidential value.

The facilities needed by doctors examining children who may have been sexually abused are described later in Chapter 14. The physical environment needed by children and families is equally important. But, however good the facilities, if the examining doctor is not sympathetic to the child's needs, or is rushed or impatient, the therapeutic contribution of the examination is lost.

The medical examination begins with a history. This may have been presented by the child's general practitioner in a referral letter, by a parent or by a social worker or police officer. Older children may give their own medical history but younger children should (almost) always be accompanied by a parent, otherwise the medical background inevitably will be incomplete.

Forensic aspects of the medical examination

The entire medical examination is in essence a forensic one in that all aspects from the history to the physical examination to any investigations performed, for example to screen for sexually transmitted disease or the presence of semen, may be used as evidence in court.

The term 'forensic examination' has become associated with the taking of swabs for evidence of sexual assault, for example looking for the presence of saliva, sperm, blood or fibres. As most abuse is ongoing and intrafamilial abuse such 'forensic tests' are uncommonly positive, and one study of 205 girls resulted in 2 positive swabs (Muram & Elias 1989). Another study performed particularly to evaluate the forensic aspects of child sexual abuse found that 40% of children had physical abnormality thought to be important evidentially and around 10% had positive swabs (Enos et al 1986). The advice given by forensic scientists in the UK (Frances Lewington, personal communication) has been to swab if there has been probable abuse within 48–72 hours (or 3–4 days in older girls); the results from this selected group show that around 10% of specimens will be positive.

However, careful physical examination is much more likely to give corroborative evidence of sexual assault. The physical signs seen vary with the type of abuse and when the last assault took place (Paul 1977). There will also be a difference in the recognition of physical signs depending upon the group of children seen, and their mode of presentation. Various studies show that between 10% and 80% of children will have abnormality (Enos et al 1986, Hobbs & Wynne 1987a, 1989, Lindblad et al 1989, Muram 1989a, Muram & Elias 1989, Frothingham et al 1991).

Paediatricians will wish to build up a clinical picture based on the history, the investigations, and presence of physical signs in order to have an opinion based on probability. It is on this balance of probability that children may be protected. The concept of the 'jigsaw of sexual abuse' in medical practice is established in Table 9.2 (Butler-Sloss 1988 – letter from Professor Forfar p 203, RCP 1991). In a criminal court, however, the court will only want to hear what the physician found. What were the physical signs? What were they consistent with? The court will not listen to hearsay evidence, such as what the child said to the doctor or teacher, whereas such evidence is admissible in family proceeding courts.

The doctor should record in the notes the place, date and time of examination, the reason for the examination and at whose request it took place. In these litigious times it is necessary to say who gave consent (even if verbal) and record who was present (Steiner et al 1988). The details of history and examination, and also which investigations (microbiological, haematological or forensic) were asked for should be recorded; for forensic swabs sent to the regional forensic laboratory it should be noted to whom the specimens were given. This is the first step in the 'chain of evidence', the details of which must be maintained for court. The doctor should also label the specimens and sign the label (Paul 1984). This is discussed in more detail in Chapter 14. Clearly, forensic sampling depends upon the clinical situation. Paediatricians will usually need the assistance of a police surgeon in 'stranger rape', when a complete collection of swabs is mandatory.

Medical history

The medical history should include the usual headings:

- history of presenting complaint or allegation (see below)
- general health – include emotional well-being, appetite, urinary and bowel history, symptoms of depression and menstrual history
- drug history
- past medical history of significant illness, such as hospital admissions for unexplained abdominal pain
- developmental history or school progress
- immunisation history
- family history – do other siblings need examining?
- social history – what is known? Is the father a Schedule 1 offender (i.e. has he a previous conviction for offences against children)?

Allegations of abuse

If the allegation is one of abuse, several points should be considered.

- Has the child already made a clear disclosure, is it necessary to repeat the questioning? There may be specific information the doctor needs to know about the abuse (e.g. pain during abuse or bleeding) which is not available from the professionals who have previously interviewed the child.
- If the child has not made a clear disclosure, the doctor with paediatric skills is usually able to form a rapport with the child and may obtain a fuller history. Ideally the history includes details as to when, where, what, who, how often, over what time-span, did it hurt (this is important when interpreting signs), when was the last assault, was there anyone else there, was lubricant used, what lubricant was it, where was it kept, was there ejaculation, where? The list is considerable but the more details there are, the more likely the police are to find corroborative evidence. Doctors may also feel able to ask about masturbation, oral sex, and anal sex, which others have avoided. Leading questions such as 'Was it in your bedroom?' are to be avoided, rather 'Where did it happen?' It is, however, permissible to ask

'Did he put it (penis) anywhere else?' If the direct question is asked 'Did he put it (penis) in your mouth?' record a nod, 'Did he put it (penis) in your bottom?' record a head shake, make clear notes of what was said. It is usual to talk to the child without parents present at some time during the history taking, even for children as young as 3–4 years.

- The child may be unwilling to talk initially, but during and after the physical examination he or she may begin to talk; ask 'What made it sore?'
- For young, mentally slow or withdrawn children, the anatomically complete dolls are helpful in skilled hands.
- Use of drawing in children may allow them to explain more easily.
- Children may not want to repeat their story; they may feel they have said it once and should be believed. Pressure may lead to retraction, because children are effectively silenced by early disbelief, as they may be by threats from the abuser or even those they might expect to help them, such as their mother.
- Difficulty in history taking also arises with very young children. Although they remember the sequence of events their concept of a period of time and of number is immature. Thus a child of 2–3 years may understand 'one, two, a lot'. If pressurised to give, for example, the number of times he or she was abused, the child may guess a number which may well change and is then dubbed 'unreliable'. Similarly a week, a month, a year are all a long time to a young child. Children do know who daddy is, not all men are daddy and children under 12 months know daddy from other men. Colours are used to discredit children as witnesses – a child may helpfully guess 'red', but at 3 years old the child is not untruthful, or confused, he or she just does not know.
- If abuse has gone on over a prolonged period, particularly if the child is stressed by anxiety or fear, memories merge, especially if the abuse is by the same perpetrator(s) in the same environment. However rape by an uncle of an 8-year-old on her birthday will be fixed in time and place. If the abuse is by dad, and involves touching, masturbation, oral sex, the child may remember the time when mum caught him doing it, the first time he attempted vaginal intercourse and hurt her badly making her bleed, and so on. Children do not exaggerate as a rule. Clinical experience shows that they are more likely to understate their abuse.
- It is necessary to ask older children if they are sexually active, and what this has entailed. Often teenagers have not discussed such matters with their parents and privacy should be ensured for this interview. Ask about the use of tampons. Remember to take a menstrual history and consider the possibility of pregnancy. Is the 'morning-after pill' needed?
- Many children will only disclose months to years after the abuse has stopped, when they feel safe to tell. Children received into foster-care because of physical abuse may months later disclose sexual abuse. Children may disclose abuse by fathers when parents separate and they feel secure. Likewise children in residential schools or homes or in alternative care away from their abuser may tell, as long as they do not have to, or to avoid, return to the abusive home or school.
- Traditionally children will only tell when they are ready, and this may be after months or years, or never. An unresolved clinical problem for professionals is early recognition of the signs of child sexual abuse before the child is ready to talk. At one time it was thought that children confronted with the suspicion would be able to disclose, but this is clearly not so. The power of abusers to keep children (and wives) quiet should not be underestimated. It may be that with recent publicity abusers are using greater threats than ever to keep their victims quiet – this would correspond with the age distribution of children who do disclose, either the very young (less than 5 years old) or teenagers. The younger ones may not be aware of the significance of telling and the

older teenagers can run away, or move away, having some independence. Around 30–50% of teenage runaways say that they have been sexually abused at home (Ch. 17).

- Children may feel a doctor 'can tell' during the physical examination and so disclose; this misunderstanding can be useful in allowing the child to talk.
- If there is a history of assault with ejaculation in the last 2–3 days, it may be useful to do forensic tests: an appropriate examination should be arranged.

Past medical history

- If practicable take a history from birth. Relationship problems between mother and child may have begun very early on.
- Record any significant illnesses, hospital admissions and operations. Children have their appendices removed because of persistent abdominal pain which may, in reality, have been a psychosomatic disorder.
- Has there been any other maltreatment in the past? There is not infrequently a history of physical abuse, particularly burns, failure to thrive, neglect, emotional deprivation or previous sexual abuse. Abused children are especially vulnerable to re-abuse, and several types of abuse may coexist.
- Have there been urinary tract symptoms in the past?
- Recurrent vaginal discharge?
- Have there been bowel problems, soiling, bleeding, pain on defecation? Is there a history of other trauma: broken limbs, burns, scalds?
- Has the child had emotional problems, been referred to a psychologist or psychiatrist? The common problems of soiling, wetting, as well as school refusal, temper, anxiety, depression, anorexia and all the 'conduct disorders' – stealing, lying, fighting, glue-sniffing – have their origins somewhere.
- How is the child coping socially? Do they have friends, how do they find school or nursery, can they separate or are they clingy, do they separate too easily? How are they progressing academically?

A *developmental history* should be taken in younger children. Include in particular language development, social skills and emotional well-being – all of which may be adversely affected in child sexual abuse. Are they making progress in school?

A *family history* is important, as a picture of the child in the context of the family needs to be built up. The parents' ages, occupations and health are enquired into, followed by other children's ages, sex and well-being. Do the other children need to be interviewed and examined? It is uncommon for only one child in a household to be abused (Muram et al 1991). It is clearly of great importance if any adult within the household has a previous record of offences against children. These are designated Schedule 1 offences.

PART 2

Physical examination

Indications for examination

Issues of consent and confidentiality are discussed in Chapter 14.

Historically doctors have not routinely examined girls' genitalia or children's bottoms after an initial inspection in the neonatal period. Although the vast majority of boys' testes have descended by 3 months of age (over 96%), boys' genitalia will be repeatedly re-examined whereas girls' genitalia are only re-examined when there is a clinical indication, for example daytime wetting. The result is that most doctors, even children's doctors, have little experience of this examination and may not know the range of normal. Without this knowledge it is difficult to give an opinion on a child who may have been abused: are the physical signs those of trauma, infection, a skin disorder or within the range of normal?

Current teaching suggests that to examine a child's anus or a girl's genitalia is intrusive, although some would disagree (Meadow 1987). However, if practitioners acknowledge the many ways in which child sexual abuse may present and have a lower threshhold for examination, experience will be gained. Doctors by examining more children will quickly learn the normal variants and which physical signs should cause concern.

An allegation of child sexual abuse is clearly an indication for a full physical examination, whether there is a history of penetration or not; children commonly understate the extent of abuse. In addition, examination is usually required if there is physical abuse, wetting, soiling, vaginal discharge or bleeding and rectal bleeding. Psychosomatic disorders (abdominal pain, migraine) as well as other behavioural symptoms may be indicators. It is good practice to think about all the children in the household: may they too be abused? It is usual, unless the allegation is of 'stranger assault' to examine all the children, boys as well as girls, and sometimes friends and relatives too. The non-disclosing child in an abusing family is more likely to have abnormal signs than the disclosing siblings (Muram et al 1991).

When and why should children be physically examined?

There may be reticence on the part of parents and professionals to allow a child to be examined. Adults may wish to 'protect' the child and feel the examination is yet another intrusion into the child's privacy, or they may have unhappy memories of insensitive gynaecological examinations themselves and this experience is projected into the debate. Yet a well-conducted physical examination may have therapeutic as well as investigational attributes (San Lazaro 1995).

The examination is performed in the context of the history, and experience has shown that all children alleging sexual abuse should be seen by a paediatrician with appropriate training to ensure it is a 'whole child' examination. The examination is comprehensive, and includes an assessment of the child's growth and development, and recognition of other forms of abuse, as well as the complete physical examination. The examination is 'forensic' in the sense that the examination may reveal signs of abuse and neglect, and forensic tests may be taken, to look for semen for example.

The child's behaviour should be noted: does it change when the genitalia are examined?

- Children may be over-active and excitable, only to become passive and frightened during the examination.
- Does he masturbate or have a sustained erection; is she provocative or coy?
- Is the child supported by his or her mother or does she sit at the far side of the room appearing disinterested, even angry?

Examination in possible sexual abuse

Six main reasons have been suggested as to why the possibly sexually abused child should be examined (Bamford & Roberts 1997):

- to detect traumatic or infective conditions which may require treatment
- to evaluate the nature of any abuse
- to provide forensic evidence
- to reassure the child, who may feel serious damage has been done
- to start the process of recovery
- as the sibling of the index child

and in addition

- to reassure the carers – as appropriate
- to check the child's growth and development
- to arrange paediatric follow-up to check physical signs of healing or re-abuse
- to assess the need for therapy and refer for psychological or psychiatric support (as indicated).

When should the child be examined?

Examination should normally be arranged during the child's usual day. There is little place for evening examinations, at a time to suit the doctor rather than the child.

If the assault is recent, that is within 48–72 hours, it may be that forensic specimens should be collected and the examination is therefore arranged urgently. Otherwise there may be advantages in waiting a few days following a 'disclosure' before examining an older child or adolescent, so work can be done to prepare the child for the examination. Undue delay is to be avoided though as healing may be rapid and may be complete and corroborative evidence lost.

Where should the child be examined?

As discussed earlier, examination should usually take place at a local hospital (not a police station). Requirements for examination include:

- Quiet, child-orientated waiting room and examination rooms with appropriate toys and equipment.
- Proper equipment:
  - couch and usual examination tray
  - bright light source
  - sexually transmitted disease screening pack (Fig. 9.8)
  - forensic pack (see Table 14.8)
  - hand-held illuminated magnifying glass
  - glass rods – no longer recommended routinely in prepubertal girls
  - colposcope – increasingly available
  - refrigerator (for specimen storage)
  - camera – essential for good record keeping
  - easy access to haematology, microbiology and radiology departments.
- Nursing staff to suport the child and family, weigh and measure the child, collect urine specimens, assist in the collection of other specimens, care for the child while the doctor talks to the adults, and to chaperone the doctor (see below). Trained nurses are essential (children trained or nursery nurses) and a nurse must be available from the arrival of the family. In practice this means a doctor and nurse should work as a team with each family.
- An adequate number of rooms to separate any parties as necessary. Separate interviewing facilities are also often needed. Ideally there should be a room with a one-way screen and sound videotaping facilities. It may become good practice to videotape the examination and to record anything the child may say on tape too. Teaching may be facilitated by use of a one-way mirror and a video camera on the colposcope.

Chaperoning

Chaperones are vital for the protection of the child and doctor. This is in addition to the mother, who may make false allegations. The clinic nurse is the usual chaperone and may assist in the examination, taking swabs and also in helping the child. Sometimes a social worker or other professional may be the chaperone (GMC 1996).

False allegations

False allegations of sexual touching have to be classified as misunderstanding, distortion and misrepresentation (Silber 1994). The child or carer may be the complainant and adequate discussion before the examination may lessen the frequency of allegations of inappropriate touching. Preparation may not be adequate. Steward (1995) found that of children attending for examination following allegations of child sexual abuse when asked 'Why are you here?' 40% responded that they did not know, 26% for a 'check up' and the rest knew the examination was related to their child sexual abuse. Only 7% knew that their genitalia would be examined, and 44% of mothers said they were not fully informed. There is clearly room for improvement.

Chambers (1995) wrote

> With clear communication and sensitivity between doctor, patient and parent, they (allegations of assault) are probably avoidable in the majority of cases . . . use of witnesses, chaperones and second opinions . . . and clear, decipherable, contemporaneous notes are essential'.

Use of the colposcope

The colposcope is an instrument developed for the visualisation of the adult cervix and for the management of cervical disease, including neoplasia (Woodling & Heger 1986, Muram & Ellias 1989, McCann 1990, Hobbs et al 1995). The instrument was first used in assessing for possible sexual abuse by Teixeira, and examiners in the US have used it routinely for several years. In the UK the advantages of using the colposcope have become evident and many paediatricians are using one.

The colposcope is most valuable for detailed examination of the female genitalia including the hymen, although visualisation of the anus is also possible. The instrument consists of a powerful and adjustable light source and binocular and variable magnification. One of the most important advantages of the equipment is that an integral camera permits simultaneous photographs to be taken during the examination without the use of an additional light source. The colposcope provides a good light source, magnification and a facility for photography (including videotaping). For photography, 35 mm single lens reflex, Polaroid and video cameras can all be used. Still photographs are obtainable from the video film; 35 mm probably provides the best quality results in the form of slides or prints. A single lens reflex camera is used with a data back: the slides are used to discuss findings with colleagues, peer review, teaching, second opinions (when slides usually avoid the need for the child to be re-examined) and medico-legal work.

Colposcopy may help in subtle cases to differentiate normal from abnormal. It allows visualisation of further minor abnormality in 10% which assists in the overall assessment (Woodling & Heger 1986). Another study (Muram 1989) showed that 96% of abnormality was visible to the unaided eye and the other 4% (seen using a colposcope) was also visualised once the abnormality was described. A hand-held magnifying glass or auriscope (without speculum) is adequate but not ideal. Evaluation of the colposcope in terms of improving the clinical assessment and hence the diagnosis of child sexual abuse do not suggest that there is a significantly more precise examination using the instrument compared with a simple light source (otoscope, lamp).

The examination using the colposcope is one of inspection and allows more distance between the examiner and the child (Hobbs 1997, RCP). Essentially the children handle the examination well and are not, as is sometimes suggested, 're-traumatised'. Evaluation of the use of the colposcope in 109 prepubertal girls (Hobbs et al 1995) found the examination acceptable to children, parents and examiners. A study which looked specifically at the response of children to colposcopic examination concluded that although children were poorly prepared for the examination they were not re-traumatised and children were signficantly less stressed after the examination (Steward et al 1995).

However, it is not essential to have a colposcope (Table 9.12) and the instrument is expensive and not readily portable. Practice is necessary to achieve a good examination and photographs, especially if the child is young and does not keep still. Sometimes its use is not possible, for example when young, uncooperative children are examined. If the child has been involved in pornography, photography may be unacceptable.

Advantages of colposcopy: summary

- Good illumination and magnification are available
- An integral measuring device in the eyepiece is available on some models
- Areas of apparent minor abnormality, unusual vascular patterns or questionable scarring are likely to be seen as normal under good illumination and magnification
- The opportunity to accurately record the examination (i.e. photographically) usually obviates the need for the child to be re-examined if a second opinion is required
- The photographs may be used in peer review and to allow discussion for colleagues in training, and also for all doctors when the physical signs prove difficult to evaluate – it is already possible, given the appropriate computer and software, to transmit high-quality pictures allowing doctors who work in isolated areas to seek advice and take part in peer review (Brayden 1991)
- Follow-up examination with photography allows the further evaluation necessary in 'difficult' cases
- The colposcope puts space between the child and the examiner; the instrument is well tolerated by children (who may like to use it to examine a doll) and parents appear to find the colposcope acceptable

Table 9.12 Advantages and disadvantages of using a colposcope (Hobbs 1997)

Advantages	Disadvantages
Non-invasive technique	Expensive (but robust)
Good light and magnification	Relatively non-portable
Facilities for non-intrusive photography	May discourage unaided examination
Acceptable to child, parents, doctor	Danger of over-interpretation of minor signs

Manner of the physical examination

The child will usually be asked who they would like to be present at the examination. Many will want their mother present but older children may want to be seen on their own, with their social worker or police officer or with a friend. The doctor *must* be chaperoned (see above) if the child is to be seen alone (GMC 1996).

Older children may prefer to chose the gender of the doctor who is to examine them, and this should be accommodated if possible. For younger children it is the manner of the doctor which is more important.

While the history is taken from the carer the child has the opportunity to settle and become accustomed to the unusual surroundings. The examination should be uninterrupted and taken at the child's pace. Many children aged 1–3 years find it more upsetting to have their ears looked into than their bottoms examined. However, this changes and by 5–6 years children are beginning to be clear about privacy and, as they are no longer in nappies, have become unused to being exposed. A sheet is used to provide as far as possible for the child's modesty.

Reassurance should be given to the child during the history taking and examination. The doctor should:

- explain who he or she is, i.e. he or she is a children's doctor.
- explain the nature of the examination before beginning the examination; many mothers will be anxious about 'an internal' – this part of the examination is not needed in prepubertal girls. Digital anal examination is rarely needed. It is better not to say 'It will not hurt' as this causes apprehension.
- if appropriate, reassure that the child has been right to tell, and it is not his or her 'fault'.
- reassure that there has been no 'damage'. Children and parents often have delusions about this, even to the extent of the effect on subsequent childbearing.
- if the girl is still technically a 'virgin' (i.e. the hymen remains) say so – this may be very important socially and culturally.
- explain that unfortunately a lot of children are abused and it is never the child's responsibility
- avoid using terms such as 'scarring', which may cause unnecessary alarm.

Sedation or general anaesthetic

It is unusual to have to sedate a child although there are circumstances when it is essential. Written consent should be sought before a child is sedated or anaesthetised for the examination and photography.

Recent practice suggests that a short anaesthetic in theatre may be the better option than sedation: the child will not start to struggle before the examination, swab collection and photography is completed and is probably safer with fewer complictions than high doses of sedatives, although ketamine sedation has its advocates (Harari 1994).

Indications for sedation or general anaesthetic

- Distraught child where examination considered essential in order to further protect the child
- Painful injuries, e.g. vaginal wall tear, which need evaluation, i.e. for possible surgery
- Risk of STD and child unable to allow adequate screening (swabs)
- Strong possibility forensic swabs would be useful and child unable to comply
- Foreign body
- Older child who wishes to comply but cannot due to anxiety

Forensic specimens

The collection of forensic specimens is discussed in Chapter 14.

Physical examination

The physical examination follows the normal paediatric routine. Children are usually weighed and measured by the nurse before the examination (unless the child is distressed). The initial contact with the nurse may be very helpful to establish some rapport if specimens are to be collected later. The measurements should be taken in a standard way, on equipment that is regularly checked. The values are plotted on centile charts.

In order to gain the child's confidence, examine the child gently from head to toe. It is also useful to screen for squint, dental caries, heart murmurs and so on as the child may have been neglected medically as well as maltreated in other ways. When examining the abdomen note carefully is there are faecal masses. Does the child have dry skin, eczema or any other skin disorder? Later constipation or skin disorder may be presented as the cause of signs consistent with child sexual abuse. It is important to record the history and examination in detail on these and other points, for example bed wetting, urinary tract infection, vaginal discharge or bleeding, pain in the genitalia.

Record the stage of puberty, i.e. prepubertal; pubertal signs should be described using Tanner's classification (Tanner 1978) (Table 9.13).

If there are any signs of recent physical assault, bruises, burns or lacerations record the findings carefully. Measure any lesion in centimetres, describe colour, depth of scald or laceration and also the dimensions of any scars (see Ch. 4).

Sexually abused children may present as though they have been physically abused (see Ch 8), or with bruises suggestive of child sexual abuse: love bites, bruises on breasts, suprapubically, inner thighs or knees or of the genitalia (Fig. 9.9; Hobbs & Wynne 1990).

Record any signs of self-mutilation: usually cuts, bites, scratches or nips on arms, upper chest, face or laceration of the gums with fingernails, and hair pulling. Injury to the genitalia may also be seen in very disturbed children. Self-mutilation should always lead the physician to consider 'Would this be abuse?' rather than, as in the case of children with learning disability 'It's part of the syndrome'. Self-mutilation may be seen at any age but is more likely in adolescence.

Physical examination of prepubertal girls

The examination of a girl who has been, or has allegedly been, sexually abused, may be normal or have non-specific signs in 26–77% of the girls examined (Muram 1989, Emans 1989, Paradise 1990, Bays & Chadwick 1993, Adams et al 1994, Hobbs 1995b, RCP 1997).

The signs seen depend on the type of abuse, the length of time from the last assault (healing may be very rapid), the chronicity of the abuse and the presence of any infection.

Examination is ideally carried out on the couch in a standard way and photographs taken of each examination even if there appear to be no abnormal signs. Children of 2 years and under are not easy to examine and if distressed are usually best examined on their mother's knee.

A good light is needed and magnification is helpful as described previously. Measurement is by a tape-measure laid adjacent to the lesion or structure. Colposcopes may in the future have an integral measuring device in the eyepiece.

All girls are examined in a similar frog-legged position. The prone knee–chest position gives a better view of the posterior margin of the hymen and may be the only way to evaluate the posterior 180° of the hymen when it is folded.

Digital examination is not indicated prepubertally and few practitioners continue to use graduated glass rods which allow evaluation of the hymenal margin and the size of the hymenal opening. The rods may provide useful information, particularly in demonstrating tears, but their use has been questioned in the measuring of hymenal opening dimensions which may be

Table 9.13 Stages of puberty (after Tanner 1978)

Stage	Breast development	Pubic hair	Genital (penis) development
1	Pre-adolescent: elevation of papilla only	Pre-adolescent: the vellus over the pubes is not further developed than that over the abdominal wall, i.e. no pubic hair	Pre-adolescent: testes, scrotum and penis are of about the same size and proportion as in early childhood
2	Breast bud stage: elevation of breast and papilla as small mound. Enlargement of areola diameter	Sparse growth of long, slightly pigmented downy hair, straight or slightly curled, chiefly along labia	Enlargement of scrotum and testes. Skin of scrotum reddens and changes in texture. Little or no enlargement of penis at this stage
3	Further enlargement and elevation of breast and areola, with no separation of their contours	Considerably darker, coarser and more curled. The hair spreads sparsely over the junction of the pubes	Enlargement of penis, which occurs at first mainly in length. Further growth of testes and scrotum
4	Projection of areola and papilla to form a secondary mound above the level of the breast	Hair now adult in type, but area covered is still considerably smaller than in the adult. No spread to the medial surface of thighs	Increased size of penis with growth in breadth and development of glans. Testes and scrotum larger, scrotal skin darkened
5	Mature stage: projection of papilla only, due to recession of the areola to the general contour of the breast	Adult in quantity and type with distribution of the horizontal (or classically 'feminine') pattern. Spread to medial surface of thighs but not up linea alba or elsewhere above the base of the inverse triangle (spread up linea alba occurs late and is rated stage 6)	Genitalia adult in size and shape

inaccurate because of stretching round the rod due to elasticity of the hymen (RCP 1991).

Rarely it is necessary to pass a speculum to find the source of bleeding, but in this circumstance a general anaesthetic is usually needed. Continuing bleeding is rare but in severe injury such as rape there may be long deep tears extending proximally though the vaginal wall (there will be other signs of trauma in this case).

In older girls a full examination for sexually transmitted diseases with visualization of the cervix is needed in a high proportion of cases, up to 25% of girls will have a sexually transmitted disease.

Child sexual abuse is the usual cause of prepubertal vaginal bleeding. Vaginal tumours are very unusual and in precocious puberty there are usually other signs of puberty.

Foreign bodies when pushed through the hymen cause pain and bleeding but the child may not be presented until an offensive, perhaps blood-streaked discharge is seen. Child sexual abuse is highly correlated with the placement of foreign bodies; insertion is painful and unlikely to be a child's activity (Herman-Giddens 1994).

Further discussion as to differential diagnosis is given later in this chapter.

Signs associated with genital abuse

- Bruising, abrasions, reddening, oedema of external and internal genitalia
- Recent or healing lacerations of labia, posterior fourchette
- Lacerations or scars on hymen which may extend to posterior vaginal wall*
- Dilated hymenal opening
- Attenuated hymen with loss of hymenal tissue*
- Multiple healed hymenal tears seen as clefts, rounded remnants, deficits in margin (NB: congenital variants)
- Sexually transmitted disease*
- Vulvovaginitis (not STD)
- Dilated and/or traumatised urethra
- Labial fusion, of variable degree (usually posterior)
- Scars, e.g. at posterior fourchette, vaginal wall*
- Signs of uncertain significance are:

- hyperpigmentation of perineum, inner thighs, perianally
- periurethral and perivaginal synechiae
- adhesions to vaginal wall
- increased vascularity of hymen (Emmans et al 1987)

- Remember to look for signs of:
  - other physical abuse
  - anal abuse/oral abuse
  - self-mutilation
  - eating disorder
- Pregnancy

Signs marked * are highly correlated with abuse and in some instances diagnostic (see text).

For a more complete description by site of the physical signs associated with genital abuse see Table 9.14.

The Tanner stages of puberty as given in Table 9.13 should be recorded.

The *external genitalia* should be inspected first for bruises, lacerations, burns, scars, skin disorders or warts, vesicles and molluscum contagiosum. Is the hymenal opening visible and gaping before the legs are abducted?

The *labia majora* are gently separated and labia minora, urethra, perihymenal regions, hymen and posterior fourchette are visualised (Fig. 9.10). Is there any labial fusion (agglutination): posterior or, less commonly, anterior? Measure the length of the fusion, note if it is superficial or thick, is there any nappy rash? (See later in this chapter for further detail on fusion.)

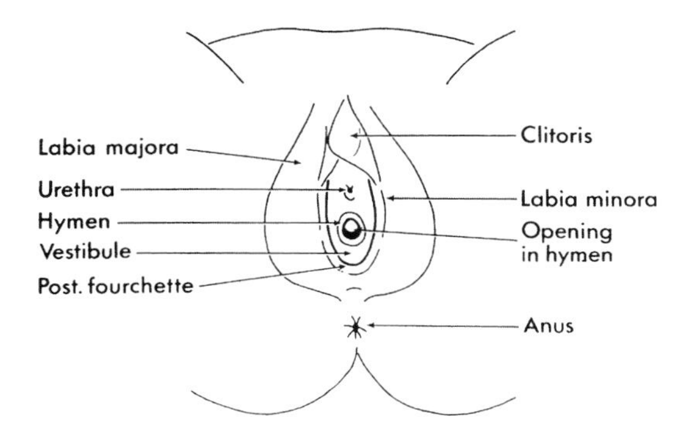

Fig. 9.10 Anatomy of normal prepubertal female genitalia.

The hymen, perihymenal tissues and *posterior fourchette* have a clear, lacy, vascular pattern. The mucosa appears much redder in pre- than post-pubertal girls. The normal introitus should be free from all scarring. Bands of tissue may be seen running across the periurethral, perihymenal tissues or within the vagina. These are called *support bands* and their significance is not clear but they are probably a normal variant.

If the child has been masturbated roughly there may be uniform erythema, swelling of the tissues and even superficial lacerations of the labia minora or posterior fourchette caused by fingernails.

Blunt trauma, as in intercrural or attempted vaginal intercourse, gives marked erythema, which may extend on to the labia majora, and oedema which may obscure the hymenal opening. There may be bruising, but this is uncommon. There may be 'scooping out' of the posterior fourchette in intercrural intercourse and also labial fusion secondary to trauma. The skin of the perineum may become thickened. Increased pigmentation has been described of perineum, inner thighs and perianally (vagabond pigmentation) in intercrural intercourse, but is a 'soft' sign particularly if the child is overweight.

Localised abrasions, often lateral to the hymen or at posterior fourchette, are seen in digital and penile abuse.

The *urethra* should be inspected. The orifice may appear to 'pout' after vigorous rubbing and occasionally abusers thread objects into the urethra, causing actual dilatation and trauma to the tissues.

The urethra may appear dilated if there is labial traction (see Fig. 9.12) and therefore the description of the urethra should be during labial separation. A prolapsed urethra is rare and appears like a doughnut (Johnson 1991).

Hymen

The hymen is the membrane across the opening of the vagina. In the newborn period and infancy all hymens are thick and redundant under the effects of maternal oestrogen but as the maternal oestrogen effect wanes the hymen changes,

Table 9.14 Signs associated with genital abuse

Site	Lesion	Description	Aetiology
Labia majora	Erythema	Reddening of skin	Inflammatory response to local irritation or skin disorder, or infection
	Bruising	Extravasation of blood into skin, initially red or reddish purple and undergoes colour change with time	Local trauma
	Burns/scald	Skin loss of varying degree, blister	Local trauma
	Oedema	Swelling of tissues	Associated with infection or trauma
	Abrasion, scratch, laceration	Superficial skin loss, initially pink or red, and moist, before healing with scab formation	Superficial trauma, e.g. fingernail scratches, frictional injury
	Scars	Area of altered skin, i.e. depigmented, thinned or thickened	Lacerations usually heal with a linear white scar which fades with time; burns or scalds, if partial thickness or deeper, scar in shape of initial lesion
	Vesicles	Small, painful vesicles surrounded by erythema – look at vulva	Is it HSV-1 or HSV-2 infection? Chicken pox?
	Warts	Soft, white, broad-based or pedunculated lesions variable in size and number – look at vulva and anus	Usually a STD (see section on STD)
Vulvovaginitis	Erythema, oedema	Swelling, reddening of vulval tissues may extend on to labia majora Discharge yellow, greenish, white, watery, sticky, scanty, profuse	Often no pathogenic organism is grown If indicated, full screen for STD should be performed Common in 2–5 year age group Increased incidence of non-specific vulvovaginitis in CSA
Labia minora, perihymenal area	Erythema	Reddening of mucous membrane	Inflammatory response to local irritation, e.g. bubblebath or infection, or trauma such as rubbing, also skin disorders
	Bruising	Areas of extravasation of blood which initially appear a darker red and after 24 hours are seen as deep red/purple	Trauma
	Oedema	Swelling of tissues	Associated with infection or trauma
	Abrasion, scratch, laceration	Loss of superficial layer of mucous membrane, appears as a red area of variable shape (NB: seen better with colposcope)	Traumatic lesions heal very quickly (1–7 days)
	Warts, vesicles	As before	
	Labial adhesions	Agglutination of labia minora at posterior fourchette	Acquired lesion due to unknown cause or trauma
Posterior fourchette	Erythema, oedema, bruising	As vulva	
	Laceration	Tear usually running vertically from below	Distinguish scar from congenital midline streak
	Friability	Tissues readily tear and bleed	
	Scarring	Altered vascular pattern. Thickened white area, irregular shape	Important area of trauma in CSA
Hymen	Erythema, oedema, abrasion, bruising	As vulva, due to trauma; or superficial infection	
	Dilatation of hymenal opening	Attenuation with loss of hymenal tissue Wider-than-expected horizontal diameter for age • 0.5 cm is upper end of normal at 5 years • 1.0 cm is not seen in prepubertal girls (labial separation, not traction)	Penetrating trauma with blunt force (RCP 1991) Stretching of hymen as in digital penetration Hymen is elastic and recovery may take place Different methods of examination important
	Deficit	Discontinuity in margin. Differentiate from notch in crescentic hymen at 11 and 1 o'clock	Penetrative tear

	Mound or bump	Seen in margin of hymen, may be multiple: • associated with disruption of hymen • often posterior	Trauma causing tears to hymen with healing causing the irregularity Often associated with dilated hymen
	Tears	If very recent (<24 hours) may see bleeding. Complete or incomplete transection of hymen, may extend to vaginal wall	Penetrative stretching
	Shape of hymen	Attenuated	Penetrative trauma (may be gradual rubbing away or more acute disruption)
		Posterior rim or heart or crescentic shape (all variants of same) Annular Fimbriate	Congenital variants
		Horse-shoe shape	May represent anterior tears, but hymen often deficient anteriorly: look for other signs – scarring, dilated hymen
		Asymmetry of shape, e.g. 'V' at 6 o'clock, sharp angle, square angles, any major distortion	May represent healed tears in hymen – look for scarring, disruption of hymen
	Scar	White, irregular, thickened area	Previous trauma – RARE
Vagina	Bruising, abrasion	Areas of darker red on vaginal wall	Penetrative trauma
	Dilated/gaping	To accommodate one or more fingers (1.5 cm–4.0 cm) at puberty	Repeated dilatation leads to widening, lengthening of vagina with eventual loss of rugae
	Loss of rugae	Flattening of rugae	
	Tears	Extending from hymen to posterior vaginal wall	Severe penetrative trauma leading to tear which may scar
	Scar	Posterior wall scarring	
Urethra	Erythema, oedema, bruising, dilatation	Reddened, swollen periurethral tissues, pouting urethral meatus	Rubbing – see as part of vulvitis Urethra may also be penetrated by foreign body
Perineum,inner thighs, perianally	Pigmentation	Increased pigmentation of skin	Due to repeated friction as in intercrural intercourse. Non-specific sign also seen in obesity

Table 9.15 Morphology of the hymen

Configuration of hymen	Newborn (%)	At 3 years (%)
Annular	72	38
Crescentic	1	55
Fimbriated	19	2
Sleeve	6	5

becoming thinner, flatter and with a sharp edge. This change has taken place in 75% of girls by 3 years of age (Table 9.15; Berenson 1995). The hymen continues in this form, thin, with a sharp edge and clearly visible vessels during childhood until puberty, when it once again becomes oestrogenised. The pubertal hymen is thick, paler, redundant, sleeve-like or fimbriated and often there is a white physiological discharge. Hymenal elasticity increases with pubertal development. The capillary network is obscured (A J Thomas, personal communication 1997).

Congenital absence of hymen is very rare. In one study in 1131 newborn infant examinations, all 1131 infants were noted to have a hymen (Jenny et al 1987). Between 3% and 4% had hymenal variants such as tags and transverse hymenal bands. The highest possible frequency of congenital absence of hymen was calculated as less than 0.3%. The authors concluded that if hymenal tissue cannot be identified traumatic disruption should be considered as the likely cause.

In prepubertal girls the *central opening* in the hymen varies in shape between thin and crescentic, annular, frilly, septate, cuff-like and punctate (Herman-Giddens and Frothingham 1987). The margin becomes smooth and thinner after infancy. The hymen is often more pronounced posteriorly and relatively deficient anteriorly.

The *annular and crescentic* (posterior rim) configurations are the two commonest variants (McCann 1990). The crescentic rim appears to be commoner in older girls (RCP 1997) with 45%, annular hymen in 27% and fimbriated 20% (Gardner 1992). Berenson (1995) in a longitudinal study of hymenal morphology from 2 months or younger to 3 years confirmed the findings in Table 9.15. Heger (1991) found that 75–80% of girls attending a referral centre for vulvovaginal complaints and abuse had crescentic hymens and postulated that gradual coercive dilatation might convert an annular or fimbriated hymen into a crescentic one in abused older girls.

Occasionally a *septate* hymen (a vertical septum) is seen and this may be in association with a septate vagina and bicornuate uterus. An ultrasound scan in older children will delineate the extent of the problem. Occasionally the septum is limited to a smoooth bump (2–3 mm vertically) at 6 o'clock, which is thought to be a minor degree of a 'septate' hymen. 'Hymenal' tags are relatively common in the newborn but are occasionally seen in older children too as a redundant tag of tissue described as hymen usually attached inferiorly.

An *imperforate* or *microperforate* hymen is very uncommon. The hymen is smooth, which distinguishes it from a secondarily imperforate hymen which has been traumatised and has a thickened disorganised appearance (Berkowitz et al 1987).

When the labia are separated the hymen may be clearly visible, but the opening is usually closed. In order to visualise the hymenal margin there is further labial separation and if necessary labial traction. Labial separation involves gentle pressure downwards and laterally and if unsuccessful labial traction is needed, the labia are lifted followed by gentle downward pressure for a few seconds (Figs 9.11 and 9.12). These manoeuvres affect the dimensions of the hymenal opening and the method of examination should be noted.

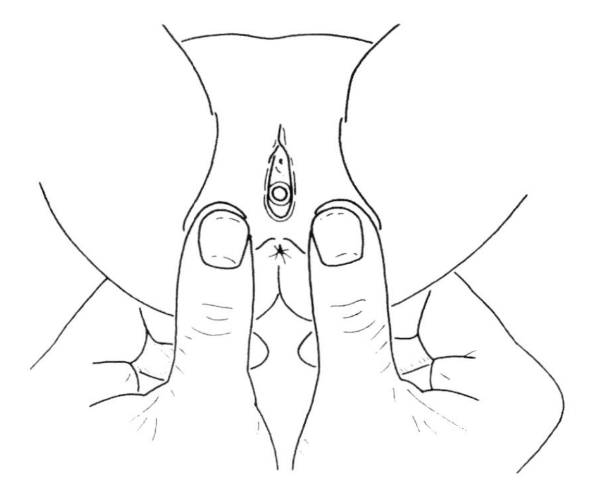

Fig. 9.11 Separation as a means of achieving relaxed visualisation of the hymenal opening.

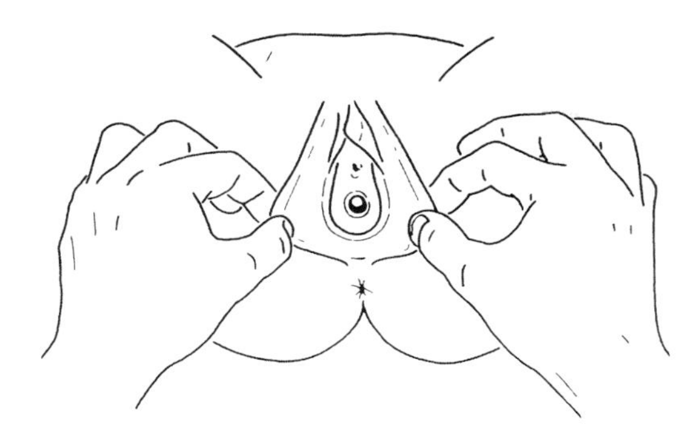

Fig. 9.12 Labial traction as a means of achieving relaxed visualisation of the hymenal opening.

A gaping hymenal orifice on abduction of the legs, that is before any manipulation of the labia, is suggestive of abuse (RCP 1997).

If the posterior part of the hymen is not visible on traction and it appears rolled examining the child in the knee–chest position will allow better visualisation as the hymen unfolds.

McCann (1990) found, by using a combination of examination methods in 172 prepubertal girls aged 10 months to 11 years, that in only two children did the vaginal introitus not open. Labial traction was more successful than labial separation and the knee–chest position was the most successful.

The *dimensions* of the hymenal opening depend on the method used to examine the child (McCann 1990) and the measuring device. A rigid tape measure placed adjacent to the child's genitalia gives an adequate assessment of the horizontal dimensions. Photographs taken using a colposcope may be accurately measured. Graduated glass rods are not routinely used to measure the hymenal opening as given the elasticity of the hymen the measurements are thought to be inaccurate (RCP 1997).

The hymenal orifice increases only a little with age, up to 0.4 cm at 4 years (Woodling 1986). The opening in a girl of 5 years is rarely more than 0.5 cm (Huffman et al 1981). When early signs of oestrogen effects are visible the hymenal orifice 'will measure 7 mm or more in diameter by the time a reaction to oestrogen is grossly visible' and is around 1 cm when puberty is complete (Dewhurst 1988).

The above figures are from standard gynaecology texts. More recent research findings are summarised in Table 9.16.

A summary by Heger and Emmans (1990) of current ideas is helpful:

- Healing is rapid, and the hymen if stretched rather than attenuated may recover and even in cases where there has been penetration (usually digital) there may be normal findings (Muram 1989b).
- A horizontal diameter of >4.0 mm is associated with abuse (Cantwell 1987, White et al 1989).
- Care must be taken in overemphasis of measurements of only a few mm (Paradise 1989).
- The size of the hymenal opening depends on:
  - age of the child
  - stage of pubertal development
  - position of the child (supine or knee–chest)
  - degree of labial traction
  - relaxation of the child
  - obesity of the child – increased vertical diameter only (Kerns et al 1992).
- The usual shape of the opening is annular (i.e. it encircles the hymen) or crescentic (absent 11–1 o'clock).
- Healing may lead to contraction of the opening as a result of scar formation (Berkowitz 1987).
- Healing may take place when the child is protected from further child sexual abuse (Cantwell 1987) unless the hymen is attenuated, when it cannot recover.
- A normal hymenal opening does not exclude child sexual abuse and minor abnormality does not prove child sexual abuse.
- A diagnosis of child sexual abuse is made on all the evidence, not one single sign.

The *hymenal opening* may appear to wink during examination: this is normal. The hymenal opening is usually *symmetrical* in mid-childhood. Marked asymmetry, for example a small notch at 11 o'clock and a marked notch at 1 o'clock or other sharp angles, square angles or distortions of the hymenal margin should be noted as signs of possible previous trauma.

Table 9.16 Research findings in prepubertal girls

Study	Subjects	Findings
Cantwell (1983)	Children with a vaginal introital opening > 0.4 cm	74% had a history of child sexual abuse
Herman-Giddens & Frothingham (1987)	Children with a vaginal introital opening > 0.4 cm	4% denied a history of child sexual abuse
White et al (1989)	Children with an introital diameter > 0.4 cm	94% had a history of sexual contact
Goff et al (1989)	373 girls at routine health checks	In supine frog-leg position the mean diameter in the first year of life was 0.17 cm, rising to 0.25 cm at 7 years
Emans et al (1987)	3–6-year-old girls ('normals')	Measurements of 0.29 + 0.13 cm (with a range 0.1–0.6 cm) recorded
McCann et al (1990b)	Girls selected for non-abuse	*2–4 years* Labial separation 0.39 ± 0.14 cm (range 0.1–0.55 cm) Labial traction 0.52 ± 0.14 cm (range 0.2–0.8 cm) *5–7 years* Labial separation 0.42 ± 0.17 cm (range 0.1–0.8 cm) Labial traction 0.56 ± 0.18 cm (range 0.1–0.9 cm) *8 years – Tanner Stage 2* Labial separation 0.57 ± 0.16 (range 0.3–0.8 cm) Labial traction 0.69 ± 0.20 cm (range 0.25–1.5 cm) (Measurements in knee–chest position are greater)
McCann et al (1990a)	Girls in a child sexual abuse evaluation clinic	*Pre-school* Labial separation 0.35 ± 0.14 cm (range 0.1–0.7 cm) Labial traction 0.57 ± 0.16 cm (range 0.1–1.0 cm) *Early school* Labial separation 0.40 ± 0.16 cm (range 0.25–1.0 cm) Labial traction 0.59 ± 0.17 cm (range 0.25–1.0 cm) *Pre-adolescent* Labial separation 0.50 ± 0.20 cm (range 0.2–0.9 cm) Labial traction 0.65 ± 0.21 cm (range 0.3–1.0 cm) (Measurements in knee–chest position are greater)
Paul (1990)	Commentary on his experience as a police surgeon	Diameters of 0.2–0.9 cm may be normal
Bamford & Roberts (1997)		Unstretched hymenal orifice in most young girls is no more than 0.5–0.6 cm
RCP (1991, 1997)		Suggests that at puberty the horizontal diameter is approximately 1 cm, that a diameter of more than 1 cm is not commonly seen in normal pre-pubertal children but quote 9/79 non-abused girls having an opening of more than 1 cm (Gardner 1992). A hymenal opening of 1.5 cm in a pre-pubertal girl in association with other trauma would be highly suggestive of abuse. The report emphasizes that this is supportive evidence of child sexual abuse but not diagnostic on its own
Berenson (1992)	Non-abused girls	Horizontal diameter using labial traction: 01–12 months mean 2.5 mm range 1.0–3.5 mm 13–24 months mean 2.9 mm range 1.5–6.5 mm 25–48 months mean 2.9 mm range 1.0–6.5 mm 49–81 months mean 3.6 mm range 2.0–6.8 mm
Hobbs & Wynne (1995)	109 prepubertal girls referred for assessment of possible child sexual abuse	Mean hymenal orifice transverse diameter: 20–59 months 4.23 mm 60–99 months 4.26 mm >100 months 6.17 mm 37/90 girls had an opening <4 mm 45/90 girls had an opening >4 mm

Minor bumps in the margin are probably normal variants, but bumps in association with a distorted hymenal margin and a disrupted vascular pattern seen especially posteriorly and laterally are seen in association with abuse. The non-traumatised hymenal rim is usually thin and smooth with a clear vascular pattern.

Vaginal ridges running vertically down the vagina are normal and may cause a smooth bump at the hymenal margin.

Hymenal tears (transections or lacerations) may occur at any site:

- Those caused by penile or attempted penile penetration are likely to cause greater damage than those caused by digital penetration and are commonly found at 5–7 o'clock (Herman-Giddens & Frothingham 1987, Emans et al 1987, Muram 1989b) and may extend on to the posterior fourchette and occasionally the posterior vaginal wall. Synechiae or bridging scars may be seen following these penetrative injuries.
- Berenson (1995) described notches in 8% in a cohort selected for non-abuse. No notches were seen in between 4 and 8 o'clock. See Table 9.17.

The current position is that a notch in the posterior half of the hymen is not found in non-abused children and is an abnormal sign, being supportive of a diagnosis of abuse (RCP 1997). There is debate around notches which are lateral or anterior. The authors of this book consider these notches if deep, asymmetric (if anterior), or associated with distortion or scarring are consistent with abuse. A single, shallow notch at 12 o'clock is usually normal.

Attenuation of the hymen is described '. . . as a sign of damage due to hymenal tissue being rubbed or worn away due to chronic abuse' (RCP 1997). The loss of tissue may be asymmetric and is often posterior or lateral. Scarring is uncommon but if present indicates abuse. Attenuation of the hymen with resultant enlargement of the hymenal orifice is a diagnostic sign of penetrating injury (RCP 1997). Attentuation does not 'heal': the hymen will always remain deficient and the orifice wide. Even after puberty the hymen will remain deficient, unable to develop into characteristic petals over the attenuated area.

If there has been stretching of the hymen without loss of tissue, healing will take place (if the abuse stops) and the orifice will become smaller again.

There have been attempts to refine the examination of the hymen by measuring the width of the posterior rim: a standard range would be useful in defining posterior attenuation. Unfortunately this is not as easy as it sounds and it is not always clear how the measurements are made and where exactly the endpoint is (Hobbs 1995b). The range of findings is shown in Table 9.18.

Scars are very unusual but may be seen at the posterior fourchette after a '. . . splitting or shearing injury' (RCP 1997). The scar is seen as a thickened, white irregular area, which disrupts the usual lacy vascular pattern. Scars are to be differentiated from the congenital flat, white, midline streak (Herman-Giddens & Frothingham 1987) or the area of relative pallor seen in the midline in some non-abused girls (McCann 1990). Vulvar coitus may cause a split which scars or results in labial fusion.

Hymenal *tears* caused by digital penetration may be seen circumferentially but are said to be seen mainly between 9 o'clock and 3 o'clock anteriorly. Penile penetration or attempted penetration is likely to cause more damage and tears are likely to be posterior and may extend to the posterior fourchette or the posterior vaginal wall.

Table 9.17 Hymeneal notches: research findings

	Position of hymenal notch	Neonate (%)	3 years (%)	Prepubertal
Berenson (1995)	11–1 o'clock	6	19	—
	2–4 o'clock	3	10	—
	5–7 o'clock	0	0	—
	8–10 o'clock	4	11	—
Hobbs (1995b)	12 o'clock	—	—	3
	11–12 o'clock	—	—	8
	6 o'clock	—	—	25
	Elsewhere	—	—	25

Table 9.18 Measurements of the posterior rim of the hymen

Study	Subjects	Findings	
		Mean	Range
Berenson (1995)	Normals		
	age 1 year	2.4 mm	2.9 ± 0.7 mm
	age 3 years	2.5 mm	3.2 ± 0.4 mm
Berenson (1992)	Normal prepubertal girls to 80 months	2.8 mm	0.9–5.0 mm
McCann (1990)	'Normal' prepubertal girls to 120 months	2.3 mm	2.3 ± 0.6 mm
Adams (1994)	Abused mean age 9 years (8 months–17 years 11 months)	48% ample posterior rim, 6% narrowed < 1mm (ample is 1–2 mm but <1 mm is a 'suspicious' sign)	
Kerns et al (1992)		Also found hymenal rim narrowing to be an abnormal sign	

Tears may heal in 1–3 days but 'acutely' may be seen in association with a gaping hymen, an oedematous hymen and perihymenal tissues and localized abrasions.

Synechiae or bridging scars may follow severe injury in association with scars at the posterior fourchette or labial fusion (as above).

When tears heal they may leave:

- V-shaped notches in the hymenal margin
- clefts: note that the hymen is often deficient anteriorly and clefts at 12 o'clock at usually a normal variant, likewise the symmetrical clefts of a crescentic hymen
- a bump: where a tear has healed and the opposed sides have not been accurately aligned there is often some thickening and disruption of the hymen – ensure the bump is not a vaginal ridge or just a minor irregularity
- an asymmetrical, square or distorted shape to the hymenal orifice
- concavities of the hymenal ring (Kerns 1992): posterior/lateral location, angular or irregular features, hymenal ring narrowing were all associated with abuse.

Physical signs and the reported abuse do not always correlate as expected (Muram 1989b). Tears are the most common finding in girls who describe penile or digital penetration. If the disruption of the hymen is more forcible, causing multiple tears, only remnants or tags of hymen may remain. However, even if there has been a history of vaginal penetration, up to one-third of girls have no abnormality on examination (57% if digital penetration, 3.5% if penile; Muram 1989b). With continued healing fewer and fewer signs are evident. Definite scars in the hymen are rare, but a thickened, irregular margin of a distorted hymen is seen – the changes are usually laterally or inferiorly.

Earlier teaching based on gynaecolgical practice suggested that hymenal tears do not heal. Experience of child sexual abuse shows that if abused girls cease to be involved in sexual activity healing does take place unless the hymen is attenuated (rubbed or worn away by chronic abuse). An attenuated, scarred hymen is never seen in normal children (RCP 1991). Attenuation is highly correlated with abuse, scars in the hymen are rare but distortions are seen frequently in a damaged hymen.

Occasionally a traumatised hymen will heal to obliterate the orifice, hence the term 'acquired' imperforate hymen (Berkowitz et al 1987). This is differentiated from a congenitally imperforate hymen as the latter is smooth and the traumatised imperforate hymen is thickened and has a disorganized appearance.

Labial fusion

Labial fusion, the partial or complete adherence of the labia minora, is commonly seen in infancy and early childhood, often in association with nappy rash. It occurs secondary to denudation of the upper squamous epithelial layer of the labial mucosa with the formation of a thin connective tissue bridge (Rimsza & Feingold 1989) and is caused by inflammatory disorders, including vulvitis and nappy rash, or trauma.

McCann et al (1988) described adhesions seen in non-abused children aged 2 months to 7 years as very superficial, semi-transparent and easily ruptured by lateral traction. The majority were diagnosed under the age of 2 years, disappearing by puberty. The incidence of these adhesions was 1.4%. In a later study of girls selected for non-abuse (McCann 1990) the incidence of labial fusion was reported as 39% but in 19/35 girls the fusion was 2 mm or less and only seen on magnification using a colposcope.

The incidence of labial fusion in sexually abused girls has been reported in 3–18% of girls (Berkowitz et al 1987, Emmans et al 1987). McCann et al (1988) described injury to the posterior fourchette by intracrural or intralabial intercourse causing trauma to the tissues which varied in severity from reddening to deep laceration, leading to labial fusion.

Labial fusion in child sexual abuse often follows trauma which is more violent that the irritation or infection associated with nappy rash, but the adhesions may be indistinguishable clinically. In child sexual abuse, labial fusion may be:

- longer, 0.5–1.0 cm or more
- superficial, semi-transparent and easily ruptured
- thick, irregular and, if there has been severe injury, scarring (McCann 1988)
- associated with a disrupted vascular pattern
- in older girls (Bays & Jenny 1990)
- indistinguishable from the 'innocent' labial fusion seen in infancy in association with nappy rash (RCP 1991).

Other signs associated with genital abuse

Some other signs are associated with abuse.

- *Vulvitis* (erythema and oedema) is a non-specific sign and is caused by infection, trauma (e.g. vigorous rubbing) or contact with irritant soap, bubble-bath).
- *Vulvovaginitis:*
  - non-specific infection
  - sexually transmitted disease, e.g. gonorrhoea.
- *Pouting or dilated urethra* caused by rubbing or, occasionally, dilatation due to insertion of a foreign body, urethral intercourse is rare.
- *Urethral prolapse:* is not well understood but may be associated with child sexual abuse, but is not diagnostic of child sexual abuse.
  - The child presents with a history of blood in the nappy, difficulty in micturition and in addition there may be constipation.
  - On examination there is a swelling protruding through the labia which is usually purplish-black in colour and has the shape of a doughnut or rosette. The swelling is 0.5–3.0 cm in diameter and as the swelling settles is seen to encircle the urethral meatus.
- Urethral prolapse is rare and is seen more often in girls with Afro-Caribbean origins, and in the 3–6 year age group.
  - The aetiology is unclear but constipation, trauma and child sexual abuse have been cited (Johnson 1991, Giardino et al 1992, Shah 1996, M Rossiter, personal communication 1996).
  - Urethral prolapse is a sign and not a diagnosis but child sexual abuse may be the cause.
- *Masturbation* is universal, may begin in infancy, and involves rubbing of the clitoris, rocking and rubbing thighs together. The child may develop a glassy stare and look pale. Children soon learn that it is socially unacceptable to masturbate in public and if a child masturbates obsessively against, for example, an adult's knee, a chair or manually, child sexual abuse or emotional abuse should be considered. Children who have been sexually aroused by an adult masturbating them (boys and girls) may be so sexually excited that even during a medical examination a boy may have a sustained erection or a girl may rub her thighs together (Sauzier 1989). Other children who have been hurt and/or frightened during child sexual abuse may dissociate and are 'absent' during the examination and even sleep. There is no association between damage to the hymen

(tears and dilatation) or the posterior fourchette and gymnastics, horse-riding and other sports. Gynaecological examination does not cause damage and even tampon use has little effect: the mean hymenal opening in postpubertal girls was 1.2 cm in girls not using tampons, compared to 1.5 cm for tampon users (Emans et al 1994).

Vaginal foreign body

- In children referred because of genito-urinary complaints it is rare to find a foreign body, around 4%, and foreign bodies are also uncommonly seen in girls referred for assessment of possible child sexual abuse (Paradise & Willis 1985, Paul 1986).
- The history is of a persistent, offensive vaginal discharge which may be bloody.
- The complaint is often long-standing and previous foreign bodies may have been removed.
- Herman-Giddens (1994) in a retrospective study of 12 girls found
  - the average age was 6.3 years
  - five were seen more than once
  - two had a sexually transmitted disease (gonorrhoea)
  - the foreign body was paper, plastic, hair, cotton wool
  - in eight girls child sexual abuse was confirmed, in three girls child sexual abuse was suspected and in one child the child sexual abuse status was unknown.
- Freidrich et al (1991), in a review of the sexual behaviour of children, found that insertion of objects into the vagina or anus is rare. Not only does the insertion of objects through the hymen cause pain, but young girls are unaware of the orifice and masturbatory activity does not include penetration, with damage to the hymen, in non-abused pre-pubertal girls.

Physical examination of pubertal and post-pubertal girls

Children do not like being examined for signs of child sexual abuse, but up until the age of 3 years it is often easier to examine a child's bottom than his or her ears. Once a child goes to school pants are 'rude', but as long as a child has not been hurt examination is often very straightforward and to ask '. . . is it alright if I examine your tuppence?' is reasonable; younger than 3 years the response is likely to be no.

As children mature they understand the enormity of what has happened, boys from seven to eight years onwards may be very embarassed, and the older a child the more upset the child is likely to be as he or she understands the consequences of what has happened and consent becomes increasingly informed.

Professionals must think through their position on this, particularly colleagues who talk about the examination as being 'as abusive as the abuse'. This should be challenged: is it 'abusive' to examine the genitalia of a 4-year-old wetter? Isn't it negligent not to examine?

Timing of a paediatric assessment

- If a child alleges sexual assault within 72 hours for children and 5 days for post-pubertal girls forensic tests may be positive, i.e. vaginal swabs. Rectal, oral and skin swabs are ideally done within hours of the assault
- Bruising ('love-bites'), grip marks, scratches and lacerations, burns should be documented as soon as possible: within 24 hours
- Where there is vaginal or rectal bleeding immediate referral is needed for assessment as to possible surgery
- If pregnancy or genito-anal infection is possible, same-day referral is needed
- It is now known that healing is rapid and children understate rather than exaggerate their abuse; the combination of these factors means that delayed examination may be negative even where there has been penetration, described as 'a bit of touching'

Manner of the paediatric assessment

It is important to take time and help the child to relax: who would he or she like to be present, does the doctor need a chaperone (see above) or assistance in collecting specimens? Maintain as much privacy as possible by the use of screens, a sheet and a minimum of adults.

Before the examination time spent in talking with the child and carer will establish some rapport and make a successful examination much more likely. A well-conducted examination may also have therapeutic attributes (San Lazaro 1995).

Teenagers in particular may decide not to comply, or allow examination of 'love-bites' on his or her neck but no more. An appointment for a further examination in 2–3 weeks may be accepted, and in this period of time the social worker may help the child prepare him- or herself. Teenagers are at particular risk of sexually transmitted disease if their behaviour is sexually promiscuous (reported at 25%), and professionals counselling them should be aware of long-term complications, for example infertility, despite few symptoms or signs in some instances.

In pre-pubertal girls the incidence of sexually transmitted disease is much lower: one study found gonorrhoea in 2.8%, warts in 1.8%, chlamydia in 1.2%, with an overall prevalence of 5% (Ingram et al 1992).

The examination begins with the nurse weighing and measuring the child. The nurse should be available during the appointment for several skilled tasks, including giving support to the child, chaperoning, collection of forensic, microbiological samples, etc. The examination begins with a look at the child from head to toe, finishing with the genitalia and anus, by which time many children will have relaxed.

If a colposcope is used it may be helpful to let the child look through the eyepiece to examine a doll; this helps the child and carer to understand the use of the equipment before the examination takes place, and the 'identification card' may be photographed. Remember to seek consent before photography. Explain the use of the colposcopic pictures – see later.

It is desirable to carry out a complete sexually transmitted disease screen, using a speculum with visualisation of the cervix. A 'teenage clinic' with appropriately trained doctors and nursing support is ideal for this, as genito-urinary physicians working with paediatricians complement skills.

Position for examination of the genitalia

- Frog-legged position with the hips abducted, knees flexed and the soles of the feet touching.
- Knee–chest position is used to view the posterior hymen in selected circumstances, usually where the hymen is redundant and there are folds giving the appearance of possible transections.
- On mother's knee – in infancy or young children if distressed. An unreferenced point in the RCP report (1997) says that this method of examination makes the 'shape of the hymenal opening different'. If the child lies along the length of the mother's thighs distortion should be minimized.

Method of examination

- Height and weight.
- During the examination note the child's demeanour and that of the carers, record any changes in behaviour, e.g. becomes passive when genitalia examined.
- Any spontaneous comments are reported verbatim. Is the carer supportive, distanced, distressed?
- Complete physical examination with recording of any bruises, bites, lacerations, burns. NB secondary sexual characteristics (breasts, pubic hair, genitalia).
- Genito-urinary examination is usually left until the end of the examination.

Genital examination

- *Inspection*: for erythema, oedema, bruising, burns, laceration, scars. Is the hymenal opening gaping and visible even before labial separation? Are the labia majora wrinkled, 'scooped-out' posteriorly, is the perineum thickened – all signs consistent with intracrural intercourse.
- *Labial separation*: the labia majora are gently parted and the hymen, urethra and posterior fourchette visualised. If the hymenal opening is gaping in a young child this is suggestive of abuse (RCP 1991).

- *Labial traction*: is necessary in many non-abused children to open the hymen and the dimensions of the opening will be greater when this technique is used than for labial separation. The labia majora are gently lifted and pulled down towards the girl's feet. With experience there are few examinations where it is not possible to 'open' the hymen: this is necessary to look for tears, scars and to measure the opening.

Equipment and techniques

- *Glass rods* have have been used to measure the size of the hymenal opening and inspect the margin for tears. Recently rods have been used infrequently as it has been considered that as the hymen is 'elastic' measurements are liable to be inaccurate and cotton wool buds may be used to inspect the margin of the hymen and are disposable. In addition, the less intrusive the examination the better it is tolerated.
- A *speculum* is used in post-pubertal girls to, for example, swab the cervix for gonorrhoea. If a child is badly traumatised and there is marked vaginal bleeding it is likely that a speculum examination is needed to see the source of the bleeding. In this situation a general anaesthetic is necessary too.
- *Digital examination* is not indicated pre-pubertally but once the hymen is oestrogenised inspection alone is not adequate. When examining older children it is usual to wear gloves and having looked at the hymen, with the help of a dampened cotton wool bud, to do a gentle digital examination. The technique is simple, and each examiner will know, for example:
  - at puberty the 'usual' hymenal opening is about 1.0 cm and even the examiner's smallest finger is likely to cause discomfort and it may be inferred that penile penetration is unlikely and digital penetration infrequent, if at all. The smallest tampon is less than 1 cm and may cause a little stretching (Woodling & Kossoris 1981, RCP 1991, Emans et al 1994).
  - an index finger, 1.5 cm, inserted without discomfort would clearly be consistent with digital penetration.
  - a two-finger examination, with ease, would be 3.5–4.5 cm and consistent with penile penetration – if penetration has been infrequent the girl may complain of discomfort. Repeated vaginal intercourse leads to a widened, lengthened vagina with, it is said in older textbooks, eventual loss of vaginal rugae.
- Always take a history of *tampon/pad usage* – although it is not of great significance, lawyers may present it as 'essential'. Likewise ask the girl, in a non-judgemental way, whether she is sexually active. Around 20% of 15-year-old girls and 25% of boys will have had intercourse (Stuart-Smith 1996). Sexually abused girls are more likely to be sexually active than non-abused girls. Despite sexually promiscuous behaviour, knowledge of HIV and sexually transmitted disease may be scanty and use of contraception is low: 50% in a group of sexually active 12–16-year-olds (Clarke & Lacey 1990).
- *Anal abuse* becomes less common as the girl grows into adolescence but still occurs, probably more frequently in 'stranger rape'. The examination is decribed later.

Rape and sexually transmitted disease

The prevalence of sexually transmitted diseases amongst rape victims varies and is greater in stranger and multiple assailant attack (Forster 1992). The long incubation period, for example, of genital warts requires prolonged follow-up, as does HIV infection if it is to be excluded.

A protocol to screen all rape victims

- Complete forensic swabs
- Sexually transmitted disease screen
- HIV testing as indicated (see Chapter 11 and Table 9.19).
- Postcoital contraception offered

- Prophylactic antibiotics are not usually indicated unless it is known the assailant is infected
- Refer victim and family members for counselling

Use of the colposcope

In rape, use of a colposcope (Slaughter 1997) reveals evidence of trauma in more than 90% of victims (11–18 years) and a pattern of signs (tears of the hymen, at 6 o'clock and at the posterior fourchette, abrasions of the labia, bruising of the hymen) is described. Additionally 25% of victims were sodomised and over 50% had non-genito-anal injury.

In consensual sex, use of the colposcope showed that 11% of subjects had signs of trauma but at a single site: rape victims had signs at four or more sites.

Physical signs: genital abuse, healing and other disorders

Disclosure

Disclosure is the usual way in which child sexual abuse presents; 40% of the children in the Leeds 1989 series presented in this way and a further 20% spoke of the abuse during the initial investigation (Hobbs & Wynne 1987a,b, Frothingham 1991). Disclosure is the single most important element in building up a diagnosis of child sexual abuse (RCP 1997).

Examination

In about 50% of children examined because of possible child sexual abuse abnormality will be found. In Leeds the figure is higher (58%) and this relates to the early provision of paediatric assessments; delay allows healing which may be rapid and complete (RCP 1997). Abnormal signs also vary from non-specific, for example erythema, to diagnostic, such as a recent tear of the hymen (RCP 1997). The published series are not always comparable (see Table 9.20).

Table 9.19 Protocol for HIV testing and child sexual abuse

Risk factors in assailant	Risk factors for child
HIV infection	Multiple assailants
Intravenous drug abuser	Presence of other sexually transmitted disease
Bisexual practices	High-risk behaviours
Multiple sexual partners	Parent/child requests test

Table 9.20 Findings in cases where there has been a confession or conviction

Study	'Normal examinations'	'Non-specific findings'	'Abnormal signs'
Adams et al (1994)	28%	74%	29%
DeJong (1988)	49%	0%	26%
Muram (1989)	14%	26%	45%

Significance of physical signs

There is ongoing debate as to the significance of various physical signs (Vandeven & Emans 1995) but diagnosis is based on more than a single sign (see Fig. 9.15) and it is the pattern of the history, examination and investigations which is of greatest significance.

Attempts have been made to correlate the legal outcome and the physical signs (Adams et al 1994) but that is flawed too (Hobbs & Wynne 1995a). There may be little correlation between the abuser's confession and reality.

San Lazaro (1996) found, in a series of 160 children where child sexual abuse was diagnosed, that the majority had been penetrated and abnormal physical signs were found in 60%, or 76% of those taken to criminal court. Of the 153 alleged abusers, 57 reached trial and 86% were convicted, although 27% of the convictions were for lesser charges than initially brought. This paper demonstrated that criminal investigation can result in conviction if cases are well selected and a specialist paediatric unit works well with all the other professionals including the courts. The particular conviction does not accurately describe the crime in over a quarter of cases.

Differential diagnosis of genital signs

- Recent trauma due to sexual interference
- Accidental injury, e.g. straddle injury
- Vulvitis, e.g. threadworms, bubblebath, trauma
- Skin disorder, e.g. lichen sclerosus, eczema
- Congenital abnormality, e.g. vascular lesion

- Infection, e.g. candida after antibiotics
- Infection complicating trauma as in child sexual abuse
- Previous trauma with scarring
- Urethral caruncle, haemangioma, prolapse, polyp

Digital examination

Assessment of girls once the genitalia have been oestrogenised inevitably requires a digital examination. This is because the hymen becomes thick, pale and redundant and the folds of tissue (or 'petals') meet in the midline and inspection alone will not give information about tears or any dilatation of the hymenal ring or vagina. Differences in studies are related to examination technique. Adams' (1996) paper does not record an estimation of vaginal dimensions and if the examination is limited to inspection all may look normal, particularly once 'acute' signs (bruising, recent laceration of hymen) have healed.

There are few studies; Emans (Table 9.21) demonstrated the problem of assessing sexual activity by physical examination; there is only a relative relationship i.e. speculum examination in post-pubertal girls who are sexually active was rated as easy in 81%, in nonsexually active tampon users easy in 56%, and pad users 26%. 19% of sexually active girls had no visible abnormality of the hymen, reflecting its elasticity (Rogers 1988). All that can be concluded from the Emans study is sexually active girls have a larger mean diameter hymenal opening than non-sexually active girls. Digital examination may demonstrate a wide hymenal opening and wide vagina where inspection appeared normal.

In an unpublished study (A J Thomas, personal communication 1997) found:

- 13/14 girls presenting at a genito-urinary clinic had hymenal opening measurements of 3.5 cm or more (two digits or medium-sized speculum); there was one girl who was intolerant of examination 3 weeks after a rape.
- Of 26 girls presented to paediaticians for assessment of possible child sexual abuse 14 had notches or transections of the hymenal edge, 4 hymenal remnants, 3 loss of hymenal tissue, 9 notches at posterior fourchette and 13 had genital infection.
- For 11 girls who were examined digitally physical signs did not correlate well with the history: 3 allowed finger-tip only, 5 index finger and 3 two-finger examination. The girls had consistently understated the level of abuse. Ideally all 26 girls would have been digitally examined, and a cotton wool bud used to demonstrate the hymenal edge, as undoubtedly signs were missed.

Table 9.21 Diameter of hymeneal opening (Emans et al 1994)

Subjects	Median diameter	Range
Sexually active post-pubertal girls	2.5 cm	1.5–3.5 cm
Non-sexually active/tampon user	1.5 cm	0.3–2.5 cm
Non-sexually active/pad user	1.2 cm	0.2–2.0 cm

The *wide range* of measurements of the hymenal opening is noted: the tissues are elastic and examination techniques crude.

Inaccuracy of assessment relates also to inexperience of the examiner, and the inability of the girl to relax (anxiety, pain due to trauma or infection or fear). As with other physical signs it is the combination of signs which is important in the context of the history.

In adolescence it is *essential to screen* for sexually transmitted disease and anal abuse when girls are referred for suspected child sexual abuse.

Erythema

Erythema is a poor marker of injury in post-pubertal teenagers (Slaughter et al 1997) but although non-specific in younger girls (contact: bubble-bath, soap, infections, etc.) it may be that a girl who complains of 'soreness and stinging when I wee' and goes on to describe grandpa 'rubbing my tuppence' is giving a history consistent with the generalised erythema seen on examination.

Healing and scarring

Healing (Table 9.22) has not been adequately researched. Muram (1989b) has attempted to correlate sexual acts and genital findings and Finkel has attempted to look at the outcome for anogenital trauma (Finkel 1989). Hymenal tears are

Table 9.22 Approximate guide to healing of genital signs

Time	Stain bruises	Labia majora bruises	Vulval abrasion/ bruising/ lacerations	Vulval oedema	Tears in hymen	Deficit/scar in hymen	Scars at posterior fourchette	Dilatation of hymen
Hours	Red-purple	+	+	+	+	+	–	+
1–3 days	Purple – swollen Yellow 2+ days	+	±	+	+	+	–	+
3 days	Yellow Fading Brown	±	±	±	±	+	–	+
2 weeks	±	–	–	–	–	+	±	±
3 weeks	±				–	+	+	±
Longer	±					+	+	May reverse completely or remain fixed, gaping

Bruising of mucous membranes may be difficult to detect clinically. There is no good clinical method available; photography and follow-up may help.

the commonest persisting sign of penetrative child sexual abuse.

Healing is rapid following trauma: Adams et al (1994) found abnormal signs in 42% of girls seen less than 72 hours after the last episode of abuse and in only 8% at more than a month. Healing is also rapid in consensual sex (Slaughter 1997 et al) and scarring is very uncommon even in rape unless there has been suturing.

Scars are seen in less than 5% of sexually abused children (Hobbs & Wynne 1987a) and may be seen at the posterior fourchette (McCann et al 1988) as an area of thickened, avascular whitish tissue. Hymenal tears may heal leaving a small contracted opening or a secondarily obliterated opening (Berkowitz et al 1987).

Many authors have commented on the lack of persisting physical abnormality despite penetrative abuse, or where healing has been complete. Marshall (1988) reported normal findings in 71% of sexually abused girls including 48% with a history of interlabial penetration. Muram (1989b) in his review of sexually abused girls aged 1–17 years (mean 9.1 years) looked at the abuser's confession. He found definitely abnormal signs (vaginal tear, hymenal opening greater than 1 cm) in 16% of girls where there was an admission of digital penetration and 86% of girls where penile penetration was admitted. However, only 57% and 3.8% of these two groups respectively were felt to have normal genitalia.

Effects of puberty

Puberty may appear to mask earlier hymenal damage as the effect of oestrogen on the hymen is to cause it to hypertrophy but if the hymenal margin is inspected carefully old transsections will be evident and in areas of previously marked attenuation there may be little hymen visible or hymenal remnants only (myrtiform caruncles).

Trauma

Acute trauma causing swelling, erythema, abrasions and bruising settles over days, and even hymenal lacerations may heal rapidly in prepubertal girls if the abuse stops.

Healing involves regeneration and repair (Finkel 1989). Superficial abrasions and lacerations heal by regeneration only. The process begins with thrombosis and inflammation followed by regeneration of the epithelium with new cell formation and then differentiation into a new surface epithelium. The wound heals by 48–72 hours and differentiation is complete in 5–7 days. The superficial injury has thus healed without residue in a week.

If, however, the laceration has been deeper and healing involved repair with formation of granulation tissue, there will subsequently be scar tissue. Regeneration in this situation is followed by organisation, which is the replacement of coagulated blood by granulation tissue and wound contraction. The granulation tissue appears red initially but with time as the cellular and vascular components of the tissue decrease, its colour changes to become paler and smaller. Most scars mature in about 60 days. However, as the scar contracts it may distort the surrounding tissue in an unexpected way. The final scar is much smaller than the original injury.

Appreciation of the effects of healing by secondary intention helps to explain the distorted architecture, for example of the scarred, contracted hymen.

Lacerations may heal completely or with a 'bump' in the margin whilst other lacerations heal with remaining notches or deficits. Repeated penetration leads to a distorted hymen as lacerations fail to unite. A deep posterior/lateral notch is commonly seen and may be in association with attenuation of the posterior part of the hymen (RCP 1997, McCann 1998).

Narrowing of the posterior hymenal rim is considered the consequence of repeated penetrative abuse (Adams et al 1994).

The hymenal opening after abuse may be gaping on inspection and dilated. If just 'stretched' the hymenal dimensions will diminish over time (Cantwell 1987). If the hymen is 'rubbed away' or attenuated it will not recover.

Non-specific signs

Non-specific signs of abuse are erythema, vulvovagnitis (other than sexually transmitted disease), and labial fusion: the labial fusion will break down at puberty if not before and the former heal in days.

The posterior fourchette is the area of major damage in penile abuse and, although rare, this is the zone where scarring is seen on occasion. Friable granulation tissue which bleeds easily on examination may also be seen and is related to intracrural coitus.

A linear 'white streak' may be seen running across the posterior fourchette – it differs from a scar which is thickened, irregular and distorts the vascular pattern.

The clinical picture is complicated by:

- type of abuse, frequency and force used
- age of the child
- ongoing abuse?
- the stage of healing
- genital infection
- an ongoing disease process, e.g. lichen sclerosis.

There is also ongoing controversy as to the definition of signs and their significance (AAP 1991, RCP 1991, 1997).

Muram (1989c) found fewer than a third of children had signs specific for child sexual abuse and even these changed with time: hymenal opening greater than 1 cm, hymenal laceration, bites.

Summary of 'normal' genital findings (Hobbs et al 1995):

- Hymen present
- Configuration of hymen changes with age – variants are annular, crescentic, sleeve, septate, fimbriated
- Free margin of hymen thin with fine vessels visible
- Hymenal opening <4 mm
- Minor bump in hymen in association with vaginal ridge
- No notches in posterior rim of hymen, any anterior notch expected to be shallow, midline or symmetrical at 10 and 2 o'clock
- No attenuation or localized narrowing of hymen
- Minor degree of labial fusion
- Non-specific vaginal discharge
- Midline pallor at posterior fourchette due to paucity of blood vessels
- Post-pubertal girls have a thickened, pale hymen which is redundant, admits tip of fifth digit (1 cm) and physiological vaginal discharge)

Summary of significant signs

These lists summarize data AAP (1991) and RCP (1997).

Diagnostic signs

- Fresh laceration of hymen (digital, penile, other penetration)
- Old laceration of hymen + healed with scarring and interruption of hymenal margin (hymenal penetration)

- Attenuation of hymen, often posterior/laterally, narrow hymenal rim (chronic abuse)
- Pregnancy
- Positive 'forensic tests'

Supportive signs

- Notch in posteior hymenal edge ± scarring (penetration)
- A notch is usually normal in the ventral 180° of hymen (RCP 1997) but opinion is divided and asymmetrical notches anteriorly may also be considered traumatic
- Acute injury to genitalia such as localized erythema, oedema, minor abrasions (seen in all types of contact abuse)
- A scar at the posterior fourchette may follow a shearing or splitting injury (intra-crural intercourse may also lead to labial fusion)
- Size of hymenal orifice, >1.5 cm
- This is rarely seen in clinical practice (Hobbs 1995):
  - 82 girls mean age 70.4 months (range 12–124 months) seen for possible child sexual abuse
  - Hymenal orifice ≤4 mm in 37 girls, >4 mm in 45 girls
  - The range of transverse hymenal diameter was 1–10 mm and 3 girls measuring 10 mm were aged between 90 and 120 months.
- Foreign body in vagina
- Sexually transmitted disease (see later)
- Physical injury to external genitalia, grip marks, 'love-bites', other non-accidental injury
- Child's behaviour during examination
- Other signs of emotional abuse and neglect

Accidental genital injury

Whatever the cause, any injury will be painful, with immediate bleeding, that is, a dramatic history (Bays & Jenny 1990). West et al (1989) described three types of injury:

- straddle injury
- penetrative injury
- tearing injury.

Straddle injury

The most commonly seen are straddle injuries. The history given is of a child falling astride a climbing frame, cross-bar of a bicycle, or furniture. The injury is caused by the forced compression of soft tissues between the object straddled and underlying bone, that is the pubic symphysis and rami. The injury may affect the mons, clitoris, urethra and anterior part of the labia majora and minora. The soft tissue injury may be linear, asymmetrical, and coincide with the bone. There may be marked swelling, and bruising in the traumatised tissue, and on occasion lacerations. The hymenal opening is not dilated (Enos et al 1986; Muram 1986; West et al 1989). Of a review of 67 girls with straddle injury and complex injury (Dowd et al 1994) 79% had minor or major laceration or abrasion of the labia majora or minora, 16% had injury to the posterior fourchette. Three girls had damage to the hymen: but also a history of a complex injury involving penetration. The average age was 6.5 years.

Five girls in the Dowd study presented with 'falsified presenting histories' and had been sexually abused. Dowd acknowledges that as his was a retrospective study it may be an under-recognition of child sexual abuse.

In this study 22% girls were admitted to hospital and 15% required surgical repair.

Penetrative injury

Accidental penetration of the labia is the second most common accident (West et al 1986). It is seen more often in children aged 18 months–3 years who have a history of falling astride toys, steps. There is often only minor bruising but a small, 0.5–1.0 cm laceration of the labia minora which may bleed profusely. The laceration heals rapidly, in 2–3 days without scarring. Surgery is rarely needed.

These lacerations are indistinguishable from those caused by fingernails as in child sexual abuse.

Tearing

Tearing due to forced abduction of the legs is rare. Bays & Jenny (1990) describes the splitting of the midline structures, based on a report of Finkel (1989) when the girl's legs were forcibly parted during abuse.

Dowd describes nine girls with laceration of the posterior fourchette. Randall Bond et al (1995) also recognised 'accidental injuries' were in the main anterior 73%, but 34% were posterior; the hymen was not involved. The range of accidental injuries is wide and the differentiation of accident or inflicted injury may be difficult.

Seat-belt injury

A case report (Baker 1986) describes the injuries in a 5-year-old girl involved in a road traffic accident and found by the police 'draped over the front seat in a prone position'. The injury was unilateral and involved abrasions to the right side of the mons, right majora and minora and perineum. The hymen was intact. The injuries appear consistent with the history.

When to investigate an 'accidental injury' as possible child sexual abuse? (after Dowd et al 1994; Randall Bond et al 1995)

- Any injury in infancy
- Any injury with an incompatible or inconsistent history
- Any severe or extensive injury
- Any hymenal, vaginal or perianal injury
- Other non-accidental injury

Female genital mutilation

The United Nations has called for an end to ritual female genital mutilation: 130 million girls and women are estimated to have been mutilated (WHO 1997 estimate).

Mutilation involves partial or total removal of the external genitalia or other injury to the genitalia (Black & Debelle 1995, Hamilton 1997). The practice is cultural and seeks to reduce sexual responsiveness. The mutilation is performed by elderly women, with an old razor blade or glass, no analgesia and no sterilization. The acute complictions are pain, shock, haemorrhage, urinary retention and sepsis.

Longer term, there may be abscesses, fistulae, scarring, dyspareunia, incontinence and problems in childbirth.

In the UK the practice has been illegal since 1985, under the Prohibition of Female Circumcision Act. The practice mainly involves refugees from Eritrea, Ethiopia and Somalia, and girls may be sent there for a 'holiday' often when 7–9 years of age. In the UK 10 000 girls and young women are estimated to be at risk. mutilation should be considered as a form of child abuse in the UK. Management is complex but clearly mutilation is 'significant harm' and the child may be protected by the Children Act 1989 and a 'prohibited steps order' or some form of care order.

Masturbation

Masturbation does not cause damage unless it is part of self-mutilation, usually following child sexual abuse. 'Excessive masturbation' in a child with learning problems or a 'syndrome' should be investigated for possible child sexual abuse: what does this behaviour mean? (Muram 1986, Bays 1990).

Harmful genital care practices

Harmful genital care practices in children can be considered a type of child abuse (Herman-Giddens 1989). Such practices involves painful washing of the genitalia, frequent and ritualistic inspections, applications of creams, and various medications for 'genital soreness', discharge and perceived infection.

A suggested classification is:

- *ritualistic* with excessive focus on and handling of the child's genitalia
- *fictitious illness*: usually presenting as recurrent vaginal discharge to a variety of doctors leading to multiple examinations and investigation
- *overt sexual abuse*: the father used creams as an opportunity to touch the child's genitalia.

Clinically:

- 79% were girls
- average age 6.4 years
- examination revealed vaginal discharge, erythema, scarring at posterior fourchette, widened hymenal opening, vaginal foreign body, hymenal distortion.

Treatment is difficult and Herman-Giddens suggests that the starting point should be 'these practices should be recognised as abusive to the child'.

Skin disorders and infections

In childhoood skin disorders are common and may coexist with sexual abuse.

- *Nappy rash* is due to contact with wet or soiled nappies, exacerbated by diarrhoea. The nappy area is red with macerated skin which may become abraded or superficial, short, linear splits may be seen.
- *Atopic or seborrhoeic eczema* is associated with nappy rash, and the skin may be sensitive and split (as above).
- *Lichen sclerosus* may give an initial impression of trauma (Jenny et al 1989) but inspection shows the characteristic white atrophic plaques and speckled purpura (Ridley 1987). The ano-genital area is most often affected in young girls, in a figure-of-eight pattern. There may be bleeding from haemorrohagic blisters and purpura may look like bruises.

  The girl may complain of 'burning' or an intense itch. The differential diagnosis is with child sexual abuse, made more complicated as it is thought that trauma may be involved in the aetiology of the disorder (Priestley & Bleehan 1987, Ridley 1987, San Lazaro 1995).

Treatment is with corticosteroid cream of moderate potency until the child is asymptomatic. The condition waxes and wanes and girls should take responsibility for applying the creams themselves as they grow older, to avoid application becoming abusive. Boys do not appear to have the disorder perianally (RCP 1997), but a disorder said to be equivalent, xeroderma obliterans, involves the penis.

Congenital vascular lesion

Small vascular lesions may appear as a purple swelling on the labia minora or the perineum and look like a bruise. A follow-up appointment will clarify the situation.

Genital infections

- *Fungal nappy rash* in association with oral candidiasis – although older girls who are 'sore' are often treated with antifungal creams, it is infrequently proven an infection.
- As part of a *systemic illness* such as chickenpox, streptococcus.
- *Sexually transmitted disease* should be checked out as possible child sexual abuse.
- *Non-specific infections* occur with a discharge and signs of inflammation (erythema and oedema). If recurrent vulvitis or vulvovaginitis occurs, child sexual abuse should be considered (Emans 1998).

Bacterial vaginosis

Bacterial vaginosis is a polymicrobial infection in which there is an overgrowth of multiple organisms including *Gardnerella vaginalis*. It is diagnosed by an offensive discharge and clue cells, and a fishy odour is elicited by the addition of 10% potassium hydroxide to vaginal secretions.

Cultures for specific organisms are meaningless in bacterial vaginosis. The condition occurs in child sexual abuse more often than in controls but it does occur in non-abused girls, if uncommonly (Bartley et al 1987).

False allegations of abuse (fictitious abuse)

Fictitious sexual abuse in the context of fictitious illness has been described (Meadow 1993). This was not in the context of custody disputes, but the author does assume that 'a large proportion of allegations of abuse, particularly sexual abuse, prove to be unsubstantiated'.

Clinical experience is that false allegations of child sexual abuse are uncommon but child sexual abuse is difficult to prove and given the distorted perceptions of perpetrators of fictitious illness (by proxy) and the frequency of child sexual abuse in their past history it would not be surprising to find an association. More research is needed.

Examination of boys

Injuries to the genitalia used to be thought uncommon: 3.2%, 7%, 2.2% (Spencer & Dunklee 1986, Reinhart 1987, Hobbs & Wynne 1989, respectively) of sexually abused boys. However, it is appparent that doctors have been slow to acknowledge genital injury, and even now fail to name the injury, for example a ligature round the base of the penis may be explained away as 'punishment for bed-wetting' or aggression on behalf of the abuser (Feldman 1997).

Genital abuse

- Genital abuse may be associated with anal abuse, physical abuse, neglect and always emotional abuse.
- Injury may be
  - sexual abuse
  - physical abuse
  - self-mutilating/self-inflicted
  - peer inflicted (Erickson 1991)
  - accidental.
- Boys need treating with the same respect as girls during the history taking and examination.
- Boys aged under 6–7 years often express no preference as to the gender of the examining doctors, and although older boys may prefer to be seen by a male doctor this is not invariable particularly if the boy has been hurt or humiliated by a male abuser.
- Accompanying the boy is a known, trusted adult – there should be a chaperone (GMC 1996).
- Ideally the boy is examined on the couch but younger boys may, of necessity, be seen on their mother's knee; sedation is rarely needed.
- The examination follows a usual pattern with measurement of height and weight and a general examination finishing with a record of any non-genital injury and finally an inspection of the genitalia and anus.
- A urethral discharge is abnormal: do a sexually transmitted disease screen.
- The boy's behaviour should be noted: was he cooperative, angry, sad, frightened? Did he have a sustained erection? Did he masturbate? Why is he so sexually excited?
- Note the Tanner stage of puberty (Table 9.13).

Physical abuse

The commoner injuries seen are (Hobbs & Wynne 1995b) (Fig. 9.13):

- *bruising*, which may include petechiae and swelling in a sucking injury
- *torn frenulum* due to forced retraction of the foreskin
- *incised wound* to the penis, usually proximal and dorsal but may extend from an arc to circumferential (Lukschu & Bays 1996, Feldman 1997)
  - An 'accidental traction injury' is said to occur and the 'thin penile skin is torn to give a ragged wound' (Jumbelic 1997). It is not clear how adequate force is applied to

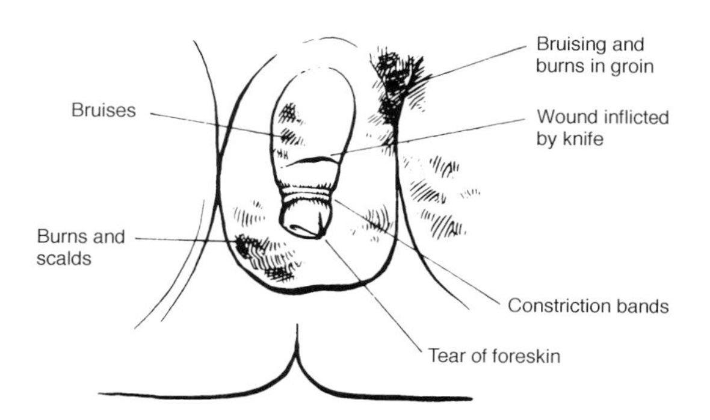

Fig. 9.13 Injuries of the male genitalia encountered in abuse.

the distal end of a (small) penis to cause this lesion and there is only anecdotal evidence that it occurs

- red, linear, *circumferential mark* due to a ligature
- *contact burn, scald*
- *damage to urethral meatus* due to insertion of foreign body as part of abuse or self-mutilation (Bays & Chadwick 1993)
- urethral discharge – sexually transmitted disease
- bite
- bruising or swelling of the scrotum due to intra-abdominal trauma.

Self-inflicted injury (Lukschu & Bays 1996)

- Insertion of urethral foreign body.
- Injection of water into urethra leading to urinary infection.
- Masturbation causing damage to frenulum in adolescence – this based on anecdotal evidence only.
- Vacuum cleaner injury.

Accidental injury

- *Straddle injury* occurs following a fall where the soft tissues are compressed against the pelvic bone. The usual injury is caused on a cross-bar or climbing frame but there are reports of unusual accidents in break dancing, go-carts, and banana-seat bicycles (Dowd et al 1994). In a series of straddle injuries, Dowd et al reported the injury site 16/28 scrotum (laceration, swelling), 12/28 penis (laceration, bruising) – the lacerations were mainly superficial but 10/17 required suturing; there were no perianal injuries. The boys complained of pain. Sexual abuse was 'not a documented concern of the examiner or parent'.
- *Zip injury* – mainly young boys.
- *Dog or horse bite.*
- *Toilet seat injury* – this is often quoted as giving a crush injury but as a mechanism for injury requires more research.
- *Harmful genital care practices* (Herman-Giddens 1989) has been addressed above in some detail; however, no boys were included in that study and this may be another area where with current practice this form of abuse is not recognised (Elliott & Peterson 1993).
- *Circumcision* is legal in the UK and is performed primarily for religious reasons by members of Islam and Jewish faiths. There are quasi-medical reasons for the operation (Duckett 1995) but 'the need to be like the others' appears to hold sway in North America and Australia whereas in western Europe the rate of operating has fallen.

Causes for concern about circumcision include:

- Issues of consent: the child cannot consent and an essentially unnecessary surgical procedure is performed.
- The lack of analgesia and evident pain suffered by the boy.
- Complications: in the UK in 1949 there were 16 deaths due to infection and unrecognised clotting disorders.
- In 1989 seven cases involving 'traumatic' amputation of the penis in 8-day-old babies from New York were described (Horowitz et al 1995): the rate of complications for neonatal circumcision in the US is 0.2% and 1.7% of older boys.
- In 1996 it was reported that 26 young men in eastern South Africa had reconstructive surgery after their penises were mutilated during traditional circumcision rites. 62

young men were injured and 3 died (*Guardian* 1996a).

- The General Medical Council (GMC 1996) has given clear advice to doctors who carry out this operation concerning informed consent, expertise and the use of anaesthesia and analgesia.
- The complication rate in Western Europe and North America is low.

Examination of the anus and perianal region

The examination of the anus comes at the end of the examination and the child is hopefully relaxed and is able to curl up quite comfortably in the left lateral position, older children covered by a sheet.

Young children and babies are also ideally examined on the couch but if distressed the child may be better on the mother's knee lying on his or her back with legs lifted vertically.

A proportion of children when asked to turn on their side turn prone: was this how they were abused? Other children may go quiet and passive, even appear to sleep; this is probably a learned, dissociative behaviour. Others are angry, embarrassed and distressed.

A knee–chest position allows good visualisation of the anus but is undignified and may be humiliating if the child has been abused in this posture.

The position of the child and the method of examination must be recorded: the evaluation of some signs, notably reflex anal dilatation (RAD) and the appearance of dilated veins have been studied on children in the left lateral position, but buttocks are gently parted and the anal sphincter observed for 20–30 seconds (Hobbs & Wynne 1986). The findings of other researchers, notably McCann et al (1989), are not comparable (RCP 1991), as the children were placed in knee–chest position for up to 8 minutes. The UK recommendation is that the child should be in the left lateral position and the period of perianal examination should not exceed 30 seconds (RCP 1991).

The Cleveland Inquiry directed that doctors should agree a consistent vocabulary to describe the physical signs associated with child sexual abuse (Butler-Sloss 1988). Table 9.23 gives a description of signs and Table 9.24 an approximate guide to healing from experience in Leeds.

- The anal and perianal abnormalities associated with child sexual abuse are due to:
  - trauma, which may be superficial, blunt or penetrative
  - infection, which may be sexually transmitted disease or other infection.
- Healing may be rapid (Finkel 1989, Hobbs 1993, McCann 1998).
- Scarring is uncommon (Hobbs & Wynne 1989).
- Signs may be modified by:
  - healing
  - use of lubricants
  - age of the child: in general the younger the child the more signs there are likely to be as a consequence of anal penetration, and teenagers may have no obvious abnormality (Muram 1989)
  - some children appear able to 'make my bottom big' i.e. exhibit RAD as a learned behaviour: RAD is a sign known to fluctuate from examination to examination in some children and Ganz (1962) described the apparently voluntary control of RAD in adults.

Examination findings

The anal sphincter is contracted, the anus is 'closed' and regular skin folds radiate out to give a puckered appearance and the skin is dry.

Reddening of the perianal skin is relatively common, particularly in children still wearing nappies, and may be due to one or a combination of factors:

- poor hygiene, soiled nappy, nappy rash
- candidiasis
- threadworms (which cause irritation and the child scratches)
- skin disorder such as infantile eczema, seborrhoeic dermatitis, lichen sclerosus

Table 9.23 Examination of anus and perianal region

Site	Lesion	Description	Aetiology
Skin	Erythema	Reddening of skin	Non-specific response to local irritation (infection, trauma, skin disorder)
	Thickening, pigmentation, lichenification	Swelling which may be associated with erythema, superficial cracks, darkening of tissues	Damage to skin as a result of skin disorder, e.g. eczema, scratching, rubbing (as in CSA) but no specific response over prolonged period
	Loss of anal skin folds	Thickening of folds, leading to smooth, often pink, shiny skin with loss of fold pattern	Uncommon in childhood. Reported in adults where long-standing anal abuse
	Scars	Fan-shaped, linear, of heaped-up skin. Distorted usual skin folds	May be secondary to fissures from any aetiology. Uncommon in childhood. NB: wedgelike smooth areas in the midline with or without depression are to be differentiated from scars
	Faecal staining	Soiling of liquid faeces about anus	Imperfect hygiene. Seepage of liquid faeces in chronic constipation. Lax anal sphincter
	Perianal warts, vesicles	As genital warts, vesicles	
	Threadworms	Cotton-like worms, cause intense local irritation, hence erythema and superficial excoriation	
Anal margin	Oedema of anal margin	'Tyre sign', i.e. swollen anal margin (see notes)	Recent trauma to anal margin by forcible stretching
	Bruising	As other skin bruising	Suggests severe trauma
	Haematoma anal verge	Discrete red swelling on anal margin	Suggests severe trauma
	Skin tag	Mound of skin on anal verge	Deep fissures may heal leaving a skin tag. Anterior skin tags or folds were found in 11% of children
	Fissure	Break in the lining of the anal canal usually extending from inside the canal to the anal verge and travelling vertically to the verge Open lesion May be narrow and superficial or deep and wide when usually chronic, and often posterior Variable number and position Occasionally heals with scarring if deep	Due to stretching of anal margin as in severe constipation or anal penetration Occasionally inflammatory bowel disease is seen in childhood and associated with fissures and other skin signs Uncommon even in constipation, when usually children 1–3 years and single fissure seen Multiple fissures, especially in absence of constipation, strong possibility CSA Fissures commonly seen at 6 or 12 o'clock in CSA or other causes
	Anal verge deficit	Indentation covered with skin in anal verge, i.e. not a fissure	Does it represent an old anal verge injury? Is it a normal variant? Clinical follow-up may be needed.
Perianally	Venous congestion	Purple, blue to black discolorations perianally, vary from grape-like swellings to flat areas May exist as a ring or just segmental (may be related to fissure, 6 or 12 o'clock usual site)	Mechanism unsure, seen in association with anal penetration. Do not observe anus for longer than 20–30 seconds as may be normal findings in non-physiological position, e.g. knee–chest for 5 minutes
Configuration of anus	Funnelled anus	The anus appears deeply set It is a fixed funnel shape	Recorded in older forensic texts Is occasionally seen usually mid-childhood or teenagers; reflects chronic anal abuse
	Shortening or eversion of anal canal	The ano-rectal junction with its characteristic star-shaped folds becomes approximated to the anal orifice	Seen in first 2–3 years of life and likely to reflect repeated anal abuse Associated with laxity and reduced anal tone
External sphincter	Laxity (open anal canal)	On gentle traction or merely parting the buttocks the anus appears open and gapes	The anus should be shut on inspection A patulous anus is described in neurogenic disorder Digital assessment of anal tone is unreliable, unnecessarily intrusive and should be abandoned

Table 9.23 continued

Site	Lesion	Description	Aetiology
	Gaping	A widely gaping anus, up to 2 cm, may be seen shortly after anal abuse	Within hours of abuse the anus may dilate widely, but this is a transient phenomenon
	Twitchy	External sphincter alternately contracts and relaxes every 2–5 seconds	Manipulation of the anus, for example repeated digital penetration or use of suppositories
External and internal sphincter	Anal dilatation	When the buttocks are separated the external and internal sphincters relax and a central hole is seen which allows the observer to look through the anal canal to the rectum The relaxation is such that the orifice is roughly round, of 0.5–2.0 cm in A-P and horizontal planes. The opening may close, only to reopen, sometimes repetitively. The opening is smooth and the anal skin folds are clearly visible Faeces may be clearly visible in the rectum. Occasionally children will demonstrate the sign, 'I can make my bottom get big'. The sign will go after days to months, once the abuse ceases	Passage of wind during the examination may demonstrate anal dilatation – but the dilatation is usually seen once, i.e. it is not repeated Manual evacuation of faeces, instrumentation may, theoretically, give transient signs (RAD, laxity) but there are no clinical studies Theoretically use of suppositories may cause twitchiness Anal dilatation has been described in inflammatory bowel disorder, haemolytic uraemic syndrome Severe chronic constipation may give a 'visibly relaxed anus' If associated with anal abuse there will usually be other physical signs evident Whether the sign is due to damage by stretching of the internal sphincter or a learned behavioural response or other mechanism is not known

Table 9.24 Approximate guide to healing of anal signs

Time	Bruising erythema, perineum, perianally	Abrasions anal verge	Oedema anal verge (tyre sign)	Spasm anal sphincter	Anal fissures	Dilated veins	Anal dilatation	Laxity	Gaping anus
Hours	Red-purple +	+	+	+	+	+	+	+	+
1–3 days	Purple-swollen + Yellow 3+	+	+	+	+	+	±	+	±
7 days	Yellow + Fading – Brown	±	±	+	±	+	±	+	–
2 weeks	±	–	–	–	±	±	±	+	
3 weeks	±			–	±	±	±	+	
Longer	±				Deep fissures may remain unhealed for months	± May be seen over months	± Usually disappears in few weeks if child separated from abuser	±	

Other signs include haematoma at the anal verge, skin tags, scars (take up to 2 months to organise), thickening of perianal skin and loss of skin folds (chronic abuse).

- excessive washing, cleaning and inspection as a form of child sexual abuse (Herman-Giddens 1989)
- occasionally a β-haemolytic streptococcal skin infection presents as an angry, swollen, red ring of infected skin perianally, the skin may split in superficial linear cracks, there may be an associated vulvovaginitis with a purulent discharge
- trauma, as in intracrural intercourse where the erythema extends forwards to involve the perineum, labia (posterior fourchette may

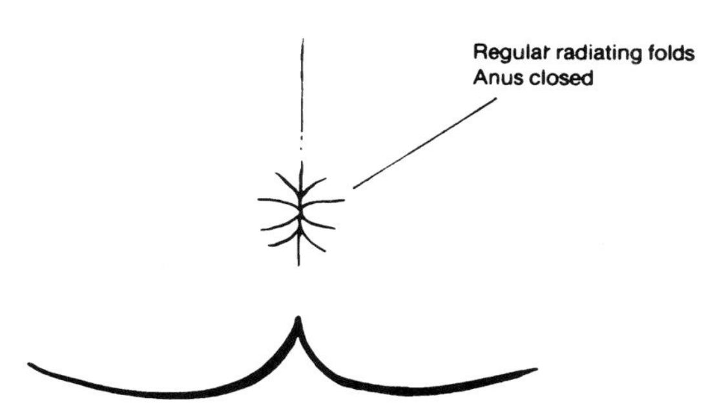

Fig. 9.14 Normal anus.

be erythematous with friable tissue) and scrotum, and upper inner aspect of the thighs (RCP 1997).

If there is faecal soiling or seepage, erythema is common:

- constipation with overflow (large faecal masses may be palpable in the abdomen and visible at the anal sphincter)
- encopresis occurs in emotionally disturbed children: child sexual abuse may be the stress which is causing this behaviour
- a patulous, lax anus, as in chronic anal abuse, is said to occur (Reinhardt 1987); this is not UK experience.

The constant irritation of faeces causes perianal erythema, but all skin signs are reversible except scarring (Butler-Sloss 1988).

Other skin changes in child sexual abuse

- Repeated friction of the perianal tissue leads to the skin thickening, there may be loss of skin folds and the skin looks pink, smooth and may be shiny (Goff et al 1989).
- Hyperpigmentation of the inner thighs and perianally may occur in long-standing intracrural intercourse, but is a non-specific sign and is more common in pigmented skin and obesity.

Healing and scarring

- The perianal skin should be free of scars, and a midline raphe should be differentiated from scarring. Superficial fissures usually heal without permanent scarring, but deeper fissures may scar (McCann 1992).
- Healing may be delayed by infection, continuing constipation and further anal abuse.
- Scars may be fan-shaped, linear, or in association with heaped-up skin or definite tags. Fan-shaped scars should be differentiated from the depressions seen at 6 and 12 o'clock in some non-abused children (McCann et al 1989, Berenson et al 1993).
- Scars are unusual and seen in fewer than 10% of anally abused children (Hobbs & Wynne 1989).
- Scars outside the midline were not found in children selected for non-abuse (McCann et al 1990b).

Note: Paul (1986) described the chronic skin changes which are listed above, and the assumption is that they are thickening of the skin due to friction and anal laxity due to repeated stretching.

Skin tags

Skin tags may form at the end of a healing fissure but it is thought that some may be congenital: a study of neonates is required.

- Berenson et al (1993) found tags in 3/89 children ('normal') of 18 months or less, and McCann et al (1989) in 11% of children selected for non-abuse: all were in the midline.
- Muram (1989a) described tags in 14% of sexually abused children but few children attending a clinic for gastrointestinal complaints.
- Hobbs & Wynne (1989) described tags and scars in 8% of 337 children thought to have been abused, in the 0–5 year group 3% had tags or scars.
- McCann (1993) described the healing process in four anally abused children: in one child a tag was formed due to 'avulsion of the perianal skin'.
- Tags, thickening of skin folds and scars are found more frequently in sexually abused children than non-abused children, and should be noted but although scarring is indicative of previous trauma (a deep

fissure), 'congenital tags' should not have signs of scarring, the significance of tags and tears requires critical assessment.

Swelling of the perianal tissues

- There may be an oedematous ring around the anus which results from acute trauma to the anal sphincter as in forcible penetration (penile or digital) and is seen 24–48 hours after abuse (Hobbs & Wynne 1989) and called the *tyre sign*.
- Bamford & Kiff (1987) described muscular hypertrophy of the external sphincter as the 'tyre sign' and surmised that it was caused by the child trying to maintain continence in spite of a dilating internal sphincter. Bamford has preferred the 'Hobbs' causation of the sign in later work (RCP 1997, Bamford pers. comm.).

Bruising

- Bruising to the perianal canal is uncommon but bruising to the neck, breasts, lower abdomen, and grip marks to the arms, thighs, and knees are common (Reinhardt 1987, Hobbs & Wynne 1990).
- Bruising and other injury (bites, laceration, burns and ligatures) to the genitalia are less common, but penile/scrotal injury has been under recognised.
- Certain sadistic injuries such as burns, bites, and the use of ligatures to the neck, genitalia) or suffocation are extremely dangerous, in terms of risk, if the child has not been protected.

Fissures

- Fissures are tears (discontinuities) in the lining of the anal canal usually extending from inside the canal to the anal verge and travelling vertically to the verge. They are *not* cracks in the skin seen perianally in scratching due to threadworms or eczema. A fissure is an open lesion, which may bleed and heals, sometimes with a scar, which may be visible and there may be a skin tag (Butler-Sloss 1988). Deep fissures are more likely to scar, form a tag and there may be a sentinel vein at either side of the fissure. Paul (1986) described linear and fan-shaped scars.
- Fissures are described with reference to position (12 o'clock is anterior and 6 o'clock posterior), number, length, depth and state of healing. Is the fissure acute or chronic?
- Be careful to differentiate fissures from folds in the mucosa lining of the anal canal.
- Fissures are caused by stretching of the anus (by a large, hard stool, implement, penile penetration) and the causation is not evident from examination.
- McCann et al (1989) found no fissures in 267 children selected for non-abuse and Berenson et al (1993) in another normative study found only one fissure in 89 children of less than 18 months.
- Constipation is a common cause of fissure formation but most constipated children do not have fissures. Clayden (1992) running a tertiary constipation clinic found 17% gave a history of previous fissure, and fissures were seen infrequently in a study of 171 children with gastrointestinal complaints (San Lazaro 1989). Agnarsson et al (1990) did a study of children with mild to moderate constipation and their results differ in that nearly 26% of children had fissures, mainly anterior, including 14% with two or more fissures and two children had multiple fissures.
- In a study of anally abused children, under 5 years, 59% had fissures and 53% of the total group had fissures (Hobbs & Wynne 1989).
- Fissures are caused by stretching and are not diagnostic of abuse but particular note is taken:
  - if there is no history of constipation and there are no signs of constipation on examination
  - if there are multiple fissures (Hobbs & Wynne 1989), but a single fissure at 6 or 12 o'clock may be highly significant given an appropriate history of anal penetration, namely bleeding, pain
  - if the fissure(s) is deep and extends on to the perianal skin (AAP 1991)

  - the superficial excoriations, seen usually as narrow, linear areas of skin loss and associated often with scratching are not fissures. Causes include nappy rash, eczema, threadworms, diarrhoea and occasionally the abuser's fingernails.

Perianal venous congestion

- It is important to note the position of the child, i.e left lateral, and to limit the period of inspection, i.e. to 20–30 seconds. Record the sign which varies from a flat halo of purple through to 'grape-like clusters', purple to black, as a ring or an arc round the anus; there may be a fissure and an associated sentinel vein.
- Haemorrhoids are very rare before puberty and are unlikely to cause difficulty in diagnosis (Shandling 1987, McCann 1990).
- Venous congestion is a non-specific sign and is caused by any condition which interferes with the vascular drainage in the area, for example a sacral tumour (Hobbs & Wynne 1989). There may be a temporary dilatation of veins during and after defecation, particularly in infancy (RCP 1997) but this is anecdotal and Berenson et al (1993) found 'venous pooling' in only 1/89 children aged less than 18 months.
- Timing and positioning of the child are important. McCann (1989) left his cohort of children in knee–chest position for 2 minutes or more and 52% developed venous congestion. These were 'normal children' (see later).
- 21% of anally abused children were found to have some degree of venous congestion at 30 seconds and examined in the left lateral position (Hobbs & Wynne 1989).
- Venous congestion may be the last sign to resolve after anal abuse (Hobbs 1991).
- *Note* that it is not possible to compare the work of McCann et al (1989) in describing 'normal' children with descriptions from Hobbs & Wynne (1989) looking at anally abused chiildren (RCP 1997) because examination differs:
  - in positioning the child: knee–chest compared with left lateral position
  - in timing: upwards of 2 minutes inspection (McCann 1989) compared with 20–30 seconds.
- There may have been abused children in McCann's study as he only administered the structured interview to the parents and research (Lanktree 1989) shows the proportion of children disclosing abuse to be up to 31% with directed questioning.
- Another point which needs acknowledgment is the time delay which some clinics impose, for whatever reason, before the child is examined, allowing healing to take place. The children in McCann's study were at a holiday camp and theoretically away from their abuser so healing may have occurred.
- Other clinics may only arrange a paediatric assessment if the child gives a history suggesting that there may be a physical injury, experience shows that many children minimise their abuse rather than exaggerating (the 1:4 rule, which frequently also applies to abusers who also minimize or tell of only a quarter of the abuse at any one time)
- Finally, good practice has shown if one child is being abused within a family, and he or she discloses, ideally all the siblings should be examined as the non-disclosing child is more likely to have abnormality on examination, and is more of a 'victim' than the child who has the confidence to make the allegations (Muram et al 1991).

Anal laxity and reduced anal tone

- Laxity and reduced anal tone may be associated with anal abuse due to repeated stretching (Paul 1986, McLay 1990b), given the absence of a neurological disorder, for example spina bifida.
- Gross faecal loading, as seen in severe, chronic constipation, leads to a visibly relaxed sphincter (Clayden 1988).
- Assessment of anal tone is a matter of controversy, and many paediatricians think digital examination unnecessary (Butler-Sloss 1988). Manometry is the only objective measure of tone and a clinical observation of

the anal sphincter parting as the buttocks are separated (or in minimal traction) is as valid as an individual's experience of digital examination.
- After an anal stretch operation (4 fingers) paediatric surgeons report that anal tone recovers rapidly; if after anal abuse the tone does not quickly improve this suggests the abuse was long-standing or continuing.

Shortening or eversion of the anal canal

- Shortening or eversion is associated with anal penetration in young children up to around 3 years (Hobbs & Wynne 1989).
- The ano-rectal junction with its characteristic star-shaped folds becomes approximated to the anal orifice. These folds require to be associated with reduced anal tone and laxity, and there is prolapsing of the rectal mucosa and occasionally a total rectal prolapse.

Gaping anus

- Gaping of the anus may be seen as an acute sign after sodomy.
- The anus is widely open, 1–2 cm and there may be signs of acute trauma, erythema, oedema, fissures and occasionally bruising.
- The gaping may last from hours to days.
- This sign differs from the lax, patulous anus as seen in a neurogenic disorder.

Anal verge haematoma

- These haematomata are uncommon and are associated with forcible anal penetration
- They are seen as a purple/red, localized, round swelling on the anal verge which distorts the adjacent skin folds.
- Anal verge haematoma are painful.

Anal warts

Anal warts are described on p. 213.

- They are found around the vaginal introitus, perigenitally, perineum and perianally, rarely penile in children.
- They may be condylomatous, papular or flat.
- They may be symtomless, cause soreness, irritation, bleeding.
- They are commonly seen in association with other sexually transmitted disease.
- They are associated with child sexual abuse and, except in infancy where vertical transmission occurs, should lead to a further investigation.

Other sexually transmitted diseases

- STDs may be seen particularly in older children and teenagers involved with multiple abusers.
- They may cause discharge, irritation, pain, urinary symptoms or be asymptomatic.
- Screening for STD, hepatitis and HIV is discussed on p. 210.

Rectal abscess

- Rectal abscess has been described, but rarely in association with anal abuse in childhood.

Twitchy anus

- Twitchy anus is the term used to describe the repeated, rapid contraction and relaxation of the external sphincter.
- The significance of the sign is uncertain but it may be related to repeated digital penetration.
- Clinical experience suggests that it is not uncommon for children aged 6–10 years to do this to themselves; it is perhaps initiated by child sexual abuse or peer activity.

Funnelled anus

- The term 'funnelled anus' was used in earlier literature (Mant 1960) in relation to older children and adults who have been anally penetrated over a long period.
- It is not described in young children.
- The anus appears to be deep-set, dished.
- The RCP report (1997) uses the term quite differently:

Some children are born with an anal canal that does not close at rest in its distal portion. In these children the anal canal, when viewed from the perineal aspect, does not have the usual tubular shape but funnels down from the open anal verge to its closed upper lumen.

- This anomaly was not described in more than 1000 children examined during 1985–1986 (Hobbs & Wynne 1989).

Reflex anal dilatation

Reflex anal dilatation (RAD) was a sign well known in forensic medicine before the laws concerning homosexual relationships were changed (Ganz 1962, Paul 1986, Butler-Sloss 1988). The mechanism of RAD is not fully understood (RCP 1997).

- The anal canal is 1.8 cm long at birth, 2.5 cm long at 2 years and 3 cm in the adult; the rectum is 7 cm, 11.5 cm and 14 cm long respectively. The anal canal is surrounded by the internal sphincter which is under involuntary control. The internal sphincter controls the passage of flatus and diarrhoea and when contracted closes the anal canal in conjunction with the mucosal folds of the anal canal. The external sphincter is voluntary muscle (RCP 1997).
- Weakness of the external sphincter leads to urgency to defecate, weakness of the internal sphincter leads to leakage of flatus and liquid faeces and weakness of both sphincters leads to faecal incontinence.
- Anal distension leads to relaxation of the internal sphincter (as does distension from the higher gut), penetration of the external sphincter leads to contraction but is is under higher cortical control and therefore the sphincter may be voluntarily relaxed, necessary for anal intercourse (RCP 1997).
- When a child is examined the initial response is for an increasing tightening of the external sphincter which may be partially voluntary but in addition the cutaneo-anal reflex contracts the sphincter. The child is able to maintain this contraction for 10–30 seconds, although adults are said to be able to maintain contraction for up to 3 minutes. The sphincter relaxes but the internal sphincter and mucosal folds obscure the view into the rectum unless the internal sphincter relaxes too as in reflex anal dilatation (passing of flatus, defecation, or possibly abused child).

Demonstrating RAD

- The child lies in the left lateral position and the buttocks are gently parted. It is not necessary to use more pressure than is needed to see the anus – in any event it is not possible to dilate the internal sphincter by increased tension (RCP 1997).
- The internal sphincter is observed over 30 seconds
- The external and internal sphincters relax and the anal canal opens up like a tube and the examiner may see into the rectum, in younger children the view may be obscured by prolapsing mucosa.
- The opening may close and open repeatedly and the degree of dilatation varies but may be up to 25 mm horizontally.
- Minor degrees of dilatation, 5–10 mm, may represent healing.
- An unexplained aspect of RAD is the inconsistency in demonstration, the sign may persist or vary from examination to examination even over a time-span of hours; there does appear to be a learned element to RAD as several children have described how they achieve dilatation. Colposcopic photographs are particularly helpful in recording fluctuating signs.
- If the child wishes to defecate the examination should be delayed until the bowels have been emptied; wait a further 30 minutes?
- The presence of stool should not invalidate the sign (Hobbs & Wynne 1995c), the rectum has storage of stool as a function. Clinical experience shows (Hobbs 1993) that when further investigation has continued, despite the stool in the rectum, diagnosis of child sexual abuse has been validated.

- There is disagreement (McCann et al 1989) concerning the presence of stool and RAD and also concerning constipation and RAD.
- RAD is a dynamic sign and not the 'visibly relaxed sphincter' of Clayden (1988) which is associated with severe, chronic constipation.
- RAD has been described after instrumentation to the anus (Paul 1986) and care is needed interpreting anal signs if there has been repeated use of suppositories, enemata or rectal examinations and manual evacuations.

Opinions on RAD

- Butler-Sloss (1988): 'We are satisfied from the evidence that the consensus is that the sign of anal dilatation is abnormal, suspicious and requires further investigation. It is not in itself evidence of anal abuse.'
- Police Surgeon Association (1988): 'While not pathognomic of sexual abuse it (anal abuse) should give rise to the suspicion sexual abuse may have occurred.'
- RCP (1991): 'RAD greater than 1 cm is supportive evidence of abuse, and RAD greater than 2 cm is more likely than not to be associated with abuse.'
- Bamford and Roberts (1997): 'RAD may be a pointer to sexual abuse but is not reliable as a sole diagnostic sign and its significance is currently unproved.'

See Table 9.25 for a summary of findings on the prevalence of RAD. Problems in the comparison of findings arise from:

- different definition of RAD – Clayden (1988), Agnarsson et al (1990)
- different examination technique – McCann et al (1989)
- no description of method – Stanton & Sunderland (1989)
- inclusion of unknown numbers of sexually abused children in 'non-abused cohort'– Clayden (1988), Stanton & Sunderland (1989), Agnarsson (1990), McCann (1990)
- change in definition of RAD without further research – RCP (1997), Bamford & Kiff (1987).

Table 9. 25 Prevalence of RAD

Study	Findings
Hobbs and Wynne (1989)	4% referred ?physical abuse, child sexual abuse, neglect 18% of children diagnosed child sexual abuse 42% of child sexual abuse with anal signs
Wright et al (1987)	8.5% of referred child sexual abuse to police surgeon
McCann (1989)	15% of 'non-abused' in 30 seconds
Stanton et al (1989)	14% of 'non-abused' – 5–35 mm
Priestley (1986)	4% of 'non-abused'
Agnarsson et al (1990)	8% of mild–moderate constipation

Clinically it is known that:

- RAD is commoner in anally abused groups than others.
- RAD is an uncommon physical sign (which even many children's doctors have never seen), and when seen in an otherwise normal child is a cause for concern and justifies follow-up.
- RAD may vary from day to day in some children.
- When the anal abuse ceases the sign disappears, over weeks to months, and during the period of healing lesser degrees of dilatation are seen
- RAD has been known to occur in inflammatory bowel disease and after anal manipulation
- RAD of >1 cm is supportive evidence of abuse: 'is more likely than not to be associated with abuse' (RCP 1991).
- RAD of >1.5 cm which is reproducible is a supportive sign of child sexual abuse (RCP 1997).
- RAD seen when a child is ventilated or has died is difficult to evaluate and may be significant. Children are killed in the course of sexual abuse and other signs of abuse should be sought. See case history 9.10.
- When infants or children die the anus usually remains closed (G Batcup personal communication, reviewed autopsies 1992). In sudden, unexplained death due to asphyxia

if there is a dilated anus child sexual abuse should be considered – but, clearly with circumspection.

- RAD is a sign associated with buggery but the diagnosis of child sexual abuse is made up of the entire clinical jigsaw of history, examination and investigations put in the wider context of the social services department's and police's knowledge of the child and his family (Hobbs & Wynne 1986)

Summary of the significance of RAD

- A definition, as in Table 9.23, is recommended
- Examination of a child referred because of possible child sexual abuse should be standardised, i.e. the child lies in the left lateral position, the buttocks are gently parted and the anal sphincter inspected for 30 seconds. Colposcopy with photographic (still or videotaped) recording is ideal
- Further research is needed to improve the understanding and consequently the significance of the association of RAD with respect to age, constipation, general anaesthesia, post-mortem change and neurological disorders

CASE HISTORY 9.10

A 2 years 6 months child was brought to the hospital after he had had a period of apnoea. He was badly beaten and had one fixed, dilated pupil. Emergency neurosurgery removed a large blood clot. He had been sexually abused, admitted by his assailant; his anus was lax, RAD to 1.5 cm, and there were multiple fissures.

Over the next 2 weeks his condition remained critical, he was ventilated and recovery seemed unlikely. In spite of his poor general condition his anus showed signs of healing – the slides were taken on day 2 and day 5 (see Plate 100).

Perforation of the bowel

Child sexual abuse may lead to perforation of the bowel by digital or penile penetration or the insertion of an object through the anus. Accidental perforation is rare but has been described after sitting on spikes or glass. A boy of 9 years perforated his rectum when leap-frogging over a snooker table and landing on a cue.

CASE HISTORY 9.11

A 6-week-old boy was admitted to hospital very ill with peritonitis secondary to a rectal tear. The father admitted to causing the injury by digital penetration while sexually abusing his son.

Skin disease

- Atopic eczema, seborrhoeic dermatitis and candidiasis are all common and may coexist with child sexual abuse.
- Lichen sclerosis has a characteristic appearance (see p. 209) and may affect the anus with perianal swelling, erythema and fissures.

Chronic inflammatory bowel disease

Chronic inflammatory bowel disease has been thought to mimic child sexual abuse (Hey et al 1987) but the picture as a whole enables the diagnosis to be made. The published case was of Crohn's disease asymmetrically affecting the genitalia and anus.

Haemolytic uraemic syndrome

- Vickers et al (1988) presented three girls under 3 years with bloody diarrhoea and markedly abnormal anal signs.
- It should be remembered that children with physical or intellectual disability are at increased risk of all types of abuse including child sexual abuse.

Congenital anomalies

- It is uncommon for congenital anomalies to be presented as child sexual abuse as many are recognised neonatally
- McCann (1990) noted smooth, depressed, wedge-like areas at 6 and 12 o'clock which

might be mistaken for scars, and also a prominent medial raphe. There should not be too much problem in differentiating these from scars which are thick, irregular, pale and distort the local anatomy (and are rare).
- Pronounced skin folds and skin tags may form at the end of healing fissures. Some may be congenital (Berenson et al 1993) and congenital tags are expected to be in the midline (McCann et al 1989). Tags were seen in 14% of children who had been abused (Muram 1989a). Tags alone are not evidence of abuse, but a history suggestive of a fissure (constipation, pain, bleeding is expected and perhaps tags outside the midline in the absence of an appropriate history are more significant).
- Fissures due to child sexual abuse are more commonly in the midline, which is another confounding factor although McCann thinks tags due to trauma are distinguishable because of local disruption as part of the healing process.

Rectal tumour

A rectal tumour may present with bleeding, and in the absence of fissure the child will require proctoscopy.

Assessment of anal signs

Chronic constipation

- This is a relatively common complaint and may coexist with child sexual abuse.
- Clayden (1987) suggested that warning signs of child sexual abuse in a constipated child included:
  - a history of emotional disturbance with a history of possible abuse
  - passivity during the examination
  - laxity of the anus
  - bruising perianally
  - infection with a sexually transmitted disease.
- Clayden (1987) concludes by noting that anal abuse may occur in the absence of abnormal physical signs and conversely anal abnormality may be evidence of another disorder, i.e. a differential diagnosis is part of the medical assessment.

Neurological disorder

- A child who has a neurogenic bowel and bladder will have a lax sphincter, and is likely to have repeated enemata which will add to the laxity.
- Children with other chronic disorders, e.g. cerebral palsy, have a tendency to constipation and may require enemata, so anal signs need careful assessment.
- There is an ongoing debate as to anal abnormality and myotonic dystrophy. In this condition constipation is common, and a report suggested that several children had been wrongly diagnosed as victims of child sexual abuse (Rearden 1992). Since that paper was published children who were subjects of the paper have alleged child sexual abuse and the signs may have been misinterpreted. There is a need for research in this disorder into anal signs.
- Twenty children of all ages with Down's syndrome were examined and all had normal bottoms (Dr F Bamford, personal communication 1991).

Any anal abnormality must be reviewed in the context of the wider paediatric assessment (see the 'jigsaw', Fig. 9.15).

- Anal abuse appears to be common because even at a young age it is possible to penetrate the distensible anus and rectum (oral sex is common for the same reason).
- The younger the child the more likely it is to find abnormal signs (under 5 years 60% had abnormal signs and over childhood 42% of 337 of confirmed cases of child sexual abuse had signs (Hobbs & Wynne 1989).
- Despite anal abnormalities it is uncommon for a child to have bowel symptoms, there may be a history of bleeding, pain on defecation and constipation, but it is rare for there to be any faecal leakage due to anal laxity.
- Physical examination should normally be early.

- Examination of any child who is thought to have been abused should include the anus and mouth (rarely petechiae on the hard palate or a sexually transmitted disease is found). Children may be too embarrassed to disclose oral and anal sex.
- The only diagnostic signs are: gonorrhoea, syphilis, semen/sperm on forensic testing and all other information is of relative significance.
- The relative frequency of signs associated with anal abuse are given in Table 9.26. A guide to rates of healing can be found in Table 9.21. Table 9.27 lists signs associated with acute and chronic child sexual abuse.
- The patterns of anal signs are highly significant, a gaping anus with perianal erythema and multiple acute fissures is one example as is rectal gonorrhoea. Perianal erythema with superficial excoriations is much less specific and could equally be due to threadworm infestation.
- If the child is able to give a clear, spontaneous disclosure erythema and a single fissure may be highly significant. Likewise a single, deep, acute or chronic fissure (usually at 6 o'clock) in a toddler with no history of constipation may be the only sign of anal penetration. What other aetiology is there of an anal fissure extending down the anal canal and across the anal margin and perianally other than excessive scratching?
- Outside the midline, skin tags, scars, fissures and abrasions were not found in McCann's 'normal' population (1990). Berenson et al (1993) in a study of children of under 18 months who were thought to be not abused found
  - 26% had a smooth area at 6 or 12 o'clock
  - 10% had altered pigmentation
  - 7% redness
  - 3% skin tag
  - 1% venous pooling (after 2 minutes) and fissure (the cause is not stated), i.e. there was little abnormality.
- In older children, perhaps mid-childhood onwards, there may be no abnormality after anal abuse if the assailant is careful and uses a lubricant (Bamford & Roberts 1989). A figure of 50% is quoted for the 'normal' examination of teenagers who have been buggered but the figure may be too high and related to the delay in examination which may have been of months (Spencer 1986, Reinhardt 1987).

Differential diagnosis of anal abuse

- Accidental trauma
- Skin disorder, e.g. atopic eczema, lichen sclerosus
- Congenital abnormality, e.g. midline raphe, wedge-shaped area in midline
- Infection, e.g. candidiasis, streptococcal cellulitis
- Inflammatory bowel disease, e.g. Crohn's disease
- Severe, chronic constipation causing anal laxity
- Single anal fissure, e.g. constipation
- Neurological disorder, e.g. neurogenic bowel in association with spina bifida
- Rectal tumour

Summary of the perianal signs of child sexual abuse (RCP 1997)

- 'Diagnostic of blunt force penetrating trauma – the only specific indicator of anal abuse is a fresh laceration or a healed scar extending beyond the anal margin on to the perianal skin in the absence of reasonable alternative explanation . . . contusions of bite marks are very suggestive . . . and scars are seen in less than 10% . . .'
- Supportive signs:
  - anal laxity
  - RAD greater than 15 mm and reproducible
  - acute changes, e.g. erythema, swelling, fissures, venous congestion and bruising
  - chronic changes include the triad of signs of frequent anal intercourse, i.e thickening of the anal verge skin, with resultant reduction in anal verge skin folds, increased elasticity and reduction in the power of the anal sphincter
- Lack of discernible signs
- Anal signs in children vary with the type of abuse, the frequency of the abuse, the age of the child, the use of lubricant, any sexually transmitted disease, the time since the last assault (acute signs, healing, chronic signs including scarring)

Table 9.26 Signs likely to be significant in the assessment of anal abuse

Sign	RCP (1991)	'Abused children' frequency Hobbs & Wynne (1989)	'Non-abused children' frequency McCann et al (1990)
Laceration or healed scar extending beyond the anal mucosa on to perianal skin with no reasonable history, e.g. major trauma	Diagnostic	Few	0%
Anal laxity	Supportive	38%	0%
RAD > 1 cm (30 seconds *left lateral* position)	Supportive (0.5–2.5 cm)	42%	–
RAD (30 seconds *knee–chest* position)	–	–	9%
RAD >2.0 cm	Penetrating trauma (Heger 1991)	–	1.2%
Fissures	Supportive	53%	0%
Erythema	Supportive	53%	41%
Swelling	Supportive	8%	0%
Venous congestion (30 seconds left lateral)	Supportive	24%	7%(?)
STD/warts	Supportive/diagnostic	4%	0%
Scars/tags/folds	Supportive	8%	0% outside midline 0% boys 11% anterior skin tags, folds in girls
Haemorrhoids	Very unusual	0%	0%

Venous congestion was seen at the beginning of the examination. Knee–chest in 7%.
Signs of chronic anal abuse include skin changes, with the perianal skin thickened and smooth (Paul 1990).
Many older children who have been anally abused are normal on examination (RCP 1991).

Forensic tests

Forensic tests are uncommonly helpful in child sexual abuse because of the chronicity and familial nature of the abuse – if the child has been bathed, or has defecated since the last assault, the skin and anal/rectal swabs will be negative for semen but items of clothing, bedding or furniture may be available for testing (for details see Ch. 14).

Table 9.27 Signs associated with anal abuse (Hobbs & Wynne 1989, Paul 1990, AAP 1991, RCP 1991)

'Acute' signs (within hours)	'Chronic' signs
Swelling perianally (tyre sign)	Thickened perianal skin, with loss of skin folds
Bruising	Anal laxity
Haematoma anal verge	Anal dilatation
Fissures, may bleed	Venous congestion
Gaping anus	Chronic fissures
Linear abrasions of skin	Scarring (linear, fan-shaped)
Genital signs	Skin tags
Other signs of physical injury	Warts or other STD
	Funnelling (teenager?)
	Hyperpigmentation
	Self-mutilation

Referral

Referral to other agencies depends on the level of concern; it is usually good practice to discuss uncertainties with a medical colleague initially, and having reached a consensus decide:

- whether to make a direct referral to social services department if the clinical picture is clear, e.g. a 3-year-old with gonorrhoea
- if there is a need to collect more information from the general practitioner, health visitor, school nurse. Then have a discussion with a senior social worker about the medical concerns.

What is most unhelpful (to the child) is for social services department and the police to go into an investigation not understanding the limits of the medical 'evidence'. In difficult situations a formal, face-to-face, rather than a telephone strategy meeting should be held (Figs 9.15 and 9.16; Zeitlin 1987). Although caution in the early stages may leave the child unprotected in the short term, it is much more likely that a throught-through assessment will be helpful to the child.

If the referral comes initially from the social services department or the police, following a disclosure, for example, it may be possible to give an immediate opinion, but if necessary it is possible to delay this opinion to give time for thought and discussion with medical colleagues.

The diagnosis of child sexual abuse has far-reaching consequences and there are pitfalls (Paul 1990) but if practitioners are thorough and well informed mistaken medical opinions should be avoided.

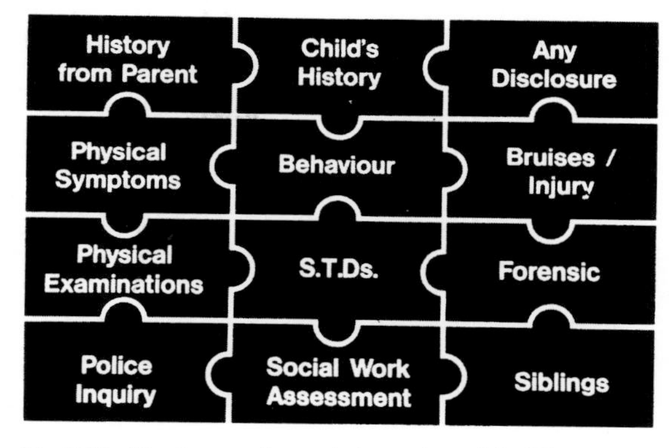

Fig. 9.15 The jigsaw of sexual abuse. A model of the complex interlocking nature of sexual abuse diagnosis. A multidisciplinary approach is implied in this model.

Summary

1. The recognition of child sexual abuse is increasing as adults are better informed and listen to children with greater understanding.
2. Child sexual abuse may present in many ways.
3. Doctors who work in this field should ensure that they are not professionally isolated and also understand the need for inter-agency co-operation.
4. Informed consent is needed before a paediatric assessment takes place, take legal advice if in doubt, e.g. is the teenager 'Gillick competent', or who has parental responsibility?
5. The diagnosis of child sexual abuse is made by building up the pieces of the diagnostic jigsaw: the physical examination is one part, albeit an important part in this process.
6. Children's disclosures of abuse should be taken on face value initially but subsequently require skilled validation.
7. Physical indicators of child sexual abuse are important as they may be the first sign of abuse. They may corroborate the child's story.
8. Normality on examination is common even if the child has been abused.
9. Follow-up examination is often helpful in the evaluation of signs: is healing taking place or a disease process, e.g. lichen sclerosis evolving?
10. Single abnormal physical signs may support the diagnosis of child sexual abuse but are rarely proof of abuse: pregnancy, sperm found in the vagina or rectum, and gonorrhoea are exceptions to this generalisation.
11. Physical and child sexual abuse are seen together in around 15% of cases: burns and bites are particularly associated with child sexual abuse.
12. All sexually abused children have been emotionally abused. Does the child/family require referral for psychological/psychiatric help?
13. Penetrative abuse in young children involves oral and anal abuse, vaginal penetration occurs in older girls, sodomy may persist.
14. Working with child sexual abuse is difficult and emotionally taxing.

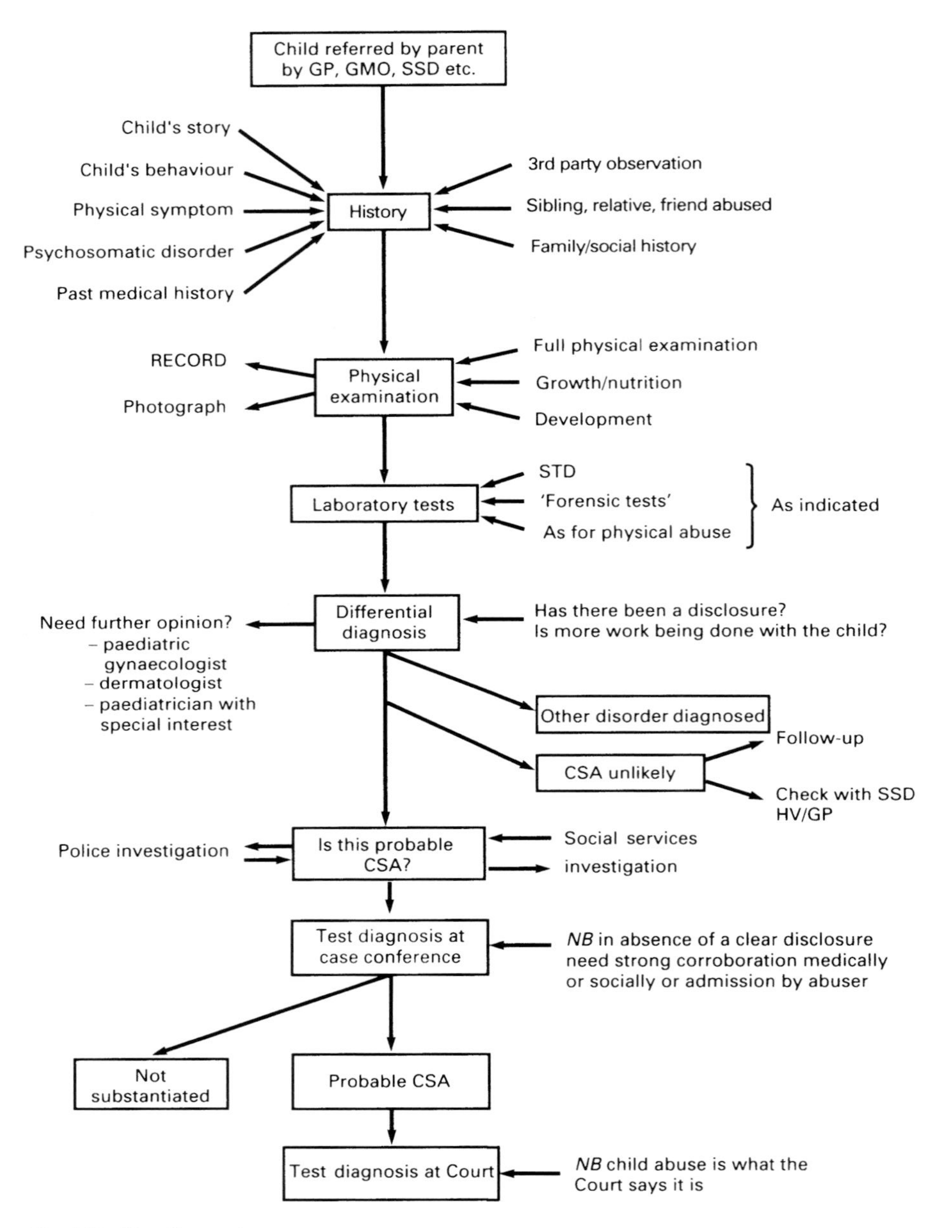

Fig. 9.16 The diagnostic process.

REFERENCES

AAP 1991 American Academy of Pediatrics Guidelines for the evaluation of sexual abuse in children. Paediatrics 87:254–260

Adams J A, Harper K, Knudson K, Revilla J 1994 Examination findings in legally confirmed CSA: it's normal to be normal. Pediatrics 94:310–317

Agnarsson U, Clayden G 1990 Constipation in children. Maternal and Child Health 15:252–256

Agnarsson U, Gordon C, Wright C et al 1990 Perianal appearances in childhood constipation. Archives of Diseases of Childhood 65:1231–1234

Anderson C 1975 Constipation. In: Anderson C, Burke V (eds) Paediatric gastroenterology. Blackwell, Oxford

Arnold R P, Rogers D, Cook D A G 1990 Medical problems of adults who were sexually abused in childhood. British Medical Journal 300:705–708

BAAF 1991 Implications for medical practitioners. Children Act 1989. Practice note 28. British Agencies for Adoption and Fostering, London

Baker A B 1986 Seat-belt masquerading as sexual abuse. Pediatrics 77:435

Bamford F W, Kiff E S 1987 Child sexual abuse. Letter. Lancet ii:1396

Bamford F, Roberts R 1989 Child sexual abuse. In: Meadow S R (ed) ABC of child abuse. BMJ Publications, London, p 31

Bartley D L, Morgan L, Rimsza M E 1987 *Gardnerella vaginalis* in prepubertal girls. American Journal of Diseases of Children 141:1014–1017

Bays J, Chadwick D 1993 Medical diagnosis of the sexually abused child. Child Abuse and Neglect 17:91–110

Bays J, Jenny C 1990 Genital and anal conditions confused with child sexual abuse trauma. American Journal of Diseases of Children 144(12):1319–1322

Benninga A M A, Buller H A, Heymans H A S 1994 Is encopresis always the result of constipation. Arch Dis Child 71:186–193

Bentovim A, Boston P 1988 Sexual abuse – basic issues – characteristics of children and families. In: Bentovim A, Elton A, Hildebrand J, Tranter M, Vizard E Child sexual abuse within the family. Wright, London, Ch 2

Bentovim A, Elton A, Hildebrand J, Tranter M, Vizard E 1988 Helping children to describe experience of child sexual abuse. In: Child sexual abuse within the family. Wright, London, Chs 5, 6

Berenson A B 1995 A longitudinal study of hymenal morphology in the first 3 years of life. Pediatrics 95:628–631

Berenson A B, Somma-Garcia A, Barnett S 1993 Perianal findings in infants 18 months of age or younger. Pediatrics 91:838–840

Berkowitz C D et al 1987 Labial fusion in pre-pubertal girls: a marker for sexual abuse? American Journal of Obstetrics and Gynecology 156:16–20

Black J A, Debelle G D 1995 Female genital mutilation in Britain. British Medical Journal 310:1590–1592

Branch G, Paxton R 1965 A study of gonococcal infections amongst infants and children. Public Health Reports 80:347–352

Brown R M et al 1989 Child abuse presenting as an organic disease. British Medical Journal 299(6699): 614–615

Butler-Sloss E 1988 Report of the Inquiry into Child Abuse in Cleveland 1987. HMSO, London

Cantwell H 1983 Vaginal inspection as it relates to child sexual abuse in girls under thirteen. Child Abuse and Neglect 7:171–176

Cantwell H B 1987 Update on vaginal inspection as it relates to child sexual abuse in girls under thirteen. Child Abuse and Neglect 11:545–546

Chambers T L, Panting G P 1996 Guarding paediatricians against allegations of assault. Arch Dis Child 75:82–85

Childhood Matters 1996 Report of the National Commission of Inquiry into the Prevention of Child Abuse. Stationery Office, London

Clarke J 1997 'How did she get these warts?' Ano-genital warts and sexual abuse. Child Abuse Review in press

Clarke J et al 1990 The sexual behaviour and knowledge about AIDS in a group of young adolescent girls in Leeds. Genitourinary Medicine 66:189–192

Clarke J, Lacey C 1990 Sexually transmitted diseases in sexually abused children. Community Paediatric Group Newsletter

Clayden G S 1981 Chronic constipation in childhood. University of London, pp 118–120

Clayden G 1987 Anal appearance and child sexual abuse. Letter. Lancet i:620

Clayden G S 1988 Reflex anal dilatation associated with severe chronic constipation in children. Arch Dis Child 63:832–836

Clayden G S 1992 Management of chronic constipation. Arch Dis Child 63:340

Corbett J et al 1977 Progressive disintegrative psychosis in childhood. Journal of Child Psychology and Psychiatry 18:211–219

Corwin D L 1988 Early diagnosis of child sexual abuse: diminishing the lasting effects. In: Wyatt G E, Powell G J (eds) Lasting effects of child sexual abuse. Sage, London, pp 251–269

Davies G, Wilson C, Mitchell R, Milson J 1995 Videotaping children's evidence: an evaluation. Home Office, London

DeJong A R 1986 Sexually transmitted diseases in sexually abused children. Sexually Transmitted Disease 13:123–126

DeJong A 1991 Legal proof of CSA in absence of physical evidence. Pediatrics 88(3):506–511

de la Haye Davies H 1987 Protocol for the forensic examination of the sexually abused child. Police Surgeon 32 (Dec 1987)

Dewhurst J 1988 Evidence. In: Butler-Sloss E Report of the Inquiry into Child Abuse in Cleveland 1989. HMSO, London

DHSS 1988 Diagnosis of child sexual abuse: guidance for doctors. HMSO, London

DoH 1991 An introductory guide for the NHS: the Children Act 1989. DoH, London

Dowd M D, Fitzmaurice Knapp J F, Mooney D 1994 The interpretation of urogenital findings in children with straddle injuries. Journal of Pediatrics 29:7–10

Duckett J W 1995 A temperate approach to neonatal circumcision. Urology 46(6):769–770

Elliot A J, Peterson L W 1993 Maternal sexual abuse of male children. Postgraduate Medicine 94(1):169–180

Emans S J, Woods E R, Allred E, Grace E 1994 Hymenal findings in adolescent women: impact of tampon use and consensual sexual activity. Journal of Pediatrics 153–160

Emans S J 1987 Genital findings in sexually abused, symptomatic and asymptomatic girls. Pediatrics 79:778–785

Emans S J 1988 Evaluation of the sexually abused child and adolescent. Adolescenct and Paediatric Gynaecology 1:157–163

Emans S J 1998 Vulvovaginal problems in the pubertal child. In: (eds) Emans S J Laufer M R Goldstein D P Pediatric and Adolescent Gynaecology Lippincott-Raven 75–107

Enos W F et al 1986 Forensic evaluation of sexual abuse in children. Pediatrics 78:385–398

Erickson P I Rapkin A J 1991 Unwanted sexual experiences among middle and high school youth J Adolesc Health 12:319

Feldman K 1997 Inflicted incision of penis. Letter. Child Abuse and Neglect 21(3):253–254

Finkel M A 1989 Anogenital trauma in sexually abused children. Pediatrics 84(2): 317–322

Finkelstein E, Amichal B, Jaworowski S, Mukamel M 1996 Masturbation in prepubescent children: a case report and review of the literature. Child 22(5):323–326

Flemming K A, Venning V, Evans M 1987 DNA typing of genital warts and diagnosis of sexual abuse in children (letter). Lancet ii:454

Forster G 1992 Rape and sexually transmitted disease. British Journal of Hospital Medicine 47(2):94–95

Forster G 1994 STDs and CSA. British Journal of Hospital Medicine 51(5):206

Freidrich F N, Grambach P, Broughton D, Kuiper J, Beilke RL 1991 Normative sexual behavior in children. Pediatrics 88:456–464

Frothingham T, Barnett R, Hobbs C, Wynne J 1992 Child sexual abuse in Leeds before and after Cleveland.

Furniss T 1991 The multi-professional handbook of child sexual abuse. Routledge, London

Ganz E 1962 Signs of sodomy. Letter. British Medical Journal 1:263

Gardner J J 1992 Descriptive study of genital variation in healthy non-abused premenarchal girls. J Pediatrics 120:251–257

Gellert G, Durfee M 1989 HIV infection and child abuse. Letter. New England Journal of Medicine 321:685

Gellert G, Durfee M, Berkowitz C, Higgins K, Tubiolo V 1993 Situational and sociodemographical characteristics of children infected with human immunodeficiency virus from pediatric sexual abuse. Pediatrics 91:39–44

Giardino A P, Finkel M A, Giardino E R, Seidel T, Ludwig S 1992 A practical guide to sexual abuse in the prepubertal child. Sage, London

Glaser D 1995 Children's evidence – state of the art? a commentary on 'Videotaping children's evidence: an evaluation'. Child Abuse Review 4:240–245

Glaser D, Collins C 1989 The response of young non-sexually abused children to anatomically correct dolls. Journal of Child Psychology and Psychiatry 30(4):547–560

Glaser D, Frosh S 1988 Child sexual abuse. Macmillan, London, Chs 4–6

GMC 1987: Annual Report 1987, General Medical Council, London, p 15

GMC 1996 General Medical Council advises doctors on intimate examinations. British Medical Journal 313:1996

Goff C W et al 1989 Vaginal measurements in pre-pubertal girls. American Journal of Diseases of Childhood 143:1366–1369

Goldsmid J, Kibel M A, Mills A E 1985 Diseases due to infection. In: Forfar J O, Arneil G C (eds) Textbook of paediatrics. Churchill Livingstone. Edinburgh

Graham P 1991 Child psychiatry. A developmental approach. Oxford University Press, Oxford

Guardian 1996a Surgeons repair penises. Guardian, London, 27 August 1996

Gutman L T 1990 Sexual abuse and human papilloma virus. Letter. Journal of Paediatrics 116(5):495–496

Gutman L T et al 1991a Diagnosis of child sexual abuse in children with genital warts. Archives of Disease in Childhood 145(2):126–127

Gutman L T et al 1991b HIV transmission by child sexual abuse. Letter. Archives of Disease in Childhood 145(2):137–141

Gutman L T, St Claire K, Herman-Giddens M E, Johnston W W, Phelps W C 1992 Evaluation of sexually abused and non-abused young girls for intravaginal human papillomavirus infection. American Journal of Diseases of Children 146(6):694–699

Gutman L T, Herman-Giddens M E, McKinney R E 1993 Paediatric acquired AIDS. American Journal of Diseases of Children 147:775–780

Hamilton J 1997 UN condemns female circumcision. British Medical Journal 314:1148

Hammerschlag M R 1988 Sexually transmitted disease in sexually abused children. Advances in Paediatric Infectious Disease 3:1

Handfield-Jones S E, Hinde F R J, Kennedy C T C 1987 Lichen sclerosus et atrophicus in children misdiagnosed as sexual abuse. British Medical Journal 294:1404–1405

Handley J, Dinsmore W, Maw R et al 1993 Anogenital warts in prepubertal children: sexual abuse or not? International Journal of Sexually Transmitted Disease and AIDS 4:271–279

Hanks H, Hobbs C J M 1992 Self abuse and suicide. Current Paediatrics 2:57–59

Heger A 1991 (in evidence to RCP) Physical signs of sexual abuse in children

Heger A, Emmans S J 1990 Introital diameter as the criterion for sexual abuse. Paediatrics 85:222–223

Herman-Giddens M 1989 Harmful genital care practices in children. Journal of the American Medical Association 261(4):577–579

Herman-Giddens M E 1994 Vaginal foreign bodies and child sexual abuse. Archives of Pediatric and Adolescent Medicine 148:195–200

Herman-Giddens M E, Frothingham T S 1987 Prepubertal female genitalia: examination for evidence of abuse. Pediatrics 80(2):203–208

Herman-Giddens M E, Garmann L T, Benson N L 1988 Association of coexisting vaginal infections and multiple abusers in female children with genital warts. Sexually Transmitted Diseases 15:63–67

Hey et al 1987 Differential diagnosis in child sexual abuse. Letter. Lancet i:283

HMSO 1992 Memorandum of good practice on video recorded interviews with child witnesses for criminal proceedings. HMSO, London

Hobbs C J, Wynne J M 1986 Buggery in childhood: a common syndrome of child abuse. Lancet ii:792–796

Hobbs C J, Wynne J M 1987a Child sexual abuse – an increasing rate of diagnosis. Lancet ii:837–841
Hobbs C J, Wynne J M 1987b Management of sexual abuse. Archives of Diseases in Childhood 62:1182–1187
Hobbs C J, Wynne J M 1989 Sexual abuse of English boys and girls: the importance of anal examination. Child Abuse and Neglect 13:195–210
Hobbs C J, Wynne J M 1990 The sexually abused battered child. Archives of Disease in Childhood 65:423–427
Hobbs C J, Hanks H I G, Wynne J M (eds) 1993 Rates of healing In: Edinburgh Ch. 9 Clinical aspects of sexual abuse Churchill Livingstone
Hobbs C J, Wynne J M 1995a Examination findings in legally confirmed CSA: It's normal to be normal. Letter. Pediatrics 95:148–149
Hobbs C J, Wynne J M 1995b The examination of the genitalia of the infant and young child – normal and abnormal. Current Paediatrics 5:236–242
Hobbs C J, Wynne J M 1995c Letter re visible stool and RAD. Child Abuse and Neglect 19(3):385–386
Hobbs C J, Wynne J M, Thomas A 1995 Colposcopic genital findings in prepubertal girls assessed for sexual abuse. Archives of Disease in Childhood 73(5):465–471 and letter p 480
Horowitz S, Glassberg K I 1995 Circumcision: successful glandular reconstruction and survival following traumatic amputation (abstract). American Academy of Paediatric Annual Meeting, Urology Section, October
Huffman J W et al 1981 The gynaecology of childhood and adolescence. W B Saunders, Philadelphia, p 25
Ingram D L, Everett D, Lyna P et al 1992 Epidemiology of adult sexually transmitted disease agents in children being evaluated for sexual abuse. Pediatric Infectious Disease 11:945–950
Jenny C et al 1987 Hymens in newborn female infants. Pediatrics 80(3):399–400
Jenny C, Kirby P, Fuquay D 1989 Genital lichen sclerosus mistaken for child sexual abuse. Paediatrics 83:597–599
Johnson C F 1991 Prolapse of the urethra – confusion of clinical characteristics of sexual abuse. Pediatrics 487(5):722–725
Jones D P H, McQuiston M G 1992 Interviewing the sexually abused child, 4th edn. Gaskell, London
Jumbelic M L 1997 Letter re: Inflicted incision of the penis. Child Abuse and Neglect 21(3):249
Kaplan K M, Fleischer G R, Paradise J E, Friedman H N 1984 Social relevance of genital herpes simplex in children. Archives of Diseases in Childhood 138:872–874
Kerns D L, Ritter M L, Thomas R G 1992 Concave hymenal variations in suspected CSA victims. Pediatrics 90:2,265–272
Klevan J L, DeJong A R 1990 Urinary tract symptoms and urinary tract infection following sexual abuse. American Journal of Diseases in Childhood 144:242–244
Lanktree C, Zaidi L, Briere J, Gutterez V 1989 Differential identification of sexually abused children in psychiatric outpatients, American Psychological Association, New Orleans, Abstract, August
Lindblad F et al 1989 Child sexual abuse: physical examination. Acta Paediatrica Scandinavica 78(6):935–943
Lukschu M, Bays J 1996 Inflicted incision of the penis. Child Abuse and Neglect 20:279–281
Lukschu M, Bays J 1997 Letter Re: inflicted incision of the penis. Child Abuse and Neglect 21(3):251
Lusk R, Waterman J 1986 Effects of sexual abuse on children. In: MacFarlane K, Waterman J, Conerley S, Damon L, Durfee M, Long S (eds) Sexual abuse of young children. Holt Rinehart & Winston, New York
McCann J 1990 Use of the colposcope in childhood sexual abuse examinations. Pediatrics Clinics of North America 37(4):863
McCann J et al 1988 Labial adhesions and posterior fourchette injuries in childhood sexual abuse. American Journal of Diseases in Childhood 142:659–663
McCann J et al 1989 Perianal findings in prepubertal children selected for non-abuse: a descriptive study. Child Abuse and Neglect 13(2):179–194
McCann J, Wells R, Voris J et al 1990a Comparison of genital examination techniques in prepubertal girls. Pediatric Clinics of North America 85:182–187
McCann J, Voris J, Simon M 1990b Genital findings in prepubertal females selected for non-abuse: a descriptive study. Paediatrics 86(3): 428–439
McCann J, Voris J, Simon M 1992 Genital injuries resulting from sexual abuse: a longitudinal study. Pediatrics 89:307–310
McCann J, Voris J 1993 Perianal injuries resulting from sexual abuse: a longitudinal study. Pediatrics 89:307–317
McCann J 1998 The appearance of acute healing and healed ano-genital trauma. Child Abuse & Neglect 22:245
MacFarlane K 1986 Child sexual abuse allegations in divorce proceedings. In: MacFarlane K, Waterman J, Conerley S, Damon L, Durfee M, Long S (eds) Sexual abuse of young children. Holt, Rinehart and Winston, New York, Ch. 7
McLay W D S (ed) 1990a Sexual abuse of children. In: Clinical forensic medicine. Pinter, London, Ch 13, 234
McLay W D S (ed) 1990b Sexual offences against adults. In: Clinical forensic medicine. Pinter, London, Ch 14, 263
Mant A K 1960 Forensic medicine. Lloyd, London, 243
Marshall W N, Puls T, Davidson C 1988 New child abuse operation in an era of increased awareness. American Journal of Diseases in Childhood 142:664–667
McCrae W M 1985 Disorders of the alimentary tract. In: Forfar J O, Arneil G C (eds) Textbook of paediatrics, 3rd edn, Vol 1. Churchill Livingstone, Edinburgh, 472–474
Meadow S R 1987 Staying cool in child abuse. Editorial. British Medical Journal 295:345
Meadow S R 1993 False allegations of abuse and Munchausen syndrome by proxy. Archives of Diseases of Children 68:444–447
Mehl A L 1990 Urinary tract infection and sexual abuse. Letter. American Journal of Diseases in Childhood 144:1073
Mok J Y Q 1996 When is HIV an issue after CSA. Archives of Diseases of Childhood 75:85–87
Molesworth A, Tookey P 1997 Paediatric AIDS and HIV infection. Communicable disease reports 7(9):R132–R134
Muram D 1986 Genital tract injuries in the prepubertal child. Paediatric Annals 15:616–620

Muram D 1989a Anal and perianal abnormalities in prepubertal victims of sexual abuse. American Journal of Obstetrics and Gynecology 161(2):278–281
Muram D 1989b Child sexual abuse: relationship between sexual acts and genital findings. Child Abuse and Neglect 13:211–216
Muram D, Elias S 1989 Child sexual abuse – genital tract findings in prepubertal girls. II. Comparison of colposcopic and unaided examinations. American Journal of Obstetrics and Gynecology 160:333–335
Muram D, Speck D M, Gold S S 1991 Genital abnormalities in female siblings and friends of child victims of sexual abuse. Child Abuse and Neglect 15:105–110
Neinstein L S et al 1984 Non-sexual transmission of sexually transmitted diseases: an infrequent occurrence. Paediatrics 74:67–76
Obalek S, Jablonska S, Favre M et al 1990 Condylomata acuminata in children: frequent association with human papillomavirus responsible for cutaneous warts. Journal of the American Academy of Dermatology 23:205–213
Paradise J E 1989 Predictive accuracy and the diagnosis of sexual abuse: a big issue about a little tissue. Child Abuse and Neglect 13:169–176
Paradise J E 1990 The medical evaluation of the sexually abused child. Pediatric Clinics of North America 37:839–862
Paradise J, Willis E 1985 Probability of vaginal foreign body in girls with genital complaint. American Journal of Diseases in Childhood 139:472–476
Paul D M 1977 Medical examination in sexual offences against children. Medicine, Science, and Law 17:251–258
Paul D 1984 Examination of the living. In: Mant A K (ed) Taylor's principles and practice of medical jurisprudence. Churchill Livingstone, Edinburgh
Paul D M 1986 What really did happen to Baby Jane? The medical aspects of the investigation of alleged sexual abuse of children. Medicine, Science and Law 26:85–106
Paul D 1990 The pitfalls which may be encountered during an exam for signs of sexual abuse. Medicine, Science and Law 30(1):3–11
Peters S D 1988 Child sexual abuse and later psychological problems. In: Wyatt G W, Powell G J (eds) Lasting effects of child sexual abuse. Sage, Beverley Hills, CA, pp 107–117
Pigot Report 1989 Report of Advisory Group on Video Evidence. Home Office, London
Priestley B L, Bleehan S S 1987 Lichen sclerosus et atrophicus in children misdiagnosed as sexual abuse. British Medical Journal 295:211
Raine P A M 1991 Investigation of rectal bleeding. Archives of Disease in Childhood 66:279–280
Randall Bond G R, Dowd M D, Landsman I, Rimza M 1995 Unintentional perineal injury in prepubescent girls: a multicenter, prospective report of 56 girls. Pediatrics 95:628–631
RCP 1991, 1997 Physical signs of sexual abuse in children. Report of working party. Royal College of Physicians, London (2nd edn 1997)
Reardon W, Hughes H E, Green S M 1992 Anal abnormalities in childhood myotonic dystrophia: a possible source of confusion in CSA. Archives of Disease in Childhood 67:527
Reinhardt M 1987 Sexually abused boys. Child Abuse and Neglect II:229–235
Richman N, Stevenson J, Graham P 1982 Pre-school–school: a behavioural study. Academic Press, London
Ridley C M L 1987 Lichen sclerosus et atrophicus. Editorial. British Medical Journal 295(21):1295–1296
Rimsza M E, Feingold M D 1989 Labial fusion. Picture of the month. American Journal of Diseases of Childhood 143:381–382
Rock B, Naghasfar Z, Barnett N, Buscerna J, Woodruff J D, Shah K 1986 Genital tract papillomavirus infections in childhood. Arch Dermatol 122:1129–1132
Rogers D J Stark M 1998 The hymen is not necessarily torn after sexual intercourse (letter) British Medical Journal 317:413
San Lazaro C 1995 Making paediatric assessment in suspected sexual abuse a therapeutic experience. Archives of Disease in Childhood 73(2):174–176
San Lazaro C, Steele A M, Danaldson L J 1996 Outcome of criminal investigation into allegations of sexual abuse. Archives of Disease in Childhood 75:149–152
Sauzier M 1989 Disclosure of child sexual abuse. For better or for worse. Pediatric Clinics of North America 12:455–469
Sgroi S et al 1988 Children's sexual behaviours and their relationship to sexual abuse. In: Sgroi S (ed) Vulnerable population, Vol 1. Lexington Books, Lexington, MA
Shandling B 1987 Surgical conditions of anus, rectum and colon. In: Behrman, Vaughan (eds) Nelson textbook of pediatrics, 13th edn. W B Saunders, Philadelphia
Silber T J 1994 False allegations of sexual touching by physicians in the practice of pediatrics. Pediatrics 94:742–745
Siran A B et al 1988 Interaction of normal child with anatomical dolls. Child Abuse and Neglect 12:295–304
Slaughter L, Brown C R V, Crowley S, Peck R 1997 Patterns of genital injury in female sexual assault victims. American Journal of Obstetric and Gynaecology 97:610–616
Smith P, Wilson A 1991 Children as witnesses. Seen and heard. Vol 1, p 25
Spencer H, Dunklee P 1986 Sexual abuse of boys. Pediatrics 78:133–138
Spencer J 1991 Reformers despair. New Law Journal 787
Spencer J, Flin R 1990 The evidence of children, the law and psychology
Stanton A, Sunderland R 1989 Prevalence of reflex anal dilatation in 200 children. British Medical Journal 298:802–803
Steiner H et al 1988 Description of recording physical signs in suspected child sexual abuse. British Journal of Hospital Medicine 40(5):346–351
Steward M S, Schmitz M, Steward D S, Joye N R, Reinhart M 1995 Children's anticipation of and response to colposcopic examination. Child Abuse and Neglect 19(8):997–1005
Stuart-Smith S 1996 Teenage sex. Leader. BMJ 312:390–391
Tanner J M 1978 Physical growth and development. In: Forfar J O, Arneil G C (eds) Textbook of paediatrics. Churchill Livingstone, Edinburgh, Ch 7

Vandeven A M, Emans S J 1995 Commentary on Hobbs et al (1995) paper
Vickers D et al 1988 Anal signs in haemolytic uraemic syndrome. Letter. Lancet i:998
Vizard E, Tranter M 1988 Recognition and assessment of sexual abuse. In: Bentovim A, Elton A, Hildebrand J, Tranter M, Vizard E (eds) Child sexual abuse within the family. Wright, London, Ch 4, pp 59–88
Warrington S A, de San Lazaro C 1996 Lichen sclerosus et atrophicus and sexual abuse. Archives of Disease in Childhood 75:512–516
West R, Davies D, Fenton T 1989 Accidental vulval injuries in children. British Medical Journal 298:1002–1003
White S T et al 1983 Sexually transmitted diseases in sexually abused children. Paediatrics 72:16–21
White S T et al 1989 Vaginal introital diameter in the evaluation of sexual abuse. Child Abuse and Neglect 13:217–224
Whitwell D 1990 The significance of childhood sexual abuse for adult psychiatry. British Journal of Hospital Medicine 43:346–352
Woodling B 1986 Sexual abuse and the child. Em Med Serv 15:17–25
Woodling B A, Heger A 1986 The use of the colposcope in the diagnosis of sexual abuse in the pediatric age group. Child Abuse and Neglect 10:111–114
Woodling B A & Kossoris P D 1981 Sexual misuse, rape, molestation and incest. Pediatric Clinics of North America 28:481–499
Working Together 1988 Working together: a guide to arrangements for inter-agency co-operation for the protection of children from abuse. HMSO, London
Working Together 1991 Working together under the Children Act 1989. A guide to arrangements for inter-agency co-operation for the protection of children from abuse. HMSO, London
Wright C et al 1987 Detection of sexual abuse in children. Letter. Lancet ii:218
Wynne J M, Hobbs C J 1995 STDs and CSA. Letter. British Journal of Hospital Medicine 53(1/2):54
Zeitlin H 1987 Investigation of the sexually abused child. Lancet ii:842

FURTHER READING

Davies G, Wilson C, Mitchell R, Milsom J 1995 Videotaping children's evidence. The Home Office, London
Kerns D L (Guest editor) 1998 Establishing a medical research agenda for CSA. Child Abuse & Neglect 22(6):453–660
Plotnikoff J, Woolfson R 1995 The child, the court and the video. Social Services Inspectorate Prosecuting Child Abuse, Blackstone, London
Spencer J R, Nicholson G, Flin R, Bull R (eds) 1989 Children's evidence in legal proceedings. University of Cambridge, Cambridge

10 Abuse of children with disability

ESTIMATES OF THE PREVALENCE OF NEGLECT AND ABUSE

WHY ARE CHILDREN WITH SPECIAL NEEDS SO VULNERABLE?

CLINICAL PRESENTATION

CONSEQUENCES OF ABUSE AND NEGLECT

In the recognition of abuse in children with disability it is now apparent that (Kelly 1992):

- abuse may be the cause of the disability
- children with disability are abused at 1.7 times the rate of other children (NCCAN 1993), but under-reporting is a major concern and there is a paucity of good data
- abuse may compound a pre-existing disability.

Until recently abuse of disabled children was ignored and several reasons for this were suggested (Marchant 1991):

- disabled children were not likely to be abused because they were not attractive or their disability aroused sympathy rather than exploitation
- abuse would not be so harmful because children would not understand it
- denial: many adults find it difficult to accept that any abuse occurs, thus abuse of handicapped children 'must be very uncommon . . .'
- children with disability would be more likely to make false allegations
- 'they' would not benefit from therapy.

Degener (1992) wrote 'any child born with disability growing up today has to survive and overcome discrimination and stigmatisation', and Sullivan (1987) in this context says 'When disabled children or adults are assumed to be less human because of their disability, then abuse is not that humane'. Krents & Atkins (1986) noted 'a disabled child may be incapable of disclosing the abuse even if he or she is upset and realises it is inappropriate. It is crucial that these children have a way to report abuse. This may be in sign and/or symbol communication in conjunction with some level of speech or speech reading. Other children use computer-aided communication systems with keyboards and/or voice simulators (Kennedy 1992). Appropriately trained professionals are required to 'hear' the child and carer attempting to disclose abuse or concerns about possible abuse. There is then the need for 'dual specialists', professionals who understand the disability and are trained in child protection and interviewing, or professionals using more relevant ways of inter-agency working to try and ensure the child is protected (Kennedy 1990, Marchant & Page 1992). The recognition of the sexual abuse of children with special needs is emerging as a major concern whether the child is at home, at school, fostered, or in residential care. It is difficult, but necessary, for professionals working with disabled children and adults to accept the unacceptable fact that it occurs (Schor 1987). Abuse may continue into adult life and the indications are that the rates of abuse in handicapped adults are higher than in the general population (Elvik et al 1990, McCormack 1991).

It has long been known that children may be damaged by abuse (Ammerman et al 1988). This has usually been described in terms of permanent neurological damage, for example, following head injury, but the disabling consequences of neglect, emotional and sexual abuse are increasingly recognised.

Abused children may present with learning difficulties which themselves make the child more vulnerable. Lynch & Roberts (1982) wrote of the vulnerability of mentally handicapped children, recognising that, because they may be difficult to parent, abusive and neglectful behaviours might be triggered in otherwise caring and competent parents. According to the Children Act 1989, children with disability are 'children in need' and they and their families qualify for a whole range of supporting services. These services are not universally available and family breakdown and/or maltreatment leads to children, as they grow older and often more difficult, to be cared for in the public care system. Unfortunately abuse in foster care and residential units is endemic as poorly trained carers are inadequately supported and are unable to provide good, alternative care (there are many examples of good practice but research is showing the extent of neglect and abuse 'in care').

Estimates of the prevalence of neglect and abuse

Estimates from America suggest that between 1 in 3 and 1 in 4 teenagers with learning problems have been sexually abused (Chamberlain et al 1984), with an even higher prevalence amongst hearing impaired children (Sullivan et al 1987); this compares with a ratio of 1 in 10 estimated for all children in the UK (Baker & Duncan 1985). (Tables 10.1 and 10.2).

Table 10.1 Estimates of the prevalence of child sexual abuse in disabled children

Study	Findings
Kohane et al (1987)	16% of boys,48% of girls under 12 years in psychiatric hospital had known history of CSA, 72% was incest
Chamberlain et al (1984)	25% of young woman with moderate learning problems in hospital had history of sexual intercourse or attempted sexual intercourse
Sullivan et al (1987)	11% of new entrants to college for deaf CSA, 17% physical abuse Ninth grade residential school for deaf, 50% reported CSA (questionaire) 150 deaf children at residential school, 50% reported CSA (interview)
Ammerman et al (1989)	39% of children with multiple disability abused, of CSA 66% 'raped'
Kennedy (1989)	50% of hearing impaired children CSA at home, transport, school, hostel
Bone & Meltzer (1989)	Of children with disability in residential care in UK, 8% due to CSA and 7% physical abuse and neglect
Cooke (1990)	5% adults with severe learning problems CSA
Sinason (1990)	50% of referrals of children with learning and emotional problems referred to psychotherapist, 70% girls, 30% boys
Hallas (1990)	50–70% children and teenagers referred to psychiatry CSA
Elvick (1990)	37% women average age 26yrs in residential care CSA

Table 10.2 Physical abuse and disability

Study	Findings
Oliver (1988)	5% of children's disabilities due to violence by parent/carer
Ammerman et al (1988, 1989, 1994)	39% of psychiatrically hospitalised multihandicapped children had evidence of current or prior abuse, 50% physical abuse, 50% combined abuse
	61% of 138 hospitalised children experienced some form of severe maltreatment
D B Cundall (personal communication 1996)	Of 38 children seen by Child Development Team, 5 'poor care', 2 fictitious disorder, 1 adopted
Verdugo et al (1995)	Of 445 mentally handicapped children 11.5% maltreated, neglect commonest
Diamond & Jaudes (1983)	Of 86 children with cerebral palsy: 9% due to abuse, 9% abused after diagnosis, 14% at risk of abuse

A preliminary study in the UK of consultants caring for mentally handicapped adults suggested that 4–5% of these adults were being abused, sexual abuse being more common than neglect or physical abuse (Cooke 1990). This is thought to be an underestimate; if selected groups of mentally handicapped adults are considered, 50% of those referred to the Tavistock Clinic in London for psychotherapy have been sexually abused (Sinason 1992). A study in Seattle (Ryerson 1984) reported over 400 cases of sexual abuse involving children and adults with special needs over a 4-year period. Chamberlain et al (1984) described a group of 87 girls aged 11–23 years, all of whom had learning problems – 14 of 41 mildly handicapped and 2 out of 23 of the severely handicapped girls were thought to have been victims of penetrative sexual abuse, and 39% of 150 multiply handicapped children admitted consecutively to a residential hospital had been or were thought likely to have been abused (Ammerman et al 1989). Physical abuse was more common than sexual abuse, but important features of the sexual abuse were:

- in 50% the abuse began under 2 years of age
- 66% involved penetration
- 40% had been abused by multiple perpetrators.

Hearing impaired children appear to be one of the most vulnerable groups, with boys involved as frequently as girls, and up to 50% of children having been abused at home, during transport to school, or at school (day or residential) (Sullivan et al 1987, Kennedy 1989).

Thorough assessment of all children with emotional difficulties will reveal a high level of abuse. It was assessed that over half the children attending a child and family psychiatric unit had been abused, sexual abuse being the main form of abuse (M Hallas, personal communication 1990). A study of a small residential school for emotionally disturbed children aged 8–12 years found that half had been sexually abused (Wadsworth & Abel 1987).

Investigation of physical and emotional abuse in a specialist autistic school has been described by Howlin & Clements (1995).

Why are children with special needs so vulnerable?

In 1986 Finkelhor & Baron wrote that any child disabled or disadvantaged is at once more vulnerable to abuse and, once abused, is more vulnerable. The vulnerability of the disabled child may begin from very early in life if attachment to his or her parents is impaired. The child was not the hoped-for child, and research shows that lack of appropriate support at this difficult time is associated with later physical abuse. Parents' relationships with their disabled child are inevitably different because of the child's added dependence and may become distorted. The sexual abuse of older sons by their mothers is an increasingly recognised example of this. Finkelhor (1984) also wrote of the preconditions of child sexual abuse:

- motivation to abuse
- overcoming societal inhibitions
- overcoming situational inhibitions
- overcoming the child's resistance.

Schor (1987) explains these preconditions with reference to the developmentally delayed child.

Why are children with special needs vulnerable to abuse? (after Schor 1987)

- Difficulty in communication:
  - learning problem
  - language disorder
  - emotional difficulty
  - hearing impaired
- Physical disability – can't get away
- Age-inappropriate dependency (for dressing, bathing, toileting) means sense of privacy meaningless
  - learning problem
  - physical disability
  - visually impaired
- Isolated and inexperienced, do not know 'norms'
- Need for affection, friendship which is exploited
- Use of transport to school, residential placements, foster-homes
  - multiple carers
  - previous abuse
- Distressed behaviour wrongly attributed to intrinsic disorder when cause is abuse:
  - 'excessive' masturbation
  - self-mutilation
- Not seen as sexually attractive (whether adult or child)
- Low self-image of disabled child compounded by guilt discourages disclosure
- Denial by abuser and disbelief by carers may precipitate psychotic breakdown and prevent further communication and provide 'evidence' of the child's unreliability

Factors of which abusers of disabled children are aware

- Easy targets: immature, dependent, inexperienced, inarticulate, needy, previous abuse
- Recognition of the low status of children and especially handicapped children: does this lower taboo levels?
- Families may become isolated, stressed, involved in inappropriate roles such as bathing sexually mature adolescents

Not only are the children available and abusers have many opportunities to abuse, but also it is easier to maintain secrecy if the child has communication difficulties. Even if the child tries to communicate he or she may be misunderstood. The child's language or behaviour may be explicit but alternative explanations are preferred. An example would be 'excessive' masturbation – is it due, as is often said, to the disability or is this a presenting sign of child sexual abuse?

The dependency of the child who relies on others for bathing, dressing and toileting makes the notion of privacy meaningless. Handicapped children are often compliant, they may fear abandonment, feel guilty at being handicapped and not the child their parents wanted, and may wish they had never been born (Sinason 1992).

There are many myths about the sexual abuse of children with disability (Marchant 1991). One important one is that they are not sexually attractive or desirable and by virtue of their handicap will be protected. This vulnerability and powerlessness may be appealing, as is their lack of assertiveness. Abusers are well aware of the low status of handicapped children and rationalise the abuse, claiming that this is inevitably the only sexual relationship the child will have – it's not harmful, it's educational and even a good experience.

A further hazard for children with learning difficulties is that if they do disclose and the perpetrator denies the abuse they are more vulnerable to psychotic breakdown. Verbal and physical symptoms may then be seen as psychotic features (Sinason 1992).

Finally, by the time the abuse is recognised it is often of long standing, the child may have accommodated to the abuse and, as with other children, they may not be able to speak of the abuse even if it has become evident to others.

The definition of the abuse of disabled children should be acknowledged and understood in the wider context of their day-to-day living (after Newport 1991, Kennedy 1995):

- force feeding (children with cerebral palsy)
- boredom – lack of social and educational opportunities
- overprotection – not allowed/available youth club, school holidays

- inappropriate medication – hyperactivity, 'challenging behaviour' (what needs challenging?)
- physical control – splints, 'strapped in chair', put in cot, 'behaviour modification' programmes (does the child's care need modifying?)
- lack of respect/privacy
  - bathing, toileting, dressing
  - medical consultations, examinations, photography
  - fitting of appliances
- 'experimental' physical or drug therapies
- special schools – segregation educationally and socially
- bullying – verbally and physically

There is in the UK (1998) severe underfunding of facilities and resources which would allow disabled children to reach their full potential; this is state neglect.

Clinical presentation

It is important to pay attention to what the child says as well as behavioural and physical signs (Vizard & Tranter 1988).

What the child says

Children with learning or communication problems, for whatever reason, have difficulty in telling of their abuse and being understood. Skilled professionals who understand the nature of the child's handicap or developmental disorder may be able to communicate with the child but must be able to use the appropriate method(s). These include play, sign language(s), use of dolls and puppets, line drawings, or the child's drawings. The child may need engaging in sessions over months to even years in the most traumatised of cases. Direct and leading questions are often needed, as for very young children, which will have implications for court purposes, but this is inevitable. As long as the entire social and clinical picture is presented and explained, the interview with its limitations should be accepted in family courts but is unlikely to be admissible in criminal courts. As Tempkin (1994) has written,

> children whose disability results in a lack of verbal skills are particularly disadvantaged in a legal culture that takes oral communication for granted and relies heavily upon it.

Added to this is a shortage of skilled interpreters or advocates and a child witness who may well lack the confidence and self-esteem which allows a witness to appear credible (NCB 1996). The guidance in the *Memorandum of Good Practice* (Home Office 1992) goes some way to make provision for disabled children to be heard more appropriately but lacks detailed advice and in practice convictions are only likely if the perpetrator has admitted the offence(s).

CASE HISTORY 10.1

A girl of 13 years with severe learning problems presented at school with a chemical burn on the back of her hand. A medical examination revealed signs consistent with vaginal penetration. There was a clear history of escalating abuse by the taxi driver who took her to school daily. The police investigation was dropped because of inconsistencies in her story; she 'named colour of curtains wrongly in room assaults took place'. She was unable to name colours reliably.

Behavioural signs

Behavioural signs to look out for are (Vizard 1989):

- sexualised behaviour
  - explicit sexual behaviour
  - 'excessive' masturbation
- change in behaviour
  - angry, aggressive
  - withdrawn, mute
- persisting anger or disturbed behaviour
  - temper tantrums which are unexplained
  - self-destructive behaviour
  - violence to others, to animals
  - destructive of toys, belongings, room, bedding

- problems associated with urination and defecation
- eating disorder.

Physical symptoms and signs

The physical signs and symptoms are not unique to children with handicaps:

- vaginal or rectal bleeding
- sexually transmitted disease
- pregnancy
- non-accidental injury
- signs of neglect.

Physical examination

There should be a full physical examination and the child should be supported by an adult with whom he or she feels comfortable. An adult in authority, such as a head teacher, is not usually this person. General anaesthesia or sedation is sometimes needed. Issues of consent should be discussed: it is usually the parent who has the authority to consent (see Ch 9). Physical abnormality may on occasion be diagnostic of abuse (gonorrhoea or pregnancy) but is more often supportive of the diagnosis of child sexual abuse (RCP 1991). When one of their number was found to be pregnant, 35 highly dependent females aged 13–35 years were examined; 13 had signs which were consistent with penetration (Elvick et al 1990).

Forensic tests should be done if there is a possibility of recent assault. Children may have a poor sense of time and be unable to say when the last abuse occurred unless the abuse occurred on a memorable day such as a birthday.

CASE HISTORY 10.2

A girl aged 16 years with severe learning problems was seen at school to have two 'love bites' on her neck. Physical examination showed signs compatible with repeated vaginal penetration. Forensic swabs were positive for semen. The father admitted to the police a long history of vaginal intercourse.

CASE HISTORY 10.3

A girl aged 14 years with Down's syndrome said to a teacher following respite care with foster-parents that she did not like it when Uncle Terry touched her 'boo-boos'. Her father, a police officer, would not make a complaint fearing that investigation would cause his daughter unnecessary upset as the complaint was unlikely to reach court.

CASE HISTORY 10.4

A boy aged 9 years with moderate learning problems and aggressive, uncontrollable behaviour was referred because of 'excessive masturbation'.

When examined he had an immediate and sustained erection. Investigation revealed repeated abuse and probable prostitution involving his mother's many male partners. Aged 12 years he sexually abused any available younger child and at 13 years was placed in a secure unit.

CASE HISTORY 10.5

A girl aged 3 years and her brother aged 6 years who were mute and thought to have severe learning difficulties were referred by the school nurse when the girl had possible burns on her abdomen. Both children had anal signs compatible with anal penetration. In an adoptive home both children have made remarkable progress. The girl, aged 8 years, attends mainstream school with support and her brother, now 11 years, attends a unit for children with moderate learning problems. The father, who had moderate learning problems, admitted the abuse, initially saying his 'finger must have slipped when he washed them' but later made a full confession of buggery to his solicitor's clerk.

The mother, who had severe learning problems, did not understand the abuse of her children.

CASE HISTORY 10.6

A boy aged 15 years with moderate learning problems presented to the paediatrician because of recent onset of soiling. He immediately disclosed sexual abuse involving a male member of staff at the assessment centre he attended. This was denied and the *boy* was transferred.

CASE HISTORY 10.7

A girl aged 10 years with moderate learning problems and some behavioural difficulties was seen to have a bruised face and burns on her hand and neck. Her stepmother was emotionally, physically, and sexually abusing her, but was not prosecuted. The girl and her brother returned to their mother's care but the court placed the other two younger children of the new partnership back home.

CASE HISTORY 10.8

A boy aged 11 years with Duchenne muscular dystrophy and his sister, 13 years, who had moderate learning problems were both sexually abused by their 19-year-old foster-brother. Previously their alcoholic father physically and sexually abused them and their mother had abandoned them.

CASE HISTORY 10.9

A boy aged 5 years was brought to the hospital Accident and Emergency department by his mother after she found on her return home that he had extensive facial bruising. The babysitter, a man aged 34 years, was the likely perpetrator. The child had a severe spastic quadriplegia and severe learning difficulties. He was admitted to a paediatric hospital because of concern regarding his mother's care – she was a known heroin addict. On the ward he was 'very hungry' and for several days opened his mouth every time a nurse passed by. He rapidly gained weight from well below the third percentile. Further investigation revealed neglect and emotional rejection and severe non-organic failure to thrive. Why was the diagnosis so delayed? – was it because all the professionals while supporting the mother did not 'see' the child?

CASE HISTORY 10.10

A severely hearing impaired boy of 9 years was seen to have 'stick marks' across his back. He and his 7-year-old brother were under the care of a paediatrician because of soiling. The family did not speak English. There was a history of partner violence and the mother and four children had been in a local refuge a month earlier. The father worked very long hours in a factory, and abused alcohol. He had never been seen by any professional. Intensive work by the hearing impaired service and social services, with the father initially living away from home, led to better understanding by the family of the boys' disability. Improved communication was the key to progress. 'Most parents cannot communicate with their deaf children' (Ridgeway 1993).

Consequences of abuse and neglect

By virtue of their coexisting disability, children with special needs respond in protean ways to the additional trauma of abuse. There is debate as to how far this trauma actually causes learning problems (Vizard 1989).

- Abuse causes anxiety and impairs the child's ability to pay attention and learn. Even when the abuse stops, the degree of recovery is uncertain; children with learning problems are particularly vulnerable to psychological damage when they are abused (Sinason 1992).
- Disclosure of abuse may engender great anxiety in the child and disbelief may precipitate frank psychosis.
- There is a continuing increased risk of mental health problems in the survivors of child sexual abuse, notably depression (Mullen 1991).
- Abuse may have an adverse effect on the child's developing personality, in particular in the ability to make stable relationships.
- Children who have been sexually abused may become abusers, and this is also true of children with learning difficulties (Dunne & Power 1990).
- Physically abused children may become violent seeing physical aggression as a method of conflict resolution/control.

- Children born as a result of an incestuous union have a 30–60% risk of inherited abnormality (Illingworth 1987).
- Specialist clinics for treating victims and abusers are few and only a minority receive adequate help.

Table 10.3 CSA in a school for children with moderate learning difficulties (6–12 years).

Gender/medical history	H/O abuse	Significant events	Long-term
F/MLD/seizures	CSA stepfather/grandfather	Became mother at 18 years, at 20 years – CSA of child by grandfather, 2nd child born CPC – neglect/CSA	Married severely disabled man 17 years older Children later foster care
F/MLD/faints or fits	Neglect	STD/abortion/daughter CSA – by cousin	SSD involved when daughter CSA
*F/MLD/behavioural problems	CSA stepfather/grandfather, court returned home on 3 occasions 2–6 years	Failed in mainstream school – overactive wilful CSA in school/ anal penetration CPC ?6.	1998 aged 11 years, sexually promiscuous and abusing younger girls/with mother
F/slow learner/quiet/ gentle/passive	'wrote that was happier at mainstream high school.'		
F/SLD/seizures/abdominal pain adopted/mo.SLD	At special school only?	Pregnant ?father of baby at 13 years, abortion	Rape at 15 years Three more pregnancies
F/MLD/pica/high lead level and behavioural problems/?seizure/sore bottom	Neglect/FTT/CSA – 10 years, 11 years, 12 years, 14/15 years i.e all childhood	CPC 1–? Mother/partner CPC 2–Police investig.? Father? school/anal penetration CPC 3–Father	CSA – father, mother, friends, teacher, care at 15 years
F/MLD	STD Trichonomas		
F/MLD		By 20 years – 6 live births, 1 still birth, 4 abortions	1st child adopted 2nd child – NAI partner
*F/SLD/adopted	Neglect/FTT 'good school & bad school'	Attractive girl – anxiety symptoms ?related to non-disclosure	Still at school
F/MLD/enuresis/sore	Neglect/FTT/emotional	CPC in foster care	Home
F/?MLD/severe scald	Neglect	Fostered by grandma CPC Mother Schd.1 offender	1st child 17 years. CPC – NAI partner
*F/MLD	Neglect/NAI/emotional deprivation	CPC ?6 Mother SLD 2sibs foster care	Fostered/still at school
M.MLD/'hyperactive'/ withdrawn/aggressive	Neglect/NAI Emotional dep.	Excluded by special – aggression	Childrens' home – 14 years – own request
D*F/MLD/wetting/soiling	Behaviour deteriorated at special school Unexplained bruises at school Signs of anal abuse	Sexualized play investig. at special school CSA ?home or school or both	Symptoms better in holidays and when changed school
F/MLD/nightmares 'get off me'	FTT/neglect		Foster care – happier, dreams ceased
D*F/MLD/wetting/sore/ language delay	??previous CSA at home Disclosed CSA by teacher, sex drawing	CPC exam. signs of CSA Explicit police video re: teacher	Behaviour improved – Mother changed school Exam. – healing
D*F/MLD/cerebral palsy/ seizures	Behaviour deteriorated, became sexualised ??CSA at home	Child discl. CSA teacher No exam. No CPC Mother did not complain – 'would take it out on child'	Sexualized behaviour stopped when changed school

F/M Female/male
M/SLD Moderate/severe learning problem
FTT Failure to thrive
CSA Child sexual abuse
CPC Child Protection Conference
* Still in school
D Disclosed abuse pre–1997 investigation
NAI Non-accidental injury

Plate Section

Plate 1

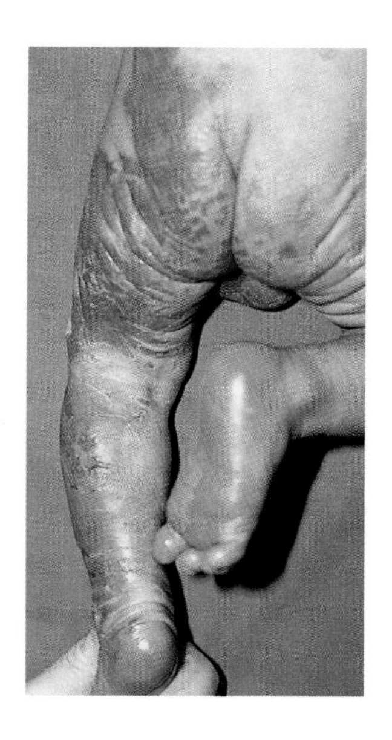

Plate 2

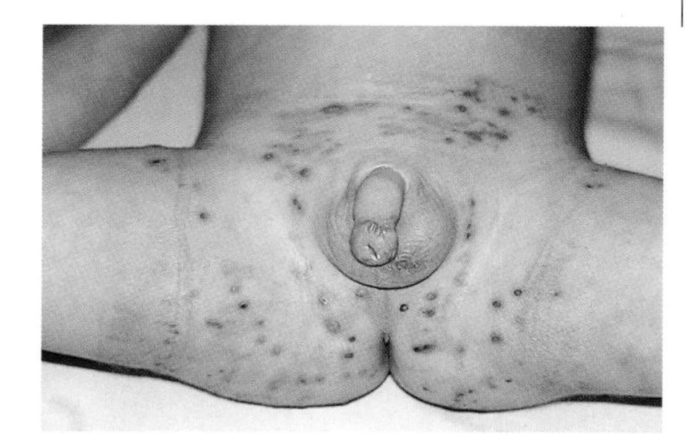

Plate 3

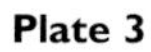

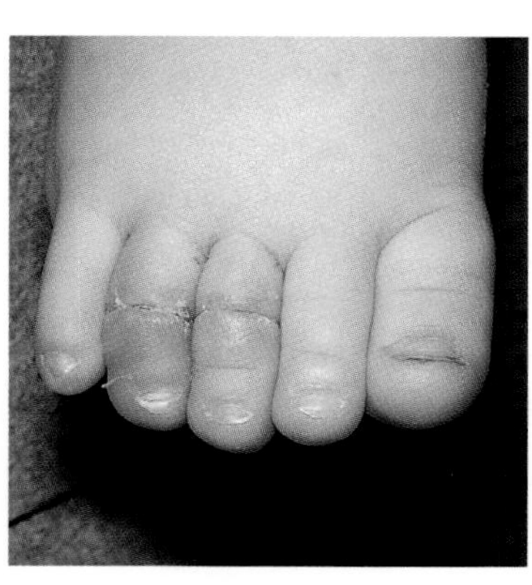

Plate 4

Plate 5

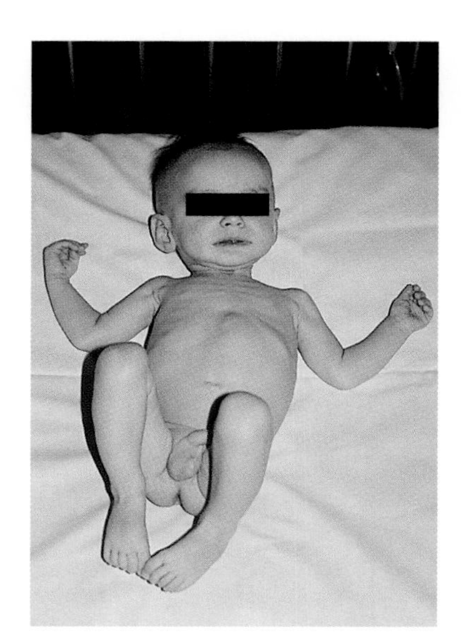

Plate 1 Neglect. Severe ammoniacal dermatitis in an infant of 4 weeks left in a wet cot for days on end. Rapid resolution on admission to hospital.
Plate 2 Severe nappy rash in 2-year-old neglected child.
Plate 3 General practitioner, called to see this infant of 8 months who was irritable and coughing, recognised a hair tourniquet partially obstructing the blood supply to the fourth toe distally. Parents were unaware of the source of the child's distress, reflecting the wider neglect in the household.
Plate 4 Grossly neglected carious teeth in a 4-year-old neglected child who presented with neglected pneumonia and empyema.
Plate 5 Emaciated appearance, flexed posture but bright and alert 6-month-old ruminating infant. Note prominent ribs.

Plate 6 (a)

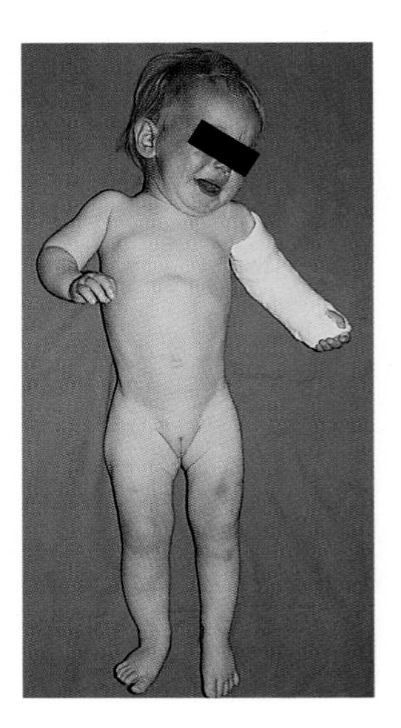

Plate 6 (b)

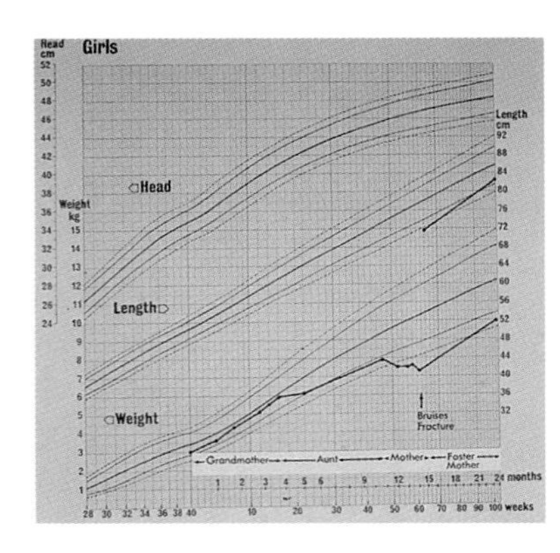

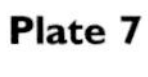
Plate 7

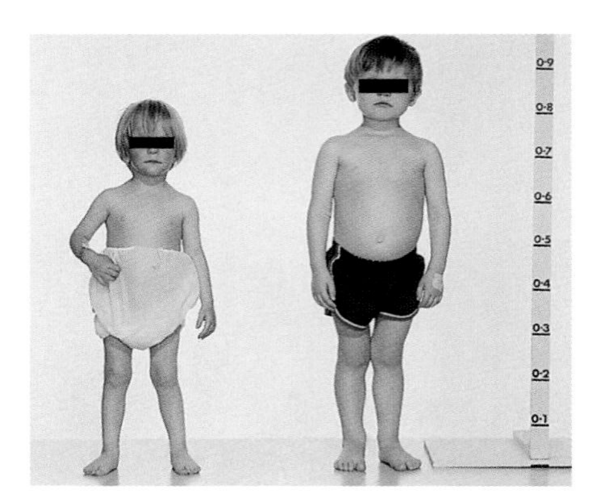

Plate 8 (a)

Plate 8 (b)

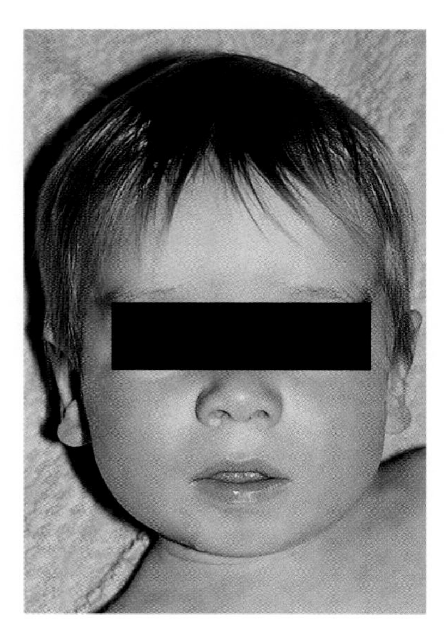

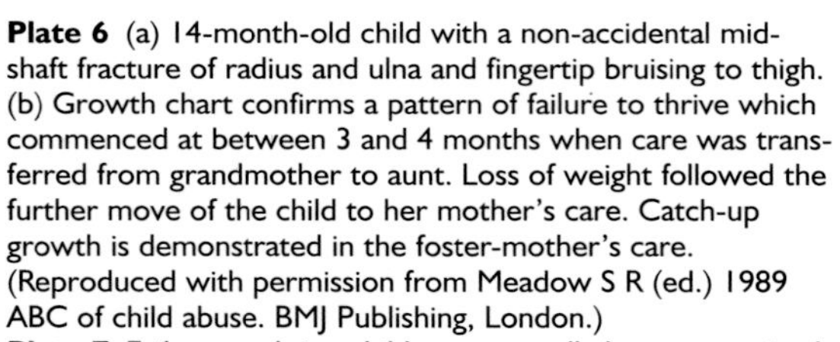
Plate 6 (a) 14-month-old child with a non-accidental mid-shaft fracture of radius and ulna and fingertip bruising to thigh. (b) Growth chart confirms a pattern of failure to thrive which commenced at between 3 and 4 months when care was transferred from grandmother to aunt. Loss of weight followed the further move of the child to her mother's care. Catch-up growth is demonstrated in the foster-mother's care. (Reproduced with permission from Meadow S R (ed.) 1989 ABC of child abuse. BMJ Publishing, London.)
Plate 7 Failure-to-thrive children are small. An average-sized 4-year-old is shown on the right in comparison with a child of the same age on the left who has failed to thrive. There is also developmental delay.
Plates 8 (a) Before and (b) after nutritional rehabilitation, facial appearance of a child at 4 and 6 months. Note difference in expression and hair.

Plate 9

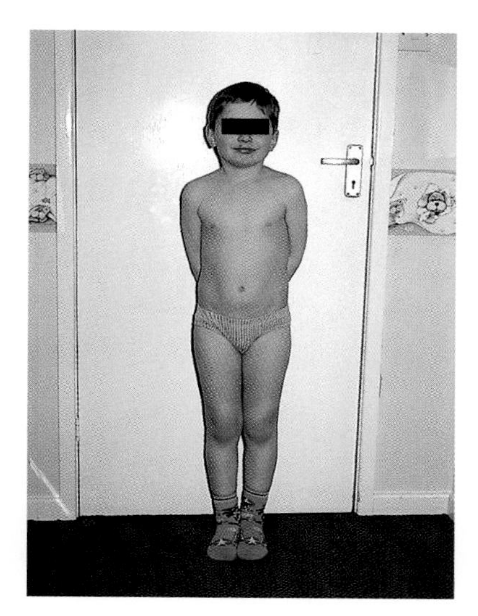

Plate 10

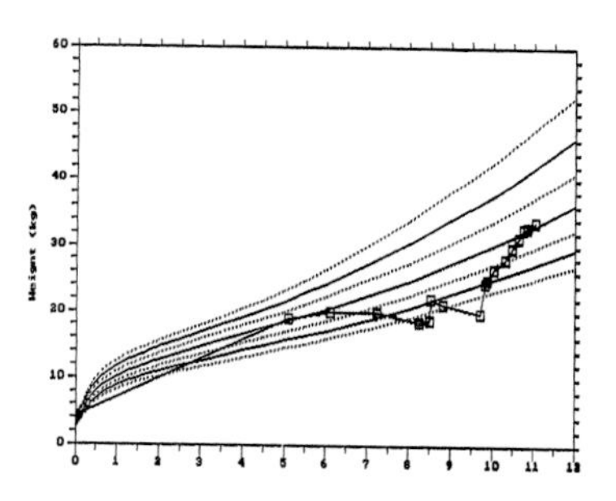

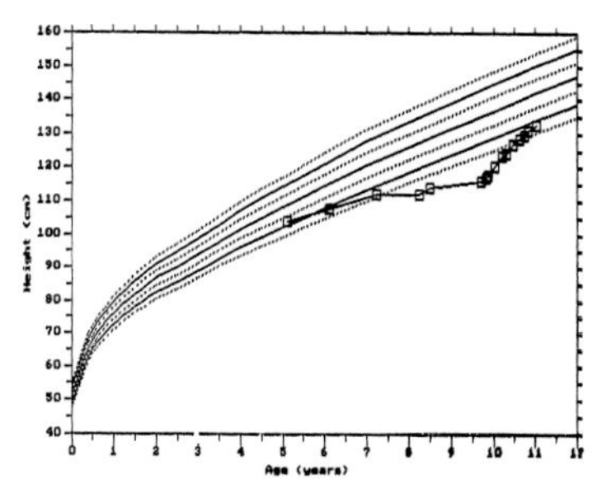

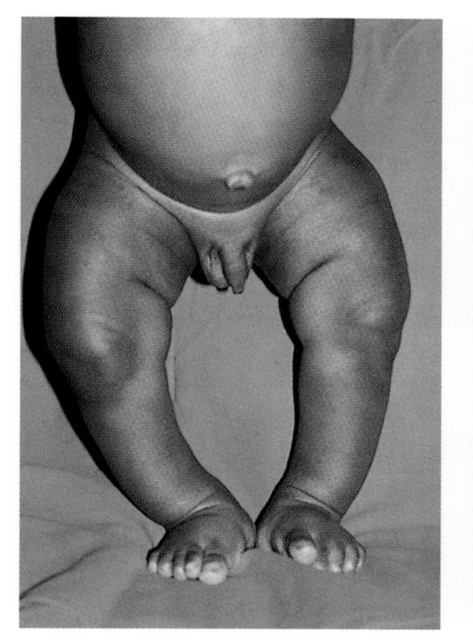

Plate 11

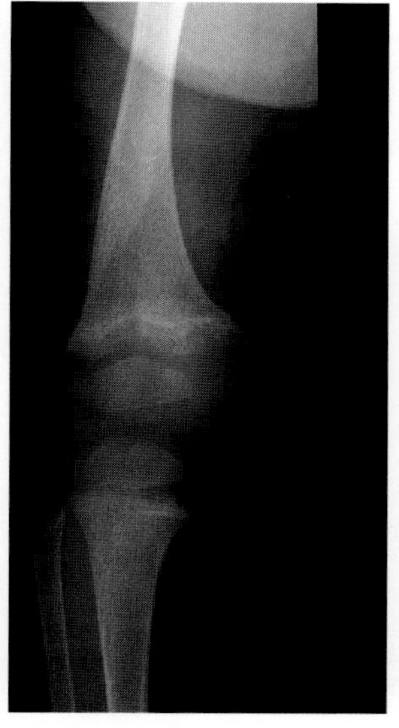

Plate 12

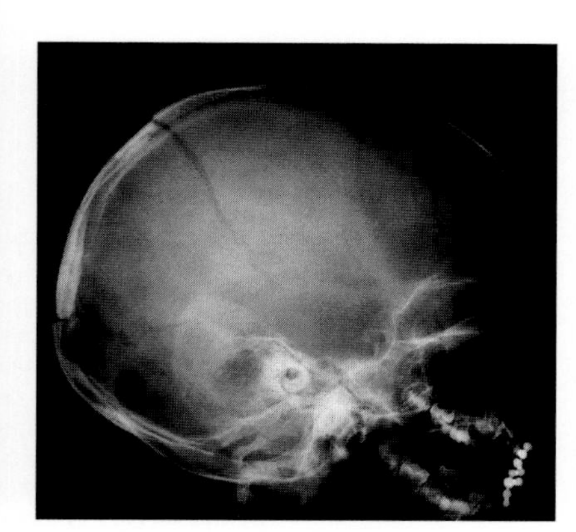

Plate 13

Plate 9 Boy aged 10 years with severe psychosocial growth stunting shortly after rejection from home and move to grandparents (see Plate 10). Note that he appears well-nourished because of his stunting.
Plate 10 Growth charts of boy with a long history of very poor growth from age 5 years when his mother remarried. Severe emotional deprivation and physical abuse not fully appreciated by many professionals involved. Growth chart shows very low growth velocity for height and zero weight gain from 5 to 9 years with catch up growth thereafter on move to grandparents' care.
Plate 11 Rickets in a 12-month-old neglected child of West Indian origin.
Plate 12 16-month-old Sikh child who presented with florid rickets. Radiograph of knee shows typical changes – wide, cupped and frayed epiphyses. Rickets is a now a rare and preventable disorder in the UK and linked to parenting difficulties.
Plate 13 Abused 18-month-old child. History of fall from chair. Depressed occipital fracture with two components. Maximum width 2 mm. Bruises to both ears, buttocks and spine. Right hemiplegia.

Plate 14

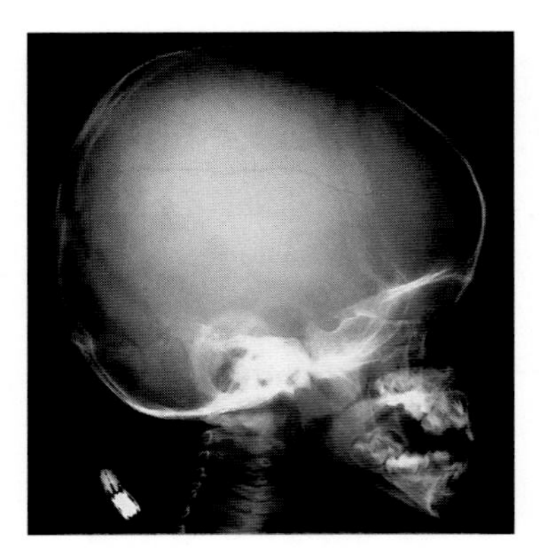

Plate 15

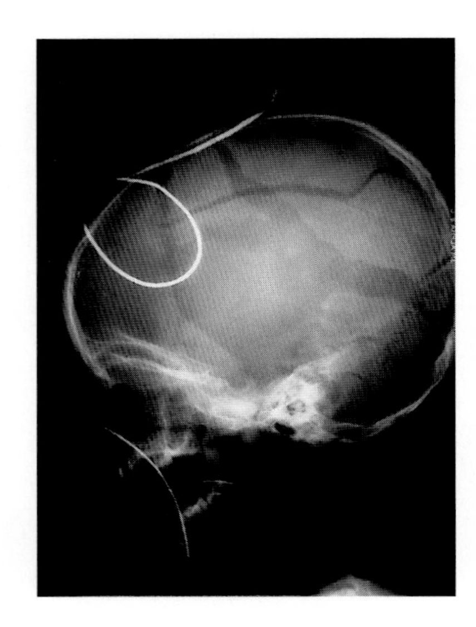

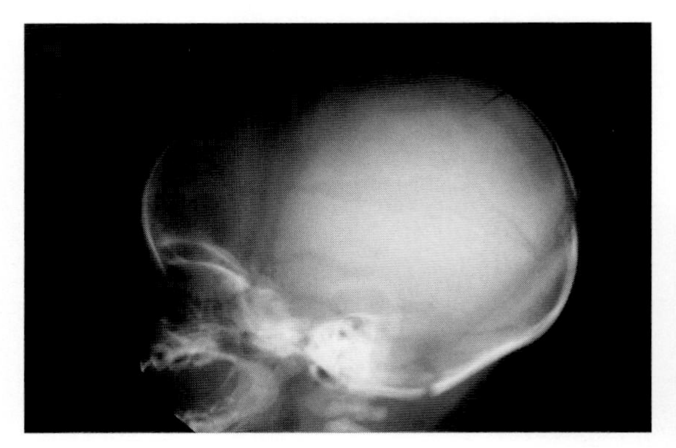

Plate 16 (a)

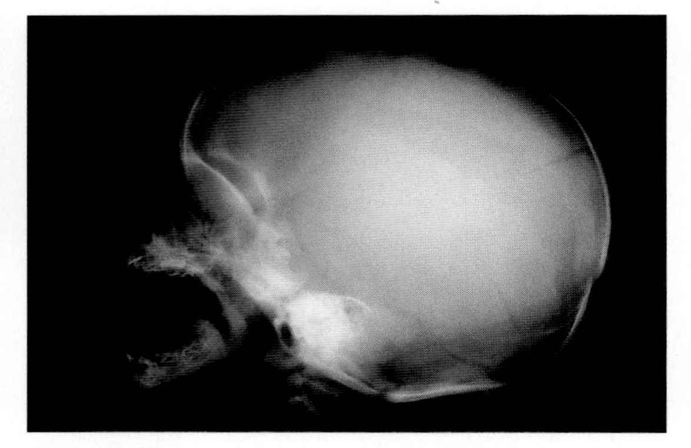

Plate 16 (b)

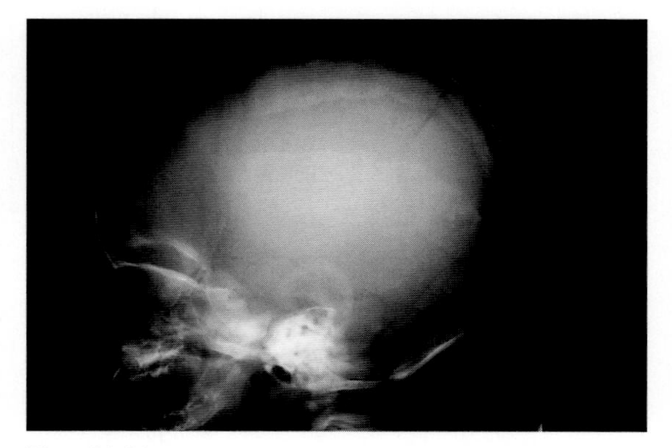

Plate 16 (c)

Plate 14 Accidentally injured 13-month-old child; fell 3 feet from kitchen unit on to concrete floor. Linear horizontal parietal fracture 10.5 cm – 1–2 mm in width. Haematoma above ear. No other injuries and no cerebral complications.
Plate 15 15-month-old fatally abused child. Failure to thrive, bilateral retinal haemorrhages, multiple bruises to forehead, ears and limbs, torn frenulum, fracture of metaphysis left knee. Large subdural haematoma evacuated through large central craniotomy. Five fractures including extensive bilateral parietal fractures, one 14 mm in width, and three occipital fractures. (Reproduced with permission from Meadow S R (ed.) 1989 ABC of child abuse. BMJ Publishing, London.)
Plates 16 7-week-old abused child with a parietal growing fracture. Child allegedly fell from father's arms on to the floor and immediately became unconscious and limp. Child developed fits and required ventilation. Fractures of ribs and femur and unilateral retinal haemorrhage present with haematoma in rectum and small bruise at top of natal cleft: (a) 11 mm at presentation. (b) 20 mm at 17 days. (c) 26 mm at 42 days. Cystic collection of fluid and underlying necrotic brain found at operation. (Plate 16c Reproduced with permission from Meadow S R (ed.) 1989 ABC of child abuse. BMJ Publishing, London.)

Plate 17

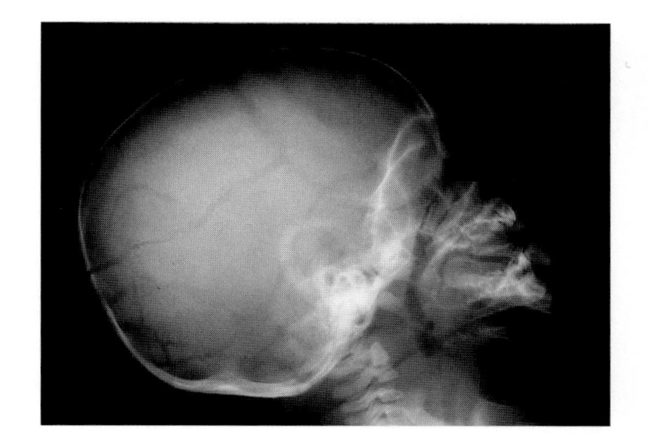

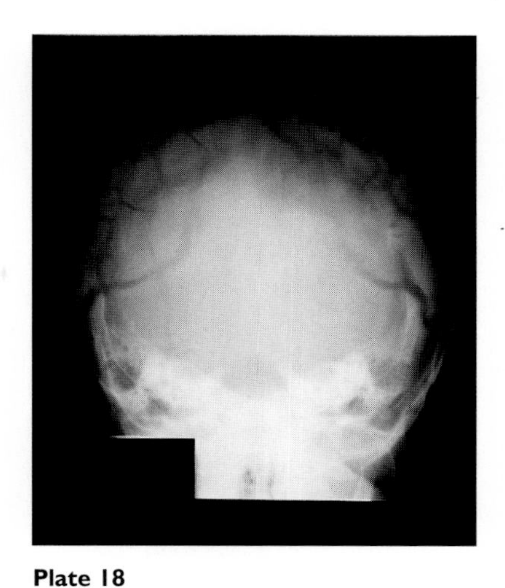

Plate 18

Plate 19 (a)

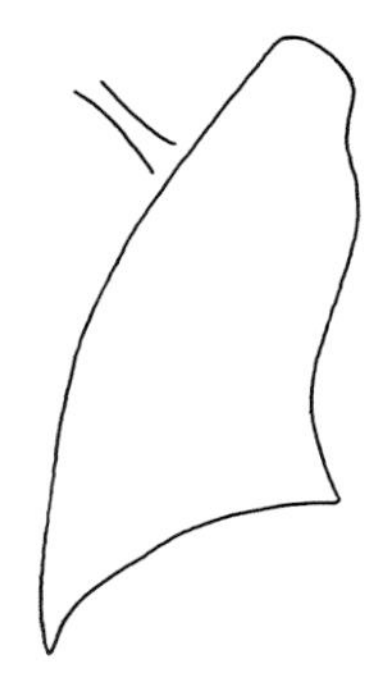

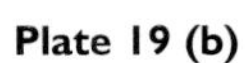

Plate 19 (b)

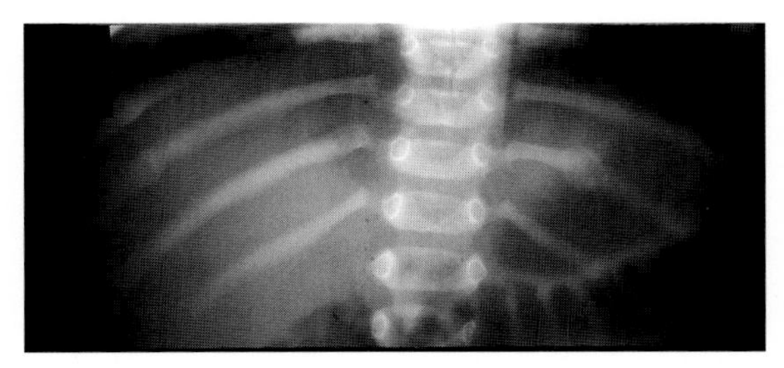

Plate 20

Plate 17 Branched parietal fracture in 5-month-old abused child (same child as Plate 20). Injury discovered on skeletal survey. History suggests it occurred several weeks earlier.
Plate 18 Multiple wide skull fractures in 'crazy paving' pattern in 11-month-old boy who allegedly fell from settee on to carpeted floor. Enlarged ventricles on CT scan. Father admitted abuse to police.
Plate 19 Radiograph (a) and line drawing to illustrate findings (b) in posterior healing rib fractures of left sixth, seventh and eighth ribs behind cardiac shadow in abused infant. Presence of callus and unclear fracture line suggests fractures are less than 2 weeks old. (Reproduced with permission from Meadow S R (ed.) 1989 ABC of child abuse. BMJ Publishing, London.)
Plate 20 Healing rib fractures of left 11th and right 10th ribs with well-developed callus (same case as Plates 17, 25 and 59).

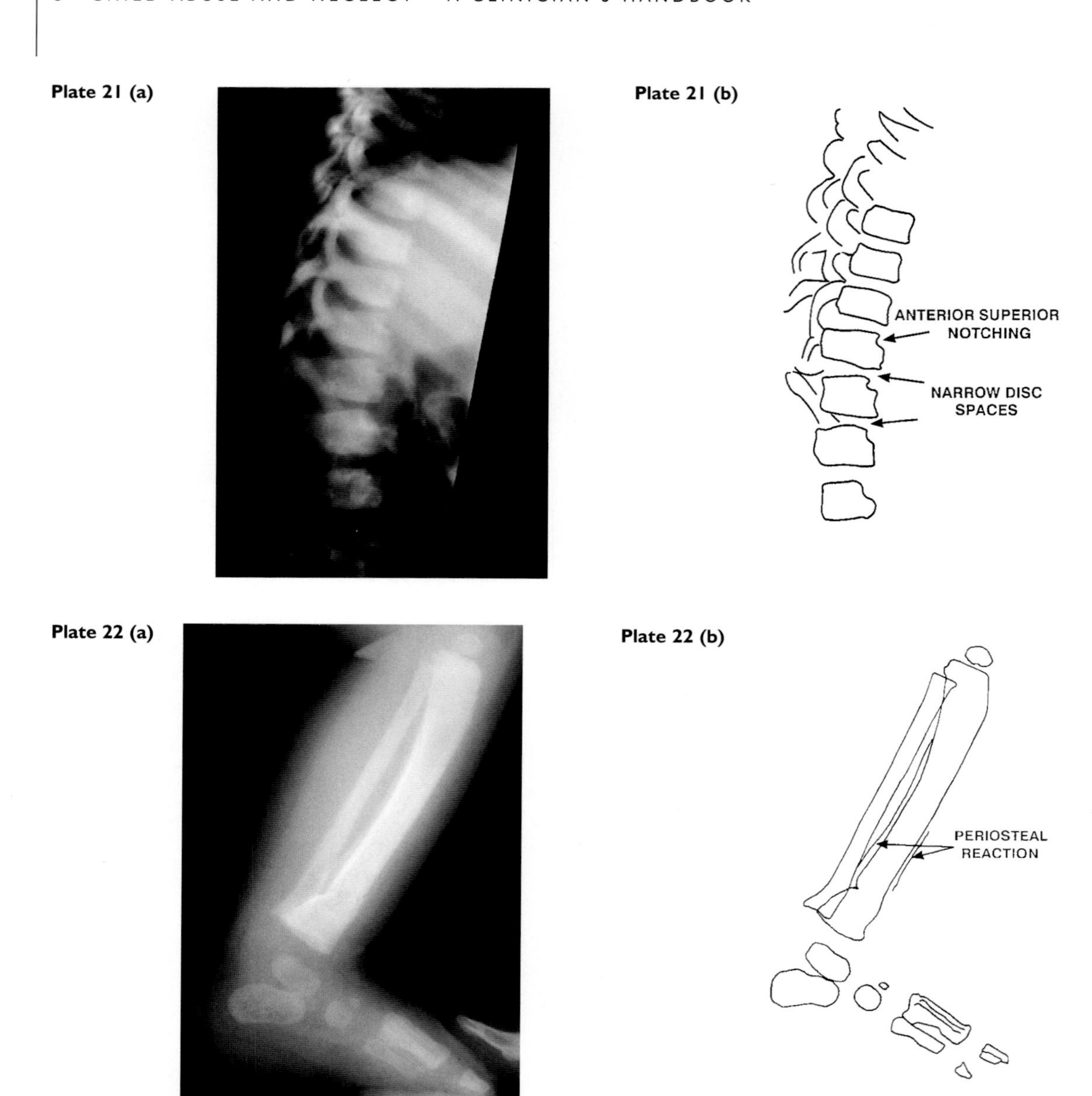

Plate 21 Radiographs (a) and line drawing (b) of spinal injury in an abused 6-year-old child who presented with chronic pancreatitis and pseudocyst. Old humeral injury also present. Characteristic notching of anterior superior surface of discs and narrowed disc spaces present. (Reproduced with permission from Meadow S R (ed.) 1989 ABC of child abuse. BMJ Publishing, London.)
Plate 22 Radiograph (a) and line drawing (b) of distal non-displaced fracture of lower shaft of tibia and fibula in an abused child of 6 months, with evidence of periosteal reaction along tibial shaft. Fracture is probably 10–14 days old. Other injuries included multiple rib and complex skull fractures. (Reproduced with permission from Meadow S R (ed.) 1989 ABC of child abuse. BMJ Publishing, London).

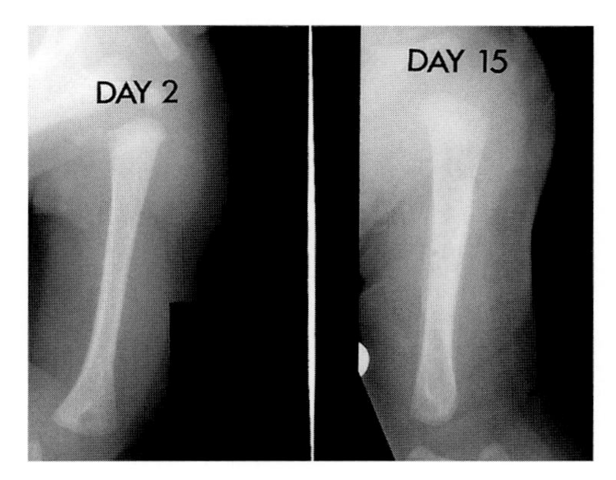

Plate 23

Plate 24

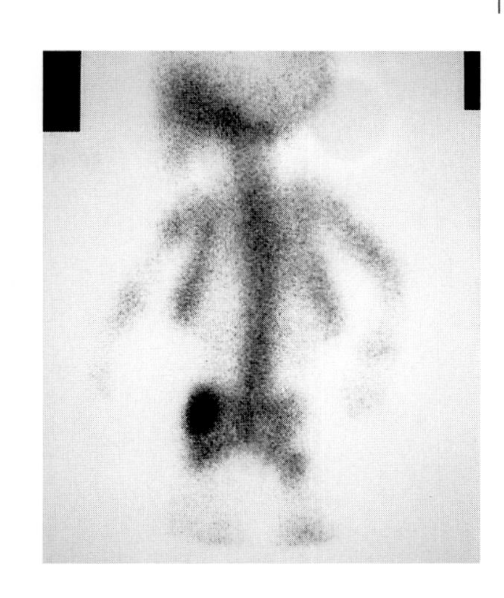

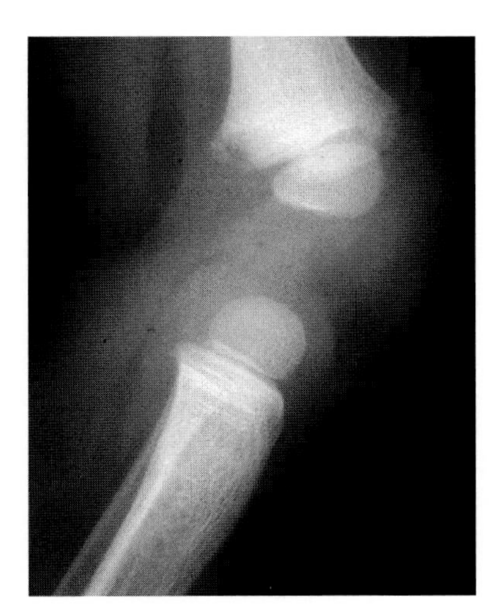

Plate 25 (a)

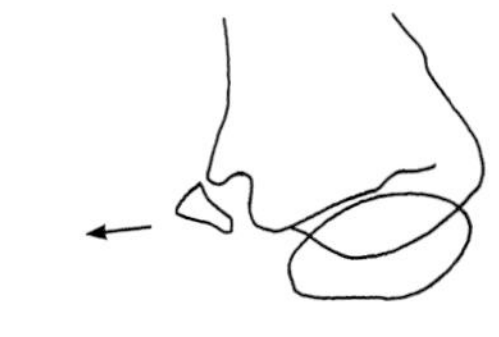

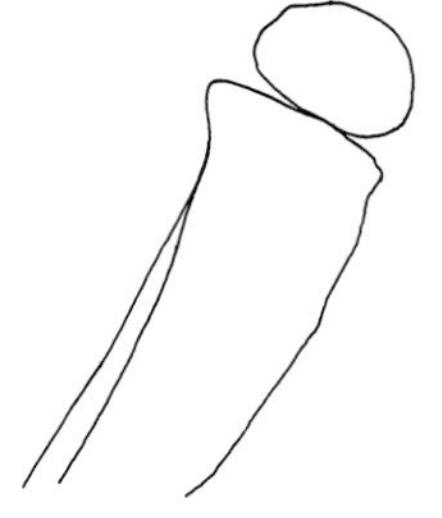

Plate 25 (b)

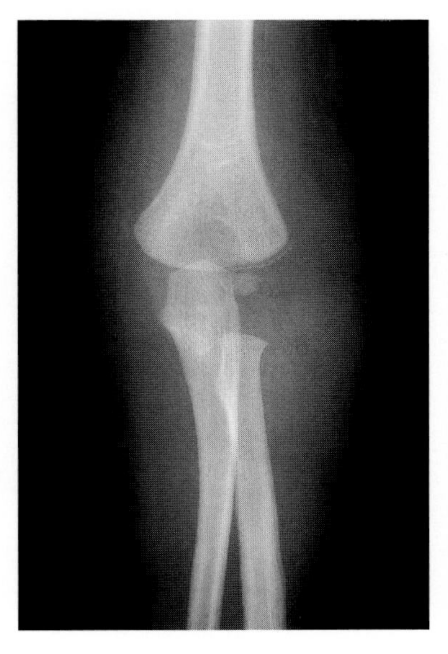

Plate 26

Plate 23 Development of radiological periosteal reaction in humerus of 3-month-old infant who presented with painful non-moving arm. No history offered. Abuse thought likely. At age 5 years, sexual abuse by father recognised when parents' marriage ended (see also Plate 24).

Plate 24 ^{99m}Technetium bone scan of 3-month-old infant (same case as Plate 23) on day 5, showing increased uptake in the left humerus relative to right.

Plate 25 Radiograph (a) and line drawing (b) of metaphyseal (corner) fracture of the lower end of the femur (same child as Plate 15). (Reproduced with permission from Meadow S R (ed.) 1989 ABC of child abuse. BMJ Publishing, London.)

Plate 26 Metaphyseal fracture of the lower end of the humerus in an abused 2-year-old boy who allegedly fell on to his elbow. Multiple bruises, penile and anal injury also present. A thin fragment of bone is seen separated from the metaphyseal end of the shaft.

Plate 27 (a)

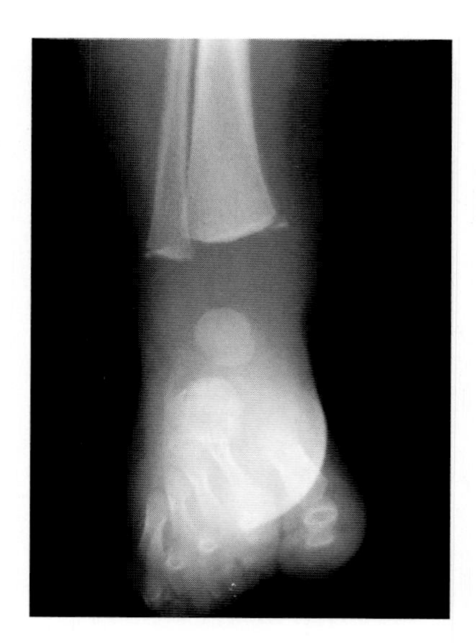

Plate 27 (b)

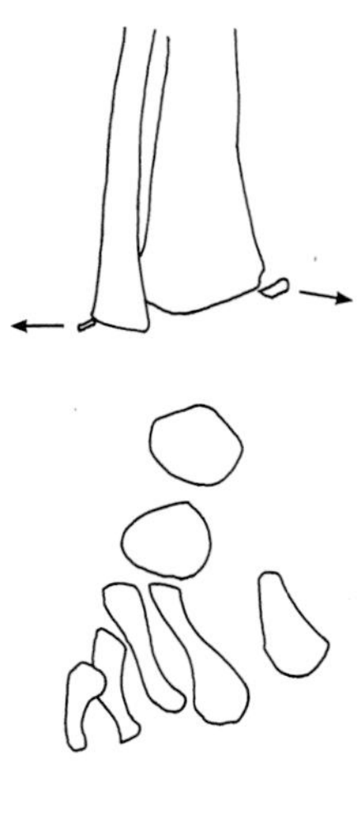

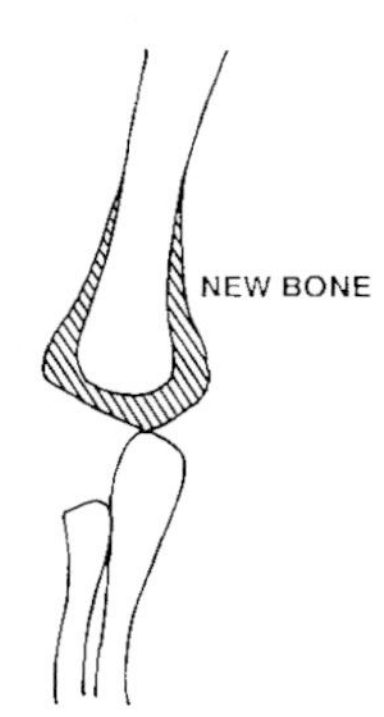

Plate 28 (b)

Plate 28 (a)

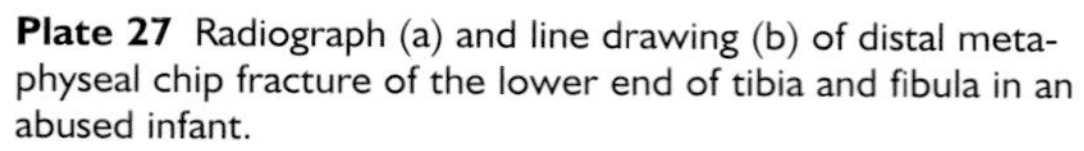

Plate 27 Radiograph (a) and line drawing (b) of distal metaphyseal chip fracture of the lower end of tibia and fibula in an abused infant.

Plate 28 Radiographs (a) and line drawings (b) of distal humerus epiphyseal separation in a 5-month-old abused infant (same case as Plates 17 and 25). Initially injury was confused with dislocation but on follow-up 4 weeks later (right-hand radiograph) extensive formation of new bone confirmed displacement of epiphysis. (Reproduced with permission from Meadow S R (ed.) 1989 ABC of child abuse. BMJ Publishing, London.)

Plate 29 Infant of 8 months taken to hospital with painful and swollen forearm after history of a fall from a settee. Skeletal survey revealed multiple fractures, at different stages of healing. Long bone shaft fractures have a low specificity for abuse but are the commonest abusive fractures encountered.

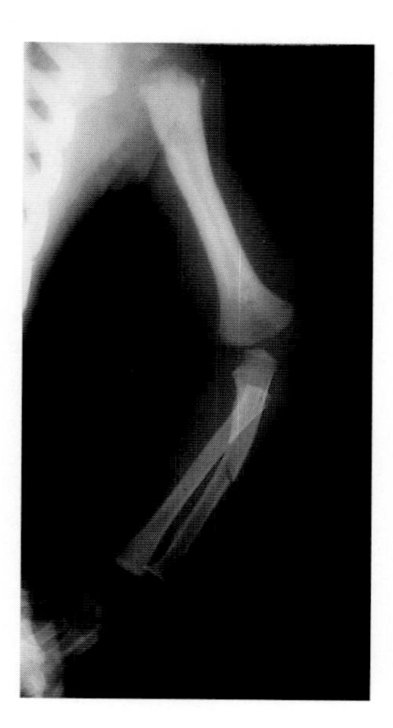

Plate 29

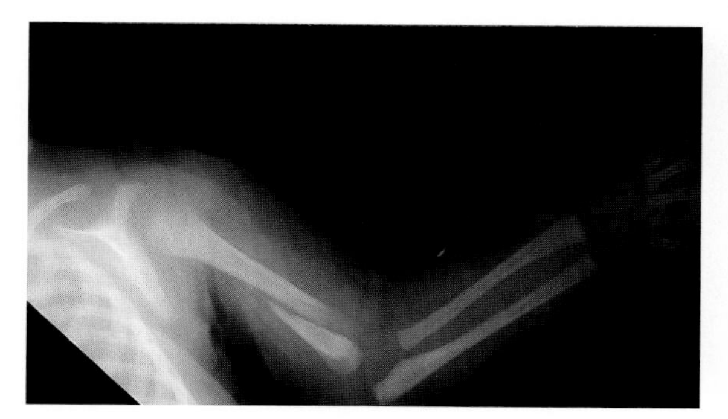

Plate 30

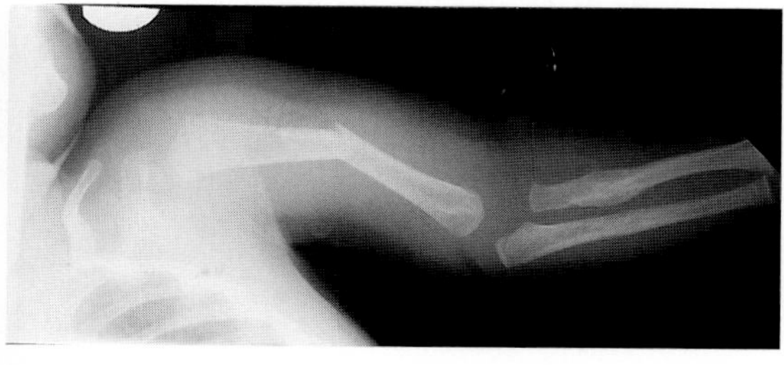

Plate 31

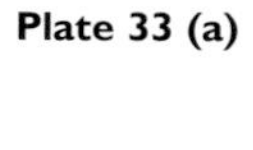

Plate 33 (a)

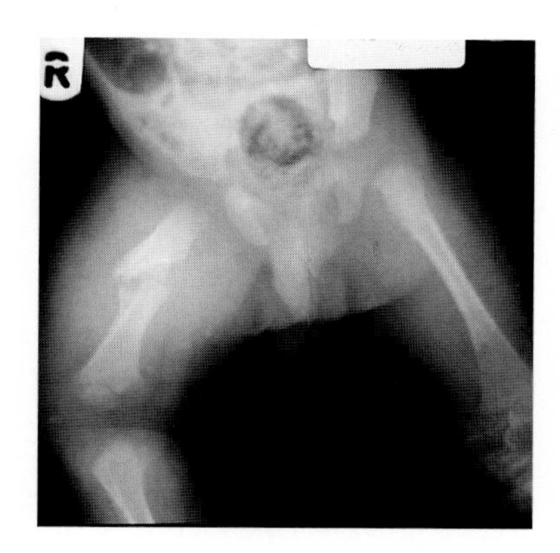

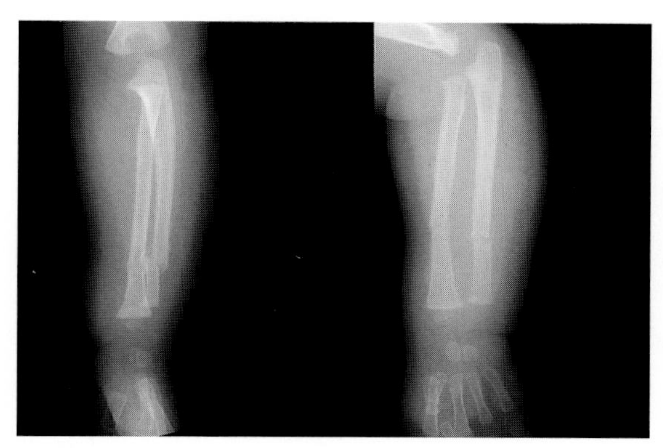

Plate 32

Plate 33 (b)

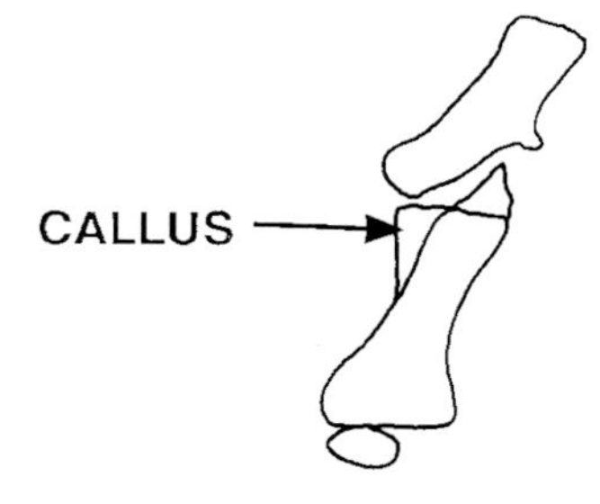

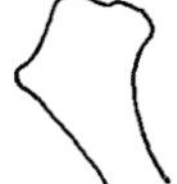

Plate 30 Spiral fracture of humerus in a 6-week-old infant whose mother said the arm broke as she dressed the child. No other injuries, so diagnosis of abuse not certainly established, but suspected.
Plate 31 Recent and old fractures of humerus, radius and ulna in a 5-month-old abused infant.
Plate 32 2-year-old boy who had extensive burns, bruises and bilateral forearm fractures of different ages and failure to thrive. Transverse fractures are usually due to direct impact.
Plate 33 Radiograph (a) and line drawing (b) of refracture of previously fractured and healing femur of a 13-week-old abused infant who presented after the second injury.

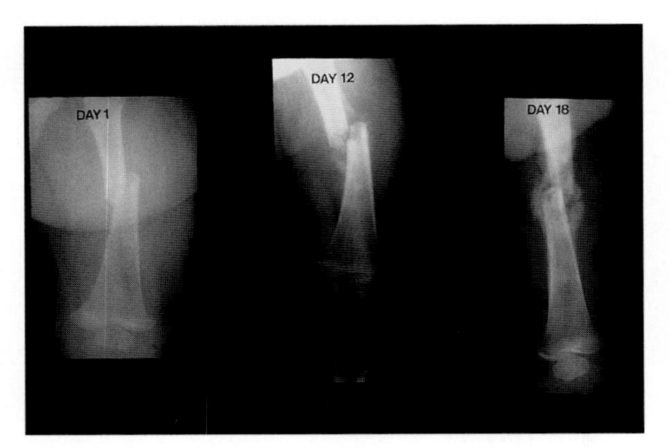

Plate 34

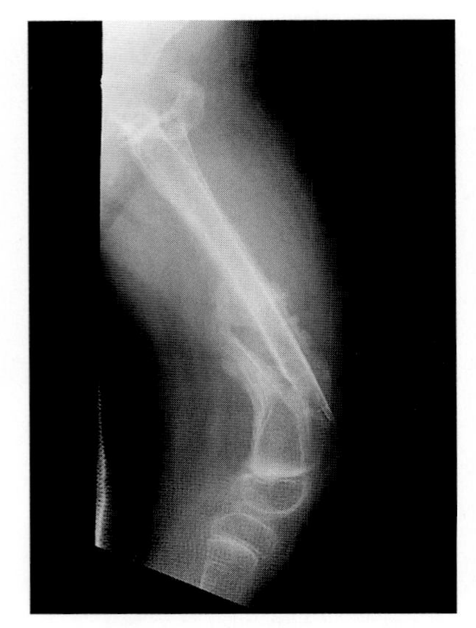

Plate 36

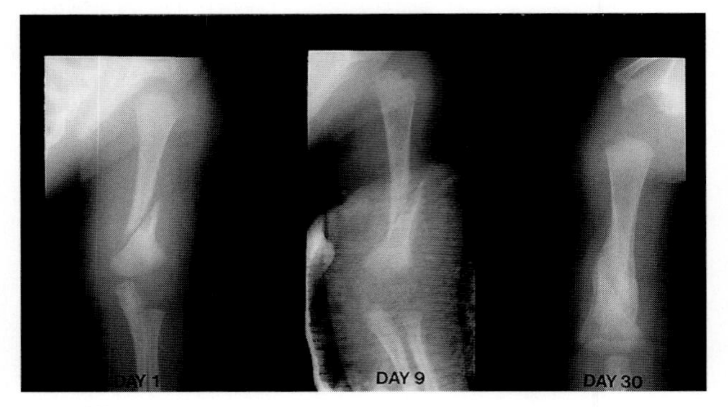

Plate 35

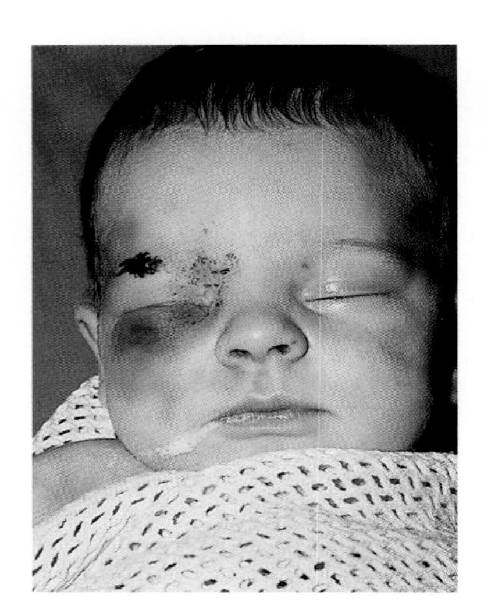

Plate 37

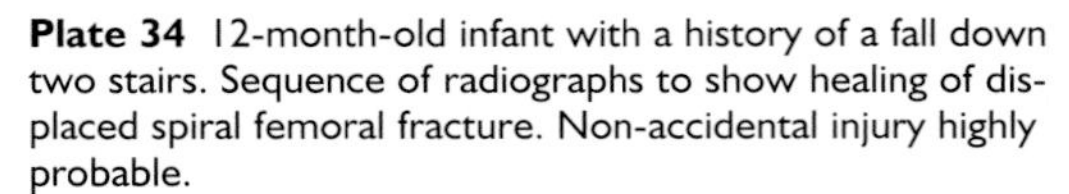

Plate 34 12-month-old infant with a history of a fall down two stairs. Sequence of radiographs to show healing of displaced spiral femoral fracture. Non-accidental injury highly probable.

Plate 35 Infant of 2 months presented with apparent pain on movement of arm. Father, a drug abuser, said he grabbed his son to save him falling out of a Moses basket. Sequence of radiographs to show healing of displaced spiral humeral fracture. Non-accidental injury highly probable.

Plate 36 Girl aged 8 years with cerebral palsy and severe learning problems, admitted to hosptial with a chest infection. Mother thought she was sitting in an unusual position when visiting and seemed to be in pain. The radiograph was taken some time later and showed a fractured femur and osteoporotic bones. Osteoporotic bones fracture more readily but a history of trauma is required.

Plate 37 Battered baby aged 2 months. Facial, ear and mouth bruising. Fractured skull, corneal burn.

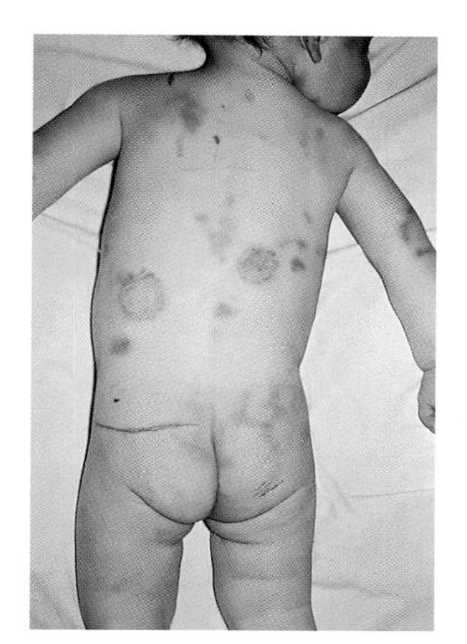

Plate 38

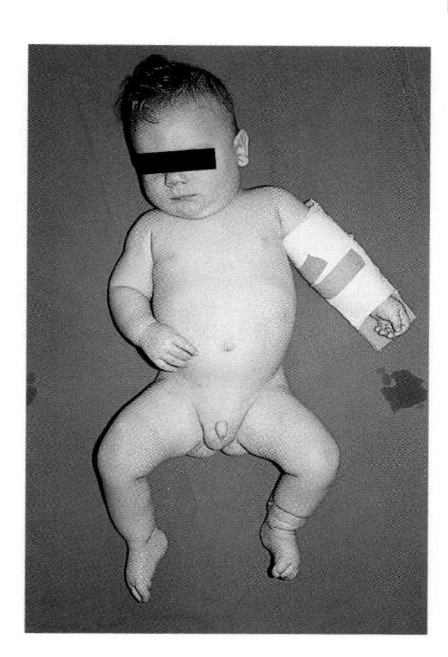

Plate 39

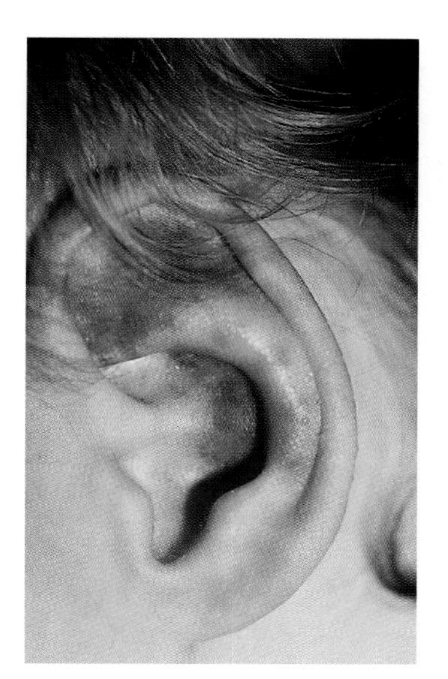

Plate 40

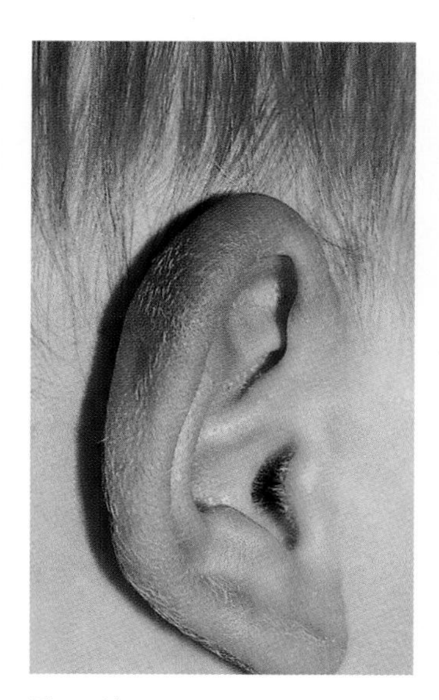

Plate 41

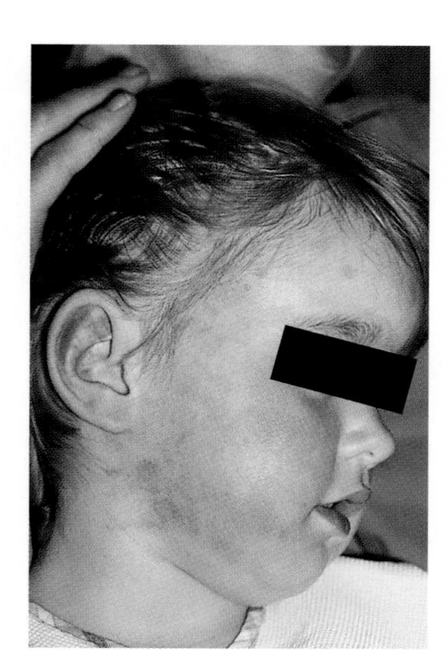

Plate 42

Plate 38 Battered baby. Various lesions including bites, bruises and healing laceration.
Plate 39 Battered baby with over 20 individual injuries. Presentation with injured elbow. Fractures of skull, ribs, humerus, tibia, of various ages on skeletal survey. Faint bruises on arm, fingertip bruising to chest and face just visible. Nappy rash. Nutrition good.
Plate 40 Bruising to ear from blow to the side of the head in a 12-month-old boy.
Plate 41 Bruising to rim of ear resulting from ear being forcibly pinched in a 15-month-old baby.
Plate 42 Diffuse recent bruising to side of face, including lower jaw and neck with linear pattern, and ear. Admitted hand slap. Child of 3 years.

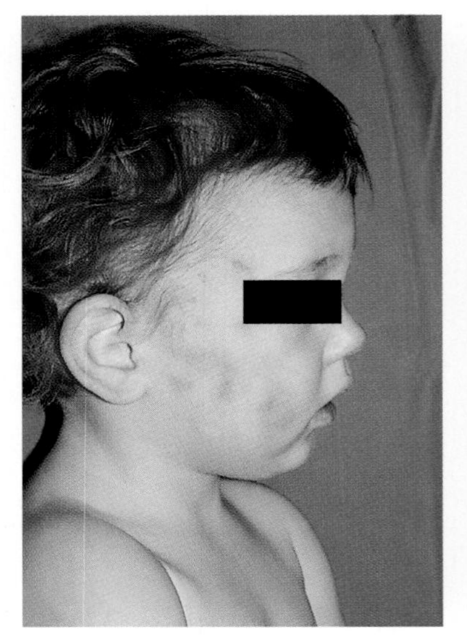

Plate 43

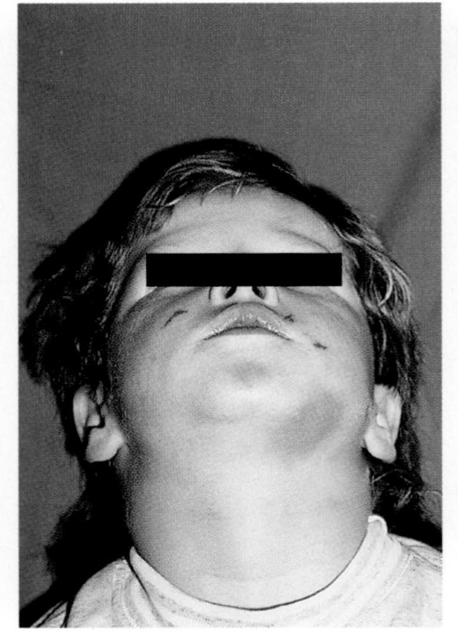

Plate 44

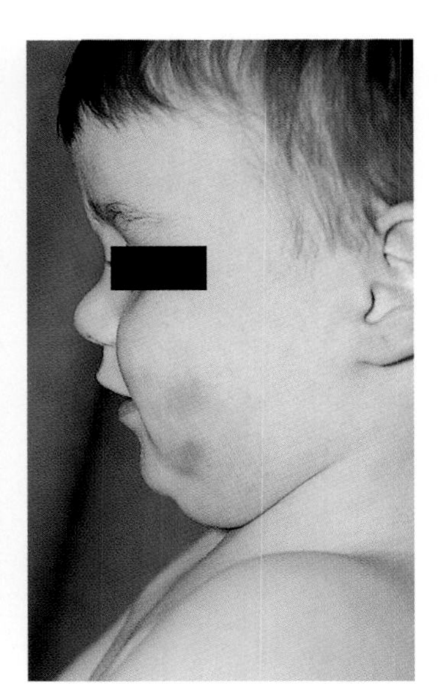

Plate 45

Plate 46

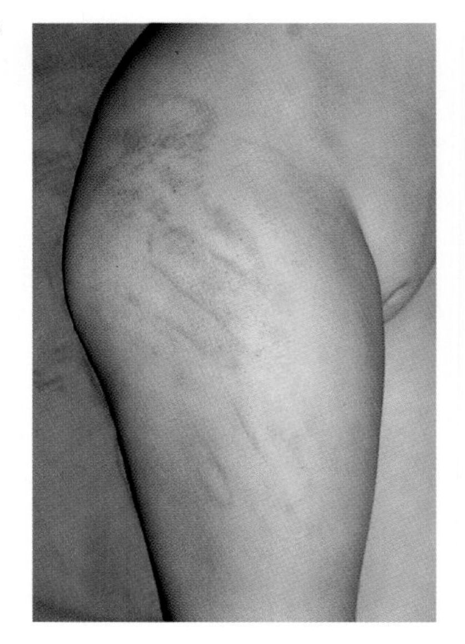

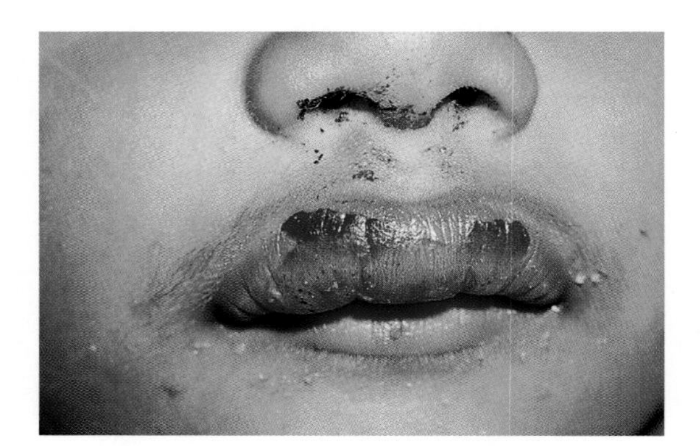

Plate 47

Plate 43 Patchy bruises, several days old, over the side of the face of a 20-month-old abused boy.
Plate 44 Jawline bruise in a 3-year-old abused girl. Several fingernail scratches are present on her face.
Plate 45 Fingertip facial bruising in a boy of 11 months.
Plate 46 Hand marks on the thigh of a 4-year-old repeatedly abused girl. Mother admitted causing the injury.
Plate 47 Swollen, bruised lip from a punch in the mouth in an older boy.

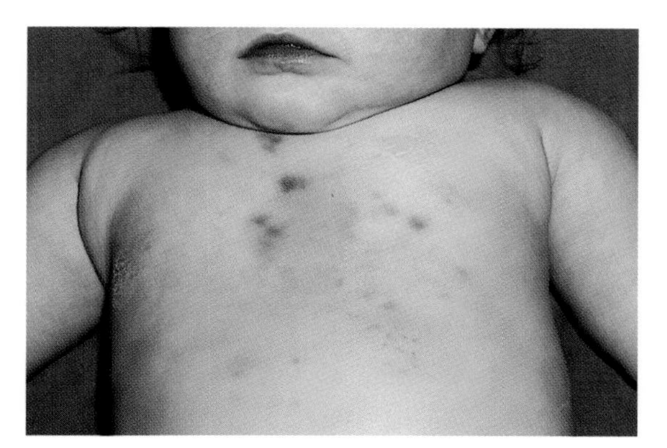

Plate 48

Plate 49

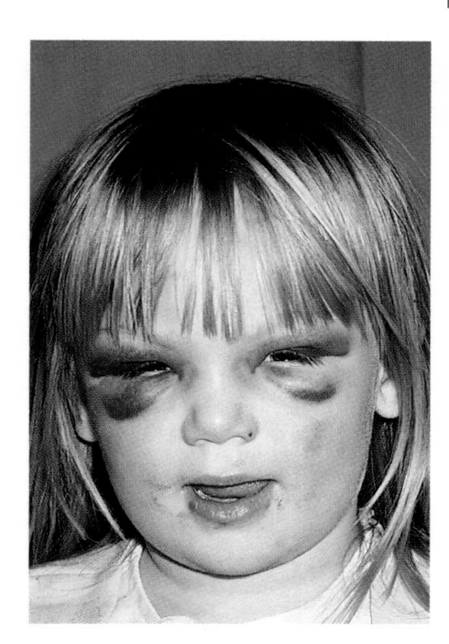

Plate 50

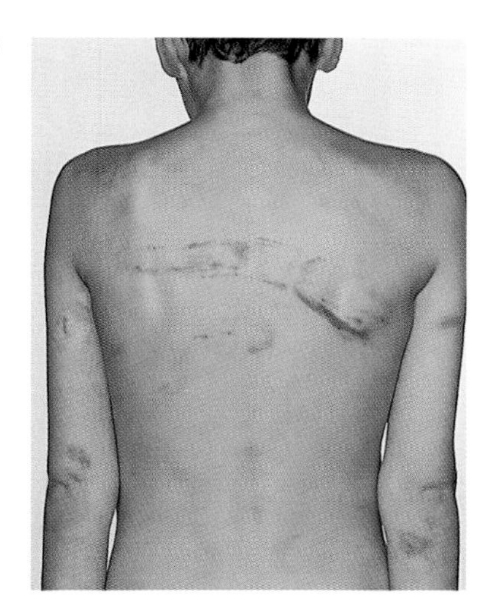

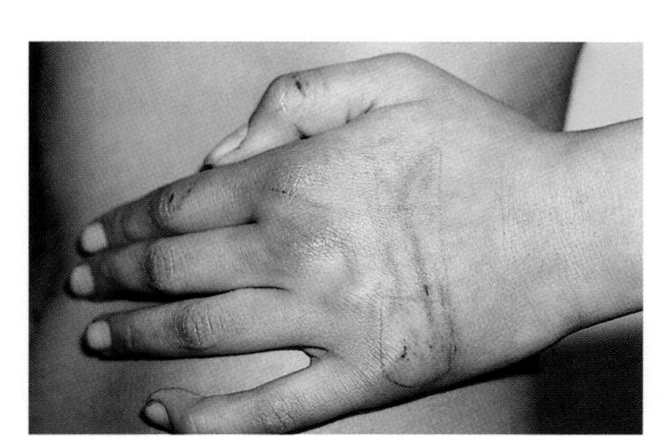

Plate 51

Plate 48 Pinch marks on the chest of a fatally abused 5-month-old infant. The bruises are paired and may be of varying ages.
Plate 49 Bilateral periorbital haematoma in a 3-year-old girl resulting from a blow to the forehead where fainter bruising and swelling was also noted. A total of 60 bruises were found on the child's body. History of an unwitnessed fall downstairs.
Plate 50 Belt mark in 11-year-old boy.
Plate 51 Mark caused by a stick beating in older Asian boy. Hand held up to protect face.

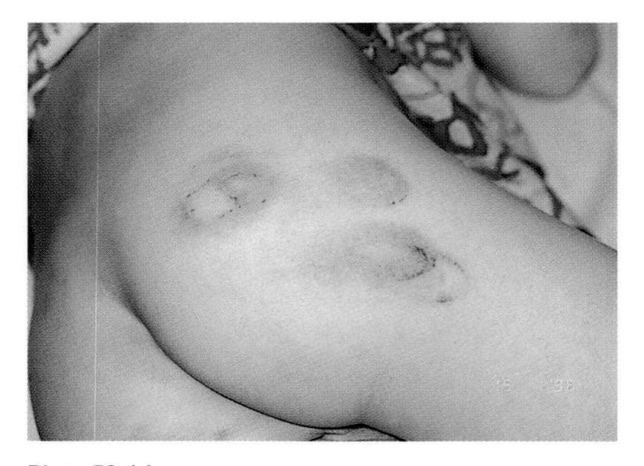

Plate 52 (a)

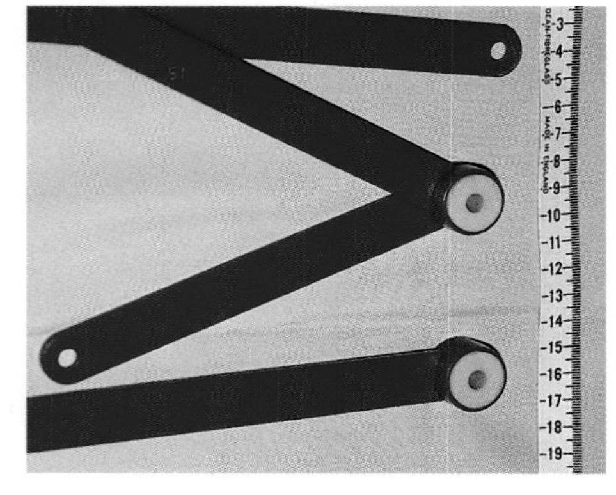

Plate 52 (b)

Plate 53

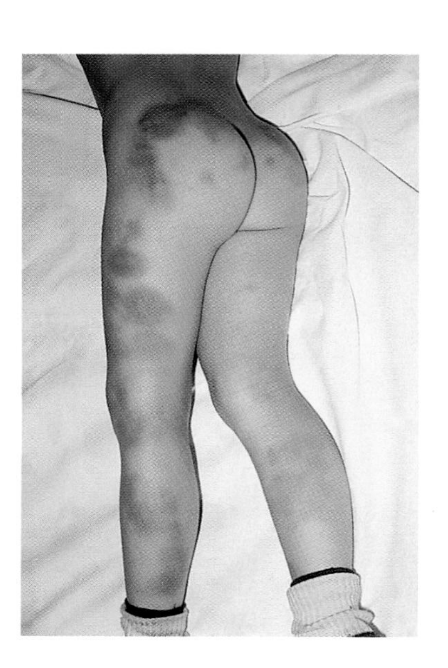

Plate 54

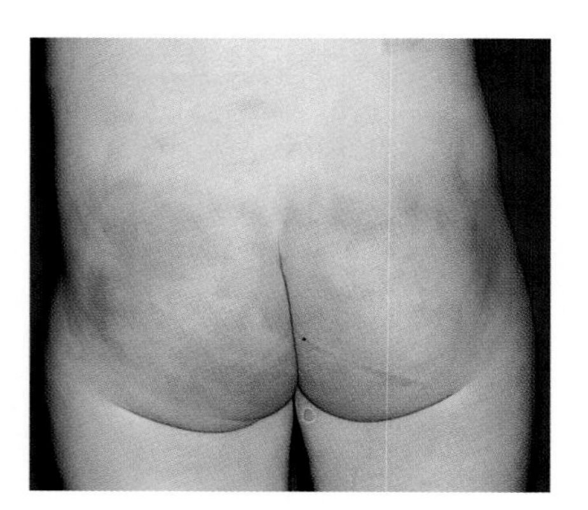

Plate 55

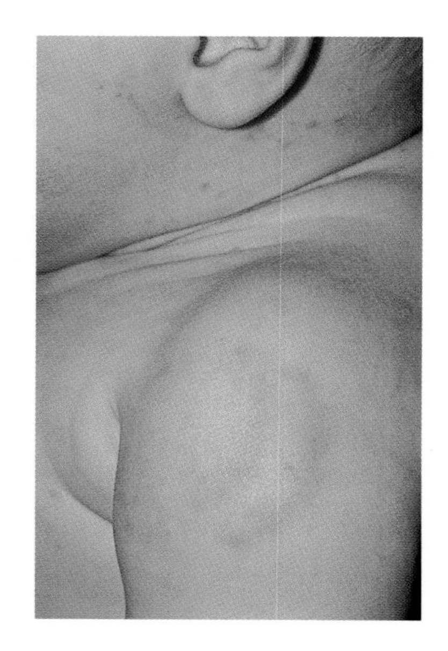

Plate 52 (a) 6-year-old boy told his teacher that his stepfather had hit him. He was brought to the examination by his mother, carrying the implement used – (b) a construction toy.
Plate 53 Bruises resulting from kicks in 5-year-old boy.
Plate 54 Bilateral fading buttock bruises in 3-year-old child from slipper beating, admitted by mother.
Plate 55 Large radius double bite mark of recent origin. Individual teeth marks can be made out. Father admitted biting this 12-month-old girl.

Plate 56

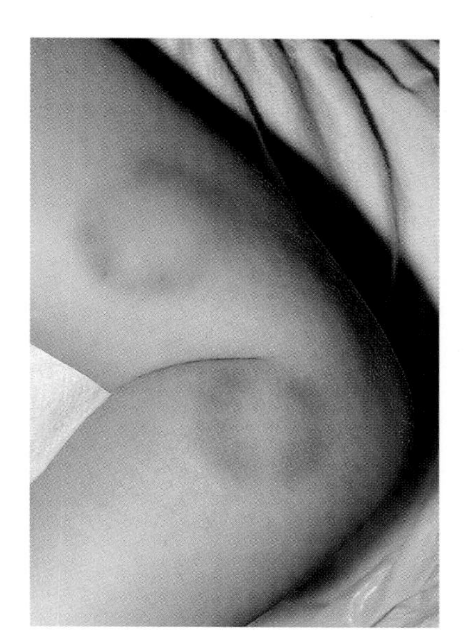

Plate 57

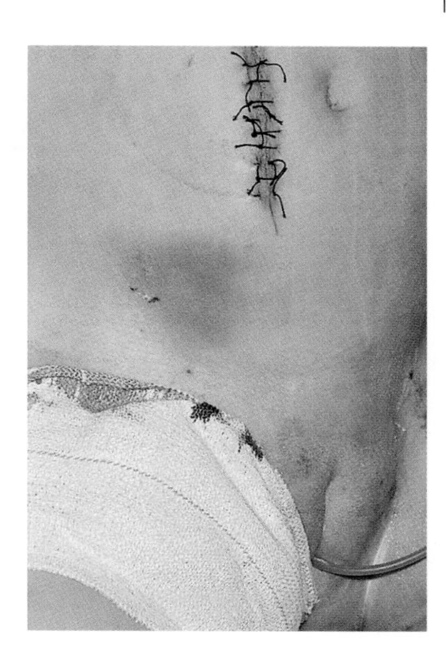

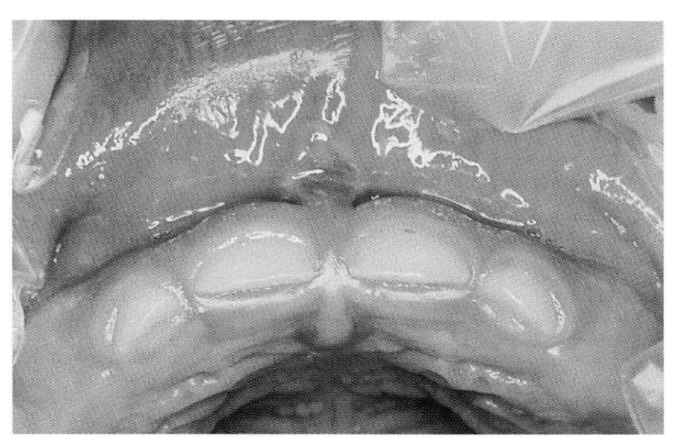

Plate 58

Plate 59

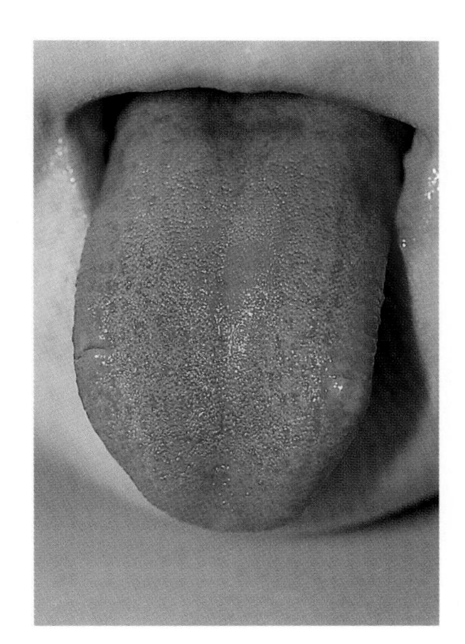

Plate 56 Two child bites witnessed in day nursery on a 4-year-old.
Plate 57 Abdominal bruising in an infant who sustained duodenal rupture. History that child had fallen across a table seemed unlikely to be true.
Plate 58 Torn frenulum in an 18-month-old girl who presented with a 2-day-old fracture and bruises to buttocks and face.
Plate 59 2-year-old boy with unexplained laceration to penis (see Plate 110). Bilateral lacerations to tongue caused by forcible mouth closure by mother's violent partner.

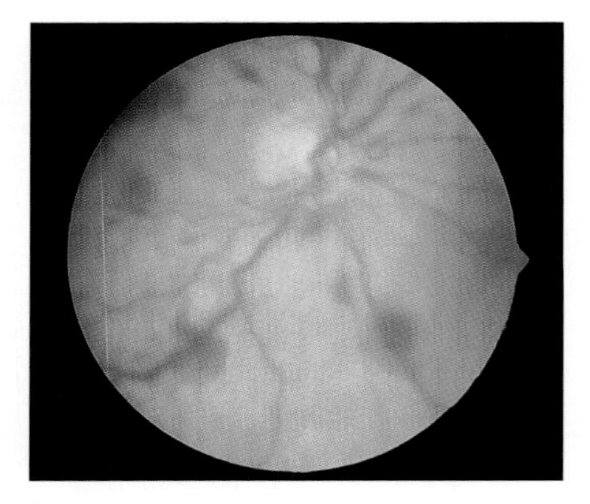

Plate 60

Plate 61

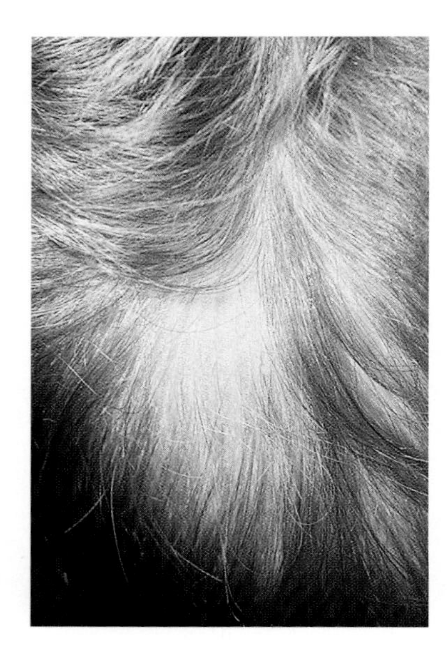

Plate 62

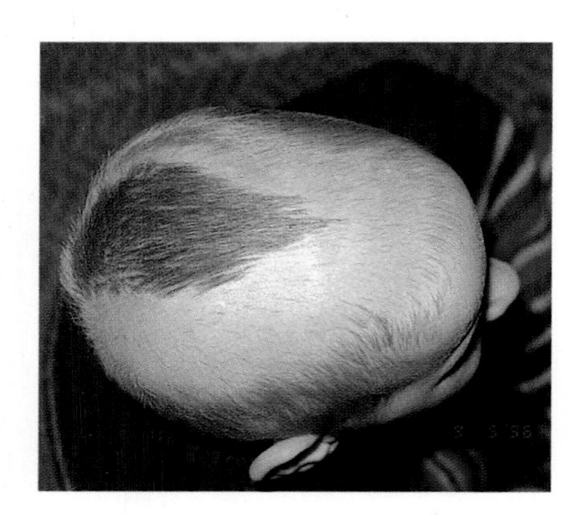

Plate 63

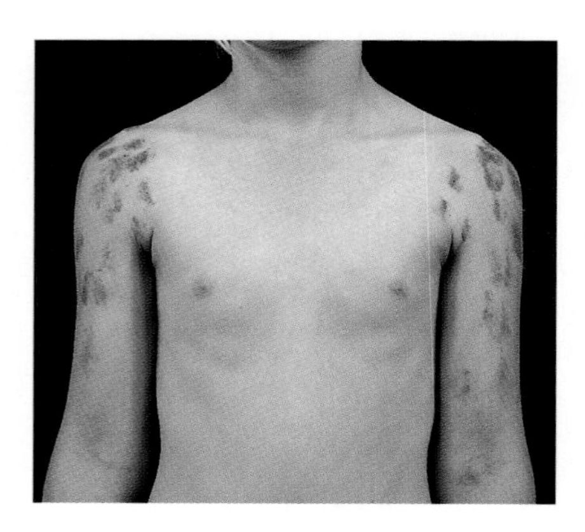

Plate 64

Plate 60 Retinal haemorrhages in a 4-year-old boy shaken to death. Evidence of anal abuse and bruises to back and face. No skull fracture.

Plate 61 Traumatic hair loss in abused 2-year-old boy.

Plate 62 Grossly denuded scalp in 4-year-old child referred by general practitioner to child psychiatrist. History of child pulling own hair out. It became evident that she was being sexually abused (see Plate 99).

Plate 63 Child of 10 years taken by mother for medical help for these unusual marks. No history of injury given. Classical self-inflicted injury.

Plate 64 Lesion found on buttocks in a 12-month-old handicapped boy. Mother strenuously insisted that it was nappy rash. Lesion consistent with burn.

Plate 65

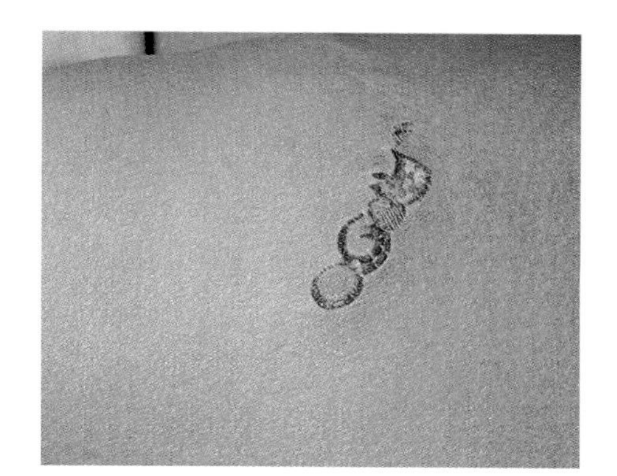

Plate 66

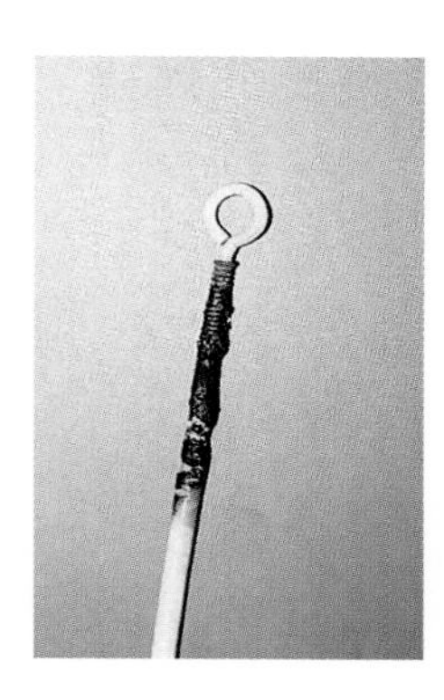

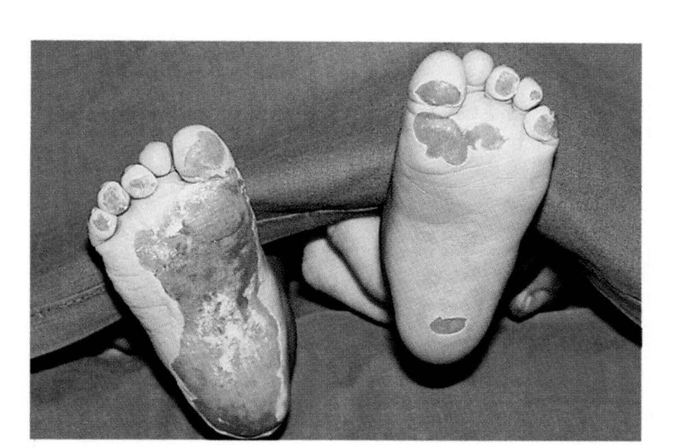

Plate 67

Plate 68

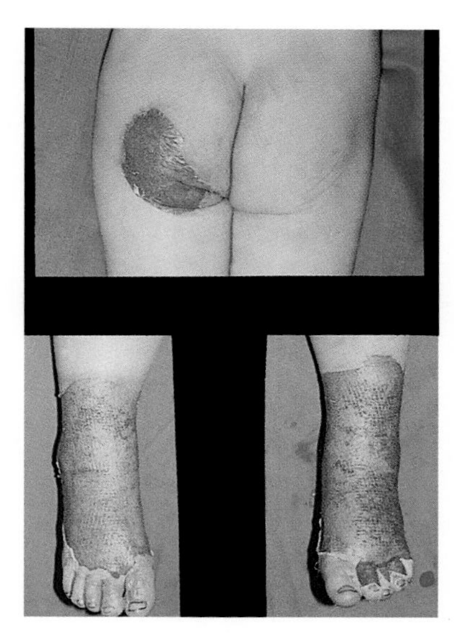

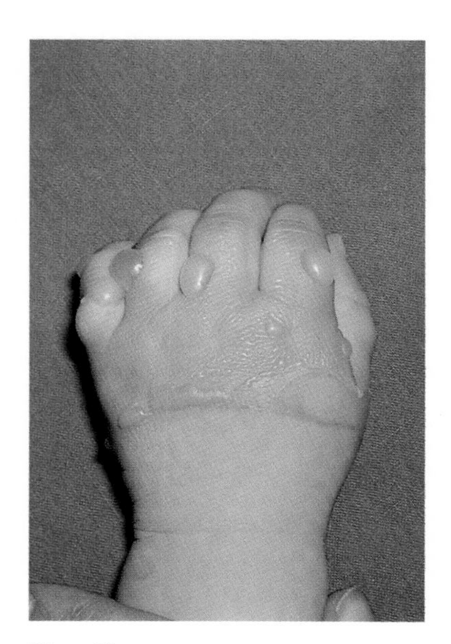

Plate 69

Plate 65 Contact burns on thigh in a 2-year-old boy with developmental retardation inflicted by his mother. Burns were also present to penis. (Reproduced with permission from Meadow S R (ed.) 1989 ABC of child abuse. BMJ Publishing, London.)
Plate 66 Curtain wire heated in fire and used to inflict burns shown in Plate 65. (Reproduced with permission from Meadow S R (ed.) 1989 ABC of child abuse. BMJ Publishing, London.)
Plate 67 Contact burns in a 9-month-old who, when left with father, allegedly crawled against a central heating radiator. Story not consistent with explanation. Delay in presentation.
Plate 68 Forced immersion scald with deep areas around both ankles in 4-year-old abused child. Stocking distribution, no splash marks. Mother admitted to holding child in the bath. (Reproduced with permission from Meadow S R (ed.) 1989 ABC of child abuse. BMJ Publishing, London.)
Plate 69 Forced immersion scald of the hand of a 3-year-old who 'sat in a bath of hot water'. No scalds were found elsewhere.

Plate 70

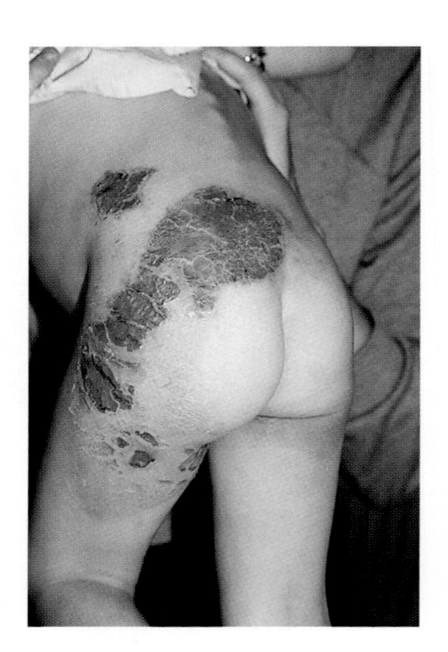

Plate 71

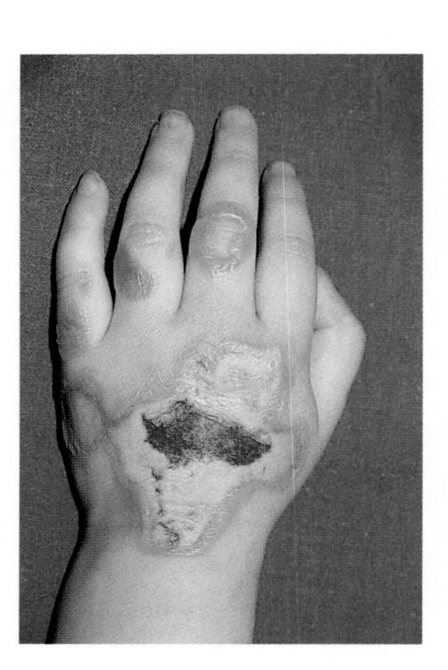

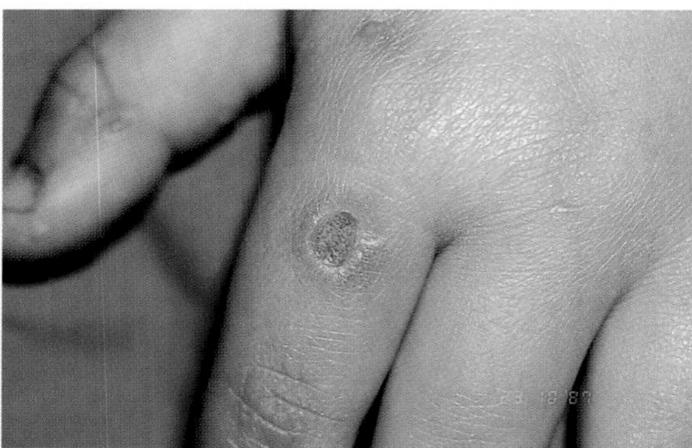

Plate 72

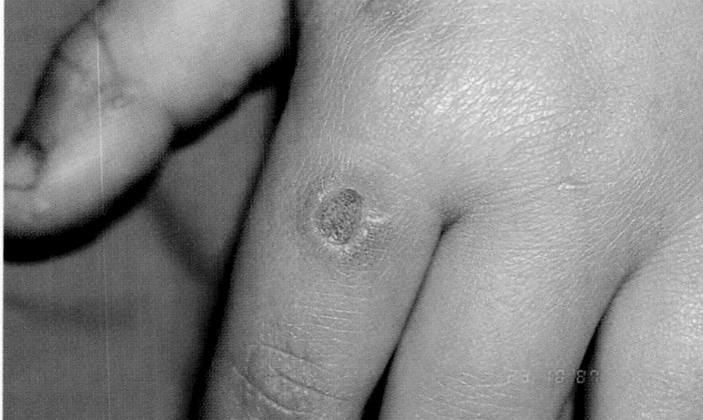

Plate 73

Plate 70 Extensive bath scalds in 3-year-old girl failing to thrive. Central part of buttock spared where pressed onto cool base of bath – 'hole in doughnut' effect. Abuse suspected but not proven. (Reproduced with permission from Meadow S R (ed.) 1989 ABC of child abuse. BMJ Publishing, London.)
Plate 71 Full thickness burn from an iron in a 2-year-old child. Alleged that older brother was responsible. Incident unwitnessed by mother. Labial fusion and multiple anal fissures present.
Plate 72 Cratered deep cigarette burn in typical site on the back of the hand of a 5-year-old boy who also said 'Mummy put her fingers in my bottom'. (Reproduced with permission from Meadow S R (ed.) 1989 ABC of child abuse. BMJ Publishing, London.)
Plate 73 Depressed scars in a 4-year-old boy. Both he and his brother had multiple cigarette burns of varying ages over their foreheads.

Plate 74

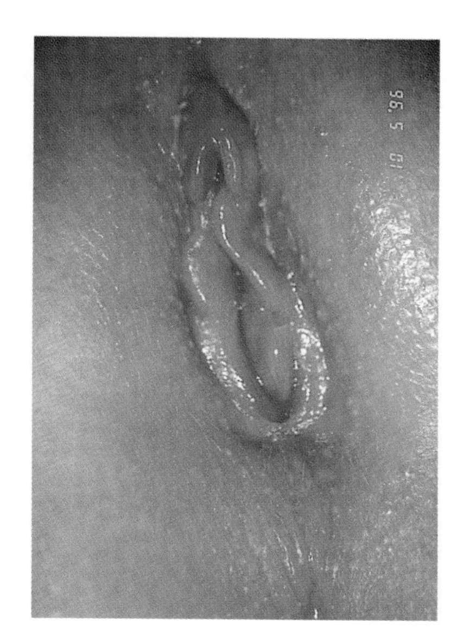

Plate 75

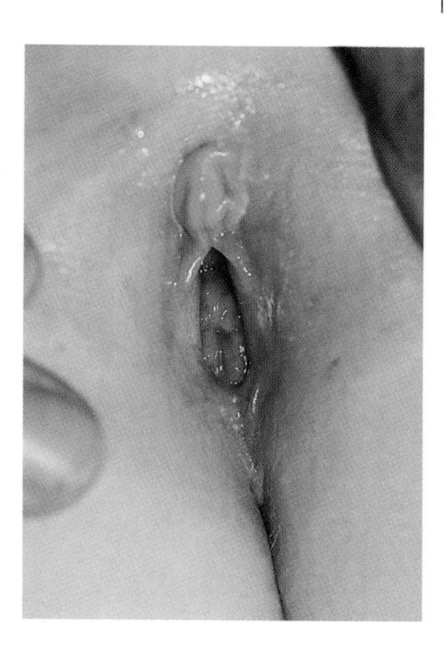

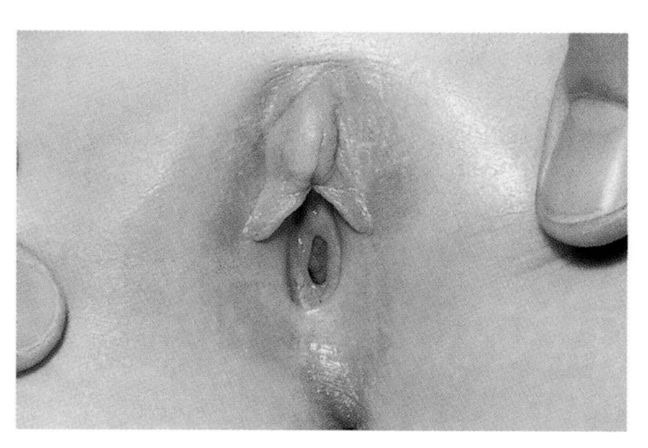

Plate 76

Plate 77

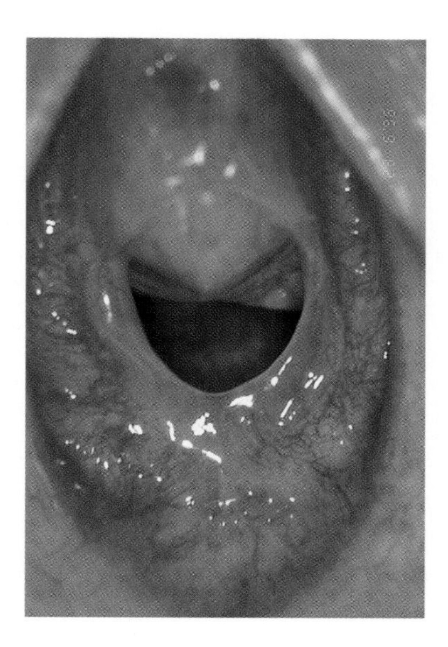

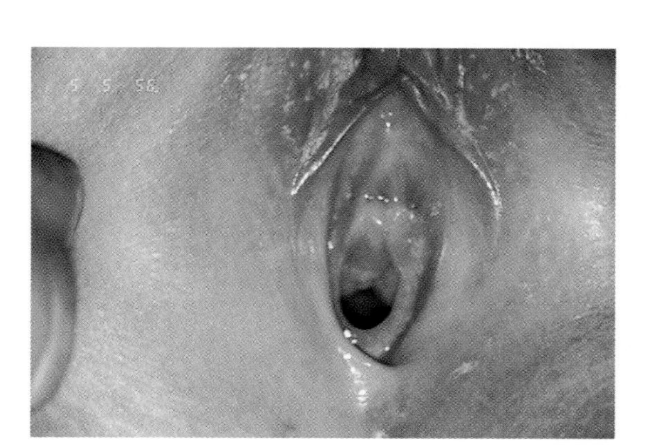

Plate 78

Plate 74 Normal infantile genitalia at 6 months. Note redundant hymen.
Plate 75 Normal infantile genitalia at age 15 months. Note fleshy hymen.
Plate 76 Normal genitalia at age 3 years. Annular hymen.
Plate 77 High magnification normal genitalia in 7-year-old. Note fine smooth margin to hymen with lacy vascular pattern.
Plate 78 Normal genitalia at age 6 years. Configuration of hymen somewhere between annular and crescentic.

Plate 79

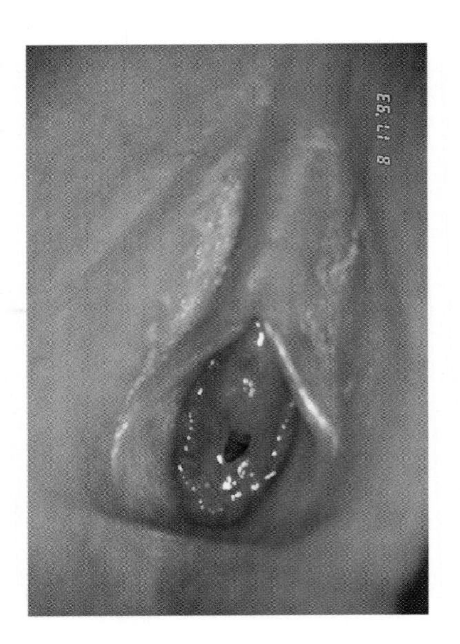

Plate 80

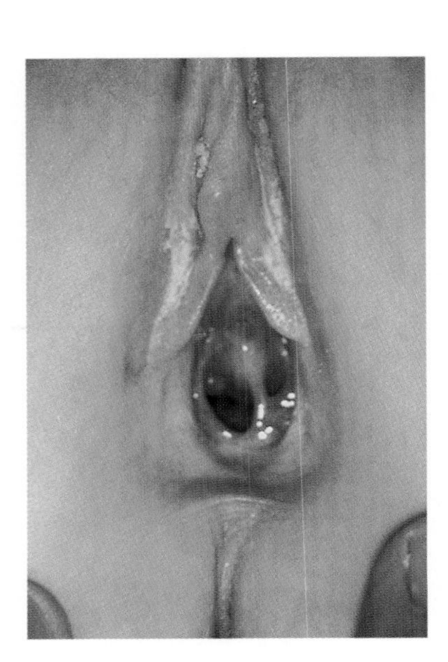

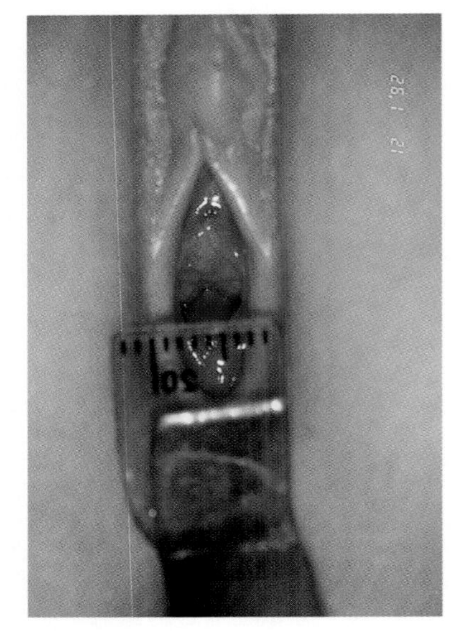

Plate 81

Plate 82

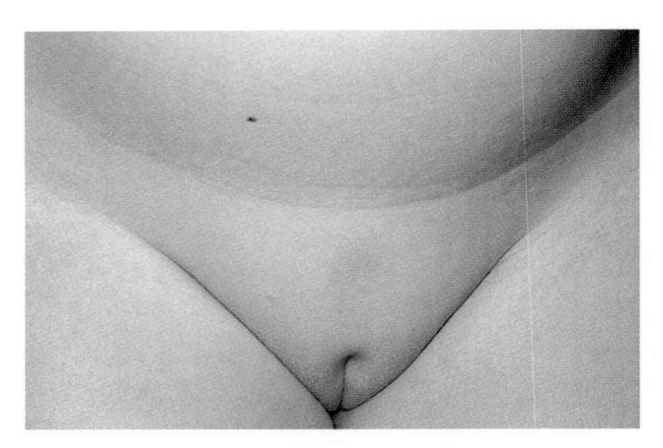

Plate 83

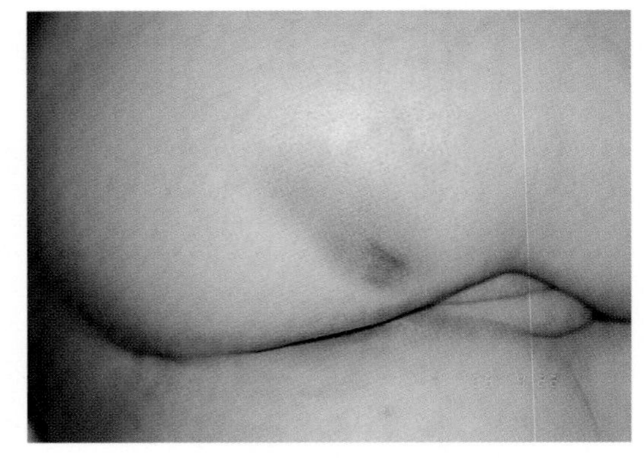

Plate 79 Normal genitalia at age 4 years. A crescentic hymen with semi-transparent smooth margin with vascular pattern preserved.
Plate 80 Hymenal septum in a 5-year-old.
Plate 81 Measuring device.
Plate 82 Suprapubic bruise in 6-year-old who disclosed sexual abuse by 15-year-old brother when returned from children's home at the weekend.
Plate 83 5-year-old girl with large unexplained bruise on right buttock discovered incidentally during examination after older sibling disclosed sexual abuse.

Plate 84

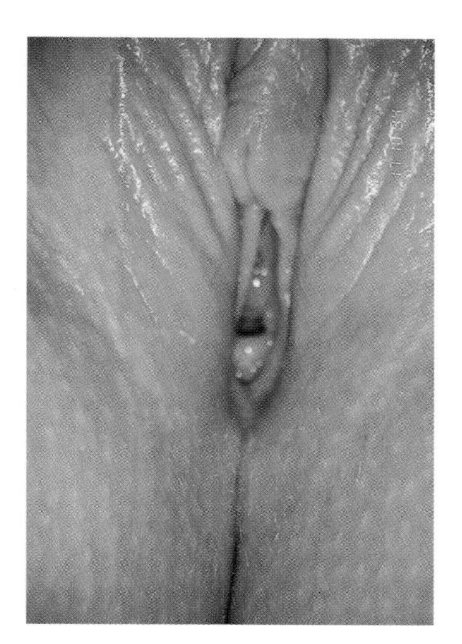

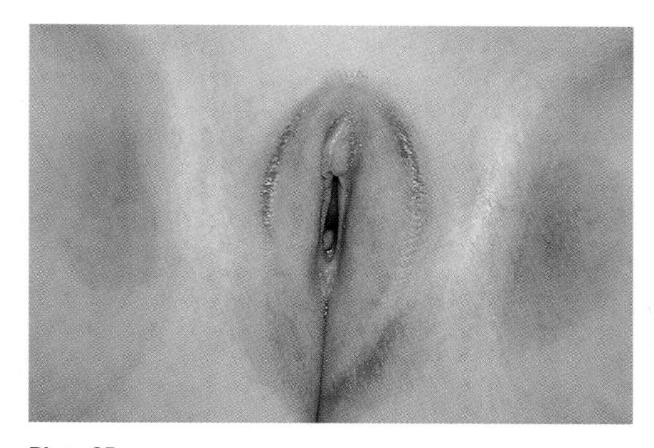

Plate 85

Plate 86

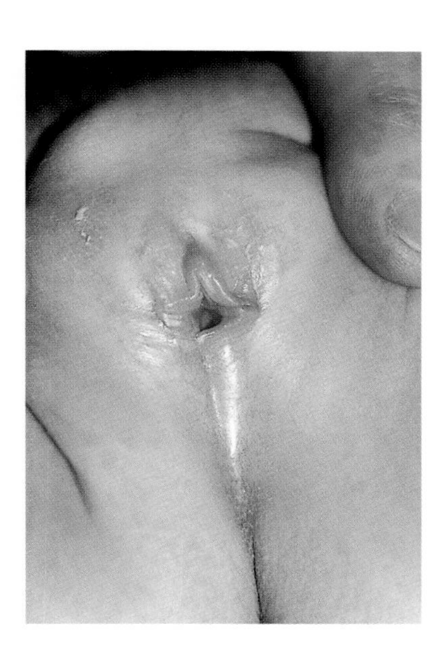

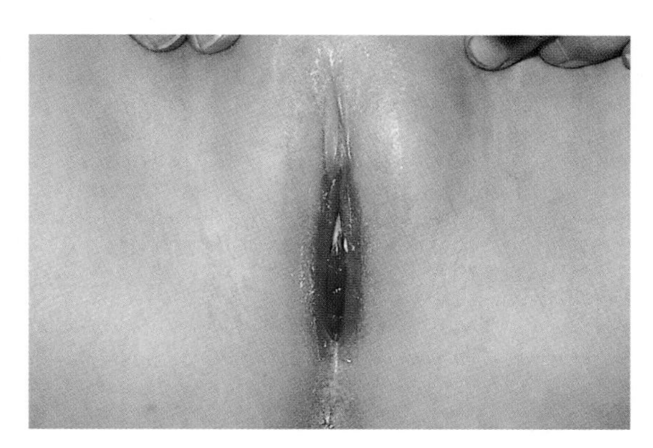

Plate 87

Plate 84 9-year-old referred because of vaginal discharge. Child said she did not like her father washing her genitalia in the bath. Previous history of rectal prolapse aged 5 years and continuing anal abnormality. Note markedly flattened and wrinkled labia, square, gaping hymenal opening and thickening of posterior hymen. Has there been intracrural intercourse?
Plate 85 Patchy tram-line reddening of both labia majora and inside of thighs in a 7-year-old. Gaping hymenal opening is visible without separation of labia. History of intracrural intercourse (penis between thighs) and digital penetration.
Plate 86 Extensive posterior labial fusion in an abused 2-year-old with anal findings and an old burn on the thigh (see Plate 120).
Plate 87 Marked reddening of labia minora and tissues of introitus in 4-year-old who disclosed digital vulval interference.

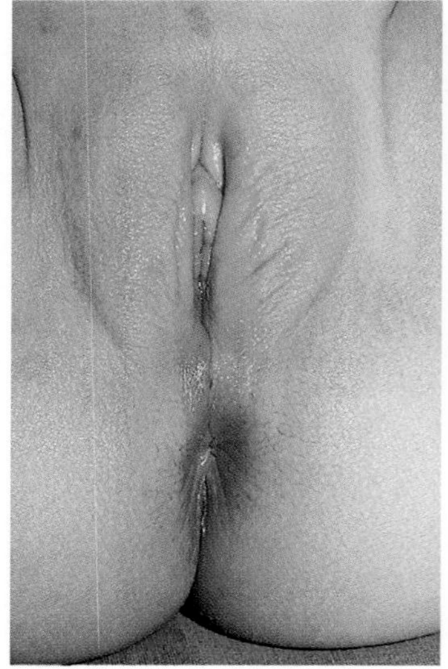

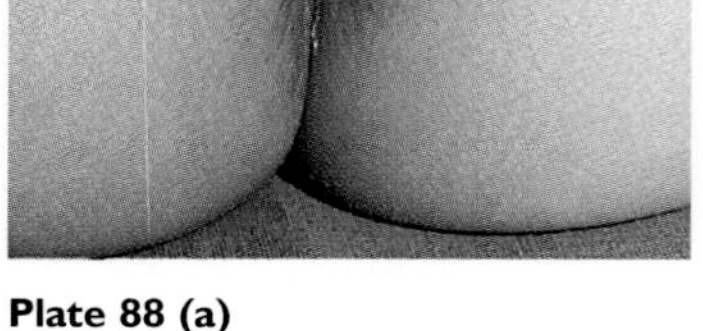

Plate 88 (a)

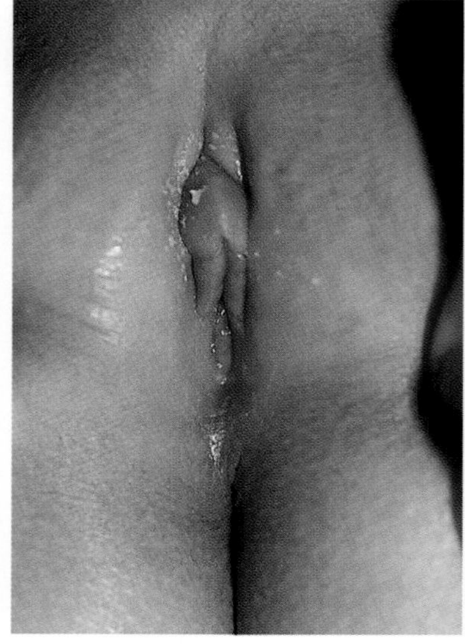

Plate 88 (b)

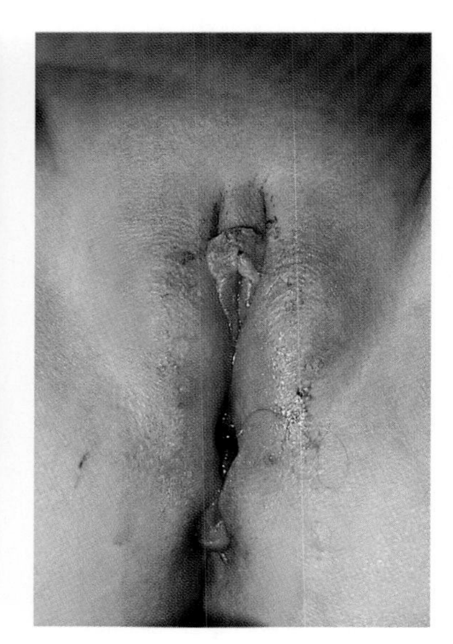

Plate 89

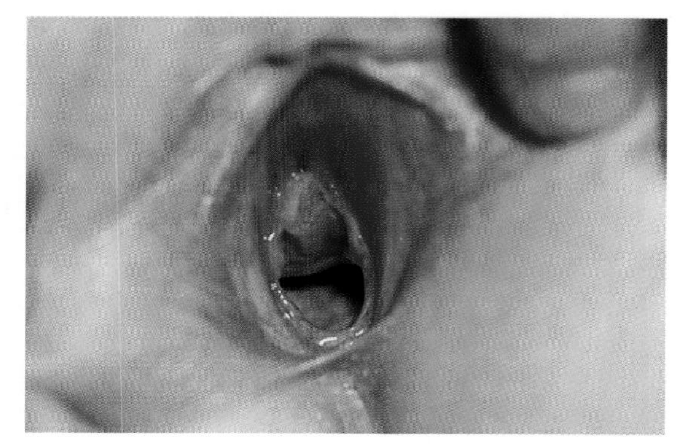

Plate 90

Plate 91

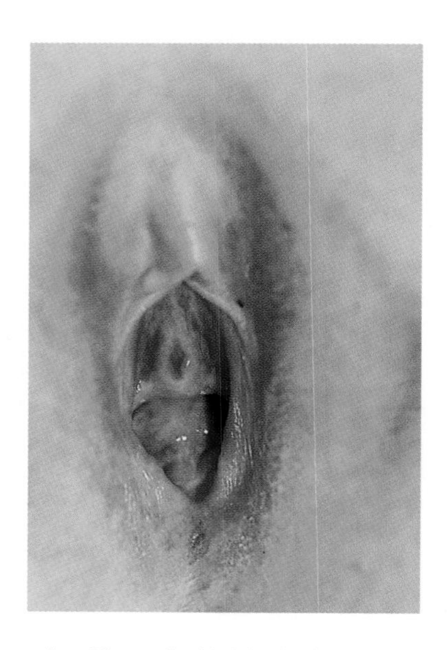

Plate 88 (a) Fresh unexplained midline tear through posterior fourchette, abuse presumed, in 20-month-old child. (b) Same child 3 weeks later. Pale midline scar now present. Hymen appears normal.

Plate 89 4-year-old abused child with recent bruising, reddening and swelling of labia majora and a midline tear extending posteriorly through the vaginal wall, perineum and as far as the anus. Anterior anal haematoma. Findings consistent with violent penetration of vagina.

Plate 90 10-year-old girl who presented with day-time wetting in school. Child flirtatious and overweight, living in the care of her father following marital breakdown. Excessive reddening of hymenal orifice and vagina with extensive healed posterior and probable anterior tears in hymen which is also attenuated. Father convicted of rape after clear disclosure by child. (Reproduced with permission form Hobbs C J, Wynne J M 1987 Child sexual abuse – an increasing rate of diagnosis. Lancet ii: 839.)

Plate 91 9-year-old girl with history of anal warts at age 4 years, history of vaginal wall tear following alleged fall at age 7 and persistent soiling, self-mutilation and emotional problems. Generalized reddening, prominent urethra, dilated vagina (1.5 cm). There is virtually no hymen visible with few remnants posteriorly. The posterior fourchette is poorly defined and a superficial abrasion is present in the skin in the midline at 6 o'clock. Child made clear disclosure of repeated abuse, but court found the child's evidence inadmissible.

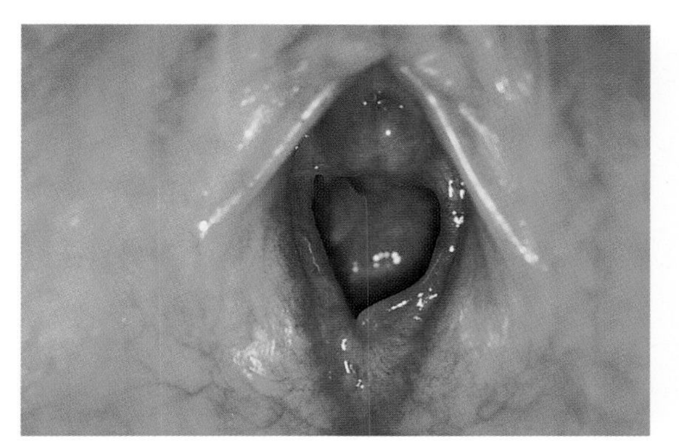

Plate 92

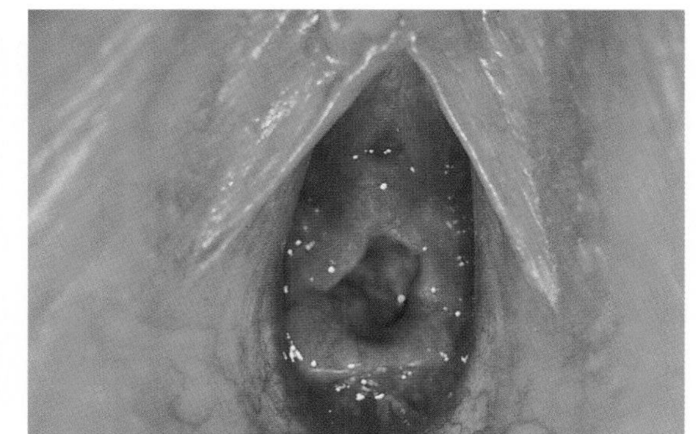

Plate 93

Plate 94

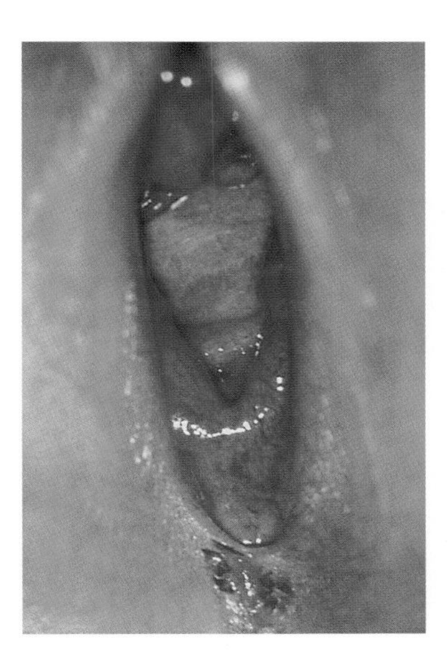

Plate 95

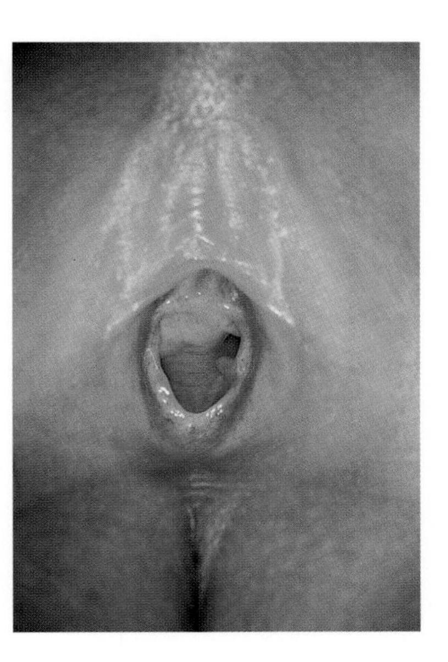

Plate 92 5-year-old with intermittent vulval soreness, withdrawn behaviour and fluctuating physical signs, both anal and genital. Hymenal opening is dilated, 1 cm horizontal diameter and there is a sharp V at 6 o'clock. The hymen is reddened, its edge is irregular, rolled and there is anterior asymmetry. The symptoms and signs regressed when the child's stepfather left the family home. The parents accepted that abuse had taken place, but by another child in the street.
Plate 93 4-year-old girl with a history of vaginal abuse. There is a healed transection of the hymen at 9 o'clock.
Plate 94 Fresh tear of fourchette in a 4-year-old child with a clear history of penile/vaginal abuse. The hymenal opening is enlarged with a deep posterior notch at 6 o'clock.
Plate 95 7-year-old girl was seen after father discharged from prison after serving a sentence for manslaughter of a child. Mother concerned about possible sexual abuse. Note gaping, attenuated hymen with irregular rolled margin and vaginal ridge at 3 o'clock. This latter is a normal structure but easily visible due to the attenuation of the hymen.

Plate 96 (a)

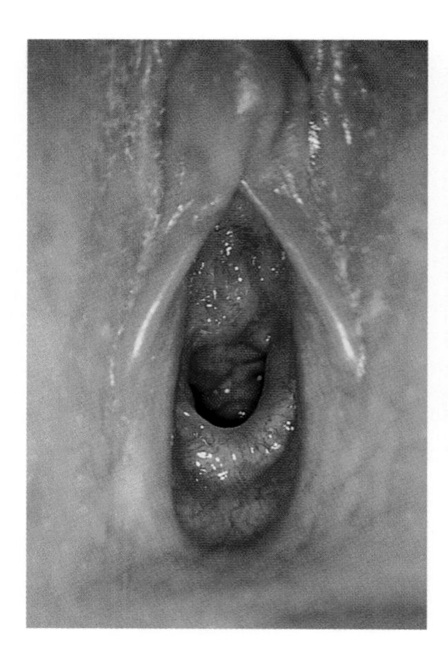

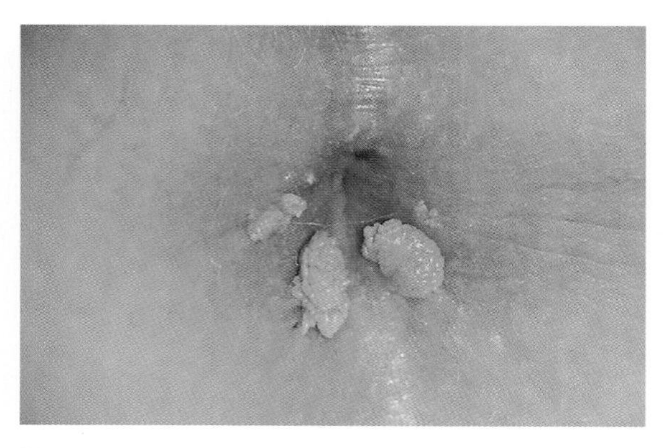

Plate 96 (b)

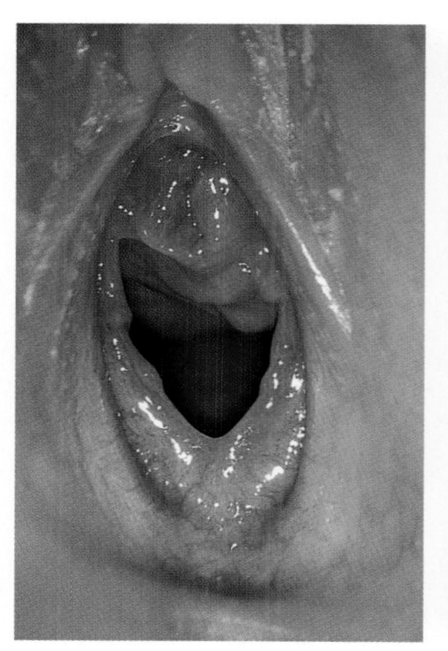

Plate 97

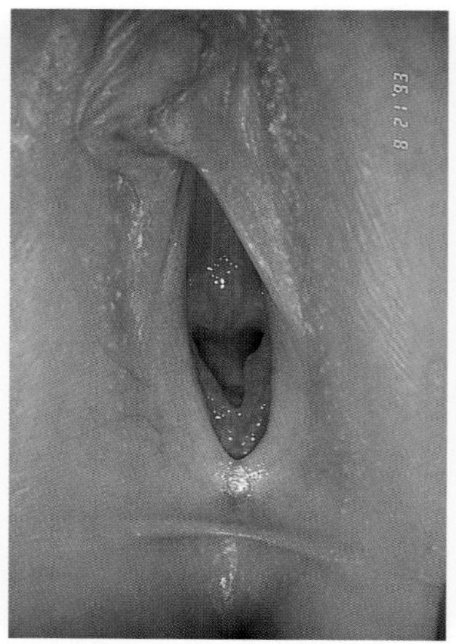

Plate 98

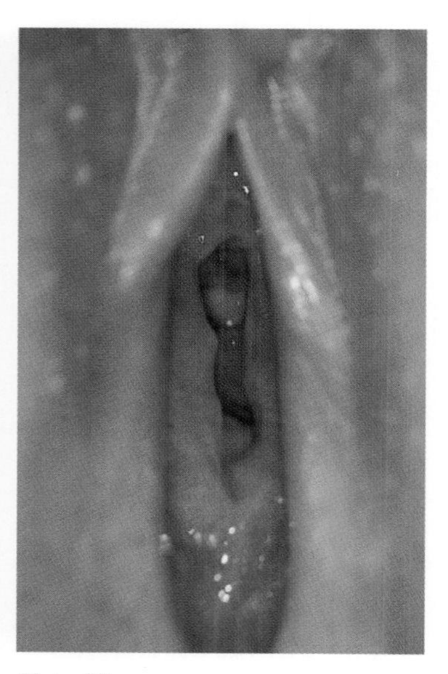

Plate 99

Plate 96 (a) 7-year-old who presented with anal bleeding from anal warts. A solitary genital wart is visible. Hymen appears thickened although the edge is smooth. There is a tear at 1–2 o'clock. (b) Multiple perianal warts. Note venous congestion.
Plate 97 9-year-old girl whose younger sister (Plate 96) presented with bleeding from anal warts. Widely gaping hymenal opening with irregular hymenal margin, with bumps at 4, 8 and 9 o'clock. Hymenal configuration likly to be the result of posterior and possibly anterior tears.
Plate 98 10-year-old girl with sexualised behaviour. Previous history of vaginal bleeding following unfortunate accident when child fell against a nail. Some generalised reddening, large posterior hymenal tear which has healed to give a rounded notch.
Plate 99 4-year-old with history of pulling her hair out and other disturbed behaviours. She made clear disclosures of sexual abuse by both parents and grandmother. Examination shows a healed extensive posterior tear.

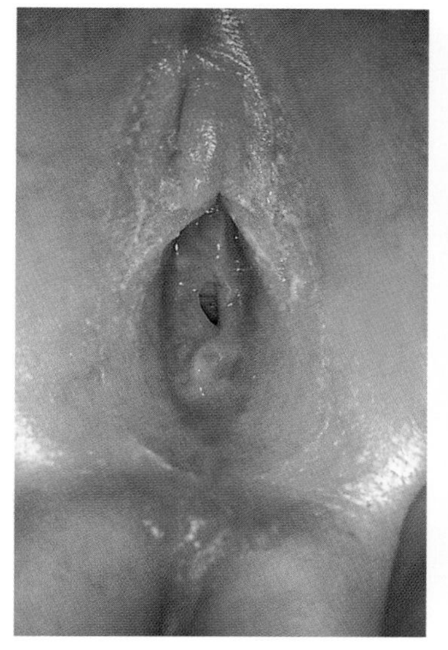

Plate 100

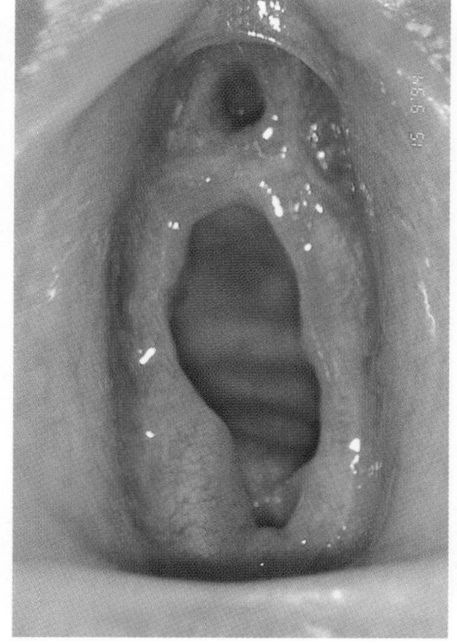

Plate 101

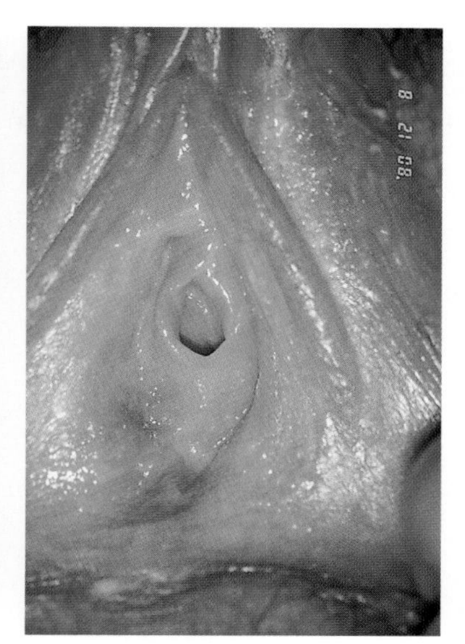

Plate 102

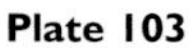

Plate 103

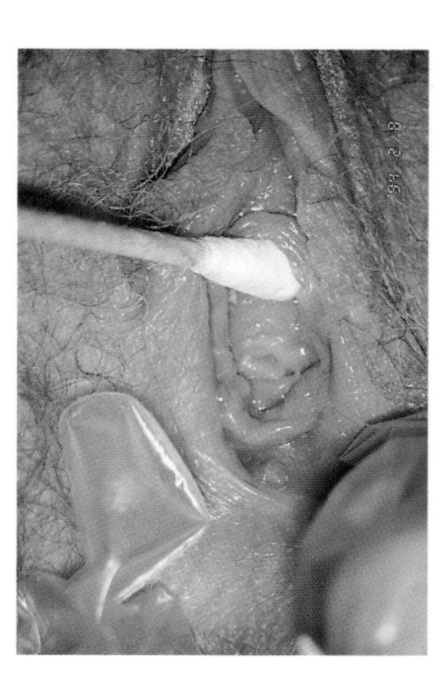

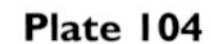

Plate 104

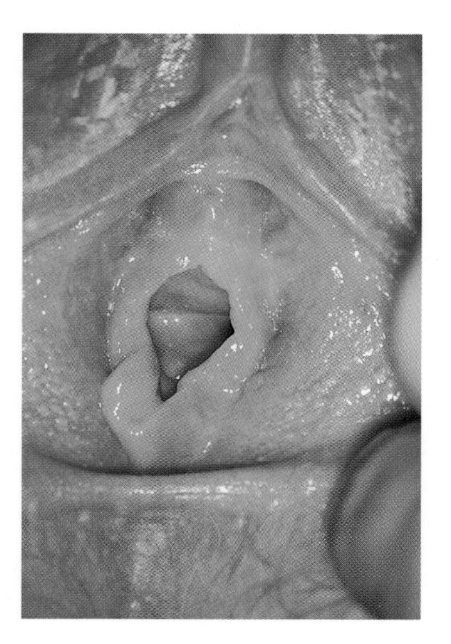

Plate 100 3-year-old examined following discovery of large bruise on thigh. Younger sibling in care following attempted suffocation by mother (fictitious illness). A distorted asymmetrical hymenal opeing is seen with thickened scarred tissues posteriorly at 7 o'clock.

Plate 101 High magnification genital appearances of urethral dilatation in prepubertal child. Healed posterior hymenal tear. The urethra is sometimes penetrated as part of sexual abuse.

Plate 102 Normal oestrogenised hymen in a 12-year-old.

Plate 103 Oestrogenised hymen with two warts visible inferiorly. The hymenal margin is demonstrated by means of a cotton wool swab. A transection is visible at 3 o'clock.

Plate 104 Oestrogenised hymen in 10-year-old. Notch visible at 6 o'clock. There is a normal physiological discharge.

Plate 105

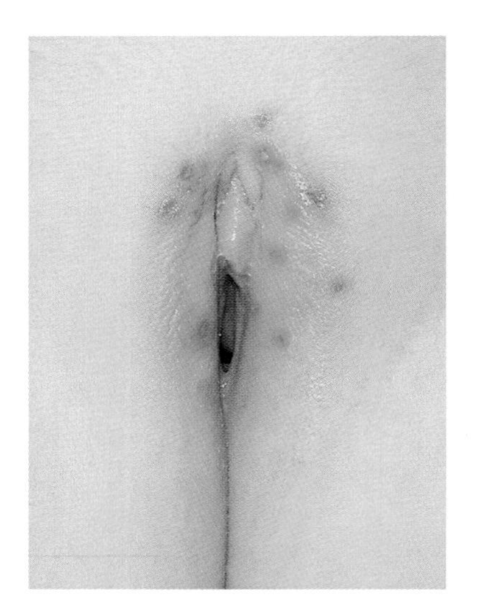

Plate 106

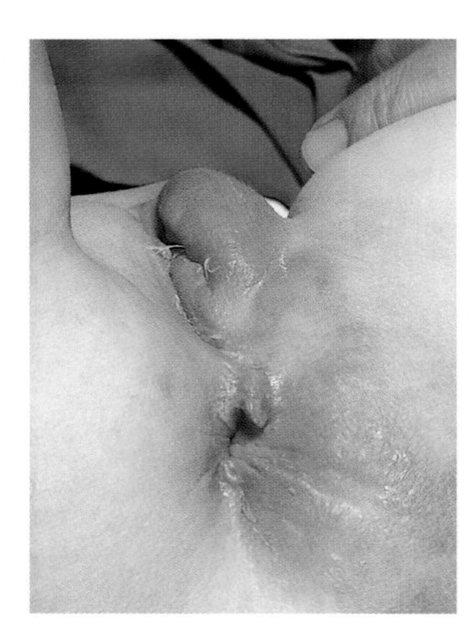

Plate 107

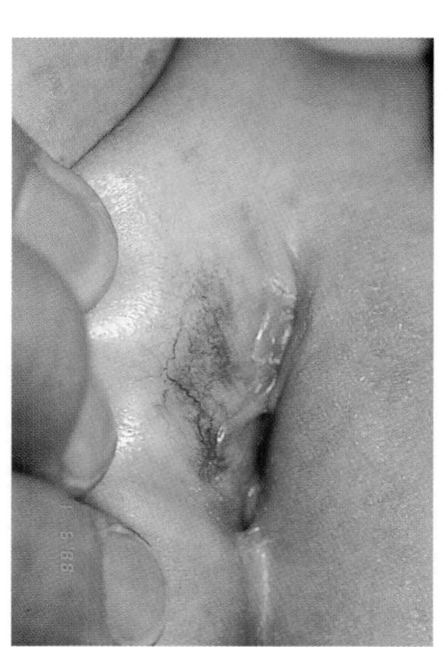

Plate 108

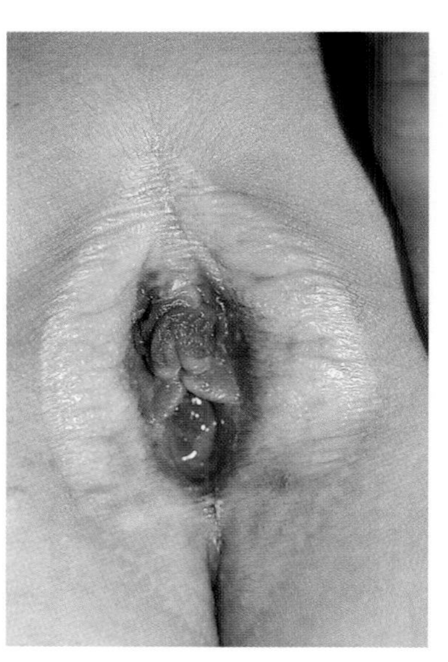

Plate 109

Plate 105 Previously sexually abused 7-year-old girl taken to general practitioner because of painful genital rash. Multiple vesicles. Type 1 herpes simplex infection.
Plate 106 Crohn's disease of vulva and anus in a 10-year-old girl. (Courtesy of Mr P C Buchan and colleagues.)
Plate 107 Vascular naevus of right labium majus in a 2-year-old child with suspicious anal findings and a worrying family history. On follow-up these findings were persistent.
Plate 108 Lichen sclerosus et atrophicus of vulva in 6-year-old girl who presented with persistent irritation, scratching and bleeding of the anogenital area. Pale atrophic skin surrounds normal mucous membrane.
Plate 109 9-year-old boy disclosed sexual assault (forced masturbation) in a public swimming pool by a stranger. Child complained of painful penis. Examination showed red, swollen penis with small tear at base of glans.

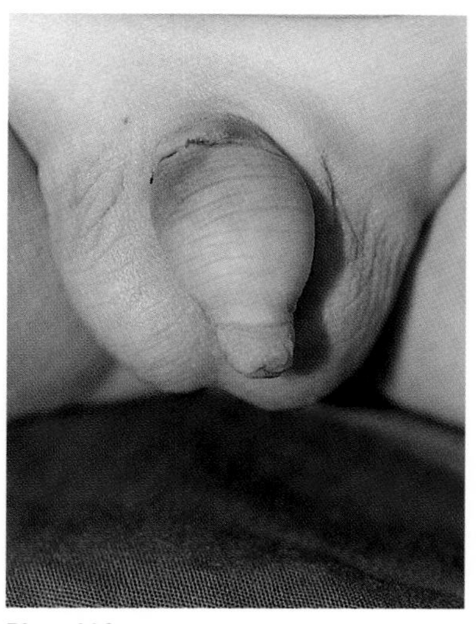

Plate 110

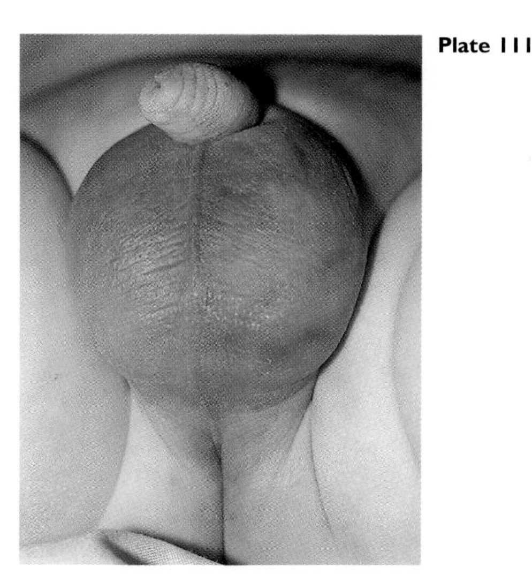

Plate 111

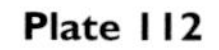

Plate 112

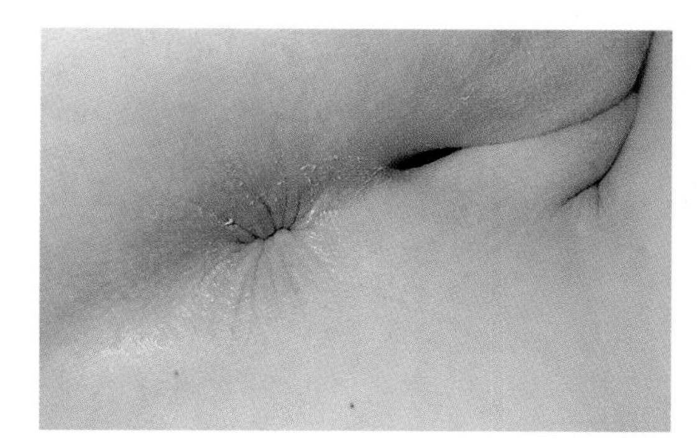

Plate 113

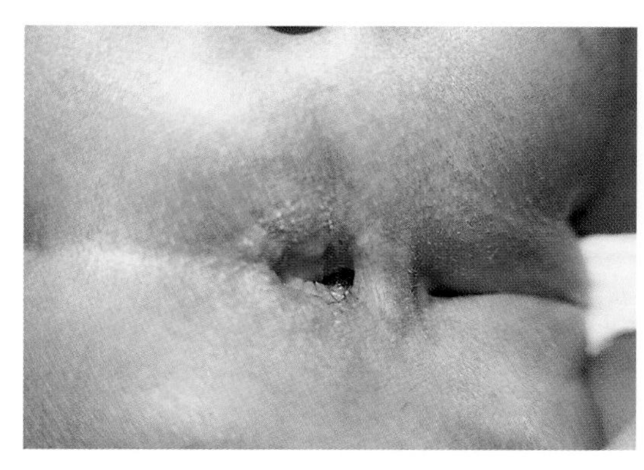

Plate 114

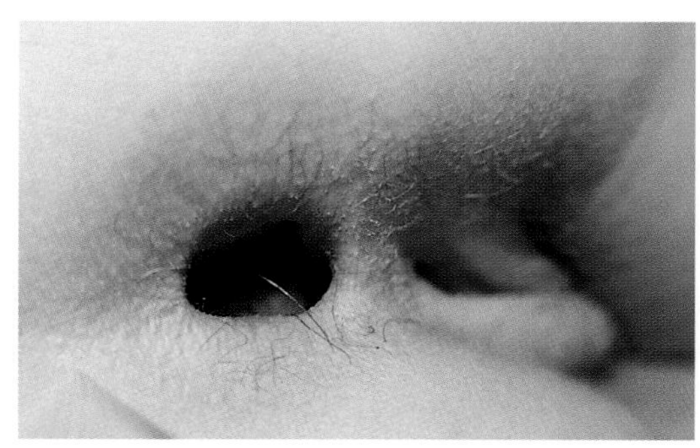

Plate 110 2-year-old child taken to Accident and Emergency department by anxious parents who discovered this unexplained injury. Deep laceration proximally on dorsum extending around a third of the circumference which required suture.
Plate 111 6-month-old taken to Accident and Emergency department with extensive old bruising to face and recent bruising to lower abdomen and scrotum. Investigation showed extensive damage to left testis and von Willebrand's disease. A diagnosis of non-accidental injury was made.
Plate 112 Normal anus in 2-year-old child, out of nappies. Note line of anterior–posterior closure with smooth regular radiating folds.
Plate 113 2-year-old black girl with sudden onset of nightmares, wetting and clinginess noted at home and in day nursery. Anus shows dilatation, 'tyre sign' and some perianal venous congestion. Signs had healed in one week. Child said 'Daddy's snake bited my bottom'. (Reproduced with permission from Hobbs C J, Wynne J M 1986 Buggery in childhood – a common syndrome of child abuse. Lancet ii: 795. Hobbs C J, Wynne J M 1989 Sexual abuse of English boys and girls. The importance of anal examination. Child Abuse and Neglect 13: 201–202.)
Plate 114 Wide dilatation in a 12-year-old girl who had a history of anal intercourse with father over a 6 year period. Resolution of signs was gradual over about 12 months. (Reproduced with permission from Hobbs C J, Wynne J M 1986 Buggery in childhood – a common syndrome of child abuse. Lancet ii: 795.)

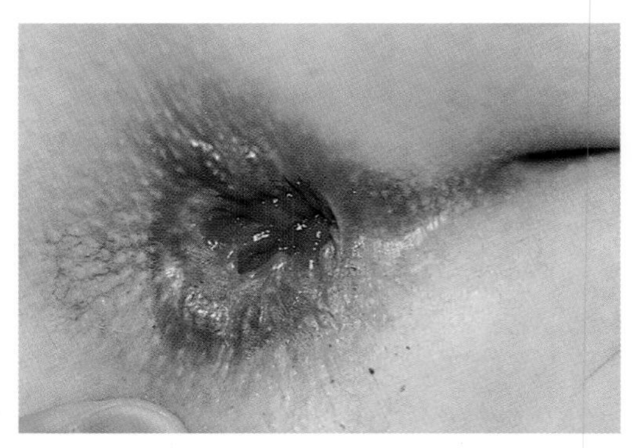

Plate 115

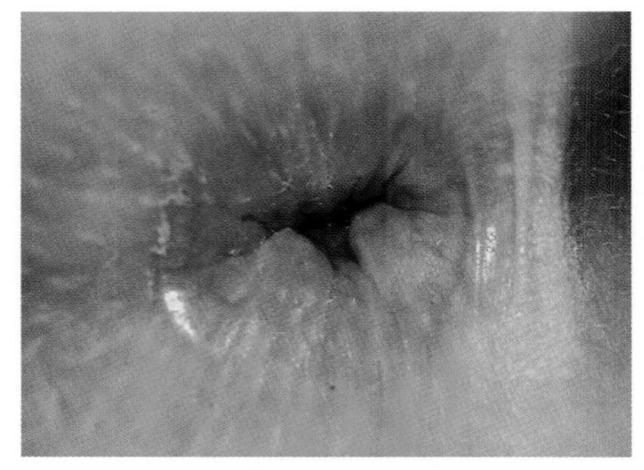

Plate 116

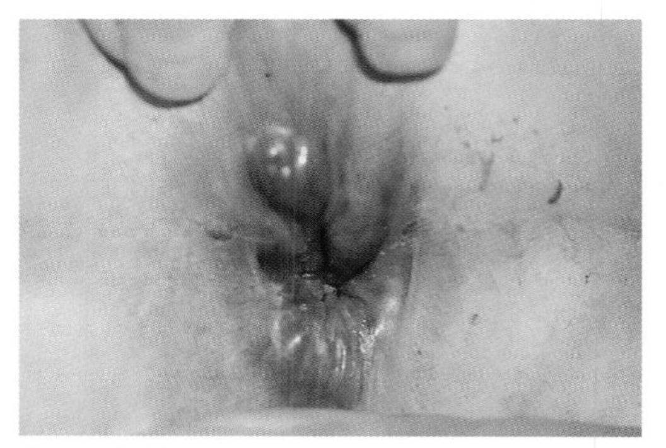

Plate 117 (a)

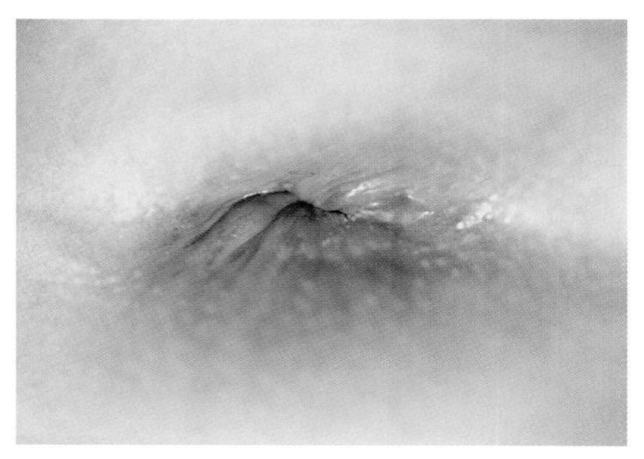

Plate 117 (b)

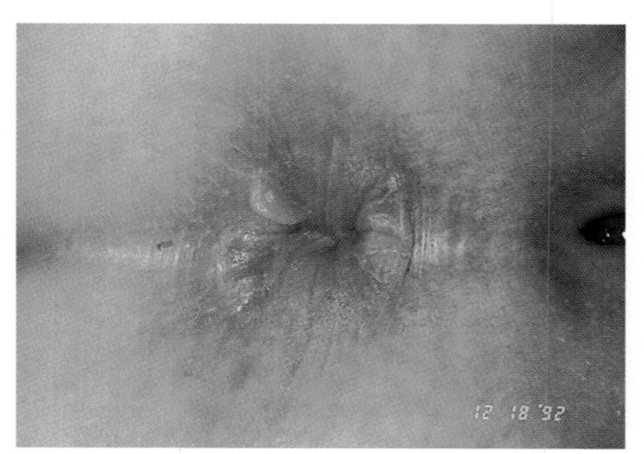

Plate 118

Plate 115 Gross anal abnormality in 3-year-old girl who had exhibited aggressive biting of younger brother. Lax dilated anus with deep fissures, swollen rim and venous (dark) congestion in a half-circle around the posterior anus. Prominent skin papillae are noted suggesting oedema of the tissues. Two other children in family with similar findings discovered. (Reproduced with permission from Hobbs C J, Wynne J M 1989 Sexual abuse of English boys and girls. The importance of anal examination. Child Abuse and Neglect 13: 201–202.)

Plate 116 Anal verge deficit at 3 o'clock in a chronically abused child aged 4 years.(same child as Plate 115). There is also a ring of veins around the anus.

Plate 117 (a) Gross venous dilatation, multiple anal fissures and reddening in a 5-year-old boy with scalds in his groins, bruised ear and frozen watchfulness. He disclosed physical and sexual abuse by his father. (b) Follow-up examination at 6 weeks demonstrates healing but persisting irregular folds and venous dilatation(Plate 117a reproduced with permission from Hobbs C J, Wynne J M 1987 Child sexual abuse – an increasing rate of diagnosis. Lancet ii: 839. Hanks H, Hobbs C J, Wynne J M 1988 Recognition of sexual abuse in the preschool child. In: Browne K, Davies c, Stratton P (eds) Early prediction and prevention of child abuse. J Wiley, Chichester.)

Plate 118 2-year-old with a past history of non-accidental injury (fracture and burn) and sexual abuse in infancy. After admission to foster-care referred to a paediatrician because of aggressive behaviour. Examination showed no recent signs of anal abuse but dilated veins, tags at 12 and 7 o'clock and possible scar anteriorly.

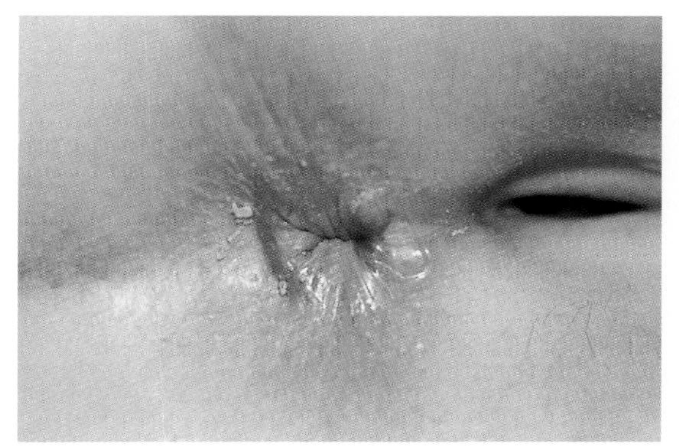

Plate 119

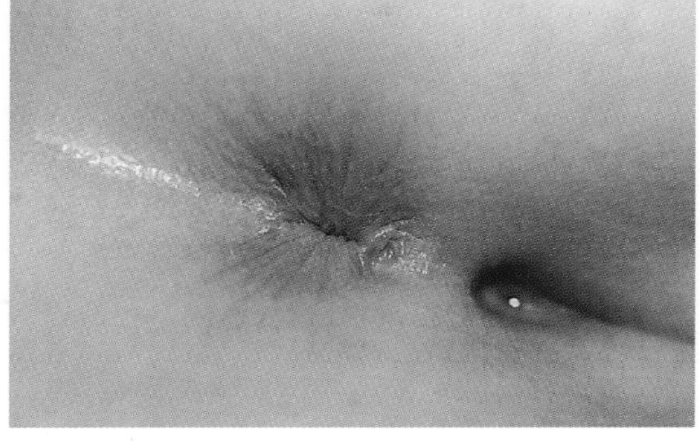

Plate 120

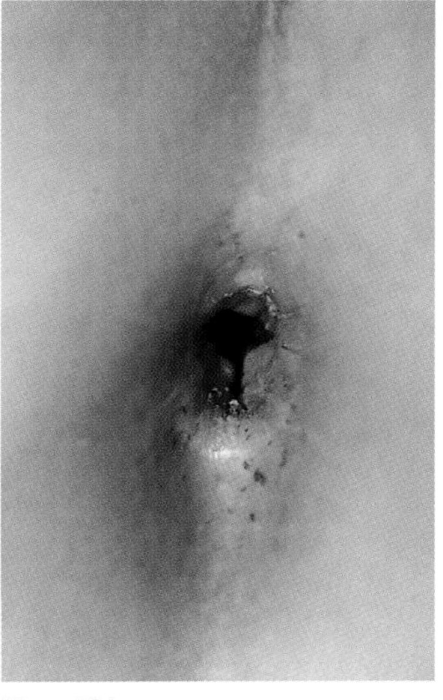

Plate 121

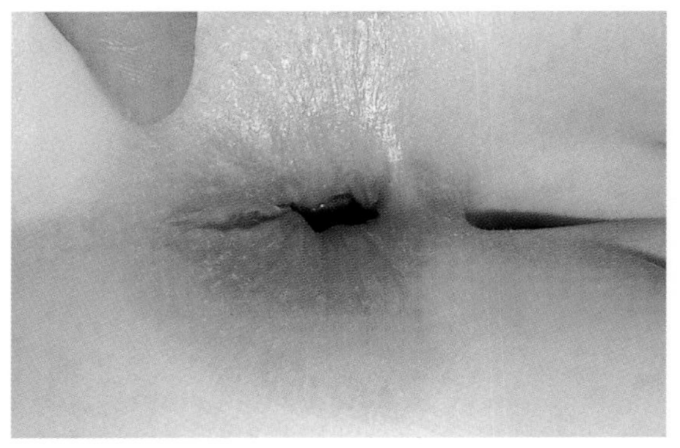

Plate 122

Plate 119 8-year-old girl with abnormally dilated hymenal opening. Anus shows pale, wide, deep anterior tear with swollen prominent fold adjacent to it. The anus is closed and the other folds are reasonable normal. There is a posterior band of dark venous congestion and the whole of the anus is darkened by venous discoloration. (Reproduced with permission from Hobbs C J, Wynne J M 1987 Child sexual abuse C an increasing rate of diagnosis. Lancet ii: 839. Hobbs C J, Wynne J M 1989 Sexual abuse of English boys and girls. The importance of anal examination. Child Abuse and Neglect 13: 201–202.)
Plate 120 Same child as Plate 86, 4 months later, to demonstrate healing. Anterior scar with prominent V-shaped ridges present. Dusky colouration but no evidence of localised venous congestion present.
Plate 121 Anal appearance in a 9-year-old boy with previous history of failure to thrive, non-accidental bruising, toddler scald following neglect, severe behavioural and learning difficulties requiring residential special education. There is anal dilatation, a deep chronic posterior fissure and smooth pink skin around the anal margin. Venous discoloration and funnelling are also present. (Reproduced with permission from Hobbs C J, Wynne J M 1986 Buggery in childhood – a common syndrome of child abuse. Lancet ii: 795.)
Plate 122 7-year-old girl described anal bleeding to doctor during boarding-out medical. She had been left in care of older brothers while her mother was admitted to hospital to give birth to her seventh child. The child quickly disclosed anal abuse the previous night. Examination showed perianal reddening, gaping anus and extensive posterior fissure. The signs are compatible with recent buggery.

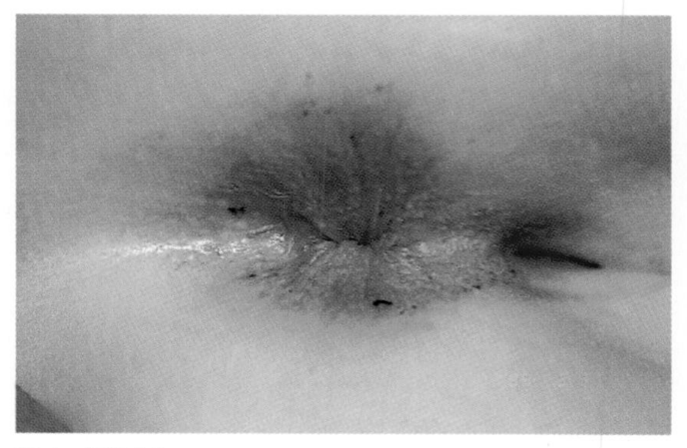

Plate 123 (a)

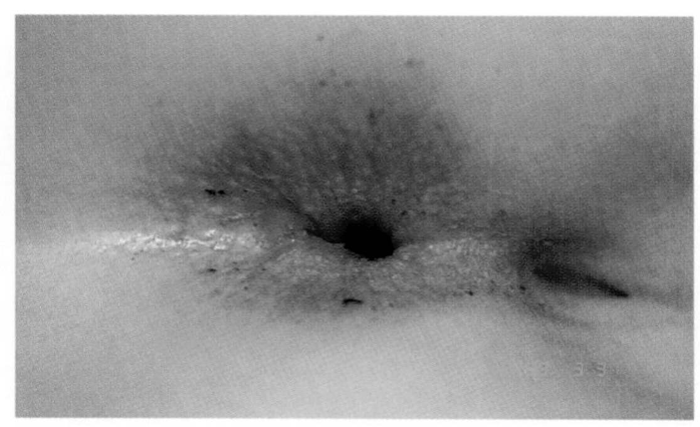

Plate 123 (b)

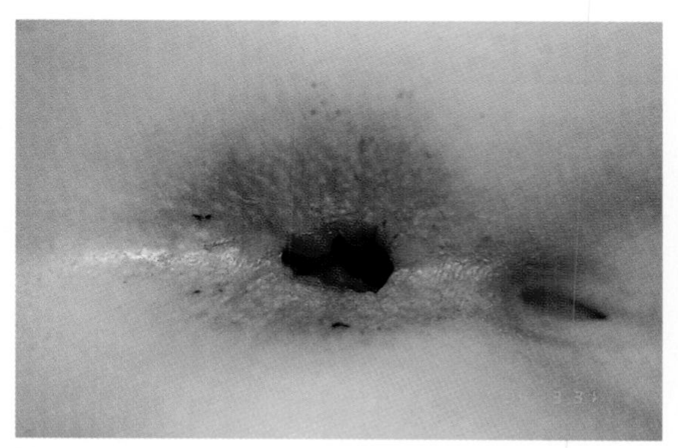

Plate 123 (c)

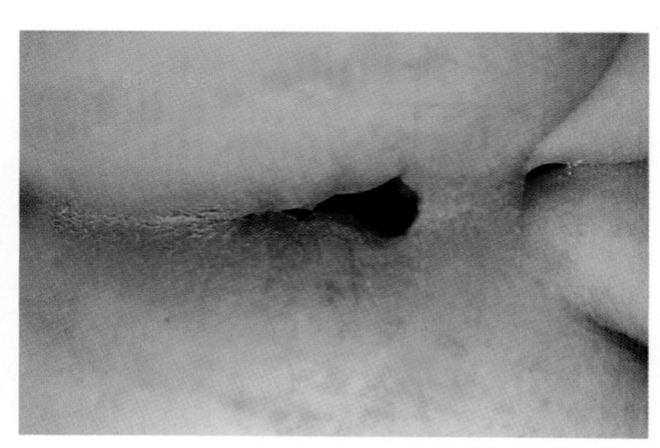

Plate 124

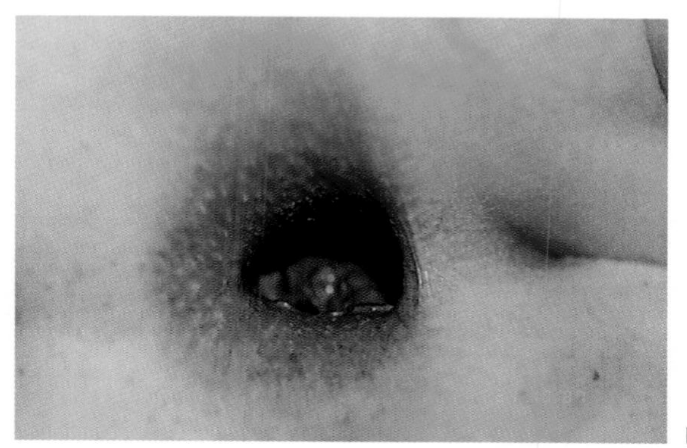

Plate 125

Plate 123 Plates a–c demonstrate the sign of reflex anal dilatation. They were taken in succession with brief intervals between them. Following dilatation the anus will usually close again. 5-year-old child sexually abused by her older teenage brother. The anus is reddened. Vulva showed evidence of multiple abrasions, swelling and reddening.
Plate 124 Lax gaping anus in an 18-month-old left in the care of an alcoholic violent cohabitee while mother had her child in hospital. The child had suffered serious non-accidental injury at the hands of her natural father, who was imprisoned. There was a vulval abrasion and these anal findings, which resolved fully within 7 days. (Reproduced with permission from Hanks H, Hobbs C J, Wynne J M 1988 Recognition of sexual abuse in the pre-school child. In: Browne K, Davies C, Stratton P (eds) Early prediction and prevention of child abuse. John Wiley & Sons, Chichester.)
Plate 125 Skin tags in a 5-year-old girl involved in sexual acting-out at school. History of sexual abuse by grandfather who also abused the child's mother. There are no signs of recent abuse.

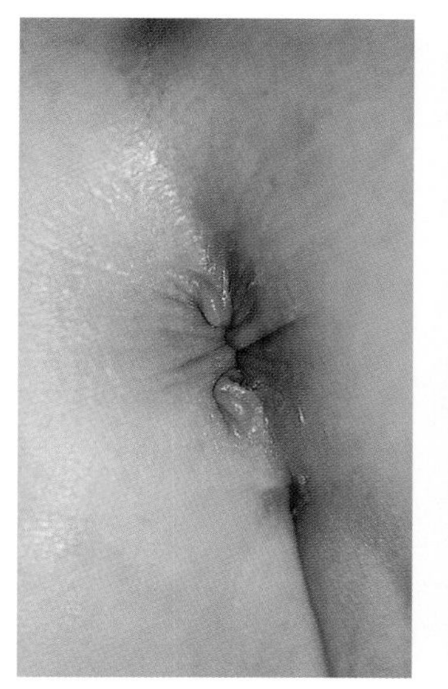

Plate 126

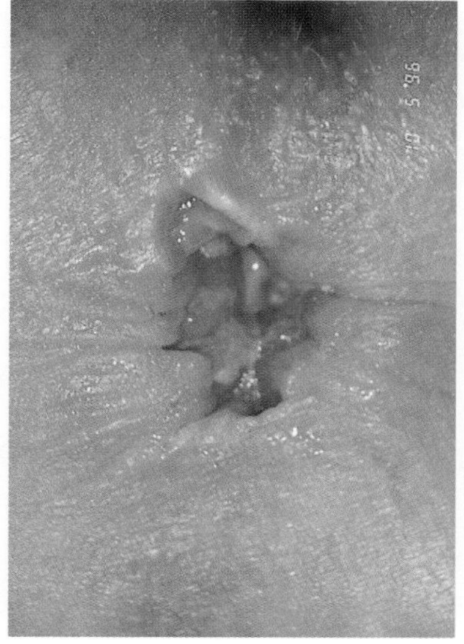

Plate 127

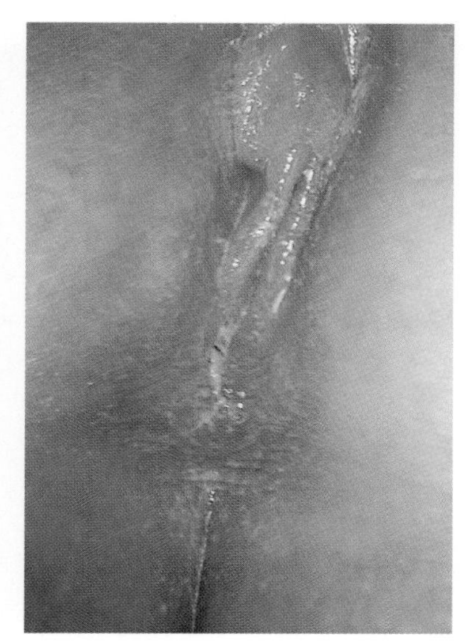

Plate 129 (a)

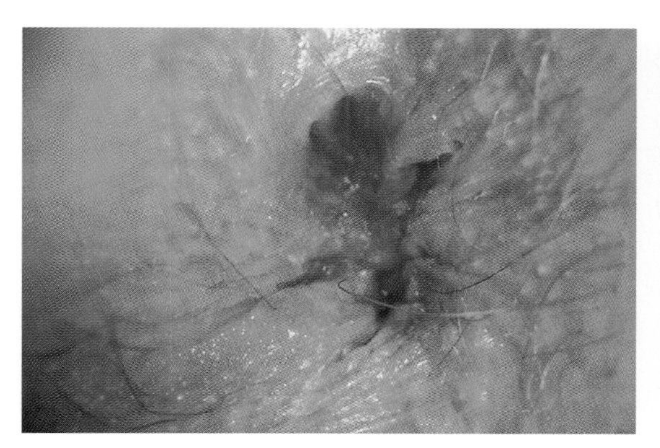

Plate 128

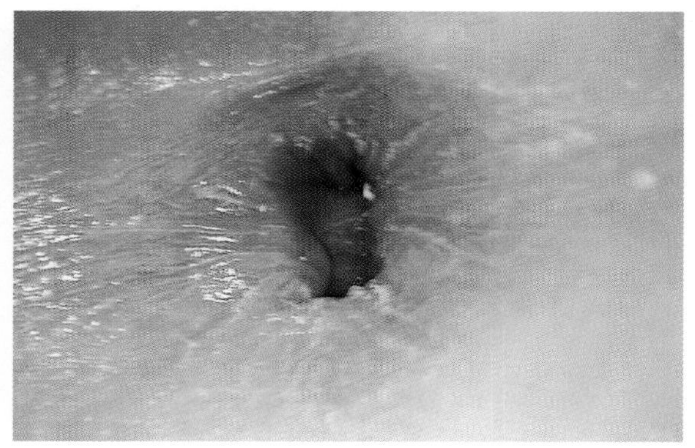

Plate 129 (b)

Plate 126 Dilated anus in a soiling, grossly constipated 5-year-old child who disclosed anal intercourse by her older (teenage) brother. Signs of anal dilatation, soiling and constipation fluctuated together over a 2 year period at home while attempts were made to protect her by removing her three brothers, who all in turn abused her. Signs and symptoms settled entirely in a residential home. This plate shows reddening around a smoothly dilated anus with faeces present in the lower rectum.

Plate 127 6-month-old baby admitted to hospital after widely gaping anus noticed by general practitioner. Infant had been taken to the general practitioner because of intercurrent illness. The mother had noticed the baby's bottom gaping 2 months earlier but it resolved spontaneously. On examination, disrupted very lax anus with prolapsing mucosa. Note extensive V-shaped tear at 10–12 o'clock.

Plate 128 Multiple fissures in a lax disrupted anus in a 12-year-old girl with multiple abusers. The examination was undertaken 3 weeks after she was taken into protective care and after abuse was thought to have stopped.

Plate 129 (a) Presented at the Accident and Emergency department by her mother with a 5-day history of unexplained abdominal bruising in the form of a wide band around her lower abdomen. Previous history of extensive labial fusion surgically treated. Examination showed extensive labial fusion and (b) markedly abnormal anus with perianal reddening, oedema and gaping anal sphincter with prolapsing rectal mucosa. A clinical diagnosis of sexual abuse was made.

Plate 130

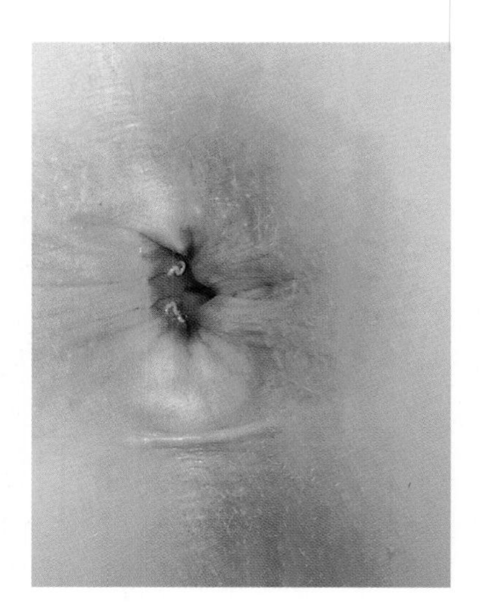

Plate 131

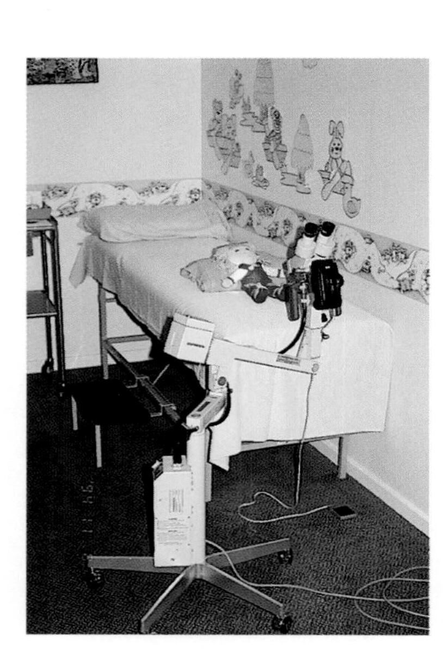

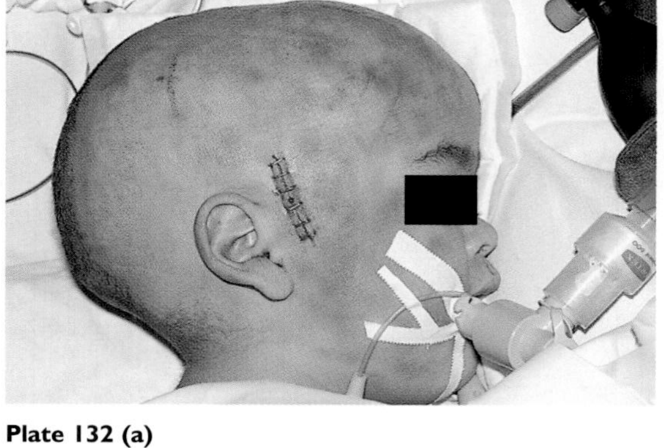

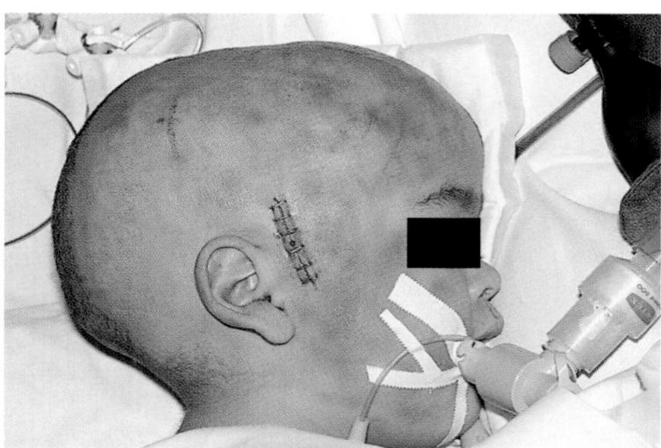

Plate 132 (a)

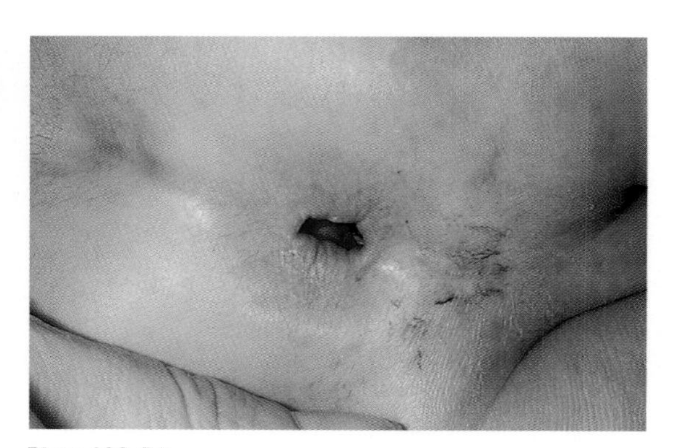

Plate 132 (b)

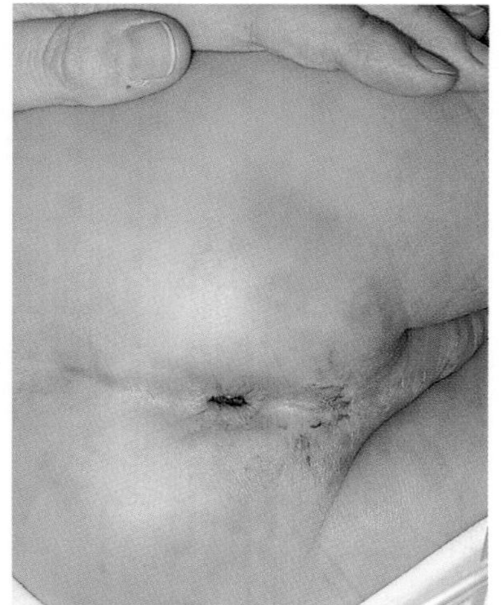

Plate 132 (c)

Plate 130 Anal scarring in an abused boy of 5 years. Two threadworms are also present.

Plate 131 Olympus OCS Colposcope with 35 mm camera attached. The camera shutter can be fired by remote release, e.g. by foot.

Plate 132 Healing of anal signs in a deeply unconscious 2-year-old boy: (a) facial signs; (b) anal signs at 2 days; (c) anal signs at 5 days.

Summary

1. The neglect and abuse of children with special needs is emerging as a major concern.
2. The prevalence of abuse in disabled children and adults is greater than for the general population. Data is not collected systematically in the UK. In the UK there are 360 000 children under 16 years who are disabled: 5000 live in residential care and 16 000 in residential schools. It has been estimated that 15% of those living away from home do so because of abuse, 8% child sexual abuse and 7% physical abuse (Bone & Meltzer 1989).
3. How much neglect and emotional abuse occurs at home? What is the incidence of all abuses in alternative care?
4. Particular groups such as the hearing impaired are at especial risk, but no group is exempt from abuse.
5. Children may be abused at home, on transport, at school, in foster or respite care, in a hospital or hostel, or anywhere.
6. In particular, child sexual abuse will only be recognised if parents and professionals are prepared to see and hear.
7. Why is so little neglect, emotional abuse and non-organic failure to thrive recognised?
8. Disabled children are particularly vulnerable because of their low status, dependency, difficulties in communication and need for companionship.
9. Traditionally, sexually explicit behaviours have been considered as part of the disorder rather than learned ones.
10. Abusers recognise disabled children as easy targets of low status with whom they may have sex with relative impunity.
11. Children are distressed by the abuse but their attempts to communicate may be misinterpreted as fantasy or challenging behaviour; disbelief may lead to psychotic breakdown in the children with learning disorders.
12. Skilled professionals with particular communication skills are needed, and usual methods of interviewing are not always appropriate. Direct questioning and leading questions may be necessary if the child is to be understood.
13. Criminal proceedings are rare unless there is an admission by the abuser or there is additional corroborative evidence.
14. Family Courts are able to hear evidence not admissible in other courts in order to ensure the welfare of the child.
15. Child victims may become abusers, in older childhood and adolescence. The abusive behaviour warrants urgent assessment *and* treatment.
16. Children with severe or multiple disability can be successfully placed with substitute families but support and planning is essential (BAAF 1996).
17. Prevention lies in:
    - implementation of the Children Act 1989 to assist families to adequately meet the needs of their disabled child
    - acceptance that disabled people have ordinary needs of respect, dignity, privacy and development socially (including sexually)
    - understanding – appropriate sex education for all children
    - education and support of carers and professionals including foster carers and residential workers
    - conviction of abusers
    - therapeutic services, with priority for young abusers.

REFERENCES

Ammerman R T, Van Hasselt V, Hersen M 1988 Abuse and neglect in handicapped children: a critical review. Journal of Family Violence 3:53–72

Ammerman R T, Van Hasselt V, Hersen M, McGonigle J J, Lubetsky M J 1989 Abuse and neglect in psychiatrically hospitalised multihandicapped children. Child Abuse and Neglect 13:335–343

Ammerman R T, Hersen M, van Hasselt, V B, Lubetsky, M J, Sieck W R 1994 Maltreatment in psychiatrically children and adolescents with developmental disabilities: prevalence and correlates. Journal of American Academy of Child and Adolescent Psychiatry 33(4):567–576

BAAF Hedi Argent 1996 The placement of children with disabilities. Practice Note 34, Skyline House, 200 Union Street, London SE1 0LX

Baker A W, Duncan S P 1985 Child sex abuse: a study of prevalence in Great Britain. Child Abuse and Neglect 9:457–467
Bone M, Meltzer H 1989 The prevalence of disability among children. HMSO, London
Chamberlain A, Rauh J, Passer A, McGrath M, Burket R 1984 Issues in fertility control for mentally retarded female adolescents. Sexual activity, sexual abuse and contraception. Pediatrics 73(4):445–450
Cooke L B 1990 Abuse of mentally handicapped adults. British Medical Journal 300:193
Degener T 1992 The right to be different: implications for child protection. Child Abuse Review 1:151–155
Dunne T P, Power A 1990 Sexual abuse and mental handicap. Preliminary findings of a community based study. Mental Handicap Research 3:111–125
Elvick S L, Berkowitz C D, Nicholas E, Lindley Lipman J, Inkelis S H 1990 Sexual abuse in the developmentally disabled: dilemmas of diagnosis. Child Abuse and Neglect 14:497–502
Finkelhor D 1984 Child sexual abuse. New theory and research. Free Press, New York
Finkelhor D, Baron L 1986 High risk children. In: Finkelhor D (ed) A sourcebook on child sexual abuse. Sage, London, p 83
Home Office 1992 Memorandum of good practice on video recorded interviews and child witnesses for criminal proceedings. Home Office and Department of Health, London
Howlin P, Clements J 1995 Is it possible to assess the impact of abuse on children with pervasive developmental disorders? Journal of Autism and Developmental Disorders 25(4):337–354
Illingworth R S 1987 The development of the infant and young child. Normal and abnormal. Churchill Livingstone, Edinburgh, pp 20, 342
Kelly L 1992 The connections between disability and child abuse: a review of the research evidence. Child Abuse Review 1(3):157–168
Kennedy M 1989 The silent nightmare. Soundbarrier: March.
Kennedy M 1992 Not the only way to communicate: a challenge to voice on child protection work. Child Abuse Review 1(3):169–168
Kennedy M 1995 Perceptions of abused disabled children. in Wilson K, James A (eds) The child protection handbook. Baillière Tindall, London, Chapter 7
Kohane M, Pothier P, Norbeck J 1987 Hospitalized children with a history of sexual abuse: incidence and care issues. American Journal of Orthopsychiatry 57(2):258–264
Krents E J, Atkins D V 1986 Guide to 'No-Go-Tell' New York. Lexington Center, New York
Lynch M, Roberts J 1982 Ill health and physical handicap. In: Lynch M, Roberts J (eds) Consequences of child abuse. Academic Press, New York
McCormack B 1991 Sexual abuse and learning difficulties (leader). British Medical Journal 303:143–144
Marchant R 1991 Myths and facts about sexual abuse and children with disabilities. Child Abuse Review 5(2):22
Marchant R, Page M 1992 Bridging the gap: investigating the abuse of children with disabilities. Child Abuse Review 1(3):179–184
Mullen P E 1991 The consequences of child sexual abuse (leader). British Medical Journal 303:144
NCB 1996 Highlight 143. Children with disabilities and child protection. National Children's Bureau, 8 Wakley Street, London EC1V 7QE
NCCAN 1993 Maltreatment of children with disabilities. Information sheet. National Centre on Child Abuse and Neglect, 63 Inverness Drive East, Englewood, CO 80112–5117, USA
Newport P 1991 Linking child abuse with disability.
RCP 1991 Report. Physical signs of sexual abuse in children. Royal College of Physicians, London
Ridgeway S M 1993 Abuse and deaf children: some factors to consider. Child Abuse Review 2:3;166–173
Ryerson E 1984 Sexual and self-protection education for disabled youth: a primary need. SIECUS Report XIII(1):1–7
Schor D P 1987 Sex and sexual abuse in developmentally disabled adolescents. Seminars in Adolescent Medicine 3(1):1–7
Sinason V 1992 Therapy. Paper presented 7 January 1992 in study day on abuse of young people with learning difficulties to Paediatrics Child Abuse Interest Group, Salford
Sullivan P M, Vernon M, Scanlan J M 1987 Sexual abuse of deaf youth. American Annals of the Deaf 3:256–262
Verdugo M A, Bermejo B G, Fuertes J 1995 The maltreatment of intellectually handicapped children and adolescents. Child Abuse and Neglect 19(2):205–215
Vizard E 1989 Child sexual abuse and mental handicap: a child psychiatrist' perspective. In: Brown H, Craft A (eds) Thinking the unthinkable. FPA Educational Unit, London
Vizard E, Tranter M 1988 Recognition and assessment of child sexual abuse. In: Bentovim A, Elton A, Hildebrand J, Tranter M, Vizard E (eds) Child sexual abuse within the family: assessment and treatment. John Wright, Bristol
Wadsworth D J, Abel K 1987 Some aspects of the primary identification of sexual abuse in children: experiences from a residential setting. Child Abuse Review 1(6)

RECOMMENDED READING AND RESOURCES

ABCD (Abuse and Children who are Disabled) training and resource pack. Available from NSPCC, 3,Gilmour Close, Beaument Leys, Leicester LE4 1EZ
Brown H, Craft A (eds) 1989 Thinking the unthinkable. FPA Education Unit, 27–35 Mortimer Street, London WIN 7RJ
Craft A (ed) 1994 Practice issues in sexuality and learning disabilities. Routledge, London
Kennedy M, Kelly L (eds) 1992 Special issue on abuse and children with disability. Child Abuse Review 1(3)
Morgan S R 1987 Abuse and neglect of handicapped children. College Hill Press
Sinason V 1993 The special vulnerability of the handicapped child and adult: with special reference to mental handicap. In: Hobbs C J, Wynne J M (eds) Child abuse. Baillière Tindall, London, Chapter 4
Westcott H, Cross M 1996 This far and no further: towards ending the abuse of disabled children. Venture Press,

11

Fetal problems

Damage in utero

A fetus may be damaged in utero by acts of omission or commission. For a pregnancy to have the best outcome it should be planned, the parents should be healthy and mutually supportive and the mother's diet should be good.

Factors that affect fetal health

- Mother's abuse of drugs (non-therapeutic)
- Mother's abuse of alcohol
- Mother's abuse of tobacco
- Physical abuse
  - directed at mother
  - directed at fetus
- Mother's non-attendance at antenatal clinic
- Mother's age (teenager)
- Father's neglect of mother's needs
- Poverty, poor housing, poor nutrition of mother
- Unwanted, unplanned, uncared-for pregnancy

All mothers and babies need to receive good obstetric and neonatal care. The principal adverse factors affecting outcome are maternal poverty, youth and unmarried status. Fetal abuse (physical or substance) is theoretically preventable. Education and increased social support are required to begin to eradicate substance addiction: the reasons why women abuse drugs are many and often socially determined. Partner violence increases during pregnancy and is intolerable. The fetus may be harmed as a direct consequence of physical assault of the mother or harm directed at the fetus (Condon 1987).

Being the fetus of a woman who regularly abuses alcohol or drugs is clearly risky, but definitions of fetal maltreatment are difficult to formulate. The effects of substance abuse, often compounded by cigarette smoking and adverse lifestyle are well described and include:

- increased mortality, prenatally and postnatally
- pre-term birth
- teratogenicity
- growth retardation
- short- and long-term neurobehavioural problems.

The direct and indirect effects of drugs and alcohol misuse are listed in Tables 11.1, 11.2 and 11.3.

Prevalence of drug and substance abuse

In the UK drug and substance abuse is rapidly increasing, mirroring the experience of the US where in 1992 36% of the entire population had used an illegal drug in their life and 11% in the last year (Bell 1995). There is a difference between substance misuse and recreational drug and alcohol use (Coleman & Cassell 1995). Alcohol or cannabis use is widespread and research shows little overlap with, for example, the use of crack (Mirza et al 1991). Cocaine use may be recreational and does not inevitably lead to addiction and all the adverse consequences associated with drug dependence (Ditton).

In the UK 15–16 year olds (Miller & Plant 1996) in a self-reported questionnaire were using drugs, cigarettes and alcohol. In the previous 30 days 42.3% had used an illicit drug (mainly cannabis), 36% had smoked cigarettes, and almost all had drunk alcohol. A study of young people reported in 1994 that 42% of 16–19 year olds living in inner-city areas had taken drugs at some time (IDD 1994).

Of 54 pregnant women attending the Leeds Addiction Unit in 1995–96, 33 used opioids, 6 stimulants, 2 alcohol, 1 solvents, 12 unspecified. This is similar to the total population attending the unit (Annual Report 1995/6). The outcome for 10 drug/substance abusing mothers attending a community paediatric clinic as part of routine follow-up/support (over 2–18 months) was as follows (Wynne 1997: unpublished).

In assessing the consequences of addictive behaviour on child rearing it is necessary to define the various factors in each case (Figs 11.1 and 11.2, Table 11.4 and Appendix, p. 447).

Table 11.1 Intrauterine effects of drug and substance abuse

Drug	Congenital malformation	Impaired intra-uterine growth	Abortion, pre-term labour	Neonatal withdrawal symptoms
Alcohol	+	+	+	+
Cigarettes	–	+	+	–
Cannabis	–	+	–	+
Opiates	–	+	+	+
Cocaine	+	+	+	+
Amphetamine	–	–	–	+
Benzodiazepine	–	+	+	+
Barbiturates	–	–	+	+
Phencyclidine	+	+	–	+
Heroin	+	+	+	+
Methadone	–	–	–	±

+, Present; –, absent.

Research and the legal rights of the fetus

It is not clear why so few alcoholic mothers are recognised and referred compared with other addicted women. Research in this field is made difficult because of unreliable histories, the complex interaction of the drug(s) taken, when, how

Table 11.2 Deaths

Parent	Drug	Consequences
Father	amphetamine	Overlay 18-month-old son on settee and child found dead in morning. First child died in similar way
Mother 17 years old	heroin	Neglected 15-month-old daughter who was found dead in cot, she had been dead sometime
Mother 26 years old Single	heroin	Heroin abuse at beginning of pregnancy, mental health problems, baby died 'SIDS' at 3-months-old

Table 11.3 Consequences of intrauterine intoxication for infant

Drug	Respiratory distress	Jittery, hyperactive	Lethargic	Poor feeding	Irritable	GI upset	Fits	Congenital malformation	Behavioural abnormality	Developmental abnormality	SIDS	Failure to thrive	HIV
Alcohol	+	+	–	+	++	–	+	+	+	+	+	+	–
Cigarettes	–	–	–	–	–	–	–	–	–	–	+	–	–
Cannabis	–	+	–	–	–	–	–	–	–	–	–	–	–
Opiates	+	+	–	+	+	–	+	–	+	+	+	+	+
Cocaine	+	+	+	+	++	–	+	+	+	+	+	+	+
Amphetamine	–	+	+	–	–	–	–	–	–	+	–	–	–
Benzodiazepine	+	–	+	+	–	–	–	–	+	–	–	–	–
Barbiturates	+	+	–	+	+	–	+	–	–	–	–	–	–
Phencyclidine	–	+	+	–	–	+	+	+	–	–	–	+	–
Heroin	+	+	–	+	+	+	+	+	+	+	+	+	+
Methadone	+	–	–	–	–	–	+	–	+	–	+	–	–

+, *Present*; –, *absent*.

much, socio-economic status (poverty, education, nutrition), and prenatal and post-natal care.

The law in the UK permits research on embryos up to the age of 14 days and elective abortion until 24 weeks (in some circumstances 28 weeks). The rights of the fetus as a separate being may thus be considered to begin at 28 weeks or when the mother has decided to continue with the pregnancy.

The situation under the law is complex. In 1987 Berkshire County Council sought to remove at birth a child, who was the victim of drug withdrawal, from her heroin-addicted mother (D [a minor] v Berkshire County Council 1987). The case was eventually heard in the House of Lords who found that 'X is being neglected or ill treated' could be interpreted under the Child and Young Persons Act 1969 to include the intrauterine phase of life. The argument was that child care was a continuum and that, if neglect was part of this continuum, the court could consider conditions occurring before the child was born.

An Appeal Court judgment in 1995 (*Guardian* 1995) has further clarified the law with reference to the fetus. A woman who was 24 weeks pregnant was stabbed in the abdomen by her drunken partner. Initially it was thought that the fetus was unharmed but at delivery 2 weeks later there were stab wounds which had injured the fetus with resultant small bowel damage requiring several operations. The infant died 3 weeks later of respiratory complications secondary to her prematurity (Puntis et al 1995). Conviction for murder or manslaughter was not possible on the grounds that the fetus was not 'a person in being'. In addition, murder requires an intention to cause death or serious bodily harm but under the doctrine of 'transferred malice' a person may be convicted of murder if he intends to kill A but kills B instead. A doctor carrying out an abortion at 24 weeks under the Abortion Act 1967 would not be acting unlawfully, as murder requires an unlawful act: this had been the defence's argument. The judgment was that the defendant could have been, in law, charged with murder or manslaughter of his daughter in addition to wounding his partner.

In the US state of South Carolina it has been ruled that a viable fetus is a person. A 33-year-old woman was successfully prosecuted because her son was born with traces of cocaine in his system. This is the only US state where this example is extant (McCready 1997).

Effects of substance abuse

Ongoing substance abuse will affect the carer(s) ability to meet the infant's needs. How the drug(s) affects the mother/carer will depend on

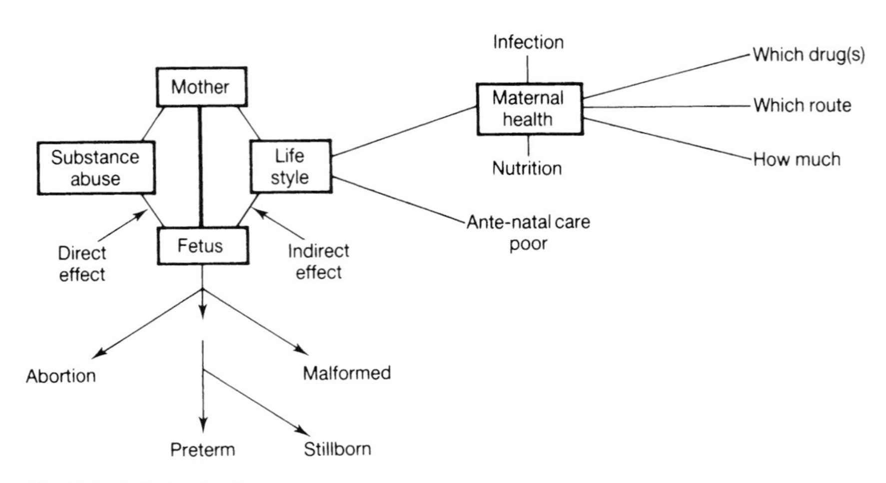

Fig. 11.1 Relationship between substance abuse and lifestyle.

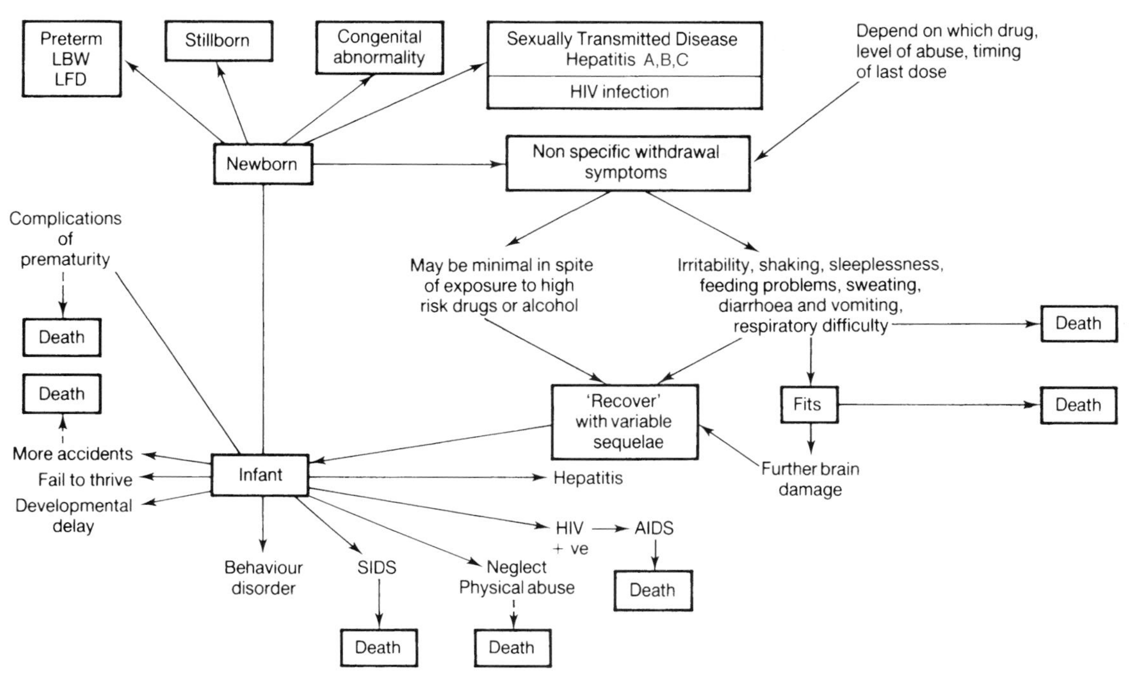

Fig. 11.2 Possible effect of substance abuse on newborn and infant.

the drug, amounts used and, indirectly, on the cost of her habit. She may have to earn up to £100 a day, and for most women this inevitably means theft or prostitution. The direct effects of individual drugs and alcohol have been listed with particular reference to their influence on fetus, child and child rearing (Coleman & Cassell 1995) (Tables 11.2, 11.3 and Appendix, p. 447).

Ideally drug addiction is recognised at the initial antenatal booking clinic and referral made to the local addiction unit (if it is not already involved) with complex programmes of antenatal care in an attempt to minimise the ill-effects of substance abuse (Boer et al 1994).

Babies born in the UK to a mother who abuses alcohol or drugs may, when well, go home with their mother after a multidisciplinary assessment, started antenatally if possible, with continuing support (midwife, health visitor, addiction unit staff, general practitioner and paediatrician). This is not always possible and depends on the baby, family and level of risk.

Assessment of family and child care (after Swadi 1994, Coleman & Cassell 1995)

- Is there a good child–parent attachment?
- Are standards of parenting 'good enough'? Is the child safe?
- Does the child have learning or behavioural problems secondary to fetal damage? Are these special needs being met?
- How much does the drug habit cost – are other bills paid?
- Is the home adequately clean and is there enough food?
- Do other substance misusers live in the same house?
- Are the child's carers dependent on other drug abusers for support?
- Is the house used for selling drugs/prostitution?
- What is the pattern of abuse: which drug, frequency, method?

Table 11.4 Direct effects of drugs and alcohol (Coleman & Cassell 1995)

Drug	Pharmacological effects	Effects on parenting
Depressants: alcohol, sedatives, tranquillisers, solvents	Depresses CNS which relieves anxiety but impairs performance	Disinhibition, loss of self-control, drowsy Withdrawal symptoms
Opiates: heroin, DF118, codeine, methadone	Reduces discomfort or anxiety. In high doses sedation	'Copes' with regular doses, problems withdrawing, irregular amounts
Stimulants: amphetamines, cocaine, ecstasy	Increased wakefulness, elevated mood, increased performance	Withdrawal causes anxiety, depression, paranoia
Hallucinogenic: cannabis, LSD	Affects perception, distorted reality	Unpredictable 'trips' Flashbacks
Perinatal problems	Complications during pregnancy, labour, postnatally	Infant needs extra care low birthweight, congenital abnormality, jittery, fits, feeding problems

- Is the disposal of needles safe, are children at risk – HIV, hepatitis?
- Is there stable drug/alcohol misuse or swings/binges with intoxication/withdrawal?
- Are there alternative childcare plans to cover periods of intoxication?
- Has treatment been offered, failed, refused, is ongoing?
- What childcare plans are available for the carers' absences: procuring drugs, thieving, prostitution, prison?
- Does the carer(s) have other mental health problems?
- Are the children involved in drug/alcohol abuse?

Care of children with drug withdrawal symptoms

Babies may be very difficult to care for in the early stages of drug withdrawal (screaming, feeding poorly, 'jittery', seizures) and may need hospital care for several weeks and be 'difficult' thereafter (Table 11.3). The position may be complicated by ongoing drug or alcohol abuse, and maternal illness such as hepatitis, AIDS related illness or mental ill health. Alternative care is inevitable for some babies.

In the US the situation is now so critical that many babies remain in institutional care owing to the difficulty in finding foster-parents who are able to cope not only with the risk that the baby may be infected with HIV or hepatitis but also the fact that babies of addicts may be extremely difficult to care for due to brain damage sustained in utero (see later).

Male violence and fetal maltreatment

Men may be involved in fetal maltreatment by physically assaulting the mother. Family violence

Table 11.5 Indirect effects of drugs and alcohol abuse (Coleman & Cassell 1995)

Activity	Consequence
Drug-related activity	Maintaining an expensive habit – unless wealthy leads to fraud, theft, prostitution, drug dealing, prison, children in care
Aggression and violence	Children exposed to crime, sexual activity, violence
Accidents and illness	Children suffer separation and loss as drug abusers have high morbidity and mortality HIV may affect carers and child Mental illness more common in abusers Accidents > in child and adult SIDS: 17 times risk
Family life	Children become carers Lack of available adult to supervise so accidents, behavioural problems Lack of routines, e.g. being in time for school Unable to meet child's emotional needs
Child maltreatment	Alcoholism and drug abuse related to greater risk of care proceedings and 'care' Physical, sexual, emotional abuse and neglect

studies show that spouse abuse occurs with increased frequency and intensity during pregnancy (Gelles 1987, Bewley 1994).

Condon (1987) investigated the frequency of physical fetal abuse. In a study of 112 pregnant women 8% of women and 4% of fathers '. . . acknowledged the urge to hurt or punish their unborn child' and, for example, hit the fetus through the abdominal wall in response to fetal movement.

CASE HISTORY 11.1

A woman, aged 22 years, 24 weeks pregnant was admitted because of multiple stab wounds to her abdomen. Her partner, in a temper, had sought to injure her and her unborn baby. The abdominal wounds were explored and although initially it was thought the fetus was unharmed, subsequent radiology and premature delivery of the baby 2 weeks later revealed that the fetus too had been stabbed, causing extensive intra-abdominal injury. The baby died aged 3 weeks of respiratory complications secondary to her prematurity.

Men may also be emotionally abusive or negative about the pregnancy. They may facilitate the mother's access to drink or drugs. They may fail to provide materially. A woman who is anxious or depressed (as many drug abusers are) needs emotionally supportive friends and family about her if she is to cope with her own drug withdrawal to better preserve the pregnancy. Unfortunately her partner and friends often also abuse alcohol or drugs, which makes it all the more difficult for the pregnant woman to alter her lifestyle. Women who abuse alcohol are also notoriously secretive in their habits and frequently do not seek help. Society appears to be more disapproving of women who drink, which may also inhibit some women from asking for help; certainly there are few facilities for alcoholic women.

Maternal alcohol and drug abuse

Drug and alcohol abusing women who become pregnant have several characteristics in common which make it difficult to assess the importance of the various factors involved in damaging the fetus.

- It is difficult to obtain a clear, accurate history as to which drugs have been abused, at what dose and how often.
- Many women abuse several drugs and in addition drink too much alcohol and smoke tobacco.
- They tend to neglect their own health and their nutrition is suboptimal.
- They are frequently poor attenders at antenatal clinics.
- There is often a history of several previous pregnancies ending in spontaneous abortion.
- They may have abused drugs for several years, be anaemic and have sexually transmitted diseases, hepatitis or HIV (Fig. 11.1).

The effect on the pregnancy may be

- early miscarriage
- fetal damage
- pre-term delivery
- stillbirth
- neonatal illness or death.

Consequences reaching into infancy include

- increased risk of SIDS
- developmental delay and learning problems
- behavioural disorders
- neglect
- physical abuse (Fig. 11.2).

However, some infants appear to survive unscathed. There are recognisable clinical patterns relating to the drug which is abused. These are listed in Tables 11.4 and 11.5.

Alcohol abuse (DOH 1995, Day 1995)

In the UK, alcohol abuse is the commonest form of substance abuse. One in 20 adults is dependent on alcohol, compared with 1 in 45 addicted to drugs (legal and illegal).

- 2% of women are drinking at levels likely to damage their health (more than 35 units per week)

- 40% of domestic violence includes alcohol, witnessing this violence causes emotional distress to children
- 30% of physical abuse of children is alcohol related
- child sexual abuse may be enabled by alcohol use (RCP 1995, Alcohol Concern 1997)
- alcoholic parents cannot supervise their children, leading to accidents as well as physical and emotional neglect.

Fetal alcohol syndrome

Fetal alcohol syndrome (FAS) was initially recognised in 1968 by Lemoine et al and re-described independently in 1973 in the children of chronically alcoholic women by Jones et al (1973). The syndrome represents a clinical continuum from the severe cases described by Lemoine to those less seriously damaged (Smith 1982).

Fetal alcohol effects (FAE) describes the consequences of alcohol abuse without the morphological features listed in Tables 11.2 and 11.3 (Murray-Lyon 1989). They include

- learning problems
- increased risk of perinatal death
- increased risk of epilepsy.

The learning problems in FAE and FAS vary from mild difficulty to mental retardation. The severity of the intellectual handicap is correlated to the severity of the physical characteristics. Infants may be hypotonic and irritable; older children have learning problems, poor coordination and are hyperactive. The growth deficiency may be marked, and catch-up growth is not generally achieved post-natally. Microcephaly also persists.

Long-term effects of fetal alcohol syndrome

The dysmorphic features of FAS become less obvious over time, but growth failure and learning problems are permanent even when subsequent child care is good. The continuing high level of psychosocial problems includes, in addition to learning difficulties (average IQ 63 in the 'classic form of FAS'), hyperactivity, impulsiveness and antisocial behaviour.

Summary of signs and symptoms of fetal alcohol syndrome (FAS)

- Growth deficiency, pre- and post-natally
- CNS defects: microcephaly, learning problems
- Distinctive facies: short palpebral fissures, flat midface, indistinct philtrum, short upturned nose
- Congenital anomalies: heart, eye, renal, skeletal defects
- As fetal alcohol effects

'Safe' drinking in pregnancy

Drinking patterns amongst women are changing in the UK. As women drink more, the effects of increased consumption are seen in the number of women where excessive drinking is a problem (around 10% of all drinkers), the increased death rate from alcohol-related disorders and admissions to mental hospital due to alcoholism (increased by 23% in 7 years).

How much alcohol is 'safe'? For non-pregnant women 14 units per week is considered non-toxic and 26 units per week is thought to be harmful. (A unit is equivalent to 10 g of alcohol, 1/2 pint of beer or 1 glass of wine, sherry or whisky.) During pregnancy, consumption of more than 8 units a day is associated with FAS. More moderate consumption is reported to result in an increased rate of spontaneous abortion, fetal malformation and fetal growth retardation. Moderate consumption was defined as up to 10 units per week, although there are reports of problems at lower levels of alcohol intake.

How many pregnant women do drink more than 10 units (100 g) of alcohol per week? This varies between 6 and 20% in different parts of the UK. In one study (Barrison et al 1985):

- 20% of mothers drank more than 10 units a week in the early stage of pregnancy
- 5% of mothers drank more than 5 units a day and were at risk of liver damage
- very few drank 8–10 units a day and were at risk of delivering a child with FAS
- consumption of alcohol falls in pregnancy except for heavy drinkers, and once

pregnancy was confirmed only 6% of women drank more than 10 units a week.

The prevalence of FAS in different countries – 1 in 100 live births in northern France, 1 in 600 in Sweden, 1 in 750 in Seattle and 1–2 per 1000 in the UK – reflects drinking patterns. In the UK women from ethnic minorities drink less than Caucasians, but not uniformly so (Barrison et al 1985).

The picture is not clear-cut; there are variable effects even for heavy drinkers – for example, one sibling of a chronically alcohol-abusing mother may be severely affected while other siblings are unharmed.

The frequent association of cigarette smoking and poor maternal nutrition also complicates the clinical picture. Education is important. Around the time of conception women should ideally drink no alcohol; this is difficult unless pregnancies are planned. It is not known whether persistent heavy drinking or peaks (binges) or both are more teratogenic. Logically, alcohol abstinence around conception is advisable, with only a limited amount of drink throughout the rest of pregnancy.

Cigarette smoking (Miller 1996)

Cigarette smoking is even more common than alcohol consumption and young women have been smoking more whilst the overall trend in the UK is towards a decrease in smoking. Smoking of five cigarettes a day has been associated with symmetrical growth retardation in the fetus (Wieburg et al 1985).

Babies may be light for dates for many reasons but the additive effect of alcohol and cigarette smoking has been noted. However, up to 30% of the low birthweight has been attributed to cigarette smoking. It has also been suggested that cigarettes are associated with spontaneous abortion, stillbirth and prematurity.

Heroin abuse (Bays 1993)

The effects of heroin abuse are given in Tables 11.3 and 11.4. Infection with HIV is prevalent amongst intravenous drug users (see later). There are high rates of fetal death, stillbirth and increased neonatal death, the latter due to respiratory distress and seizures. Withdrawal symptoms may persist for months. The neonate may have a coarse tremor and a shrill cry, be very irritable, have diarrhoea, vomiting and fever, be hyperactive, sneeze and yawn (Soepatmi 1994).

The shrill cry, feeding and sleep problems make the baby difficult to care for; developmental and behaviour problems persist. Children born to heroin-abusing mothers are described as hyperactive, having temper tantrums and a low threshold for frustration. They are clumsy, cannot concentrate, and have delayed language development and later learning difficulties at school. These problems continue through adolescence, with persisting behavioural and learning disorder.

Cocaine abuse (Bays 1993)

Cocaine abuse has overtaken heroin abuse in the USA and is rapidly rising in the UK, with crack (cocaine that has been modified so it may be smoked) being increasingly available. The effects on the fetus are just as serious as those due to heroin, if not more so. The drug is used intranasally, intravenously and in cigarette form. As with all drug abuse, several drugs may be abused simultaneously, and HIV infection is common in intravenous drug abusers. The effects of maternal abuse of cocaine are shown in Tables 11.4 and 11.5.

Cocaine causes a ten-fold increased rate of haemorrhage or placental abruption, around 30% spontaneous abortion rate, premature labour and fetal distress. Cocaine-induced vasospasm may be responsible for the placental effects as well as the congenital anomalies seen in the infant (Bays 1990, Scafidi et al 1996). The neonate is small with microcephaly, lethargic and may have considerable respiratory problems (respiratory distress syndrome and meconium aspiration).

Congenital malformations have been associated with cocaine abuse, including cerebral, renal, cardiac and skeletal anomalies (Larson 1989).

Withdrawal symptoms may be delayed, so that only after discharge from hospital does the baby become irritable, jittery and cry uncontrollably. These symptoms may persist day and night for weeks or longer. There may also be an increased risk of infection in infancy. As many as 15% of such babies are said to succumb to SIDS.

Crack makes the adult abusers more aggressive, and the level of family violence and child abuse and death has risen markedly in the USA.

Behaviour and learning problems persist through childhood and beyond, much as for the offspring of heroin addicts. The extreme hyperactivity in association with poor understanding makes children damaged by cocaine difficult to care for even in good social circumstances. It is thought that structural damage occurs in utero and causes brain damage including other severe neurological deficits such as hemiplegia and Parkinsonian dystonia (Bays 1990).

Consequences of addiction for the family

As has been described, affected neonates may not only have serious physical problems but also behavioural patterns which make caring for them difficult. Like any children, these babies need care, attention and physical comfort but the carers find it difficult to look after a child who will not feed or sleep and cries endlessly.

If the parents are still abusing drugs or alcohol they will not cope, but neither do many foster-parents who are driven to total exhaustion by the child's behaviour. Breakdown with change of carers occurs and the damaged child has further suboptimal care.

In an addicted mother, if the pregnancy was wanted, and she intends to withdraw and remain off drugs or drink, rehabilitation may be successful. If she has a partner or friends around her who are still abusing, the task is virtually impossible. The older the woman, and the longer her history of abuse, the less likely is she to succeed in staying off drugs or drink. Some cope for months but then relapse, and the child is received back into care. If this happens repeatedly the child will suffer harm.

If parents are trying to manage their baby, but both they and the child have withdrawal symptoms together, it is very hard. The child is unwell and the parents feel guilty, then angry, as they are tired and stressed. The parents are then seen not to be coping but foster-parents may equally be very stressed by dealing with such an infant.

The child may have been damaged in utero, then neonatally (especially by seizures) and finally post-natally if care is inadequate. However, not all babies are so severely affected and many have been well cared for and eventually adopted.

HIV infection in children

Although acquired immune deficiency syndrome (AIDS) was only recognised in 1981, it is a major health problem worldwide. The World Health Organisation estimated in 1996 that over 20 million adults and 1.5 million children had been infected. Not all babies born to HIV-positive mothers will become infected with HIV, but over 1000 children a day are born with HIV infection (Quinn 1996).

Vertical transmission from HIV infected mothers to fetus could be reduced from 25% to 8% by use of zidovudine (AZT) during the second and third trimester and treating the infant for 6 weeks with AZT (Connor 1993).The cost of treatment is high, but is probably less than that of treating a child with HIV infection and AZT is used in developed countries.

In the UK the clinical picture has been that children infected have been from 'at-risk groups', as described below, but this is likely to change. In Africa, heterosexual transmission is widespread and the effects are already devastating. Infants may be born infected and become ill in infancy or childhood whilst their parents are also ill from the complications of AIDS which will become an increasing cause of morbidity and mortality (Lissauer 1991).

In the UK less than 20% of pregnant women infected with HIV know their state, and consequently are not available for treatment for themselves or their fetus (Nichol 1997). The rates of HIV infection in the UK look stable but this is because of a significant mortality and it is thought that in 1996 there was the highest rate of newly diagnosed cases of HIV since 1985 (Nichol 1997).

Rates of HIV infection in the UK (Bower 1997)

- 1.5% of injecting drug misusers
- 10% of homosexual and bisexual men in London (2.5% across the UK)
- 0.6% of heterosexual men attending genito-urinary clinics in London (0.1% across the UK)
- 0.3% of pregnant women in inner London (200 pregnancies/year) (0.001% across the UK)

The projection for the incidence and prevalence of AIDS in England and Wales, 1995–99 (Day Report 1996), is for a 25% rise in the heterosexual acquisition of AIDS and a 60% increase of AIDS in children of HIV-infected mothers. The numbers of known vertically infected children in the UK is 380, 80% in London and 7% in Scotland. The majority of infected children in London are born to women from sub-Saharan Africa (Sharland 1997).

Cases of AIDS in children account for less than 2% of the total number of reported cases, and 80% of these cases arise through vertical transmission (Mok 1990). The risk of HIV transmission from infected mother to child varies from 10% to 40% (Mok et al 1989). Factors influencing the risk may include more advanced HIV disease in the mother, prematurity, first-born of twins, vaginal delivery (slight effect?) and breast feeding (7–22%) (Sharland 1997).

Risk factors

The majority of cases of paediatric HIV infection in the UK are the children of mothers from high-risk groups, that is intravenous drug users, prostitutes or women from countries where the prevalence of HIV infection is high. Around 20% of initial cases were children with haemophilia or recipients of blood transfusions. This group should reduce as donor units have been screened for HIV antibodies since 1985.

The clinical situation is changing as the pool of HIV infection increases in the general population. However, although currently the majority of HIV-positive teenagers have haemophilia, as their numbers fall the number of teenagers who are positive due to sexual abuse, intravenous drug use and unprotected sexual activity will rise.

HIV infection and child sexual abuse

HIV infection has been reported in Australia and the USA as a consequence of sexual abuse, and the question of testing sexually abused children is increasingly raised (Berkowitz 1986, Leiderman 1986, Hobbs & Wynne 1987, Mok 1996). It is probable that a significant proportion of young adults who have HIV infection have been sexually abused as children: even if they were not infected as children the behavioural consequences of child sexual abuse, including sexual promiscuity and the teenage runaway lifestyle, put them at high risk.

A series of 96 children who tested positive for HIV were followed up and 14 (14.6%) were confirmed as having been sexually abused (Herman-Giddens 1991). Three children acquired HIV infection vertically and two from contaminated blood. The abused children had multiple risk factors, for example parental drug or alcohol abuse, prostitution (by parent), neglect and poverty. A later review (Rimza 1993) commented on the barriers to making the diagnosis of HIV infection in sexually abused children.

Clinical features

The clinical manifestations of HIV infection are extremely variable. They are summarised in Tables 11.6 and 11.7. A diagnosis of possible HIV infection should be considered in any child with these non-specific or more specific symptoms, and a history of maternal or other risk factors for HIV infection.

Management

Specific therapy for children with HIV infection should be discussed with units where there is experience of treating infected children as the drugs used are toxic and the outcome uncertain.

Table 11.6 Clinical spectrum of HIV infection

Variable course	May remain asymptomatic Mild symptoms for several years Rapidly deteriorating course and death in months
Presenting symptoms	Failure to thrive Generalised lymphadenopathy, hepatosplenomegaly Oral thrush Frequent URTI, otitis media Weight loss, anaemia, fever
Symptomatic phase	Bacterial pneumonia – usual childhood pathogens but also opportunistic infections: *Pneumocystis carinii*, CMV (lung biopsy often needed) Septicaemia, osteomyelitis, septic arthritis Neurodevelopmental abnormalities: poor development, dementia, ataxia, due to infection and HIV encephalopathy or brain tumour Skin, renal, hepatic and haematological abnormality Lymphoma, Kaposi's sarcoma is rare
Prognosis	Uncertain: children who develop opportunist infection in early life have a mortality of 60–80%

General management involves aggressive treatment of infections and maintenance of nutrition.

All HIV-positive and high-risk infants should be followed up carefully. The first symptom of HIV infection may be a life-threatening illness. However, as in all chronic disorders of childhood, an attempt should be made to ensure that the child has as ordinary a life as possible. Practical issues of caring for children with HIV infection are described in BPA (1989).

Table 11.7 Clinical categories of the paediatric HIV classification system (Sharland 1997)

Category	Symptoms
N	Asymptomatic
A	Mildly symptomatic, at least two of: lymphadenopathy, hepato- or splenomegaly, rash, ENT infection
B	Moderate symptoms, a single episode of severe infection, anaemia, cardiomyopathy, , nephropathy hepatitis, candidiasis, zoster infection
C	Severely symptomatic (AIDS), two serious infections, encephalopathy, wasting syndrome, opportunistic infections, cancer (Kaposi's sarcoma, lymphoma), disseminated mycobacterial disease

The medical care of children with HIV infection is well reviewed by Sharland (1997).

Immunisation for HIV-positive children

- *Live vaccines* should be given for measles, mumps, rubella, polio
- *Inactivated vaccines* should be given for whooping cough, diphtheria, tetanus, polio, hepatitis B (if appropriate)
- *BCG vaccine* should not be given to HIV-positive people
- The *hepatitis* of seropositive mothers should be tested and the infant given vaccine and gamma globulin where appropriate
- If there are doubts the consultant in public health or infectious diseases will advise

Testing

HIV testing is a contentious issue and involves issues of confidentiality, consent and counselling (Swinburne 1989). Understanding of HIV infection in the community is limited and many myths exist as to the mode of transmission. Initially, infected people were advised to tell their general practitioner, dentist, school and nursery. The consequence was that treatment was sometimes refused, and children were, for example, excluded from nursery.

Parental consent is usual before testing a child for HIV infection; older children should also be asked (Gillick Principle; Gillick v. West Norfolk and Wisbech Health Authority 1986). The British Medical Association has stated (on the basis of General Medical Council advice) that children can be tested without parental consent if this is essential (even though in practice this means testing the mother's status too).

Who else should know the result? Again, current advice is:

- tell parents
- tell the child's general practitioner
- think before informing school or nursery, and do so only with the parents' consent (see later).

Counselling is necessary before any test for HIV infection is undertaken, and this is a particularly difficult and sensitive task (see below).

Testing for HIV-positive children

- Testing has improved with the introduction of more sensitive and specific techniques
- Immune complex dissociated p24 antigenaemia is very specific after 1 week of life, and levels of >100 pg/ml are associated with a poor outcome. The polymerase chain reaction (PCR) has a higher sensitivity
- HIV culture is ideal for diagnosing HIV infection but is very expensive and not widely available
- In the first week of life only 50% of infected infants have a positive PCR, rising to 95% by a month
- A positive test should always be confirmed on another blood sample
- To confirm that a child is not infected requires an absence of maternal antibodies (may take up to 18 months). Two negative tests by PCR or viral culture after 3 months suggests the child is not infected

Consequences for fostering, adoption and schooling

In the UK 3000 children, the majority under 10 years, are thought to be affected by HIV, mostly because of parental illness and early death (Imrie 1995). Many affected families are poor and socially disadvantaged. Emotionally the children have to cope with loss, poverty, discrimination, social isolation and illness. Teenagers frequently are ill-informed as carers dissemble because they too are distressed by the reality of AIDS.

Education is the initial step when working with foster-parents and pre-adoptive parents willing to care for HIV-positive children. They must understand the risks, the potential course and outcome of HIV infection in childhood (Batty 1987). In practice, emphasis is placed on good personal hygiene – handwashing with soap and water and covering open lesions. Health care issues such as immunisation and seeking early medical care if the child is ill are discussed. Household bleach (sodium hypochlorite), diluted 1:10, is used to clean up spilled blood from cuts, vomit and so on.

Day nursery, play or nursery school are a necessary part of a young child's social life and development and should not be denied to at-risk or HIV-infected children. Most institutions already have measures for dealing with hepatitis B control and these should be adequate.

Children who bite are the subject of much concern. However, the risk of transmission is extremely low (Swinburne 1989) and effective management of the behaviour rather than exclusion of the child is preferable. Likewise, children should attend ordinary day school. The educational needs of a child who becomes unwell should be reviewed in the light of the illness.

The Department of Education and Science (DES 1986) has stated that there is no need for school staff to be informed of the HIV status of a child. All schools should have advice on infectious disease and hygiene matters and the school health service should be involved in this aspect of education. The problem remains, when to tell the school or nursery? Ideally, if all personnel were trained and a uniform response could be assured, sooner rather than later would be the answer. If a child is ill and has increasing needs this is probably the time to discuss his condition, but all cases are different.

Sexually abused children are currently at low risk from HIV infection, although the clinical picture should be monitored (see above). There are clear exceptions to this, such as a boy of 13 years working as a rent boy. Foster-parents may thus generally be reassured. Routine testing of all victims of child sexual abuse is not currently advisable. A recent paper has suggested a protocol for testing for HIV in sexually assaulted children (Table 11.6; Gellert et al 1990, Mok 1996).

Foster-parents usually do need to know if a child they have been asked to care for is at risk of HIV infection or is HIV-positive. Foster-parents take children into their own homes; they may have children and grandchildren, and they should be informed of the risks, even if minimal, that they and their family are being asked to

Table 11.8 A suggested protocol for HIV testing of children who have been sexually abused (after Gellert 1990, Mok 1996)

Child	Assailant
Testing usually indicated if:	
Symptomatic? HIV infection	HIV-seropositive
Adolescent with high-risk behaviour (drugs, prostitution)	Symptomatic? HIV infection High-risk behaviour Multiple assailant
Parent/adolescent insistent on test	
Testing may be indicated if:	
Pre-pubescent with STD	Single unknown assailant
Adolescent with STD	
Anal or vaginal or oral penetration	

The main purposes of early diagnosis are to allow the potential use of therapeutic drugs, and for public health reasons.

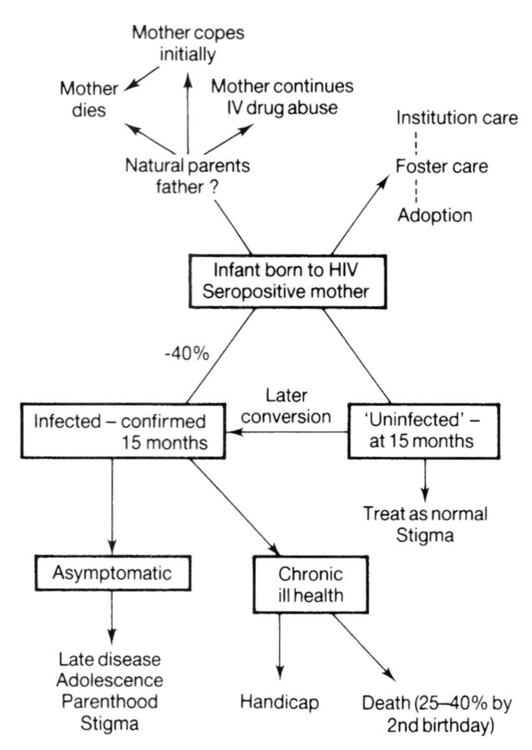

Fig. 11.3 What does the future hold for HIV-positive children? (after Mok 1987).

undertake on behalf of the child. With training and good selection of foster-parents, placements are found and are often successful given good support.

Adoption is a difficult issue, especially when the child is an infant born to a HIV-positive mother. Only by around 15 months will diagnosis of HIV infection ordinarily be confirmed and even then an HIV-positive child may remain well for many years (Fig. 11.3). The baby needs a mother and a home, whether with his or her family or in care, from day 1 – not from 15 months or 3 years. Experience in the UK is primarily in Lothian, Scotland, because of the high incidence of intravenous drug users in Edinburgh coupled with their high HIV infectivity rate (50–60%). Contrary to experience in the USA, both foster-homes and adoptive placements have been found for these babies.

For those babies who go home there must be support from all agencies. Their families are often severely disadvantaged, live in poverty, may be homeless and if the parents continue to abuse drugs the outlook for the child is even worse. Even when the mother is well motivated the prognosis is uncertain as she too has HIV infection, as probably does her partner. Parents receive prison sentences, or become ill and die. Not surprisingly the risk of neglect and physical abuse of the baby, who may also be damaged by drug intoxication in utero, is high. The uninfected children in such households are also at risk of neglect and maltreatment and should be monitored.

In the USA many children remain in hospital beds, unwanted by their families (if they still exist) with failure to attract adequate foster-parents. This may also happen in the UK if the numbers of infected babies rise rapidly and there is not adequately resourced planning.

Counselling of children

The situation for older children who are HIV positive is very difficult. Younger, asymptomatic children should be able to live as normal a life as possible, given the complication that their parent(s) may be ill. Generally it is reasonable for the family of a well child not to disclose that their child has HIV infection. Stigmatisation is inevitable given current attitudes, and this will clearly cause the child and family unnecessary additional distress.

However, as HIV-positive children reach adolescence they will have to have understood the implications of their condition. These children should understand why they, especially, should have a healthy lifestyle, preferably before sexual maturity and teenage rebellion ensue. It is particularly important that they do not abuse drugs intravenously as this will contribute to the development of symptomatic disease, but it is in sexual relationships and parenthood that there will be the greatest upset and conflict. It is difficult for a teenager to come to terms with 'safe sex and no children'. The teenager too will be party to whether his or her HIV status should be kept confidential.

For symptomatic children decisions will be taken variably as to what to tell the child and when, as with any child with a chronic disorder. When older children realise the severity of their illness they will ask about death. Carers must be prepared for these questions and answer truthfully.

Summary

1. The fetus is vulnerable to a wide range of adverse influences which relate to the mother's health and lifestyle, including drug and alcohol abuse, and physical assault on the mother and/or fetus (Kent et al 1997).
2. Additional harm to the infant may occur with ongoing accidental or purposeful intoxication of the child (Bays 1993).
3. Cigarettes are the most commonly used substance and affect birthweight.
4. Alcohol and other drugs of addiction cause fetal damage, and drug addicts often abuse alcohol and tobacco too, i.e. there is a cumulative effect on the fetus.
5. Alcohol and drugs affect parenting skills, they may precipitate mental ill health, physical illness (including hepatitis, HIV, direct toxic effects) or death, and lead to neglectful styles of parenting. Criminality leads to incarceration and loss of a parent.
6. Ongoing poor care in infancy is frequently compounded by poverty.
7. Child abuse, i.e. some degree of neglect, occurs in virtually all addicted families, and overt physical or sexual abuse in 40–60% (Bays 1993, Jaudes et al 1995, Wolcock & Magura 1996).
8. Brain damage caused in utero leaves infants with persisting behavioural and learning difficulties. They may be difficult to care for with attachment problems requiring special parenting skills. Cot death is 17 times the usual rate in the infants of addicts.
9. HIV or hepatitis infection is an increasing problem. Most cases result from infection acquired in utero. The social consequences are complex.
10. Specialist facilities are needed for families but compliance is poor and relapse to addiction common.
11. Legal interventions are required if the parents are unable to care adequately for their child.

REFERENCES

Alcohol Concern 1997 Measures for Measures. Report. Alcohol Concern, London

Barrison I, Waterson E J, Murray-Lyon I M 1985 Adverse effects of alcohol in pregnancy. British Journal of Addiction 80:11–22

Batty D (ed) 1987 The implications of AIDS for children in care. BAAF, Skyline House, 200 Union Street, London SE1 0LX

Bays J 1990 Substance abuse and child abuse. Pediatric Clinics of North America 37(4)

Bays J 1993 Substance abuse and child abuse: the impact of addiction on the child. In: Hobbs C J, Wynne J M (eds) Child Abuse. Baillière's Clinical Paediatrics 1(1). Baillière Tindall, London, Chapter 7

Berkowitz C D 1986 Sexual abuse of children and adolescents. Advances in Paediatrics 34:294

Bewley C, Gibbs A 1994 Coping with domestic violence in pregnancy. Nursing Standard 8(56):25–28

Boer K, Smit B J, van Huis A M, Hogerzeil H V 1994 Substance abuse in pregnancy: Do we care? Acta Paediatrics 83(Suppl 404):65–71

BPA 1989 HIV infection in infancy and childhood. Report of a BPA working party. BPA, 5 St Andrew's Place, Regent's Park, London NW1 4LB
Coleman R, Cassell D 1995 Parents who misuse drugs and alcohol. In: Reder P, Lucey C (eds) Assessment of parenting. Routledge, London, Chapter 12
Condon J T 1987 The battered fetus syndrome. Journal of Nervous and Mental Disease 175:722–725
D (a minor) v. Berkshire County Council 1987 1 All ER20
Day W L 1995 Research on the effects of prenatal alcohol exposure. Am J Public Health 85:1614–1615
DES 1986 Children at school and problems related to AIDS. DES and Welsh Office
DOH 1995 Sensible drinking. DH, London
Ditton J, Hammersley R, Phillips S, Forsyth A, Khan F A very greedy drug: cocaine in context. Harwood Academic
Gellert B G A, Durfee M J, Berkowitz C D 1990 Developing guidelines for HIV antibody testing among victims of paediatric sexual abuse. Child Abuse and Neglect 14(1):9
Gelles R J 1987 Family violence, 2nd edn. Sage, Newbury Park
Gillick v. West Norfolk and Wisbech Health Authority 1986 AC112
Guardian 1995 Judge wrong over 'killing' of baby. *Guardian*, London, 28 November
Herman-Giddens M E 1991 Human immunodeficiency virus transmission by CSA. Am J Dis Ch 145(2):137–141
Gutman L T, Herman-Giddens M E, McKinney R E 1993 Pediatric acquired immunodeficiency syndrome. Amer J Dis Child 147:755–780
Gutman L T, St. Claire K K, Weedy C 1991 Human immunodeficiency virus transmission by child sexual abuse. Amer J Dis Child 145:137–141
Hobbs C J, Wynne J M 1987 Management of sexual abuse. Archives of Diseases of Childhood 62:1182
IDD 1994 Drug misuse in Britain. Institute for the Study of Drug Dependence, London
Jaudes P K, Ekwo E, Voorhis 1995 Association of drug abuse and child abuse. Child Abuse and Neglect 19(9):1065–1076
Jones K L, Smith D W, Ulleland C N, Streissguth A P 1973 Pattern of malformation in offspring of chronic alcoholic mothers. Lancet i:1267
Kent L, Laidlaw J D D, Brockington I F 1997 Fetal abuse. Child Abuse and Neglect 21(2):181–186
Larson E J 1989 Intoxication in utero. In: Mason J K (ed) Paediatric forensic medicine and pathology. Chapman & Hall, London
Leiderman I Z 1986 A child with HIV infection. JAMA 256:3094
Lemoine P, Harrousseau H, Borteyro J P 1968 Les enfants de parents alcoholique. Crest Med 21:476
Lissauer T 1991 Infectious diseases. In: Harvey D, Kovar I (eds) Child health. Churchill Livingstone, London
Macready N 1997 US state rule that a viable fetus is a person. British Medical Journal 315:1488
Miller P, Plant M 1996 Drinking, smoking and illicit drug use among 15–16 year olds in the United Kingdom. British Medical Journal 17:394–397
Mirza H S, Pearson G, Phillips S, 1991 Drugs, people and services in Lewisham. Final Report of the Drug Information Project. Goldsmith's College, London
Mok J 1987 HIV seropositive babies – implications in planning for their future. In: The implications of AIDS for children in care. BAAF, London
Mok J 1990 HIV infection in children. Leader. British Journal of Hospital Medicine 43:247
Mok J Y 1996 When is HIV an issue after child sexual abuse? Archives of Disease in Childhood 75(1):85–87
Mok J Y Q, Haque R A, Yap P L et al 1989 Vertical transmission of HIV: a prospective study. Archives of Diseases of Childhood 64:1140–1145
Murray-Lyon I M 1989 Adverse effects of alcohol in pregnancy. Gastroenterology in Practice: June/July
Puntis J WL, Green M A, Thornton J G, Beck J M 1995 Perinatal death as a consequence of fetal stabbing: was it murder? J Clin Foren Med 2:89–91
RCP 1995 Alcohol and the Young. Report of the Royal College of Physicians and the British Paediatric Association. Publications Department, Royal College of Physicians London
Rimza M G 1993 Words too terrible to hear. (Editorial) Amer J Dis Child 147:711–712
Scafadi F A et al 1996 Cocaine-exposed preterm neonates show behavioral and hormonal differences. Pediatrics 97(6):851–855
Sharland M, Gibb D, Tudor-Williams G et al 1997 Pediatric HIV infection. Arch Dis Child 76(4):293–296
Smith D W 1982 Recognizable patterns of human malformation. W B Saunders, Philadelphia, p 411
Soepatmi S 1994 Development outcomes of children of mothers dependent on heroin or heroin/methadone during pregnancy Acta Paediatrica 83(Suppl 404):36–39
Swadi H 1994 Parenting capacity and substance misuse: an assessment scheme. ACPC Review and Newsletter 16:237–244
Swinburne L M 1989 Medico-legal implications of HIV infection in childhood. In: Mason J K (ed) Paediatric forensic medicine and pathology. Chapman & Hall, London
Wieburg P, Marks J S, McLaren W M, Remington P L 1985 The fetal tobacco syndrome. Journal of American Medicine 253:2998–2999
Wolock I, Magura S 1996 parental substance abuse as a predictor of child maltreatment re-reports. Child Abuse and Neglect 20(12):1183–1194

12

Poisoning, suffocation and factitious illness

Confused terminology and serious outcome

Poisoning, suffocation, factitious illness (Munchausen by proxy syndrome, MBPS), are related forms of child maltreatment. The recognition of factitious or fabricated illnesses and medical conditions induced by parents in children has been increasingly recognised and described in the literature (Southall et al 1987, Samuels & Southall 1992, Samuels et al 1992, Schreier & Libow 1993, Clure et al 1996, Gray & Bentovim 1996, Yorker 1996, Schreier 1997), and of course Meadow's (1977) much quoted paper. Though Asher (1951) described fabricated illness in adults it was Money & Werlas (1976) who first described a case of 'Munchausen by proxy'.

The story of how this term was chosen is somewhat, maybe fittingly, bizarre. Asher (1951) discussed a disorder in which adults described fictitious illness. He named it after Baron K F H von Munchhausen, a German eighteenth-century mercenary who described his adventures in a way which bore little semblance to reality. Munchhausen was compelled to tell the most incredible lies about his adventures. The secondary gains for him were in that he became well known, liked and even revered for his story telling, which lifted his spirits and increased his self-esteem. He also became (psychologically) addicted to the 'fixes' he received from such admiration and had to continually repeat the experience – tell these stories, persuade his audience that they were true, and increase the bizarreness factor each time. Another interesting distortion took place in the English-speaking world which changed the spelling of the name Munchhausen to Munchausen. The obscurity of the origins of the term in medical history and its distortion in spelling are some of the compelling reasons why we would suggest that the term is abandoned and the descriptions of whatever the child is suffering from is clearly made.

There have been attempts to describe the various presentations of the conditions. Schreier & Libow (1993) proposed 'Munchausen by proxy syndrome', Gray & Bentovim (1995) suggest that 'illness induction syndrome' may be a more appropriate term. Others, including Fisher & Mitchell (1995) and Schreier (1997) would support the term 'factitious illness by proxy' with added clear descriptions.

The tragic outcome for children of this syndrome can be life-threatening and indeed become fatal. It is essential to take the manifestation of symptoms seriously and act in a way that includes the parents in the search for clues and reasons. The condition is always linked to the crucial factor that a parent or care giver, usually the mother, fabricates an illness in a child and misleads a physician into believing that the child has an illness which needs investigation. 'Doctor shopping' is a frequent occurrence in these cases. Often the stories escalate so that ever more serious medical investigations are undertaken which include invasive procedures, even surgery, multiple radiography, laboratory investigations, poisoning, etc.

A difficult thing to acknowledge is when tampered laboratory samples are presented which may lead to further invasive procedures. It often seems so improbable that such attentive parents can tamper with the blood or urine (or other) sample of a child in an effort to achieve a confusing laboratory result. The parents work incredibly hard to gain access to medical professionals and they often also appear so desperate that they involve the media or other public forums to gain recognition of their unstinting care and to receive glowing acknowledgement of their parenting and care giving. The intense need for medical care and nurturing in the mother which drives her to seek more and more such attention should not be underestimated.

Maintaining the cycle of abuse

It is sometimes bewildering to think that highly intelligent physicians and other professionals have been persuaded to investigate and treat these children without recognising that they may be doing something which they would otherwise see clearly as not being in the interest of the child. Schreier & Libow (1993, p. 129 ff.) give a detailed explanation and many writers agree with this perplexing situation. We have seen a very similar picture and agree that doctors, social workers, therapists, professionals in the 'caring professions', usually have as part of their make-up an unresolved special need to be cared for which has also grown into a need to care for others. Mothers with children where a factitious 'by proxy' illness has been created are themselves in great need to be cared for and tap into this need of other's (professionals') need to care. A somewhat paradoxical situation. An almost symbiotic and enmeshed relationship is created in which the child's real needs and rights are not remembered or taken into account.

It needs to be understood that though the parent appears loving and caring, a vital process between mother and child is not taking place. This process relates to the age-appropriate separation that has to occur between mother and child, where the child becomes an independent person in their own right. Winnicott (1982, p. 91) described the baby learning in the first few months of life that it is separate, not a part of the mother any more: the explorations the baby makes with his or her hands, discovering for instance where 'me' ends and the blanket begins – the 'me/not-me' position. Something similar takes place between every baby and mother in terms of becoming independent, but the mother has to be the instigator and guide to this process. The baby begins the developmental progression of the sense of self. This starts with a physical recognition of self. The parents, in situations of factitious illness by proxy, often have no sense of allowing the baby and child to have this emergent 'self' develop but view the baby in terms of an extension of the mother/parent.

CASE HISTORY 12.1

A mother suffered from pains, symptoms and conditions for which she sought medical help for years; no diagnosis of her symptoms was found. She had a baby in her early thirties and stopped complaining about her symptoms. She said all her symptoms had disappeared. However the baby was frail, sickly and ill almost continually with the mother admitting that she did want to keep this child as an infant as long as she could. Feeding the baby was one of the central issues and something the mother found extremely difficult. As the baby grew older the mother refused to feed the child solids. Eventually the child went into foster care and the mother's symptoms reappeared within days.

Mothers such as these are manipulative indeed and driven by their need to be acknowledged. The parent may go to any length to gain attention, endangering the children in the process. But the professionals in these situations play their part and have to be aware of the role they play.

CASE HISTORY 12.2

A 'security alert' went out throughout a large hospital stating that a mother had reported that her child, aged months, had been snatched from her. The mother gave a very clear description of the man who had taken the child; 'white male, 5 feet 8 inches tall, of slim build, short dark hair, wearing a green top, jeans and white trainers'. The child was found in the grounds, on her own, having toddled across the road. The two were reunited. Five days later another letter came to all departments saying that the mother retracted the statement, saying it had not happened. She had received tremendous attention, sympathy and praise for her care for the child in the face of such adversity. It was suggested to her that she might have fabricated the story, which did not make sense at closer scrutiny, by professionals working with her who had previously had suspicions that the failure to thrive of her child could have been maintained because of the secondary gains she made from her involvement with medical staff.

As Schreier & Libow (1993, p. 130) put it, the parents

> create a veritable mine field for a physician faced with the skilful manipulations of the MBPS mother when she creates an 'unsolvable' clinical problem. The far reaching knowledge of matters medical exhibited by these mothers and the support they express for the work of the doctor ('Doctor, I know you are doing your best, stay with it, let's work together. We'll support you') combine to encourage the paediatrician's empathic identification with the mother. She begins to look like an appreciative colleague *and* like an ideal mother.

The professionals appreciate the supportive position of the mother, but by the same token they also feed the doctors' self-esteem and entrap them. There is another dimension to this which involves the doctors being driven to consider ever more intensive investigations, cleverer tests and more obscure diagnoses in order to prove their expertise. All of this goes on alongside the mother's criticism of other professionals, setting them off against one other. If professionals don't examine this 'criticism' they can quickly find themselves agreeing with the parent and in conflict with their colleagues.

> If it were just the issue of the paediatrician's competency, knowledge, and autonomous decision making, things would be difficult enough. But add the issue of the doctor's 'caring' and the bold and sometimes even bald manipulation of 'adulatory support' that these parents often express, and a situation is produced in which the question of his *caring* is now tied to his medical/clinical *performance*. Now, when things are not going well clinically, the doctor is left vulnerable to the *self*-accusation of not caring enough and the feeling that he needs to try harder. And this step seals 'the trap'. It is this intense inward focus by the physician, the self-blame for whatever is going wrong clinically in the case (the kind of doubt doctors and clinicians too frequently do not share with their colleagues), that is

transformed into self-doubt. These self-doubts in turn cause otherwise competent doctors to miss or misinterpret obvious clues concerning MBPS behaviour. Moreover there may well be an element of truth to the self-blame and self-doubt if the physician finds him/herself fleeing from the demands and needs of an 'engulfing' MBPS mother through actual avoidance or the desire to 'get rid of' the problem. (Schreier & Libow 1993, p. 130)

However, when a halt is called to this and a doctor does have the courage to confront the issue (and courage it does take) then the mother will leave and assign that doctor to the worthless, criticised 'bunch of useless professionals' only to move to someone else who will, with her, repeat the cycle. The parents will consolidate their beliefs and positions and the child is usually subjected to further 'illness creating' situations, challenging the next doctor to ever more efforts.

Children can be in immense and imminent danger when this situation is recognised, either by a single professional or by a group. The mothers at this point become very desperate to prove they are right, and may increase their activity to produce ever more serious or different symptoms in their children. This can lead to the death of the child and needs to be considered in any planning.

We feel it is important for professionals to recognise these intensely enmeshed situations in which they can easily lose themselves, however experienced. Their role becomes crucial in prolonging the plight for the child. The more professionals are aware of the role they are going to play in such cases the more able they are to protect the children from often life-threatening situations. Talking with others and acknowledging one's vulnerability is an essential first step.

It is, of course, not only doctors and health professionals who are likely to be involved. It is well known that those in the legal profession, particularly solicitors and judges, are equally vulnerable and will perform in almost identical ways. Yorker (1996) describes the legal scenario in some detail.

Definitions

Clear definitions for the different presentations of factitious illness are important, particularly since this form of child maltreatment is now better understood and formulations as to how to protect the child are being developed. Schreier & Libow (1993) give an invaluable account of the dynamics involved in these situations. It is also of the utmost importance that clinicians are clear about the range of presentation and that highly anxious and overprotective parents, who do want the best for their children but may appear difficult in the process, are distinguished from those who are at the other end of the spectrum and actually fabricate symptoms and create fictitious illnesses in their children (see below and page 308).

The American Psychiatric Association defined DSM-IV 'Factitious disorders by proxy' as follows.

- Intentional production of physical or psychological sign and symptoms in another person who is under the individual's care.
- The motivation for the perpetrator's behaviour is to assume the sick role by proxy.
- External incentives for the behaviour (such as economic gain) are absent? initially only.
- The behaviour is not better accounted for by another mental disorder.
- The motivation for the perpetrator's behaviour is to assume the sick role by proxy – this is the key discriminator. The carer is addicted to medical care.
- Child protection registers classify it as physical abuse.
- Pervasive and continuing emotional abuse.

However, we have seen some cases of factitious illness by proxy where financial gains were an important part of the presentation. The symptoms were highly exaggerated or simply not relinquished by the parent. For example, a mother with a child in callipers was insistent that her daughter could not walk or do things for herself. However, if staff removed the callipers from her legs at school the child was well able to exercise her muscles and walk. Attendance allowances and maintenance from the ex-husband were all assessed on the basis that the child had a disability. Epilepsy and reported fits may also fall into this category and of course there are other examples. What is important is that a doctor should discuss the motivational factors both with the family and colleagues in order to establish a picture which serves the child's interest best. This may include doubting the parents' intention when they present with a request for support for social benefits. Nevertheless it must also be stated that it is important to distinguish genuine cases and to have some empathy for those who struggle but are trapped in a negative cycle.

Factitious illness by proxy: definition

- Illness which is fabricated by the child's carer
- The child is presented repeatedly for medical assessment and care
- The perpetrator denies the aetiology of the child's illness
- Symptoms and signs cease when the child is separated from the perpetrator

The majority of children with factitious illness by proxy are cared for by their natural mothers, although there have been cases involving adoptive mothers, foster mothers, nurses, nursery nurses or teachers. The Beverley Allet case is one of the most widely publicised cases in England. Grandmothers and in a few cases fathers have also been known to be the perpetrators. Meadow (1997) described 15 cases where fathers were the perpetrators of factitious illness, poisoning and suffocation of their infants and children. These fathers also showed self injurious behaviours and invented bizarre accounts about their own and their children's injuries.

As part of defining these conditions it may also be useful to conceptualise it in terms of parental behaviours. Parents divide into different groups.

- Parents who 'doctor shop' moving from one doctor and professional to another seeking treatment for their children for non-existent illnesses. These parents fabricate illness in their children or deliberately induce illnesses into their children by, for instance, feeding them poisonous substances, mixing creams or lotions with toxic chemicals and rubbing them on the children's body to create skin irritation and poisoning, allergies, seizures; or they present children who are failing to thrive non-organically.
- Mothers who are so enmeshed with their children they keep them away from school claiming that the child has a chronic illness when in fact the mother is unable to separate from her child.
- One part of the diagnosis relates to the fact that a child who is separated from the perpetrator may stop having symptoms altogether.

Eminson & Postlethwaite (1992) developed a useful dimensional scale on which to place any given case and thereby recognising the range of concerns professionals need to have and the range of parental behaviour from normal to classic presentations of factitious illness by proxy (Fig. 12.1)

As already mentioned, factitious illness by proxy, including suffocation and poisoning, occur not only in the medical and psychological field but also in the legal arena and in education.

Poisoning

Poison is defined as a substance causing illness or death when eaten, drunk or absorbed into the body by other means. The definition of poisoning is commonly recognised, but in cases of fabricated illness the children can be presented in such a way that the poisoning is simply not perceived.

Poisoning may be accidental, neglectful or due to single acts of omission; deliberate poisoning, suffocation or the fabrication of illness by a parent are clearly forms of child abuse. Although a depressed mother may leave her pills within the reach of her exploring toddler, other mothers deliberately poison or asphyxiate their child – either as a single event or over time as in factitious illness. Gray & Bentovim (1996) describe 11

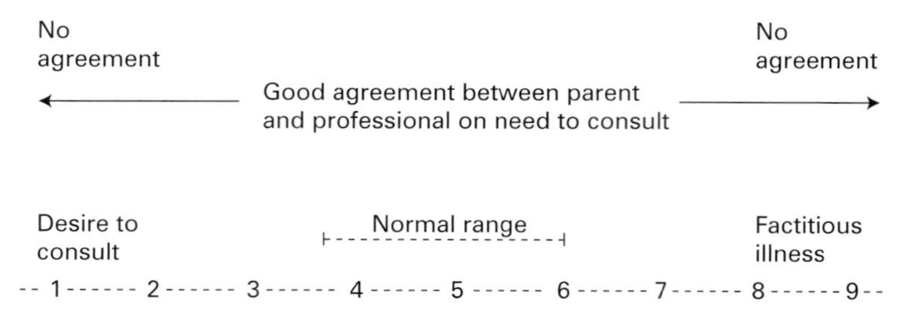

Fig. 12.1 Parents' desire to consult for their child's symptoms (reproduced with permission from Eminson D M, Postlethwaite R J 1992 Factitious illness: recognition and management. Archives of Disease in Childhood 67:1510–1516).

cases with children ranging from 4 weeks to 12 years and 3 months where a carer had 'actively administered substances which were harmful to the child or where a parent had been actively interfering with the child's medical treatment'.

A relationship between these abuses is suggested in Figure 12.2. Current research clearly demonstrates that, as in other forms of child abuse, the very young are at greatest risk. It is also evident that if a previous child in a family has died an 'unusual or suspicious death' or from sudden infant death syndrome (SIDS), recurrent apnoeic spells in the new baby must be viewed very urgently as possible suffocation or factitious illness (Emery 1985, Meadow 1990).

Repeated poisoning may be due to negligence but the consequences for the child may be equally as catastrophic as poisoning by intent or in order to fabricate illness and should be assessed as possible abuse.

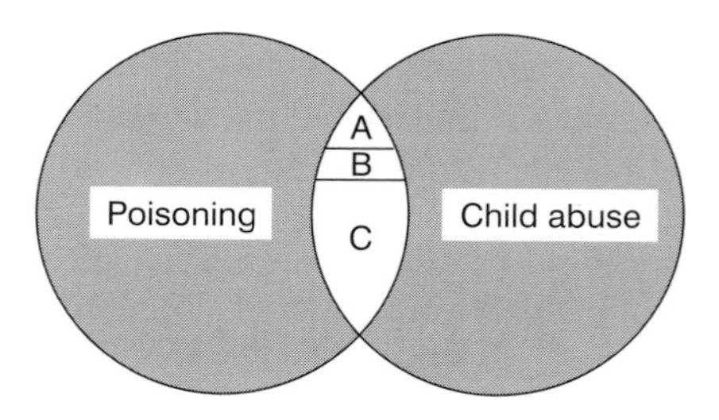

Fig. 12.2 Overlap of population of poisoned and abused children. (Adapted from Kresel & Lovejoy 1981.)

Accidental poisoning

Accidental poisoning is a major child health issue in the UK. Although it is seldom fatal, 15% of children develop symptoms related to the ingestion and many children are seen in a hospital Accident and Emergency department, made to vomit and have a very unhappy few hours which may include a brief admission to hospital.

A large multicentre study (Wiseman et al 1987) was set up to look at the causes of accidental poisoning, the outcome and also the type of packaging used by manufacturers. The peak age for ingestion was 2–3 years, adult supervision was faulty and ingestions took place at home. In 60% of cases the substance ingested was not in its usual storage place and 60% of substances were not in child-resistant containers; 22% of children were admitted to hospital, < 10% needed intensive care and there were no fatalities.

Research has also been directed to consider the circumstances in which the ingestion took place (Sibert 1975). Environmental factors such as failure to use locked drug cupboards, bleach and turpentine stored under the kitchen sink and poor parental supervision with parents stressed by marital discord, poverty, several small children in the house and/or recent house move are commonly recorded.

Accidents may occur even in well-regulated homes but repeated ingestion should be looked at as neglectful, and deliberate poisoning considered. It is also appropriate to look at parental behaviour: is the mother depressed, or impaired by the use of drugs or alcohol? Are there other signs of neglect within the family?

The drugs ingested are those often available at home – analgesics, anxiolytics, the contraceptive pill, cough medicine and iron. Bleach, detergents and petroleum products account for most of the household substances ingested.

If symptoms are severe – for example seizures, coma, intractable vomiting – consider whether an unusual substance such as salt, insulin or anticonvulsants has been administered. Laxatives, easily available, are also often used.

The age of the child is also important. Toddlers aged 18 months to 3 years explore, test and taste whatever they find; by 4–5 years most children will know not to eat pills, although if weedkiller is kept in a lemonade bottle even much older children may be poisoned. When a young infant (not yet at the crawling stage) is brought, the facts of the story need to be very carefully obtained and a vigilant stance adopted.

Parents may misread instructions on a bottle and overdose a child but then the history is clear, whereas if parents deliberately overdose their child they will conceal the history. Children from 3 years are able to give a history and tell if they 'ate grandpa's sweeties' or if mummy gave them herself. Children as young as 6 years do deliberately overdose, but this is rare under 10 years. If any child or adolescent does overdose a careful evaluation is necessary: what is making life so unbearable?

Intentional poisoning

Kempe et al (1962), in their original description of the battered child syndrome, recognised deliberate poisoning by parents as a form of serious child abuse (Rogers et al 1976, Dine & McGovern 1982). Table 12.1 lists features of poisoning, whether due to accident, neglect or wilful intent by care giver. Gray & Bentovim describe a case of a 2.5-year-old child with the highest ever reported salt levels in her system for which 'only active administration of salt could account for this finding'. Rogers et al (1976) described deliberate poisoning of infants by salt, barbiturates, and other drugs. Two of the children in that study died of salt poisoning. There is considerable overlap, but the more bizarre the clinical situation the greater the likelihood of intentional poisoning, whether as an attempt to kill the child or factitious illness. Meadow's (1993) study of deliberate salt poisoning described 12 children with this condition. The children in this study presented below the age of 6 months. Ten children did well in alternative care; several of them additionally suffered from fabricated symptoms. Two of the children died. Meadow (1993) described 12 children who were diagnosed as having non-accidental salt poisoning: seven out of the 12 mothers admitted to the poisonings and explained how they had done this and two of the children died as a result.

Drugs are also used to keep children quiet, for example the use of sedatives at night, or to make the child compliant, with high doses of anxiolytics. This has also been used to allow sexual abuse to occur. Adults who abuse drugs may also involve even very young children in their habit, and a child may present to hospital stuporous on the parent's heroin. There are many examples of children of all ages dangerously intoxicated with alcohol. This may be deliberate poisoning, or unsupervised drinking, often in a house where heavy drinking occurs. The number of deaths from solvent abuse increases annually in the UK and is nearing 200 per annum. Children as young as 8–9 years become involved in alcohol, drug and solvent abuse, usually with older teenagers (hence unsupervised) or at home with addicted parents.

Recurrent poisoning as part of factitious illness by proxy syndrome is discussed later in this chapter.

Suffocation

As a form of physical assault on a baby, suffocation is difficult to detect because, in spite of the violence of the act, there may be no signs of injury, even at autopsy (see also Ch. 18, Fatal child abuse). Differentiation from SIDS may not be possible in the absence of any external sign of injury or foreign material in the mouth or airway

Table 12.1 Poisoning: is it accident, neglect or deliberate?

	Accident	Neglect	Deliberate
Age	2–3 years Rarely older child	2–3 years Rarely older child	Infancy–3 years May be any age
History	Usually clear, makes sense	Variable, due to social chaos	None, but ill child History of accidental ingestion Recurrent symptoms
Symptoms	Uncommon <15% <1% need intensive care	Uncommon <15% <1% need intensive care	Common Seizures, drowsy, vomiting diarrhoea Dead
Outcome	Rarely fatal	Rarely fatal	
Substance			
Drugs	Analgesics, anxiolytics, cough medicine, oral contraceptive, iron		Analgesics, antidepressants, anxiolytics, anticonvulsants, insulin, etc.
Household or other	Bleach, detergent, petroleum product		Salt, bicarbonate of soda, corrosives, etc.
Past history	Nil	Repeated ingestions Increased incidence of SIDS Known to social services	Other unexplained child deaths in family including SIDS Other abuses
Diagnosis	History equates with clinical signs Confirm if necessary by toxicological investigation	As accidental	History usually at variance with clinical signs Ask advice of toxicologist: blood, urine samples **Think of possibility: parents' behaviour may be bizarre although they present as caring and concerned**

(Pullar 1984, Bowen 1989). The clinical features of suffocation have been described (Meadow 1989a, 1990). Table 12.2 lists the history.

Clinical features of babies who are suffocated and those who died of SIDS: physical examination

- Suffocated infant
  - may appear well nourished with no signs of injury
  - may have signs of physical neglect, bruising, scratches, healing fractures
  - may be underweight (check clinic growth chart)
- Signs of suffocation:
  - petechiae on face, especially eyelids
  - bruises on lips and gums
  - bruises around neck, part of neck, pressure marks at back of neck, upper chest and arms
  - nail marks around face and neck
  - foreign material stuffed in nose and throat
- Infant dying from SIDS
  - usually well nourished, no signs of injury

If suffocation is by use of a pad of material the child may not be injured. A hand across the child's face or around the neck would usually cause bruising but there may be just a few petechiae of the upper eyelids which disappear in 24–48 hours (in 'near-miss' or a non-fatal episode of strangulation).

Sudden infant death syndrome (SIDS)

SIDS is defined as

> the sudden death of an infant or young child which is unexpected by history, and in which a thorough post-mortem examination fails to reveal an adequate cause of death (Bergman et al 1970).

Suffocation and SIDS largely involve very young infants. The older the child, particularly if there has been a history of recurrent episodes of apnoea, the more thought should be given to the possibility of deliberately induced asphyxial episodes.

Table 12.2 Clinical features of suffocation in infants and sudden infant death syndrome (SIDS)

	Suffocation	SIDS	References
Incidence	Not known[a]	2/1000 live births	Emery (1985)
Age	Infant <12 months (but up to 3 years and rarely older)	Infancy, peak 3–4 months old, 90% before 8 months	
History			
Presentation	Maybe as 'near-miss cot death' or dead	Occasionally 'near-miss cot death', usually as SIDS	
Previously	Episodes of cyanosis or floppiness accepted as apnoea or seizure	Healthy	
Investigations	All negative Other unexplained symptoms of ill health		
Family			
Siblings	Unexplained disorder or death Other evidence of abuse in family, especially physical abuse or Munchausen by proxy	Recurrence of SIDS (2% risk) increases possibility of abuse	(Emery 1986)
Socially	Known to social services because of history of abuse	Children from known abusing families are at greater risk of SIDS Children from socially deprived inner city areas at greater risk of SIDS and some abuses	Baldwin & Oliver (1975), Roberts et al (1980) Golding et al (1985) Taylor & Emery (1988), Creighton (1989)

[a] *Emery (1985) suggests >1/10 but <1/15 'SIDS' due to abuse.*

The association between SIDS and social factors is well established (Knowelden et al 1985). There is a strong trend which increases steeply in the poorest families. Unsupported families and unemployed families are 2–3 times more at risk than professional or managerial families. The incidence is greatest in inner city families, in areas of poor housing and social deprivation (Golding et al 1985, Taylor & Emery 1988). There is also an increased association noted in families known to social services departments because of previous abuse (Baldwin & Oliver 1975, Roberts et al 1980, Newlands & Emery 1991).

Clinical investigation and management

Clearly it is of utmost importance to recognise if a child has been murdered, not least because of the welfare of other children in the family or as yet unborn children. On the other hand a SIDS death is a major tragedy for a family and at a time of such grief, ill-considered investigation and intrusion are to be avoided.

The differential diagnosis must also be considered.

- Has the baby been ill, has there been contact with whooping cough?
- Was the baby pre-term with a history of recurrent apnoea or has the mother mistaken exaggerated periodic respiration for apnoea, in a 'near-miss' cot death?
- Is there evidence of cardiac or respiratory disorder?
- Does the child have marked gastro-oesophageal reflux?

If the child is still alive, and there are features suggestive of factitious illness, management is as described on page 313. The ultimate investigation is video monitoring of the parent, most often the mother (Southall et al 1987, Hilton 1989, Samuels et al 1992). If there are other signs of child maltreatment the management is as for other cases of possible serious abuse (see Ch 14). If the final opinion is that this is a case of factitious illness or physical assault, the baby is at real risk of death and usually would not return to the parent's care. Murder or attempted murder is clearly a matter which should be urgently discussed with the police.

Nixon et al (1995) discussed the epidemiology and prevention in cases where a child was either suffocating, choking or strangled. The cases of 136 children, 99 boys and 37 girls, were reported to the Office of Population Censuses and Surveys during the year 1990–91. The children were under the age of 15 years. The girls had a modal age of below the age of 1 and the boys had two such points: one, like the girls, at below the age of 1 year and the other in the early teenage years.

Most sudden and unexpected deaths in infancy are due to SIDS and not to suffocation or poisoning. Investigation of all deaths should be sensitive; a child's death is always a tragedy. Much has been written of the support needed by parents in the short and long term to come to terms with an infant death, and to help with their distress, especially in the first 12 months. Paediatricians have a role, particularly in discussing the autopsy report with the parents and later on in planning the care of subsequent children following a SIDS death.

The police and coroner's officer are involved in all cases of sudden or unexpected death and a paediatric pathologist should ideally perform all autopsies on such infants. The details of the pathology of SIDS have recently been well described (Hilton 1989). Parents need to know as much as possible about the cause of death and any abnormality which may affect subsequent pregnancies. The pathologist will also use forensic skills in looking for signs of recent trauma or healing from previous assault.

Death by suffocation is not a rare form of child abuse. The victim is usually an infant, and differentiation from death due to SIDS is difficult.

- The aetiology of SIDS is unknown – is there an entity 'SIDS' or is it a diagnostic dustbin (Emery 1989)?
- If 5–10% of sudden infant deaths are due to infanticide, is the label 'SIDS' facilitating infanticide?

If careful and thorough investigation takes place, the proportion of deaths that are completely unexplained falls to around 1 in 5 (Emery 1989). If a neutral confidential enquiry took place in these instances, perhaps the final opinion would be more accurate and parents would be more appropriately counselled.

Repeated episodes of partial asphyxiation are likely to be a manifestation of factitious illness and are further discussed under this heading. Older children may also be suffocated; for example, a child who is screaming while her assailant sexually abuses her. A hand across her face will keep her quiet and may kill her. The physical evidence of the physical and sexual abuse as well as the child's testimony (if old enough, and still alive) will make the diagnosis.

Factitious illness by proxy

As already indicated above, Asher (1951) described Munchausen syndrome and it has since become a well-recognised medical entity. In 1977, Munchausen syndrome by proxy was described by Meadow in a girl of 6 years with apparent haematuria. The consensus seems to be that the term best used is 'factitious illness by proxy', with suffocation, poisonings and other symptoms being described and used in the diagnosis.

The definition of factitious illness by proxy (see also above) includes the following (Rosenberg 1987):

- illness in a child which is faked and/or produced by the parent (or carer)
- presentation of the child for medical assessment and care, usually persistently and resulting in multiple medical procedures and multiple medical opinions
- denial of knowledge by the perpetrator of the cause of the child's illness
- abatement of acute symptoms and signs in the child when the child is separated from the perpetrator although sequelae of the disorder may persist.

The carer involved is most often the mother, with the father playing an unusually passive role. Less often, fathers have also been known to be responsible for creating factitious illness by proxy both in their own right (Meadow 1997) and/or actively together with a partner. Though it is usually the paediatrician who makes the diagnosis in respect of the child, the parents have to be included in the equation and a psychiatric or psychological assessment of the parents, individually and together, is essential. It is also well worth recognising that these situations can occur in schools with teachers and educational specialists being the focus from which the parent seeks attention or that it applies to legal situations – lawyers and judges are at the receiving end of parental need. Psychiatric presentation in the perpetrator has been thought to be rare. However, Pope et al (1982) found that 4% of patients admitted to a research centre for psychosis were identified as suffering from factitious disorders according to the DSM-III criteria. As already described above there are discrepancies in many of the perpetrator's personalities and some will undoubtedly border on personality disorders.

Warning signs of factitious illness (after Wissow 1990)

- Persistent or recurrent illness – even a new syndrome?
- Discrepancy between child's apparent good health and history of grave symptoms or seriously disordered laboratory tests
- Overly attentive mother, will not leave child, appears surprisingly cheerful in face of grave clinical situation
- Signs and symptoms settle on separation from mother
- Routine treatment or medications never seem to work well
- Several medical opinions previously – notes are lost

Clinical features

Clinically the range of symptoms produced is wide and the child suffers the 'illness' and inevitable disruption of life both in the short and longer terms. The distress due to the fabricated illness is compounded by the increasingly complex and invasive medical investigations and associated hospital admissions which are imposed on the child. The symptoms are as varied as the insults visited on the child. Many children have several symptoms, few signs, but show contradictory and confusing laboratory tests.

Commoner clinical presentations in factitious illness by proxy

- Bleeding (haematuria, haematemesis)
- Seizures
- CNS depression (drowsy, coma)
- Apnoea
- Failure to thrive
- Diarrhoea
- Vomiting
- Fever
- Rashes
- Hypertension

A review of the literature (Rosenberg 1987) lists the commonest reported symptoms in factitious illness by proxy as seizures, followed by apnoea and unconsciousness. These are important in the morbidity and mortality associated with the condition. Diarrhoea, vomiting, fever and haematuria have also been repeatedly reported but over 65 symptoms have been recorded, from arthralgia to ventricular tachycardia (Meadow 1989b).

Clinical features, as given in Table 12.3, probably describe the severe end of the spectrum of factitious illness by proxy. Substances used to fabricate illness may be unusual, such as salt leading to dehydration and seizures, the mixing of poisonous substances, such as cleaning materials, applied to the child's skin, or sedation due to barbiturates or antidepressants have also been known to be used in such presentations. Parents may not only lie when telling the history but also falsify charts of the child's vomiting, temperature or urine output. Schreier and Libow (1993) give extensive histories. Yeo (1996) gives a tragic account of several children in one family being affected.

Emotional abuse is inevitable in this disorder and, as children become drawn into the deception, they too lie and fabricate illness and may as adults have the syndrome of fabricated illness in

Table 12.3 Clinical features in factitious illness by proxy. Data from published cases (Rosenberg 1987)

Gender	Boys and girls equally affected
Age at diagnosis	Average 3 years (1 month–21 years)
Length of illness	Average 14 months (days–20 years)
Morbidity	?8%
Mortality	?10–20% (most at risk under 3 years)
Other abuses	14% failure to thrive 1% physical abuse 1% sexual abuse 100% emotional abuse

their own right. Psychiatric disorder is well described in survivors of factitious illness by proxy, and a particular concern is of chronic invalidism (Meadow 1989b). Separation anxiety (from the mother) and school refusal may become part of the syndrome.

Many of the children have also failed to thrive and have a history of non-accidental injury, inappropriate medication or neglect. Within the families there is often also an excess of unexplained deaths. It is not unusual for more than one child in the family to have suffered from illnesses fabricated by the mother (Bools et al 1992). Sexual abuse may also occur.

There is now much more information on the relationship between the abused child and the mother. These families are clearly dysfunctional, with relationships between all family members disturbed. Other children in the family are at risk, too, of emotional and physical abuse as well as unexplained death (Table 12.4).

There is generally little understanding of the aetiology of the disorder, although much more has been written and researched about this condition (Gray & Bentovim 1996, Southall 1997). Why do apparently caring mothers injure their children in this prolonged, perverse and calculating manner? The majority do not have a recognisable psychiatric disorder, although there are now some reports (Schreier 1997) which highlight psychiatric illness as a precursor to factitious illness by proxy. It is now better understood that a high proportion of parents presenting in this way do have a history of childhood maltreatment, particularly emotional abuse, neglect, sexual abuse or difficulties in terms of attachment. They may be lonely and isolated, and certainly thrive on hospital wards with the attention their child's illness brings. But how they dissociate from their children to allow for their damaging behaviour is complex, and needs assessment on an individual basis. The most central feature of the syndrome is that the mother, but sometimes the mother and father, are driven by an intense need to be close to doctors and/or hospitals. They often have a wide knowledge of the medical condition and treatment for the child. This knowledge base leads often to the parents suggesting treatments and investigations which doctors find hard to resist. The parents appear extremely caring and devoted to the child, although on close observation they can be seen to behave in a contradictory fashion and not always in the child's best interest. Formal psychological and psychiatric assessment is necessary to recognise that many of the mothers have underlying psychological or psychiatric problems. (Bools et al 1992). The attachment between mother and child is most certainly skewed, despite the appearance of a close loving and protecting relationship between the dyad.

Table 12.4 Families in factitious illness by proxy

Mother	Father	Sibling
Usual perpetrator	<2% collude	–
'Model' parent on ward	Seen rarely in hospital	Physical abuse
Intelligent, caring, attentive	Detached, uninvolved, passive, in spite of child's serious illness	Unexplained deaths and illnesses
'Normal' psychiatrically		
Munchausen syndrome (self)		

Outcome

The outcome of factitious illness by proxy for the child varies with the history, though mostly it is poor in terms of the parents being able to change. Of the cases described in the literature (Rosenberg 1987) a mortality rate of 10–20% is given, with the greatest danger to the very young, due to maternally induced asphyxia. This figure is misleading, as clearly only the severe end of the syndrome is diagnosed and many less dramatic cases go unrecognised.

Long-term morbidity is probably underestimated, but little is known in the long term of these children: 8% are said to have significant sequelae (Rosenberg 1987) including psychiatric disorder, the gastrointestinal consequences of surgery, cerebral palsy, joint disease and chronic invalidism which may persist into adult life. Again there are insufficient studies to show the true extent of disability following a childhood of fictitious illness.

Children who suffer from this treatment have clear short-term consequences mostly induced by the parent(s) inducing the illness or condition and from the consequent medical care. As already indicated, the attachment relationships are often skewed: though it may look as if a child and mother are very close the attachment is of an anxious quality which leaves little room for developing social relationships in this child's life. The children's developmental stages are often delayed; they may be non-organically failing to thrive and therefore look much younger than they are. This leads to other people who may come in contact with the child not recognising that the child should be performing at a higher level. Because of the close and often stifling closeness between child and parents, the process of socialisation with peers is inhibited, and their education falls behind because they are often not capable of going to school. They may also develop fears and phobias.

The long-term consequences are not so well understood. For a rare condition such as this the death rate is high and has been reported. We know that if the children are taken into care they are not easy to look after. Many foster-parents struggle with children who have suffered factitious illness by proxy. The medical conditions may get better quickly, but the psychological and emotional aspects linger on. Some children are reminded of what they had to go through because they have visible physical scars or an illness that has become chronic and is not entirely reversible. Some of these children can show angry and sometimes self-destructive behaviours even if they have been discovered early on in their lives. Because the children have been at the receiving end of manipulating, lying, unpredictable behaviour from a parent (or parents) who has been withholding essential care, and delivered paradoxical and often lethal messages or doses of something that made the children ill, they are confused. They will also have internalised such models as a guideline to how they think they ought to be themselves: a complex picture, which will need long-term study.

Far-reaching consequences of factitious illness by proxy

- *Physical aspects*: resulting from injuries inflicted by the perpetrator, from chronic illness, consequences of surgery, unnecessary, often painful and intrusive, investigations
- *Emotional/psychological aspects*: including chronic invalidism, loneliness, skewed attachments, insecurity and confusion and preoccupation with illness
- *Social aspects*: poor relationships, isolations, lack of experience in ordinary social settings
- *Educational aspects*: poor education, lack of skills

Professional involvement

Professionals, mainly doctors, become enmeshed and manipulated by the mothers, who have been described as 'slick but sick'. The professionals can only avoid becoming part of the abusive cycle by talking to each other and not being piloted by the mother who will use them to abuse the child further (Fig. 12.3). The professionals have to recognise their involvement in a deceptive secretive and interactional liaison which has at its centre the child, the doctor or other professional and the perpetrator, but will include a system with many other people from all walks of life being drawn in. Rarely will they agree on the position of the child, still less agree that factitious illness by proxy is the root of the problem.

Diagnosis

The diagnosis of factitious illness by proxy is difficult to make, but for some children, for example infants where the history is one of repeated apnoea, there is considerable urgency and sophisticated investigation using video cameras may be

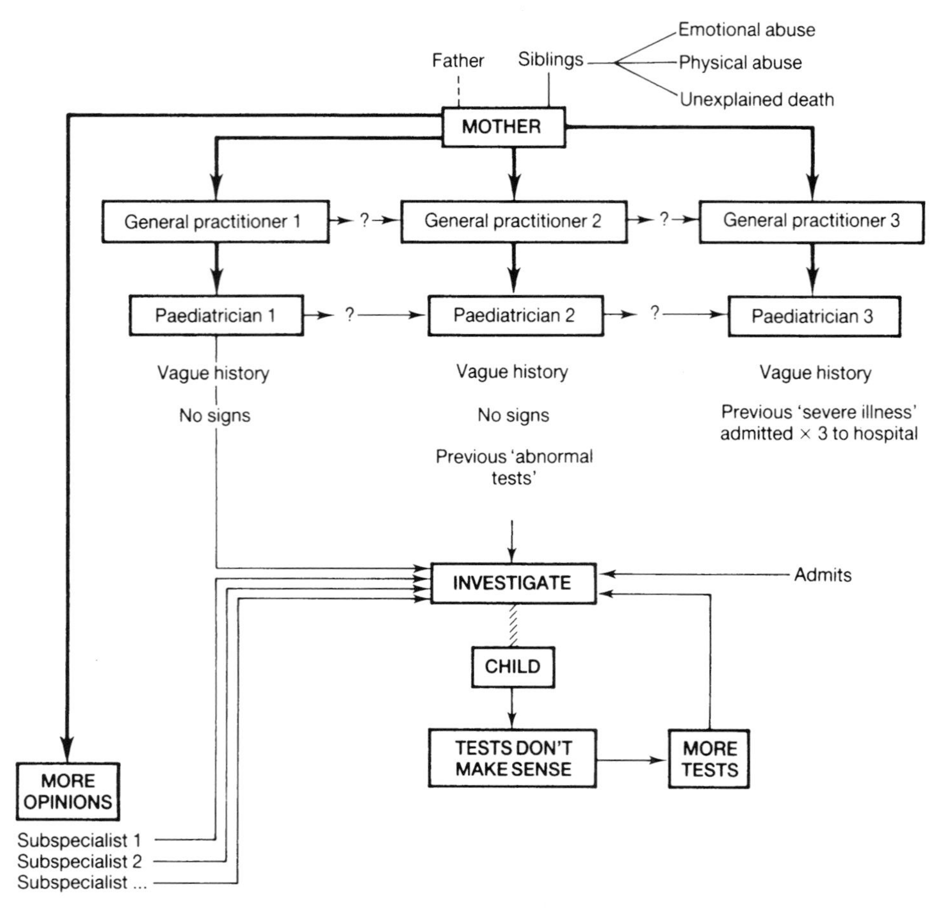

Fig. 12.3 Professional entrapment in factitious illness by proxy. The mother loves all her medical attendants until they fail to comply; then she moves to opinions new. The child is incidental but necessary for the mother's manipulation. Do the various doctors talk to each other?

needed (Southall et al 1987, Hilton 1989, Samuel et al 1992). An experienced toxicologist will advise on an appropriate toxicological screen; meticulous nursing with careful observation, checking and re-charting will reveal maternal falsification of records, for example faked pyrexia.

Because of the very nature of the situation, factitious illness by proxy is diagnosed only after a delay of months to years, or even after a child has died. Since so much more is now written about this syndrome, professionals will only make the necessary connections if they consider the diagnosis as early as possible (Kaufman et al 1989, Gray & Bentovim 1996, Schreier & Libow 1997, Southall et al 1997, Yeo 1997) despite the fact that this can be difficult. The mothers are competent, anxious and attentive but also extremely devious. Doctors do not expect parents to trick them, let alone injure their own child and allow them to suffer unnecessary, painful and sometimes dangerous investigations. Once factitious illness by proxy is considered, further management is carefully planned to collect the information necessary to make a definitive diagnosis and protect the child from further harm.

As in other forms of child abuse, management of factitious illness by proxy is not for the doctor alone. Confronting the mother with her own behaviour is not enough, as deaths have occurred after parents have been confronted and the child then allowed home (Rosenberg 1987).

Management

Rosenberg (1987) describes in detail a protocol for managing a case of suspected factitious illness by proxy.

Management protocol (Rosenberg 1987)

- Remember that factitious illness occurs and also that there is a considerable mortality – the child's safety is paramount
- Mothers may be very attentive, caring, anxious and positively enjoy being resident in hospital
- Why can't you make a diagnosis? The fabrication of disease is such that any possibility should be considered. But consider factitious illness by proxy in any 'rare' disorder
- Hospital admission is usually necessary for evaluation. Remember, a majority of mothers continue to abuse in hospital. The nursing staff must be fully involved, as the diagnosis of factitious illness is often confirmed by their observations
- Take a detailed history, check verbally where possible with general practitioner, health visitor and other family members
- Talk to the child alone. Should there be a formal psychological or psychiatric assessment?
- When the child is in hospital:
  - check all observations, e.g. temperature
  - retain samples of urine and blood for toxicology
  - you may need to supervise parental visits or even stop them, by court order if necessary
- Keep careful, detailed nursing and medical notes. Check all laboratory investigations
- Have a strategy meeting with social worker and other appropriate professionals early on to facilitate understanding and information gathering
- Arrange to meet again to ensure there is further exchange of information with continuing communication between the professionals. When the parents are confronted with the diagnosis, be prepared to take immediate action to protect the child. Parents react differently, and all will need support (including psychiatric help for some). Many mothers will deny the deception, but some will take full responsibility and others acknowledge part of their responsibility. A case conference is held to ensure that the case is fully explored. However, many children will stay in parental care, albeit with good social work support and continuing medical surveillance
- Remember the other children in the family are at risk too. They should also be examined and be involved in the social work assessment as well as any long-term family work and medical follow-up

Jones & Byrne (1996) have developed assessment and management procedures which include an important ingredient often forgotten in the tense atmosphere of such cases: the absolute necessity of a child-centred approach which is adhered to at all times through the assessment, the management and the decision-making processes.

Five stages of management (Jones & Byrne 1996)

- Interprofessional meetings – to recognise the variety of interest in the professional and other networks, etc.
- Review of the medical records of all the family's notes to look for evidence of the possibility of psychiatric disturbance or previous somatisation
- Outpatient assessment which includes a risk assessment. It is important to recognise whether the parents manage to acknowledge what has happened and whether they are willing to work psychologically on this issue
- In-patient, residential component. Jones & Byrne describe a 6–8 week period of risk assessment and therapeutic work leading to an assessment of whether it is possible to reunite the family in their home
- Discharge and plans for continued work and contact for the family and child

The assessment process is essentially that of a child abuse case. A clear picture of what has occurred to the child is a basic requirement. The individual child, and the parents, singly and together, have to be assessed. Other family members may also need assessment and a recognition of the social and professional network is appropriate.

In our experience the outcome for children in these cases is not positive when they remain, or are reunited, with the carer who perpetrated the abuse. However, a recent case study has shown that with some families treatment may be possible and a reunification acceptable (Black & Hollis 1996). However, when Davis et al (1998) investigated 119 children suffering from fictitious illness, suffocation, poisoning and other related forms of this abuse. They concluded that: since the 'mortality, morbidity, family disruption, re-abuse and harm to siblings' is so high, many of the children should not be introduced back home unless the environment is 'especially favourable' and the resources for extended support are present.

Summary

1. Factitious illness by proxy is far more common than has hitherto been acknowledged. It is part of child maltreatment and those procedures need to be followed.
2. Children in these cases need to be made the centre of concern. A child-centred approach is essential.
3. Re-abuse and sibling abuse is not uncommon.
4. The parent or carer for the child is most often the natural mother.
5. Fathers have now been firmly identified as perpetrators of this form of abuse.
6. Foster-carers, caring grandparents, nurses have also been known to be the perpetrator.
7. Deception and secrecy, together with manipulation, are the essence of these cases.
8. Doctors are the most often targeted professionals, but those working in education or law may also be sought out by a perpetrating parent. The 'caring' professions are most at risk from being involved.
9. Professionals are most likely to get enmeshed with the parent and take the side of the parent, not the child.
10. A triangular situation involving the doctor, child and parent is created, where the doctor is challenged to solve an insoluble medical problem.
11. Doctors are subjected to sometimes irresistible adoration and elevated into 'god-like' positions which are designed to make them feel good and at the same time become blind to the child's plight.
12. A doctor who challenges the parent is likely to be discarded and another doctor, a 'better' one, engaged. (Also called 'doctor shopping'.)
13. The child is very vulnerable at the point when such a parent is challenged because the efforts of the parent will be directed into increasing the symptoms and/or substituting them and so putting the child at ever-greater risk.
14. Careful assessment, working with other professionals, is vital.
15. Most paediatricians will have 'minor' cases of factitious illness by proxy on their caseloads.
16. Many of the victims suffer ongoing illness directly related to their abuse.

REFERENCES

Asher R 1951 Munchausen's syndrome. Lancet 1:339–341

Baldwin J A, Oliver J E 1975 Epidemiology and family characteristics of severely abused children. British Journal of Preventive and Social Medicine 29:205

Bergman A B, Beckwith J B, Ray C G (eds) 1970 Sudden infant death syndrome: Proceedings of the 2nd international conference on the causes of sudden death in infants. University of Washington Press, Seattle, WA

Black D, Hollis P 1996 Psychiatric treatment of factitious illness in an infant (Munchausen by proxy syndrome). Clinical Child Psychology and Psychiatry 1:89–98

Bools C N, Neale B A, Meadow S R 1992 Co-morbidity associated with fabricated illness (Munchausen syndrome by proxy). Archives of Disease in Childhood 67:77–79

Bowen D A 1989 Concealment of birth, child destruction and infanticide. In: Mason J K (ed) Paediatric forensic medicine and pathology. Chapman & Hall, London
Creighton S J 1989 Child abuse trends in England and Wales 1983–1987. NSPCC, Leicester
Davis P, McClure R J, Rolfe K, Chessman N, Pearson S, et al 1988 Procedures, placement, and risk of further abuse after Munchausen syndrome by proxy, non-accidental poisoning and nno-accidental suffocation. Archives of Diseases in Childhood 78:217–221
Dine M S, McGovern M E 1982 Intentional poisoning of children – an overlooked category of child abuse: report of seven cases and review of the literature. Pediatrics 70:32–35
Emery J L 1985 Infanticide, filicide and cot death. Archives of Disease in Childhood 60:505–557
Emery J L 1986 Families in which two or more cot deaths have occurred. Lancet 1:313–315
Emery J L 1989 Is sudden infant death syndrome a diagnosis? Leader. British Medical Journal 299:1240
Eminson D M, Postlethwaite R J 1992 Factitious illness: recognition and management. Archives of Disease in Childhood 67:1510–1516
Golding J, Limerick S, Macfarlane A 1985 Sudden infant death; patterns, puzzles and problems. Open Books,
Gray J, Bentovim A 1996 Illness induction syndrome: Paper 1. Child Abuse & Neglect 20:655–673
Hilton J M N 1989 The pathology of sudden infant death syndrome. In: Mason J K (ed) Paediatric forensic medicine and pathology. Chapman & Hall, London
Jones D, Byrne G 1996 Management of factitious illness by proxy. BASPCAN conference on child abuse and neglect, Dublin
Kaufman K L et al 1989 Munchausen's syndrome by proxy: a survey of professionals' knowledge. Child Abuse and Neglect 13:141–147
Kempe C H, Silverman F N, Steele B F et al 1962 The battered child syndrome. JAMA 181:17
Knowelden J, Keeling J, Nicholl J P et al 1985 Postneonatal mortality. A multicentre study. HMSO, London, p 12
Kresel J J, Lovejoy F H 1981 Poisonings and child abuse. In: Ellerstein N S (ed) Child abuse and neglect: a medical reference. Wiley, New York, ch 17, p 307
Meadow R 1977 Munchausen syndrome by proxy: the hinterland of child abuse. Lancet 2:343–345
Meadow R 1989a Suffocation. In: ABC of child abuse. BMJ Publications, London, p 21
Meadow R 1989b Munchausen syndrome by proxy. In: ABC of child abuse. BMJ Publications, London, p 37
Meadow R 1990 Suffocation, recurrent apnoea, and sudden infant death. Journal of Pediatrics 117:351–357
Meadow R M 1993 Non-accidental salt poisoning. Archives of Diseases in Childhood 68:448–452
Newlands M, Emery J L 1991 Child abuse and cot deaths. Child Abuse and Neglect 15:275–278
Nixon J W, Kemp A M, Levene S, Sibert J R 1995 Archives of Disease in Childhood 72:6–10
Pullar P 1984 Mechanical asphyxia. In: Mant A K (ed) Taylor's principles and practice of medical jurisprudence. Churchill Livingstone, Edinburgh
Roberts J, Lynch M A, Golding J 1980 Postneonatal mortality in children from abusing families. British Medical Journal 281(102):1215
Rogers D, Tripp J, Bentovim A, Berry D, Goulding R 1976 Non-accidental poisoning: an extended syndrome of child abuse. British Medical Journal i:793–796
Rosenberg D A 1987 Web of deceit: a literature review of Munchausen syndrome by proxy. Child Abuse and Neglect 11:547–563
Schreier H A 1997 Factitious presentation of psychiatric disorder: when is it Munchausen by proxy? Child Psychology and Psychiatry Review 2(3):108–115
Schreier H A, Libow J A 1993 Hurting for love. Guildford Press, New York
Sibert J 1975 Stress in families who have ingested poisons. British Medical Journal 3:87
Southall D P, Plunkett M C B, Banks M W, Falkov A F & Samuels M P 1997 Covert video recordings of life-threatening child abuse: lessons for child protection. Pediatrics 100:735–755
Taylor E M, Emery J L 1988 Trends in unexpected infant deaths in Sheffield. Lancet ii:1121–1123
Winnicott D W 1982 The maturational process and the facilitating environment. Hogarth Press, London
Wiseman H M, Guest V H G, Volans G N 1987 Accidental poisoning in childhood: a multi-centre study. General Epidemiology 6:293–301
Wissow S L 1990 Munchausen by proxy. In: Child advocacy for the clinician. Williams & Wilkins, Baltimore, MD
Yeo S S 1996 Munchausen by proxy: Another form of child abuse. Child Abuse Review 5:170–180
Yorker B C 1996 Legal issues in factitious disorder by proxy. In: Feldman M D, Eisendrath S J (eds) The spectrum of factitious disorder. American Psychiatric Press, Washington, DC

13

Other forms of child sexual abuse

Organised abuse

Organised abuse is a generic term for abuse which may involve a number of abusers and a number of abused children and young people, and often encompasses different forms of abuse. It involves to a greater or lesser extent an element of organisation:

> . . . some groups may use bizarre or ritualized behaviour, sometimes with a particular 'belief system' (Working Together 1991).

Bibby (1996) has developed this definition further and suggests that organised abuse is:

- the systematic abuse of children, normally by more than one abuser
- characterised by careful planning in purposeful, targeting, seduction and silencing of the children
- seen in different forms, for example institutional and ritualised abuse.

Network abuse is another way of describing the abuse of children by adults from different families, institutions or organisations; the function of the network is to ensure children are available to abuse.

Syndicated organised abuse is the term used to describe abuse with a commercial basis as in pornography and prostitution (Gough 1996).

Sex rings

The existence of child sex rings has been known for centuries, and as Wild (1989) points out, there are examples in ancient history; for instance the Roman emperor Tiberius who abused groups of children sexually on the Isle of Capri. There are also reports by Wells (1958) and by Radzinowicz (1975) which included descriptions of sex rings. Table 13.1 summarises the types of 'sex rings'.

The literature on sex rings (Burgess et al 1981, Burgess 1984, Wild & Wynne 1986, Wild 1988, 1989, Conte 1989) has highlighted the organised and sometimes extremely sophisticated methods used to gain access to and then exploit children sexually. Burgess (1984) wrote: 'Solo rings consist of one adult who is sexually involved with a number of children'. Burgess (1984) and Wild & Wynne (1986) describe this form of sex ring as one where there is no transfer of the children or of photographs, but that children may be recruited by each other and become members of groups of children involved with different adults. The sex rings described in Leeds (Wild & Wynne 1986) were discovered following the allegations of one girl (see below) and a very thorough investigation by police and the social services department including a committed specialist police unit in south Leeds. Since then several further rings have come to light but experience has shown that extensive rings do exist in the community and only if there is a commitment to undertake thorough (expensive) investigations will they be recognised.

CASE HISTORY 13.1

A boy of 5 years was taken to the Accident and Emergency department because of 'a cut on his penis'. He had a ragged laceration proximally on the dorsum of penis. The previous evening his parents had left him with a 13-year-old girl to babysit. She later described the boy masturbating whilst watching the television. She told him to 'put it away' and finally 'put it away or I'll cut it off'.

The girl subsequently disclosed sexual abuse by her step-grandfather and she was a member of a local sex ring. There were several girls in the ring aged 10–14 years who visited a single man in his 40s and in exchange for various sexual acts he gave them small amounts of money, cups of coffee, cigarettes.

Typical features of the Leeds sex rings

- Several girls (there were several 'boys' rings' too) visited a lone man
- The age of the children was usually 12–13 years but there were some younger and prepubertal girls involved too. There were also older children involved, including those with moderate learning difficulties
- The children were sometimes involved in more than one ring

Table 13.1 Forms of organised abuse (after Gough 1996)

Type of organisation	Operation	References
Solo ring	One adult involved with a number of children who may recruit others and be involved with different, lone adults The adult may target vulnerable children and be highly organised, e.g. work in day nursery	Burgess (1984) Wild (1986, 1989) Conte (1989)
Syndicated ring	Several adults in well-structured group which recruits children Produces pornography, delivers sexual services, i.e. prostitution	Gil (1982)
Transitional rings	More than one adult, not well organised, may become syndicated	
Community-based rings (boys, girls or mixed gender)	Variable number of abusers and children (cf. solo ring), often loose network, family/friends	
Day care institutions	Initially described in day-nurseries with several abusers (male and female) and many children (boys and girls)	Finkelhor et al (1988) Kelley (1994)
Residential care institutions	Children may already be vulnerable (previous abuse, disability) solo or more abusers (staff, peers) and variable degree organisation outside institution	Westcott (1991) Jones (1994)
Ritual abuse	'Abuse that occurs in a context linked to some symbols or group activity (religious/magical etc.)'	Finkelhor et al (1988)
Satanic abuse	'A specific form of ritual abuse where the ritual is related to satanic practices'	Sinason (1994) Gough (1996)

- Some of the children had been previously or were concurrently abused within their homes
- The extent of the abuse was wide, from touching to intercourse
- Children were introduced to the ring by their peers
- The men (women abusers have recently been recognised) were usually single but aged 20–80 years
- A minority of abusers had previous police convictions
- The rings were often in socially deprived areas with high levels of unemployment but not exclusively so
- The local community was often aware that 'children are always going to flat 26'
- The police successfully prosecuted many of the men in the rings discovered

CASE HISTORY 13.2

A 15-year-old boy told his current social worker that he had been abused at his previous residential school. This was a small unit run by a voluntary agency for older children with emotional problems. This boy had been abused physically and emotionally at home. He was emotionally very immature and had mild learning problems.

A male member of staff befriended the boy who had only a place in a children's' home to return to for weekends and holidays. He taught the boy to canoe and took him away, sometimes alone and sometimes with another vulnerable boy canoeing on the canal followed by a night at his cottage. There he gave the boy alcoholic drinks and probably drugs before raping him.

This boy was vulnerable because of his rejection from home, his need for 'love and attention' and his immaturity and learning problem. He was targeted and 'groomed' by a skilled paedophile who although dismissed from his job was not prosecuted because of the difficulty for children giving evidence.

Paedophiles select employment and recreational activities which allows them easy access to children. They are often 'good with children' and offer activities such as computer games, sport and excursions which are not generally available.

Syndicated rings include several adults who form a well-structured organisation for the recruitment of children, the production of pornography, the delivery of direct sexual services and the establishment of an extensive network of customers (Burgess 1984).

Transitional rings may consist of more than one adult with several children but without the organisation of the syndicated rings. The transitional rings may eventually become syndicated and, for instance, sell pornographic photographs of children. Rings are usually for male or female children. It has been recognised that girls and boys may be selected for specific rings and specific purposes and/or clients.

Links with prostitution and pornography

It was at first thought that female sex rings and female prostitution were more often connected than male rings and prostitution, but more recently it has become clear that boys are equally vulnerable to prostitution.

CASE HISTORY 13.3

A 12-year-old boy with moderate learning problems was referred to a group for young boys who had sexually abused other children. He lived in a childrens's' home following a life of sexual abuse and neglect (he had been abused by his mother and older brother and sister). He talked about a café and it soon became evident that an upstairs room there was used as a collecting place for young teenage boys for sex. Many of these children were known to each other through the 'care system'.

More recently the links with child pornography and organised crime have been described (Tate 1990) but there is little research into child sexual abuse and pornography (Kelly 1996) There is a vast international market for pornographic material (Hames 1993). There is a current debate as to how to control access to the Internet by paedophiles with pornographic material.

Many paedophiles collect and produce their own material using camcorders which are relatively cheap. They can use their films themselves, sell them, or use them to blackmail or silence children or adults. The films may be very helpful in police investigations.

CASE HISTORY 13.4

A Sunday tabloid newspaper featured the face of a young teenager and stated that they had acquired the image from a 'home-made' pornographic video. The girl was recognised and the police were involved. The girl, then aged 16, had been 13 years old when the film was made by her older sister's partner who had befriended her when she was unhappy at home. This man, a wealthy landlord, was convicted: he ran a brothel and was a paedophile abusing young girls including his partners' two small daughters.

CASE HISTORY 13.5

A family of three children under 5 years were seen when their father, a known Schedule 1 offender, was arrested for sending child pornography via the Internet. The children had minor signs – child sexual abuse was not ruled out.

CASE HISTORY 13.6

A 12-year-old boy with psychosomatic hip pain was re-admitted to the paediatric ward. He was clearly frightened of his grandfather with whom he lived. After 1 week he started to talk to the ward staff and it emerged that he bathed with his grandfather and usually slept with him '. . . frightened by the violent "18" videos he watched at night', he was worried by ghosts. Later he said he wanted to return to his mother's care – he did not like the pornographic videos he was made to watch or the way his grandfather 'touched him'. Physical examination was normal.

Prostitution is often part of syndicated rings, as children are bought for clients. The abusers have their preferences: age, gender, 'no hair or breasts' and victims are supplied. There is an international trade in children for sex (see later).

Prostitution of children is also a problem which is currently receiving attention in the UK as the children are seen as victims rather than offenders. Historically 'child prostitutes' have been arrested on the streets for soliciting and often charged, acquiring a criminal record. The adults who abuse them have been more likely to cautioned by the police. The victims are frequently vulnerable children who may have been abused, be runaways (from home or care) or are emotionally needy children who think their 'pimp' loves them (pimps are typically aged 18–25 years and trap victims often using violence and drugs to maintain control). 'Model' agencies may lure children into prostitution and children are used in 'massage parlours'. Pimps may target children's homes and work with taxi-drivers (often using CB radio) to organise their trade. In 1995 in England and Wales 364 girls 18 years and under were cautioned or convicted of loitering or soliciting for prostitution; 48 were under 16 years (Hansard 1997).

CASE HISTORY 13.6

A mother brought her 13-year-old daughter for a 'check-up' at the paediatric clinic because she was worried that she might have a sexually transmitted disease. Three weeks earlier the mother had asked social services for help as her daughter was 'out of control' and the girl was accommodated in a small children's home. She made friends with a girl the mother said was 'no better than a prostitute' and the day before the paediatric referral the two girls ran away. The mother went searching for her daughter in the red light district of Leeds and spoke to several prostitutes. One prostitute told her of the trade of young Leeds girls to Bradford and the two women travelled by taxi the 10 miles to Bradford to look for the girl. The prostitute guided the taxi to numerous cafes where there were many men and very young girls, and eventually to a cellar below a restaurant where the girl was found.

There appeared to be a network of available young girls, men and cafés but no prosecutions followed.

Links with residential care and runaways

In a 1991 study 22 young women who had spent time in care and were in the sex industry were interviewed: 4 were in the sex industry before going into care, 8 were involved whilst in care, 17 received no sex education in care (Linehan 1994).

One in seven runaways trade sex for money and over 25% of runaways are physically or sexually abused on the streets. A significant number self-harm or attempt suicide (Stein et al 1994). It is of great concern that HIV infection almost doubled in the 13–24-year-old age group between 1991 and 1993 (CDC 1994). Half the young women selling sex do so to feed a heroin addiction, and US figures suggest 50% of involved children are drug addicted too (Linehan 1997). The figures for boys are likely to be comparable and the combination of drug abuse and prostitution put these children at high risk of sexually transmitted diseases including HIV infection.

Day care abuse

Day care abuse has received much media attention, especially in the US, but in spite of the increased numbers of young children in nurseries the child remains more at risk of abuse at home (Kelly 1994) although recognition of nursery abuse is rising (in the UK too).

Finkelhor et al (1989) documented sexual abuse in day care in a detailed research study. Whether the sexual abuse took place in nurseries or family-based childcare it was found that there were multiple abusers and victims, and in a number of institutions children had been sexually and ritually abused for years. Finkelhor found that the young age of the children had posed difficult problems for investigation and prosecution, and that the reports of particularly bizarre abuse were hard to validate particularly with multiple abusers and traumatised victims (and families).

Kelly (1994) summarised the findings of her own and three other studies of the abuse of children in day care settings:

- fondling was the most frequent abuse but penetration of the vagina or anus occurred, commonly including use of implements
- pornography was common, both in showing/involving the children in making films
- children were forced to engage in sexual acts with other children
- physical abuse was common; drugs were administered to some
- threats and terrorising acts were a common aspect of the abuse
- there were two general categories of abuser, those who planned their sexual abuse of children and those who became involved because of their circumstances in the nursery (Faller 1990)
- 40% of the abusers were women
- the consequences for the children in terms of emotional trauma were comparable to other sexually abused children and families were thrown into turmoil.

Ritualistic abuse

Definitions

Child abuse has acquired yet another dimension of maltreatment in ritual abuse. This is a particularly damaging and brutal form of child maltreatment involving children, some of them very young, adolescents and adults. This form of abuse is always a part of group activity, often related to a cult, and frequently includes physical, sexual and emotional maltreatment.

A working group in Leeds (including the authors) developed the following definition in an effort to further understanding of this form of abuse:

> Ritual abuse is the physical, psychological, and/or sexual abuse of children, associated with repeated activities (i.e. ritual) which relate the abuse to contexts of a religious, magical, or supernatural kind. These activities include the use of particular language, imagery and symbols as well as the performance of certain acts (McFadyen et al 1993).

The US experience

Ritual abuse has been described in day care centres, in neighbourhoods and in nuclear and extended families; there are multiple victims and abusers (Kelley 1993). A society which has difficulties in acknowledging that child sexual abuse occurs has even more difficulty in contemplating the existence of ritual abuse. There is a continuing debate and much anger and disagreement which will only be resolved by research (La Fontaine et al 1997). A current piece of work found

> . . . The analysis of the American satanic ritual abuse day care cases does not resolve the debate (de Young 1997).

More research is needed to move the debate beyond the sterile 'belief or disbelief' argument. There is still controversy over how to define ritual abuse. Definitions have been developed, though there is confusion over distinguishing network abuse, ritual abuse and satanic abuse. Finkelhor et al (1989) defined ritualistic abuse as:

> abuse which occurs in a context linked to some symbols or group activity that have religious, magical or supernatural connotation, and where the invocation of these symbols or activities, repeated over time, is used to frighten and intimidate the children.

Finkelhor et al (1988) identified three types of ritual abuse:

- *Type I* is defined as truly cult-based, and it involves child abuse as an expression of an elaborate belief system. The abuse is part of a social system or a cult and includes physical, sexual and emotional abuse. By using children the adult reaches a mystical state, which allegedly is the goal, rather than the sexual abuse of the children. The children are indoctrinated into a different belief system which discredits parents and traditional teaching. The group is kept together as adults and children are corrupted and dare not disclose forbidden practices.
- *Type II* is defined as pseudo; here the primary motivating factor is the sexual abuse of children. Magic, costumes and animals may be part of a technique of gaining access to children and maintaining their interest before intimidating them into participation in various sexual acts and frightening them to deter any disclosure.
- *Type III* is defined as psychopathological; here the abuse is a part of an obsessional or delusional aspect of an individual or a group.

Lloyd (1992) defined this form of abuse as:

> the intentional physical abuse, sexual abuse or psychological abuse of a child by a person responsible for the child's welfare when such abuse is repeated and/or stylised, and is typified by such other acts as cruelty to animals, or threats of harm to the child, other persons and animals.

Snow & Sorensen (1990) consider ritualistic abuse in a neighbourhood setting and show that it emerges in both intra- and extrafamilial settings. They quote from research undertaken with individuals suffering from multiple personality disorder, indicating that many have been ritualistically abused as children.

The Report of the Ritual Abuse Task Force, Los Angeles County Commission for Women, September 1989 (p. 1), stated that ritual abuse is usually carried out by members of a cult. The purpose of the ritual elements of the abuse seems threefold:

- rituals in some groups are part of a shared belief or worship system into which the victim is being indoctrinated
- rituals are used to intimidate victims into silence
- ritual elements (e.g. devil worship, animal or human sacrifice) seem so unbelievable to those unfamiliar with these crimes that these elements detract from the credibility of the victims and make prosecution of the crimes very difficult

Jones (1991) examines reports of children having been ritually abused and highlights the difficulties in bringing these cases to prosecution. The description of brutal, perverse and sadistic behaviour towards children often makes the accounts sound unreal and fictitious. This is an added complication in the work of child protection for the legal profession (Lanning 1991).

The UK experience

In the UK, descriptions of ritualistic abuse have appeared in the press. The *Independent* (1990) described five criminal trials over the previous 2-year period. These trials all included the abuse of children in groups, with associated ritual, satanic and witchcraft practices.

The NSPCC have attempted to monitor the evidence for child pornography, sex rings and ritual abuse. In March 1990, C. Brown, Director of the NSPCC, said that members of seven NSPCC protection teams (out of a total of 64 teams) in England and Wales were currently working with children who were the victims of ritualistic abuse (Creighton 1993).

The Dutch experience

One of the best documented cases of ritualistic abuse in western Europe occurred in Gude Pekela, a small Dutch town with a population of 8000 people. In Spring 1987, 98 children aged 3–11 years were subject to violent and sadistic abuse, often as part of satanic rituals. The cases came to light when a 4-year-old boy presented with anal bleeding and only after several days told his parents of his anal abuse, 'sticks in bottom', which had happened to his friends too. The children were lured by men and women dressed as clowns and animals, who took them to 'parties' and gave them ice-cream and drugged lemonade. The children were told to undress and made to take part in sexual acts with adults and with each other. The children described lying naked on tables, a church, candles, headless dolls and photographs and videos being made. The adults also dressed up in white robes and threatened the children that if they told they would be killed or their house set on fire. To emphasise the threat animals were killed, a 'baby killed', 'babies' were beaten.

When the Dutch case came to light, the media response was that it could all be explained by 'mass hysteria'. Similarly, when in 1990 the NSPCC made a statement to the press, a police spokesman for the CID in London said there was 'no evidence of the ritual abuse of children in England'.

However, in Holland the Justice Ministry found that 48 statements spoke of clear sexual abuse and that two men and two women were involved in the child sexual abuse (Myers 1994). There were two arrests but no convictions.

The cases have be followed up carefully and there have now been three surveys of the children (Jonker & Jonker-Baaker 1997). From this data it is now clear that in 1987 various physical signs and symptoms as well as behavioural problems reported were wrongly rated as 'normal'. Although most of the children by 1994 had acceptable behaviour many (39%) were 'changed'. 20% had sleep problems, 8% showed inappropriate sexual behaviour, 21% were aggressive towards their parents, 20% were nervous. 7% of children had more severe behavioural disorders.

The physical signs and symptoms were inflamed genitalia/anus, dysuria, painful defecation, bleeding – possibly vaginally and rectally, itching, bruising in unusual sites and unusual sleepiness. There was an abrupt increase in these signs at the beginning of the case.

The pattern of symptoms shown by the children is therefore corroboration of child sexual abuse – what other explanation can there be? Mass hysteria does not bruise or lead to sexualised behaviour or lead young children to speak clearly of child sexual abuse.

Prevalence and presentation

Ritualistic abuse does appear to be uncommon; it represented around 1% of the total child sexual abuse cases recognised in the UK in 1988–89. In a further analysis by Creighton (1993) of children on Child Protection Registers for CSA 2% were involved in network abuse, 1% in ritual abuse and 0.2% in pornography. However, it does occur and it is likely that over the next few years the true extent of the problem will become evident. Whether the groups are linked and form a well-organised network across the country is less certain, although there is evidence for child pornography and child prostitution networks and it is likely that there are links between some groups (Itzin, 1996).

A paper commissioned by the Department of Health (England and Wales) (La Fontaine 1995) looked at the '... extent and nature of organised and ritual sexual abuse of children'. Ritual abuse was present in only 8% of cases involving organised abuse. Other attributes reported of organised abuse were:

- almost all the perpetrators were men and most victims were boys
- 75% of the families were socially disadvantaged
- many of the perpetrators had criminal records, usually for theft or violence
- many of the children were neglected
- older siblings frequently abused younger siblings.

La Fontaine's research was based on information gathered by postal ballot, 84 cases of organised abuse, (including some ritual abuse) were identified. Gallagher (1994) took the research further looking in detail at reported cases finding:

- organised abuse accounts for a small part of statutory child protection work, around 2%
- there was no typical organisation but 'a set of factors that tended to cluster'
- settings included the family, neighbours, strangers, children's homes, foster home, children's institutions
- the number of children involved was 2–20 and perpetrators 2–20 (in the rings)
- female perpetrators and boy victims were over-represented as compared with other child sexual abuse
- many of the children, or their siblings, were already known to social services before the detection of the organised abuse because of other abuse or recognised emotional and behavioural problems
- 'the sexual abuse these children suffered tended to be extreme. On occasions, they would be exposed to bizarre or sadistic practises such as being forced to eat excrement and bestiality.

The presentation of ritual abuse in the US is no less contentious but is better recorded (Finkelhor et al 1989).

The elements of the Dutch case of young children who were badly scared, the use of drugs, candles, symbols, 'killing babies', pornography and so on are repeated over and over again in disclosures by abused children but meet with scepticism by adults. In the US there is a continuing debate as to whether ritualistic abuse occurs; one side claims that it is multidimensional multiabuser sexual abuse and cannot be defined, whereas the other describes the similarities between the identified cases of ritualistic abuse and how they differ from the usual intrafamilial abuse (although there may be elements of ritualistic abuse in any sexual abuse).

Summit (1990) describes groups of very young children, 2–6 years, with multiple abusers including many women, often based in day care facilities from which the children are transported to 'big' houses, the use of pornography, video filming, drugs, violence, pain, sadism, threats and the abuse of children by children, cruelty to animals involving children too, turning the children into (albeit unwitting) abusers. Summit says that children are tricked into believing that adults have magical powers and believe what they see – babies being killed and beaten, and the more bizarre events. But by the use of drugs, fear and abnormal practices, such as smearing of faeces or eating excrement, children may be disorientated: reality and fantasy blend, they lose any sense of time and place and become confused. This does not mean that, when several children describe similar events, it is mass hysteria and because investigating authorities have not found any dead babies, nothing has happened. If adults do not understand the children, who may appear illogical and their disclosures unbelievable and contradictory, they may be suspected of false allegation.

Difficulties in investigation and resolution

While the clinical picture is disentangled the child, family and investigators (usually social worker, psychologist or psychiatrist) need support and the resources to investigate effectively. If society, the police or individual agencies 'do not believe in ritual abuse' the child, families and professionals are undermined and their credibility is attacked as the child is further damaged. The data are disturbing, but require evaluation not dismissal. Polarisation into 'believers' and 'non-believers' is unhelpful, as are concepts of 'satanists running rampant' or 'therapists generating hysteria'. An open rational resolution of the difficult problems raised by the data is needed.

Satanic abuse

Nursten (1996) wrote of satanic abuse:

> Allegations of satanic abuse involve a powerful blend of sex, secrecy, magic, domination, darkness and quasi-religious practices which leads to strong views being held on the matter.

Satanism (Kelley 1993) or elements of satanism are often described in the context of ritual abuse. The activities include (Langone 1990):

- formal or informal worship of Satan or entities equated with or associated with or associated with Satan and/or with violence, cruelty and destructiveness
- the practice of black magic for destructive ends
- preoccupation with literature, symbols, rituals or other artefacts and activities associated with Satan or related entities, or with black magic
- alternatively, attempting to enhance sexual, criminal or other activities by participation in rituals associated with the worship of Satan or related entities or with the practice of black magic.

Langone (1990) suggests four groups of satanists:

- dabblers, often teenagers
- self-styled satanists who are attracted to violence
- religious satanists in publicly acknowledged groups
- satanic cults which are clandestine and may be engaged in criminal activity.

The second and fourth groups are those where there is greater concern that children may be involved.

Characteristics of ritualistic rings in the USA (with or without satanism) have been described by Gould (1987), Finkelhor et al (1989), Summit (1990), Kelley (1993), Sinason (1994):

- many in day-care facilities
- multiple perpetrators (5% single abuser)
- women abusers are as common as male abusers
- women may be sole abusers
- abuse may have occurred over long periods (20 years)
- abuse involves all forms of serious penetrative child sexual abuse
- adult–adult, adult–child, child–child abuse
- high rate of pornography use
- drugs used to make children comply
- 'cult families'
- all have religious, magical or supernatural belief system

Ways in which children present and describe (US experience)

- May present with vomiting, nightmares, extreme anxiety, feeling 'bad'
- Aggressive behaviour – sexually abuse peers
- Extreme fear – terrorised to remain silent
- 'Supernatural powers' – magic
- Symbols used to frighten and intimidate
- Wear masks, costumes, including animal disguise
- Drink blood, urine, eat faeces
- Kill animals, 'babies', mutilation
- Dig up graves, devil worship, crosses, religious implements
- Pregnancy

Effects of ritualistic abuse (including satanic abuse)

The impact of ritualistic abuse on children is, not surprisingly, severe. The bizarre and coercive elements terrorise children and there is always severe emotional abuse, as well as physical and sexual abuse. This leads children to dissociate experiences, which may have a lasting effect on their mental health (Goodwin et al 1990, Pelcovitz 1990, Waterman et al 1990, Kelley 1993). The longer the abuse lasts, the greater the physical force used, the larger the number of perpetrators and the greater the insistence on participation between children, the more likely to lead to increased distress for the child in the future.

Children who have been in the abuser role are likely to be more aggressive and act out sexually towards their peer group or with dolls. Other children regress, become very clingy and lose toilet training skills. Some children become obsessed with monsters, death and dying. Others are deluded that they have a spider, or monster within their body. They become confused with concepts of God, the devil and evil, and their own beliefs are chaotic. Not only are the victims of ritualistic abuse more disturbed than in other cases of child sexual abuse, but their parents are upset and need considerable help.

Although much of the abuse in the USA has been described in day nurseries, various criminal trials in the UK show that teenagers are involved too and the effects on them must be equally as complex and far-reaching as sexual maturity is reached. There are particularly disturbing descriptions of teenage girls being made pregnant by cult elders, and even criminal induction of abortion. The ritualistic sex rings should be differentiated from 'historical child sex rings' (Burgess 1984). In these rings offenders are almost all male, often paedophiles, and child pornography is commonly used. Boys are abused just as much as girls and pornography is used to corrupt – particularly adolescent boys who are easily sexually aroused. Ritual abuse is not a usual component of these rings, which are focused on the seduction of children and sexual activities.

Investigation of ritualistic abuse requires meticulous planning and equal sophistication to the organisers of the ring or cult. It involves a complex multi-agency approach with practitioners and senior managers working together (Lanning 1991). The psychological strain on staff should not be underestimated.

Child pornography

Child pornography is a form of sexual exploitation of children. Pornography is an international multi-billion dollar industry, and children are thought to be featured in around 6% of the published material. There is a huge production of 'soft porn', from page 3 pin-ups in the tabloids to 'top shelf' magazines such as *Playboy* and *Mayfair*.

The distribution of such material through high-street stationers is open; clearly different outlets are needed for illegal and child pornography. Organisations such as Paedophile Information Exchange exist to manage this side of the industry.

Effects of pornography

Currently there is a debate as to the role of pornography in the abuse of women and children. Men are also affected by pornography, whether in its production or as users. The effect of a combination of violence and sex, as depicted in the particularly nasty videos, is of great concern, especially as the number of rapes and sexual assaults reported to the police rises each year. 'Snuff videos' where the hapless victim is murdered on camera have also been made – with what effect on the viewer, camera crew and so on?

Pornography trivialises sexual relationships by separating sex from its normal social context and reduces the depicted person to a recipient object. Children are therefore used in the representation of sex and sexuality with the aim of arousing sexual desire and providing or provoking sexual gratification (Ennew 1986). This material may be primarily for the use of paedophiles, but others abuse children sexually as part of their incontinent sexual behaviour. The images that are presented include a single child, or groups of children, sometimes with adults or animals. The children are variously dressed and posed in sexual acts involving other children, adults, animals or inanimate objects. One difficulty is that the appeal of child pornography lies in the eye of the beholder. Adults who sexually abuse children may find catalogues of children's clothes with child models sexually arousing. Holiday snaps of children on the beach or James, aged 2 years, naked in the bath are coveted images to some. This, however, does not alter the need for serious debate about the role of pornography in our society, including the tabloid pin-ups as well as more obviously offensive publications. Many women dislike pornography, and as men recognise the deviancy and the degradation of women such pictures portray, perhaps more men will reject it too.

It is also important to look at the role pornography plays in the sexual development of teenagers in the UK. What are teenagers learning about sexual behaviour from these publications? A study (Itzin & Sweet 1990) of 4000 women respondents to a questionnaire on pornography run by *Cosmopolitan* (a women's magazine) showed that 36% had seen pornography at less than 12 years old and 14% at under 10 years. Of this pornography 69% saw 'men only' magazines but 28% saw 'illegal magazines' depicting rape, animals or children in various sexual acts. This is abusive in itself: is this how children in the UK are to learn about 'adult' sexual behaviour? The survey indicated that 64% saw the pornography at home or in a friend's or relative's house.

More seriously, there was an association between childhood exposure to pornography and sexual experience below the age of consent (16 years). More than 25% of children who saw pornography under 12 years had sex before the age of 16 years. Does this also relate to issues of child protection? Pornography is commonly used by abusers. Offenders know that the typical adolescent is sexually curious and easily sexually aroused, if sexually inexperienced. Pornographic material may be made available in the seduction process by offenders, whether in 'historical sex rings' or intrafamilial abuse. In ritualistic abuse children have commonly described films, photographs and video-making equipment. The greater availability of camcorders has enabled amateur film makers to create their own pornography. For children involved in the making of pornographic material there are additional consequences, although these are dismissed by the children (Pelcovitz 1990). Compared with sexually abused children who were not involved in pornography this group were found to be more stigmatised, felt 'gay' or 'damaged', guilty, had greater difficulty in trusting and were angry, especially about their powerlessness.

The use of pornography by adolescent abusers is also worrying. These teenager abusers are a significant group, and the corrupting effect of pornography should not be underestimated. Neither should the 'teaching' of these immature children be of such abnormal practices which may also introduce the idea of teenager–child sexual activity. In this context teenagers as babysitters may see a video, become sexually excited, use it as a model, and then experiment on their young charges.

The law in England and Wales is represented by the Protection of Children Act 1978, which makes it an offence for a person or body to take indecent photographs (including film or video) of children under 16 years to show or distribute these, or to publish or advertise them. The Criminal Justice Bill 1988, under Section 160, makes possession of pornographic material an offence.

Pornography is not harmless, and although the evidence needs substantiating, there appear to be links between violent sex videos and violent sexual assault. It is the depiction of the misuse of power, and degradation of one person by another, usually a woman by a man, that is harmful.

A 2-year investigation of the buying and selling of boys from the age of 5–6 years was reported by two journalists (Davies & O'Connor 1997). The links between paedophiles in the UK, Holland and other European countries were established and boys were procured from London and eastern Europe. Films were made and there was evidence of violent sexual abuse and torture. Descriptions of 'snuff videos' were given.

Erotica, which is also available, is different in that love and partnership are portrayed rather than the isolation of the body from the person. It is in the former context that children and adolescents need to understand sexual relationships. When young children see pornography it appears to desensitise them to sexual activity and lead them into inappropriate behaviour. It also suggests ways of behaving which are not tolerated by ordinary social mores. In this way pornographic material may delay and distort sexual development rather than promote it. In the UK, with increasing awareness of the adverse and insidious effects of all pornography on developing children and adolescents and the misuse of sexuality by adults, there are an increasing number of campaigns, such as 'Off the Shelf', to control its production and distribution (Itzin & Sweet 1990).

Child pornography: summary (after Itzin 1996)

- Child pornography is part of the violent continuum of child sexual abuse (Kelly 1987)
- Child pornography may be part of:
  - intrafamilial child sexual abuse
  - extrafamilial child sexual abuse
  - 'rings' or organised abuse
  - institutional abuse
- The making and selling of pornographic material is highly organised
- Child pornography may be associated with child prostitution (locally, nationally and internationally)
- Child pornography sexualises children and predisposes them to:
  - abuse by strangers or known adults
  - participation as adults in pornography and prostitution

Other forms of sexual exploitation of children

Sexual exploitation of children takes many forms (Ennew 1986). All these forms of abuse exploit not only the power differential between the adult and child but also the social domination of male over female and elder over junior and, in addition, class and wealth.

Sex tourism usually involves the abuse of poor, non-white, young, non-western children by (comparatively) rich, white, western adult males.

White slavery usually implies the use of young poor women by western males. The girls are kidnapped, or forced by poverty into vice rings run for profit by racketeers. Very young girls, 8–9 years old, are used in 'kiddie porn' or 'baby prostitution'. Boys have long been known to be involved in prostitution and sex rings. Again, youth and attractiveness are valued by their abusers.

Prostitutes in developing countries may be street children, often the children of impoverished rural families who have moved to towns and are unable to care for all their children. They may also be runaways, running from abuse or exploitation at home. Girls in particular may have been hired from their fathers to work in dancing, cabaret or bar work and forced into the sex trade. Similarly, girls are hired as servants and are sexually exploited by their employers. This has been described by Filipino women employed in Saudi Arabia to such an extent their government has issued a warning to their own nationals.

There is also trading of young women from eastern Europe to the west, lured by promises of modelling or dancing jobs and a glamorous life, an escape from poverty to sexual abuse.

A particularly sinister trade has been in children adopted from poor developing countries. Some children have been adopted by paedophiles and pimps running child prostitution rings, using the cover of an adoption agency. Attempts to curb paedophilia and sex tourism through legislation in the country of origin are current in several countries. A Swedish man was convicted in Sweden in 1996 for sexually abusing children outside Sweden. Other countries including the UK have planned to enact similar laws.

Children will continue to be vulnerable to sexual abuse as long as there are gross social inequalities in society and corrupt men and women who will use powerless, available children for their own sexual gratification.

Institutional abuse

It is apparent that any abuse may occur in institutions from choir-schools to special schools to young offender's prisons to children's homes. This was recognised by Working Together (1991) and the Children Act 1989, but there are persisting gaps in legislation particularly with reference to private schools and homes.

The dynamics of institutions are characterised by their isolation and their hierarchical and unequal power relationships (Doran & Brannan 1996). Residential units make children more vulnerable and this vulnerability is greater for children in care, disabled children, and children with learning difficulties (see also Ch. 10).

Schools may be targeted by paedophiles who may take over and control the institution with systems of abuse which may include contacts with other paedophile rings. Links can then be made with child prostitution and the production of child pornography.

There have been several high profile examples of abuse in institutions, for example, Kincora Home (boys), Beeches Children's Home, Castle Hill School, Crookham Court (boarding school). In 1997 an inquiry started into children's homes in Clwyd, North Wales.

Preventive strategies and a planned approach to investigating large-scale abuse have been described (Doran & Brennan 1996).

Summary

1. Organised abuse is an increasingly recognised form of child abuse, usually found in institutions.
2. Ritual is part of much CSA but in organised abuse may involve complex belief systems and behaviours.
3. Pornography is a highly developed industry and child pornography is part of the continuum of CSA.
4. Prostitution of children is a form of abuse prevalent throughout the World. By naming the adult as an abuser there are opportunities for the child to be protected.
5. Professionals involved in the investigation and support of ritual or organised CSA need skilled support themselves.

REFERENCES

Bibby P 1996 Definitions and recent history. in: Bibby P (ed.) Organised abuse – the current debate. Arena, London, Ch 1

Burgess A W 1984 Child pornography and sex rings. Lexington Books, Lexington MA

Burgess A W, Groth A W, McCausland M P 1981 Child sex initiation rings. American Journal of Psychiatry 51:110–119

CDC 1994 1991–1993 HIV surveillance report. Centres for Disease Control, London

Creighton S J 1993 Organised abuse: NSPCC experience Child Abuse Review 2:232–242

Davies N, O'Connor E 1997 'How old?' asked the officer. Guardian, London 5 April 1997

de Young M 1997 Satanic ritual abuse in day-care. Child Abuse Review 6:84–93

Doran C, Brannan C 1996 Institutional abuse. in: Bibby P (ed.) Organised abuse – the current debate. Arena, London

Ennew J 1986 The sexual exploitation of children. Polity Press,

Faller K F 1990 Sexual abuse in day care. In: Understanding sexual maltreatment. Sage, London, pp 191–210

Finkelhor D et al 1988 The trauma of child sexual abuse: two models. In: Wyatt G E, Pomell (eds) Lasting effects of child sexual abuse. Sage, London

Finkelhor D, Williams L M, Burns N 1989 Nursery crimes. Sexual abuse in day care. Sage, London

Gallagher B, Hughes B, Parker H 1994 The incidence of known cases of organised and ritual child sexual abuse in England and Wales (1988–1991). Report to Department of Health, London

Goodwin J, Cheeves K, Connel V 1990 Borderline and other severe symptoms in adult survivors of incestuous abuse. Psychiatric Annals 20:22–32

Gough D 1996 An overview of the literature. In Bibby P (ed.) Organised abuse – the current debate. Arena, London, Ch 2

Gould C 1987 Symptoms characterizing satanic ritualistic abuse not usually seen in s.a. cases. Paper presented at a National Conference on Affirming Children's Truth, Manhattan Beach, CA

Hames M 1993 Child pornography: a secret web of exploitation. Child Abuse Review 2(4):276–280

Hansard 1997 20 January 1997

Independent 1990 Independent, London, 18 March 1990

Itzin C 1996 Pornography and the organisation of abuse. In: Bibby P (ed.) Organised abuse – the current debate. Arena, London, chapter

Itzin C, Sweet C 1990 What you feel about porn. Campaign against Pornography and Censorship, Spring 1990, Cosmopolitan Magazine, PO Box 844, London SE5

Itzin C 1997 Pornography and the Organisation of Intrafamilial and Extrafamilial CSA Child Abuse Review 6:2; 94–106

Jones D P H 1991 Commentary: ritualism and child sexual abuse. Child Abuse and Neglect 15(3):163–170

Jonker F, Jonker-Baaker I 1997 Effects of ritual abuse: the results of three surveys in the Netherlands. Child Abuse and Neglect 21(6):541–556

Kelley S J 1993 Ritualistic abuse of children. In: Hobbs C J, Wynne J M (eds) Child abuse, Ballière Tindall, London, Ch 2

Kelley S J 1994 abuse of children in day care centres: characteristics and consequences. Child Abuse Review 3:15–25

Kelley S J, Brant R, Waterman J 1993 Sexual abuse of children in day care centres. Child Abuse and Neglect 17(1):71–89

Kelly L 1987 Surviving sexual violence. Polity Press, Cambridge

La Fontaine J S 1994 The extent and nature of organised and ritual abuse. HMSO, London
La Fontaine J, Ward P, Nursten J, Smith M 1997 Re: Believe or disbelieve? with particular reference to satanist abuse. Child Abuse Review 6(2):80–83
Lanning K V 1991 Ritual abuse: a law enforcement view or perspective. Child Abuse and Neglect 15(3):171–173
Linehan T 1994 The price of independence. Community Care, 1 September, 12–13
Linehan T 1997 Who cares? Nursing Times 93(22):22–24
Lloyd D W 1992 Ritual child abuse: definitions and assumptions. Journal of Child Sexual Abuse 1(3):1–14
McFadyen A, Hanks H, James C 1993 Child Abuse Review 1:1
Myers J E 1994 The backlash: child protection under fire. Sage. Newbury Park, CA
Nursten J, Smith M 1996 Believe or disbelieve? With particular reference to satanic abuse. Child Abuse Review 5:253–262
Pelcowitz D 1990 Child pornography and extrafamilial sex abuse. Child maltreatment conference, San Diego, CA
Radzinowicz L 1975 Sexual offences: a report of the Cambridge Department of Criminal Science. Macmillan, London
Sinason V (ed.) 1994 Treating survivors of satanic abuse. Routledge, London
Snow B, Sorenson T 1990 Ritualistic child abuse in a neighbourhood setting. Journal of Interpersonal Violence 5(4):274–287
Stein M, Frost N, Rees G 1994 Running the risk: young people on the streets in Britain today. Children's Society, London
Summit R C 1983 The child sexual abuse accommodation syndrome. Journal of Child Abuse and Neglect 7:177–193
Summit R 1990 Cults and rituals: relationships to child abuse. Child maltreatment conference, San Diego, CA
Tate T 1990 Child pornography: an investigation. Methuen, London
Waterman J, Kelly R, Oliveri M K, McCord J 1990 Specificity of effects on children of ritualized and non-ritualized sexual abuse. Child maltreatment conference, San Diego, CA
Wells W M 1958 Sexual offences as seen by a woman police surgeon. British Medical Journal 2:1404–1408
Wild N J 1989 Prevalence of child sex rings. Pediatrics 83(4):553–559
Wild N J, Wynne J M 1986 Child sex ring. British Journal of Medicine 293:183–185
Working Together 1991 Working together under the Children Act 1989. A guide to arrangements for inter-agency cooperation for the protection of children from abuse. HMSO, London

RECOMMENDED READING

Barrett D (ed.) 1997 Child prostitution in Britain: dilemmas and practical responses. Children's Society, London
Bibby P (ed.) 1996 Organised abuse: the current debate. Arena, London
Browne K and Lynch M A Special issue on organised abuse (includes a literature review) 2(4):219–288
Sinason V (ed.) 1994 Treating survivors of satanist abuse. Routledge, London

ADDRESS

'Off the Shelf' Campaign, c/o Campaign against Pornography, 9 Poland Street, London W1 3DG

14

Management of child abuse

UN Convention on children's rights

The UN convention was ratified by the British government in 1991. It is relevant to the investigative procedure of child abuse in two ways. It states the basic rights of all children and these are broadly covered by the Children Act 1989.

The rights of children

- All actions concerning the child should take full account of his or her best interests; the rights and responsibilities of parents are respected
- The child has a right to express an opinion and have that opinion taken into account in any matter or procedure affecting him or her
- The child has a right to obtain and make known information and express views unless they violate the rights of others
- The child has a right to protection from interference with regard to privacy, family, home and correspondence, and from libel/slander
- The state has an obligation to protect children from all the forms of maltreatment perpetrated by parents or others responsible for their care

With the convention, the Children Act (1989) and the subsequent guidance such as Working Together (1991), the management of child abuse has been changing quite radically over the last few years. There has been an attempt to move the focus towards support of families and prevention of abuse, while not forgetting that abused children also need early recognition and support and prevention of further abuse. Therefore professionals in this field may be working in prevention, recognition or therapeutic work trying to help children and adolescents cope with the sequelae of earlier abuse.

Working documents for professionals

- Working Together (1988): a guide to the arrangements for interagency cooperation for the protection of children from abuse
- Working Together (1991): a guide to the arrangements for interagency cooperation for the protection of children from abuse under the Children Act 1989
- An introductory guide for the NHS: the Children Act 1989 (DoH 1991a)
- Diagnosis of child sexual abuse: guidance for doctors (DHSS 1988a)
- Protecting children: guidance for social workers (DHSS 1988b)
- Child sexual abuse: principles of good practice (Kolvin 1988)
- Management of child sexual abuse (Hobbs & Wynne 1987)
- Physical signs of sexual abuse of children (RCP 1991, 1997)
- Guidelines for the evaluation of sexual abuse of children (American Academy of Pediatrics 1991)
- Child protection for senior nurses, health visitors and midwives (DoH 1995)
- Child protection: medical responsibilities (DoH, BMA, Conference of the Medical Royal Colleges 1995)
- Child protection: clarification of arrangements between the NHS and other agencies (DoH 1995)
- Memorandum of good practice on video recorded interviews with child witnesses for criminal proceedings (Home Office 1992)

Inquiries into child abuse

The last major inquiry into the arrangements of the management of child abuse in the UK was the report of the inquiry into child abuse in Cleveland in 1987 (Butler-Sloss 1988). From 1973 to 1981 18 inquiries were held and from 1980 to 1989 there were 19. Reports describe working with families resistant or hostile to professional intervention, the need to see children, good supervision and support of workers and good interagency working and communication. The most recent study of inquiry reports, from 1980 to 1989 (DoH 1991b) identifies key lessons to be learned from the 1980s. It also notes the following limitations of the studies which were essentially Part 8 Reviews after the death of a child.

- Inquiries focus on child abuse as a product of family interaction and service delivery and do not analyse the associated effects of environmental disadvantage.
- Analysis of the effectiveness of services delivered excludes which services, if available, might have helped.
- Analysis of the family as individuals rather than recipients of services might give a better understanding as to why children are killed.
- The adversarial process of inquiries overseen by lawyers leads to procedural wrangles and a view as to what happened rather than why.

Inquiries do look at the relationship between policies, procedures and practices of individual agencies and how they relate to the law and how effectively they work together. The publication 'Child Protection: clarification arrangements between the NHS and other agencies' (DoH 1995) looks specifically at these relationships.

There is recognition now that at the time of the Cleveland inquiry there was minimal professional advice available in the management of child sexual abuse and little support for workers as clinical practice moved on more rapidly than the guidance was developed. As has become apparent, the practice relevant to child sexual abuse is different in some ways from that in the management of non-accidental injury, and practitioners have learned that it is often necessary to spend longer in the assessment of possible child sexual abuse in order to have as much information before the formal investigation takes place, even though this may mean leaving the child in an abusive home; in the management of physical abuse the emphasis is always on prevention of further, more serious injury and the speed of the investigation therefore is geared to safety rather than the longer term management.

- Local area child protection committees have also developed guidelines as to local practice including reviews by individual agencies and interagency inquiries by the area child protection committee.
- An integrated standard of practice is needed for child protection, integrating it with child care and monitoring it locally and nationally.
- Individual agencies should establish standards of practice, consistent with local area child protection committee procedures.
- Child protection must be seen as a priority by all the relevant agencies.
- There is a need for local and national training strategies which are coordinated to allow best training practice to be established.
- The most important recent outcome of inquiries is the need for a set of principles for professional relationships between adults and children.
- National statistics are needed – currently the only figures which are available from the government are the number of child abuse deaths, the number of child protection conferences, and the number of children on child protection registers in England and Wales.

Childcare and child protection are not the sole prerogative of the welfare agencies, and it is not the professionals who kill children. The public is ambivalent about intrusion into family life, the cost of services and the need to protect children. The professionals, the public, parents and children must work together to protect children and prevent child abuse (DoH 1991b, Working Together 1991).

Social workers carry the statutory responsibility for children in the management of child abuse but other professionals also have a role to play. Interagency cooperation is required by the Children Act 1989 not only in providing services to children in need, but also in the protection of children. Cooperation and collaboration between the different agencies is essential but is a difficult and complex process, as the inquiry reports show. With the growth of knowledge and understanding of maltreatment, policy and practice evolve and there is a need to adapt and change while still maintaining this close collaboration (Working Together 1991).

Since 1997 in the UK there has been a move towards meeting 'children's needs', as in the children's services plans. This is increasingly focusing on meeting children's needs, and to this end children's services plans are being drawn up in between city councils, health authorities and voluntary service workers.

Childcare legislation

Legislation attempts to achieve a balance between the need to protect children and respect parental responsibility while not allowing undue interference by the state in family life.

Children Act 1989

The Children Act 1989 creates a whole new framework to provide for the care and protection of children with a new range of court orders.

Principles of the Children Act 1989 (DoH 1991a)

- The child's welfare is paramount
- Wherever possible children should be brought up and cared for within their own family
- Children should be safe and protected
- Courts should avoid delay when dealing with children
- Courts should only make an order if to do so is better than no order
- Children should participate in decision-making and be kept well informed
- Parents continue to have responsibility even when their children are no longer living with them
- Parents with 'children in need' should be helped to bring up their children. Section 17 of the Act

places a duty on Local Authorities to provide a range of services to safeguard and promote the welfare of these children, or facilitate the provision of services by others, particularly voluntary agencies

- This help should be provided as a service to parents and children:
  - in partnership with parents
  - to meet the child's identified needs
  - to be appropriate to the child's race, culture, religion, language
  - to be open to effective independent representations and complaints procedures
  - to draw upon effective partnership between the local authority and other agencies including voluntary agencies.
- Section 47 places the Local Authority under a general duty to make enquiries to decide what action should be taken to safe-guard and promote the child's welfare

Children's Services Plans

The production of Children's Services Plans by local authorities is a statutory requirement with a focus on how services are provided for children in need. The definition of need does not include automatically the third of all children brought up in poverty. In line with current philosophy, plans intend to review the scope for refocusing interventions from 'crisis led' to 'needs led' at an earlier stage of difficulties within the family.

The number of children 'in need' in an industrial city in the UK, for example in Leeds, is around 6% of the population under 19 years (if poverty is excluded), or 10 000 children. If the witnessing of domestic violence is included, 20 000 children are affected. Over 30% of children are living in circumstances which render them likely to become 'a child in need'.

Priorities vary, and in Leeds 1997/99 (Leeds City Council 1997) key areas are:

- children with disabilities
- children and adolescents with mental health problems
- drug and substance abuse
- crime prevention: youth justice
- education of looked-after children
- housing for children leaving care.

Children who fall into these categories are recognised to be at high risk of abuse and re-abuse.

The children's services plan should help integrate services provided by council departments, the health authority, juvenile justice and voluntary agencies.

Child protection is a specific service in Leeds, with a child population of 170 000, and over 1000 children are on the child protection register. In 1995 there were 435 initial child protection conferences.

Looked-after children (those in care) all have special needs; in Leeds over 750 children are in foster-care and more than 120 are cared for in residential placements.

Some statistics demonstrate how children fare in Leeds compared with England as a whole (Table 14.1).

It is anticipated that children's services plans should be updated every year and that by meeting the needs of children and families via re-focused services child abuse will be prevented. This is in the spirit of the Children Act 1989 and Messages from Research (1995), work commissioned by the Department of Health.

- There are estimated to be in England 350 000 children living in a damaging environment of 'low warmth and high criticism' (Smith 1995). It is not known how many of these children are receiving help via Section 17 of the Children Act or are accommodated.

Table 14.1 Looked-after children: statistics

Parameter	England	Leeds
% lone parent (1991)	20.8	19.4
% of 'looked-after children' on orders	57	74
Children looked after/10 000 population	45	63
Children on child protection register/10 000 under 18 years	32	59
Perinatal mortality/1000 live births	8.8	9
Infant mortality/1000 live births	6.1	7.2
Childhood mortality rate/1000	17.9	18.6
Pregnancy <16 years/1000 girls	8.6	10.8
Accident mortality/<15 years/1000	4.5	5.2

- How accurate is the child protection process in recognising abuse? Thornburn et al (1995) has estimated that in England each year there are 160 000 inquiries of which 25 000 are found to be unsubstantiated.
- Which families were likely to be investigated? (Section 47).
  - 36% were headed by a lone parent, 30% had both birth parents at home, 57% had no wage earner and 54% were on income support
  - 27% gave a history of domestic violence and 13% of mental ill health, in 23% a family member had had a serious illness or accident in the previous 12 months
  - 65% of children were known to social services departments and 45% had been previously investigated for abuse
  - 14% of the parents were known to have been abused as children
  - 51% are referred by a family member, or the child, 39% by professionals working with the family, 10% were referred by professionals during an unrelated event.
- of the 160 000 referrals made, the child protection register was contacted in 2/3
- a family visit is made in around 120 000, emergency separation of the child occurs in 1500 and there is no further action in 80 000 of the referrals
- a child protection conference is held in 40 000 and in 11 000 no further action is taken, but 3000 children enter care, a further 3000 are accommodated and there are 24 500 additions to the register. In addition 3000 children are retained in the system (these figures are estimates based on 1992 figures, Messages from Research 1995).

To summarise, of the initial referrals 15% children will be registered and 96% of children stay at home with relatives. Gibbons et al (1995) found that:

- for *physical abuse* few unsubstantiated cases reached a child protection conference but some children remained unprotected
- for *neglect* few reached a child protection agency and vulnerable children missed out in receiving available services
- for *child sexual abuse* there were few unnecessary child protection conferences, and few high-risk cases were dealt with inappropriately
- thresholds vary from place to place.

The conclusion of the researchers was that the net was spread too widely and professionals might have been more effective spending more time with parents and children looking at ways of working together in partnership. It could also be argued that as professionals appear to have difficulty in recognising neglect and emotional abuse (although this may be changing), and the courts have high standards of proof (the more serious the allegation of child sexual abuse the greater the required proof), much abuse remains unacknowledged, albeit at different levels.

It is also clear to those professionals working with the whole spectrum of abuse and neglect that the 'in need' approach may be appropriate in the management of many cases of neglect and physical abuse but a different approach is needed in intrafamilial child sexual abuse with denial. The 'addicted' perpetrator of child sexual abuse is not going to stop abusing without a clear programme which initially, at least, separates him (or her) from children, and there is an acknowledgement by the abuser that there is a problem. The abuser may continue to deny that his/her behaviour is abusive and as a consequence remains a risk to children.

Area child protection committees

In order that all the agencies involved in child protection may work closely together there must be a joint forum for developing, monitoring and reviewing child protection policies; this is the area child protection committee (in England and Wales).

The area child protection committee members are accountable to the agencies they represent, and the agencies are jointly responsible for area child protection committee action. Social services, police service, health service (community and hospital, nursing and medical), education, probation, voluntary agencies and others are represented.

Functions of the Area Child Protection Committee (Working Together 1991)

- Establishing, maintaining and reviewing local interagency guidelines
- Monitoring the implementation of legal procedures
- Identifying significant issues arising from the handling of cases and reports from enquiries
- Scrutinising arrangements to provide treatment, expert advice, and interagency liaison and making recommendations to the responsible agencies
- Conducting Part 8 reviews: detailed studies carried out after a child's death or a case of public interest. Review instigated by Chair of the local ACPC and a multi-agency committeee carries it out.
- Publishing an annual report about child protection matters
- The committee may also set up working groups to:
  - carry out specific tasks, e.g. provide a training programme, review cases
  - provide specialist advice, e.g. advise in relation to specific ethnic and cultural groups

The National Health Service commitment

Each health authority is responsible for the provision of a comprehensive service for children at risk of abuse and their families. Health professionals need their own guidelines which are consistent with those of the local area child protection committee procedures. Chief officers at a district and regional level of the NHS have responsibility for ensuring appropriate arrangements are in place.

Medical responsibility

'Child Protection: Medical Responsibility' (DoH 1997) is the current advice to medical practitioners concerning child abuse. It has been prepared by the DoH, the BMA and the Conference of Medical Royal Colleges and is based on Working Together (1991) and interim guidance PLCO(93)2.

The document makes it clear that medical involvement in all aspects of child protection work is important but acknowledges that there are tensions for medical practitioners, relating particularly to confidentiality. The advice is essentially that the child's protection and welfare should be the overriding principle. However, doctors have a legal and ethical duty to maintain confidentiality and should only disclose information without consent if it is justified 'in the best interest of the child'.

The UK General Medical Council advised in 1993 that

> where the doctor believes the patient may be the victim of abuse or neglect the patient's best interests are paramount and will usually require a doctor to disclose information to an appropriate, responsible person or officer of a statutory agency.

The appointment of designated doctors in each health authority should provide a focus for discussion and advice, whether this includes a further clinical assessment or referral to social services, for example.

Designated professional (doctor and nurse) (DH 1995a)

- Each health authority should have a senior doctor and a senior nurse (with a health visiting qualification) usually based in a provider unit but with responsibilities across the health authority, to be designated as senior professionals to sit on the ACPS(s) to which the health authority relates (DoH 1995).
- Named professionals may be appointed where a health authority covers several area child protection committees. The designated professional delegates responsibility to the named colleague.
- Job descriptions should be agreed between the health authority and NHS trust.
- The designated professionals are usually expert and current practitioners in the child protection field; or will have had relevant previous experience
- The time commitment and average workload should be contracted for, i.e. as

part of the child protection contract. The elements of the contract are described in 'Clarification of arrangements between the NHS and other agencies, DoH 1985) and includes notes on general practice, NHS trusts, funding of child protection conferences, etc. (see Figs 14.1 and 14.2).

Role of the designated doctor

The main tasks of the designated doctor include:

- an *advisory role*: giving expert health advice to health professionals and other agencies
- *policy and procedures*: keeping development of interagency procedures and individual agency procedures up to date

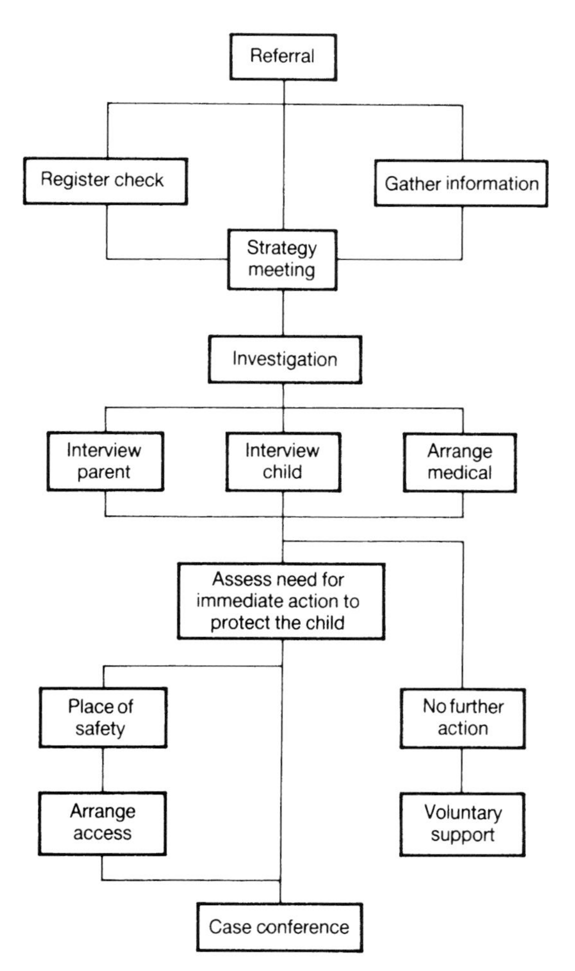

Fig. 14.1 Investigating child abuse: the inital stages.

- *training* of health professionals, and multi-agency training
- *coordination and communication*: to ensure that the health authority meets the obligations placed on it by the Children Act 1989 and to ensure that there is good communication between the NHS trusts involved, including the transfer of records
- *monitoring* the child protection contract with the health authority and an effective system of audit of agreed child protection standards
- the need for the development of support and appropriate supervision system for designated professionals should be recognised, actioned and funded (DH 1995a).

The named professional works closely with the designated professional who also gives clinical advice and support. The role of the community child health staff in the '. . . examination, diagnosis, assessment and ongoing care . . .' is emphasised, with the note that the designated doctor is likely to be a consultant community paediatrician.

Clearly all health professionals who meet children have a responsibility to recognise the various forms of maltreatment and understand the local procedures in hospital, health centre, school, etc. (which should be in line with area child protection committee procedures) and act accordingly.

Role of the general practitioner

General practitioners may be able to recognise family stress at an early stage, and at routine surveillance examinations or during intercurrent illness signs of maltreatment may be evident; and

> While general practitioners have responsibilities to all their patients (parents) the welfare of the child must come first because of the vulnerability of children (DH 1997).

The general practitioner must share his or her concerns; increasingly this is with a consultant community paediatrician who may then see the child and family or following discussion refer to one of the statutory agencies (DH 1997).

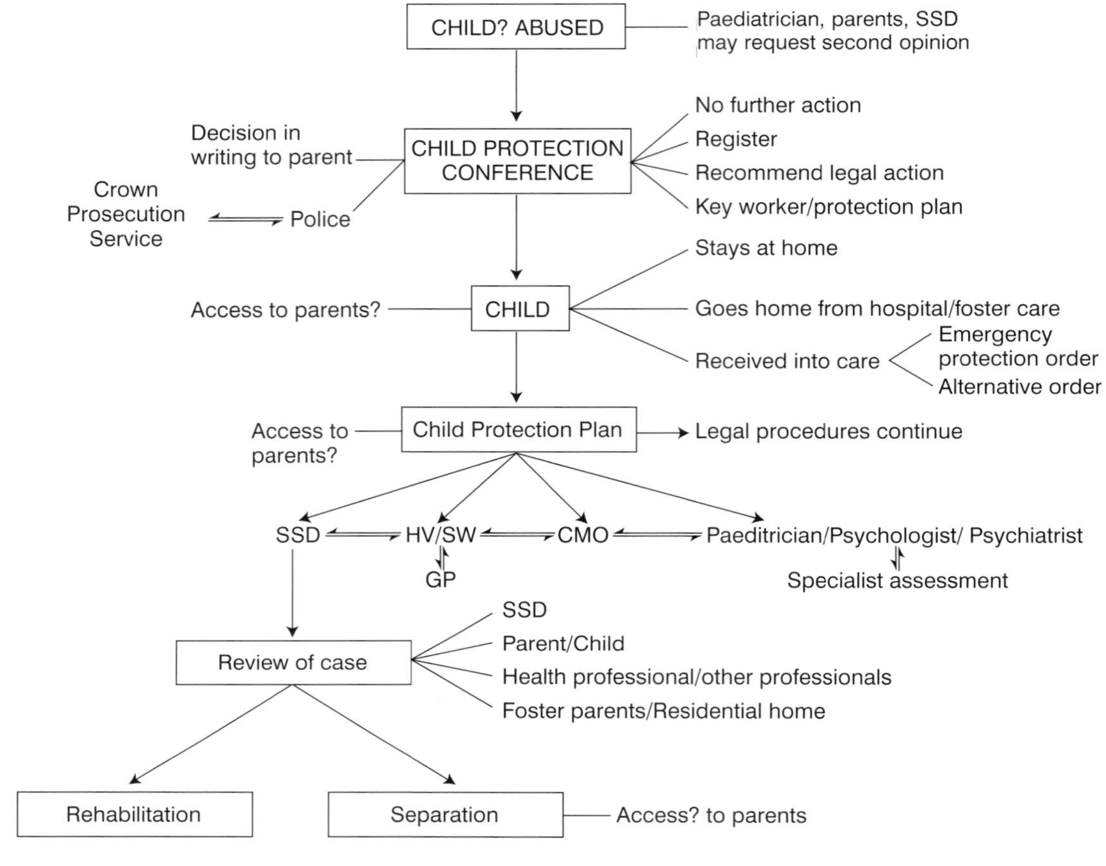

Fig. 14.2 Investigating child abuse: further management.

Family doctors may also be requested to attend court. Many family doctors will be anxious about confidentiality, and this is explored later in the chapter.

Community health service medical staff

Clinical medical officer

Under the direction of a consultant paediatrician or lead senior clinical medical officer, clinical medical officers have a particular responsibility towards neglected and abused children. Clinical medical officers who visit a social service department's day nurseries will see children who are failing to thrive, who have delayed development and are neglected. Staff will refer children with 'sexually explicit behaviour' to them and they should know how to act. As is being increasingly recognised, there are many abused children in special schools and clinical medical officers may be the only doctors with regular access to the group (Ch. 10). Clinical medical officers share the same responsibility as other doctors in recording and attending child protection conferences and court appearances. However, as with junior medical staff in hospital, there should be adequate training, supervision and support of all clinical medical officers.

Psychiatrist

Child and adolescent psychiatrists are increasingly involved in child abuse work. In the UK there is a serious lack of provision of therapeutic services and in practice only the more difficult cases are therefore referred.

Psychiatrists may be involved in two main ways. Firstly in assessment as to the probability of abuse, usually emotional abuse with or without child sexual abuse which also includes an assessment of the functioning of the family. In difficult cases it is very useful to have a child psychiatrist with an important part in making an assessment as to whether abuse has occurred. However, there is a shortage of therapeutic services for children and many psychiatric teams work with children of families following the recognition of abuse to try and help with the emotional and behavioural sequelae of abuse.

Psychologist

Clinical psychologists are increasingly involved in child protection work, and their involvement varies. Ideally there would be more psychologists involved in assessment, particularly of children with learning problems, frightened children or those with psychiatric disorder. Psychologists tend to work in a more therapeutic setting where their skills are much needed, and social workers and non-specialist police officers conduct the initial investigative interviews.

Paediatrician

All general and community paediatricians have a responsibility to work with abused children and their families. In each health district there should be a designated doctor, often a consultant community paediatrician, who serves on the area child protection committee, ensures that there is an accessible and efficient service and is actively engaged in multi- and single-discipline training in child abuse.

Police surgeon

Most police surgeons are family doctors who undertake a small number of sessions as a deputy police surgeon each week. The senior police surgeon advises the police authority. Police surgeons must work closely with paediatricians, and if police surgeons examine children alone they must understand the need for a 'whole child examination' (de la Haye Davis 1987, Butler-Sloss 1988), the use of appropriate investigations, for example to screen for sexually transmitted disease, and the need for follow-up (paediatrically or psychiatrically). Police surgeons should also write reports for and attend the child protection conference.

Nursing staff

Health visitors, midwives, hospital or school nurses and nursery nurses are well trained to recognise risk factors and warning signs of abuse but also have skills to support children and families when abuse is identified and to be able to continue to work with them subsequently.

It is important that general practitioners, clinical medical officers and paediatricians all work closely with nursing colleagues in hospital and the community.

Initial steps in the recognition of child abuse

The DoH guidelines for doctors are essentially to stop, think, and discuss concerns with medical and non-medical colleagues – unless of course there is clear evidence of abuse or an allegation has been made, when there should be no delay in referral to statutory agencies.

In cases of uncertainty it is recommended that when the preliminary consultations reach a 'critical threshold of professional concern' doctors must share these concerns with the statutory agencies for further evaluation and 'within a time frame which is not detrimental to the child's interest'. Doctors, like all other professionals in this field need training and professional support. They should also:

- keep detailed, contemporaneous notes, which may be later accessed by the patient and also used in court proceedings
- keep written records of telephone calls, discussions and any other contacts.

Continuing medical involvement following referral includes strategy discussion, investigation, writing of reports and attendance and participation in the child protection conference (if held).

Part 8 Reviews (see Working Together 1991) are held after the death of a child or a child protection concern of major public interest.

Medical tasks in child abuse (after Butler-Sloss 1988)

- Take a full medical history
- Make a thorough medical examination
- Arrange appropriate investigations for
  - sexually transmitted diseases
  - forensic tests
  - pregnancy
  - bruising
  - bony injury
- Complete full and accurate records (at the time of examination)
- Prepare medical report for general practitioner, social services or NSPCC, child health, hospital record
- Prepare a statement for police on request
- Ensure results of investigation are recorded
- Arrange appropriate referral for psychiatric, psychological or paediatric follow-up
- Attend child protection conference or court
- If there are differences of medical opinion. endeavour to resolve these differences or at least identify area of dispute (Butler-Sloss 1988)

Child protection team

There are advantages in having a child protection team based at each district general hospital. This would comprise paediatricians (hospital and community), psychologists, psychiatrists, liaison health visitor (from Accident and Emergency department, the ward, the child development team), social workers and colleagues in training.

Professional involvement

The core of professionals will provide

- an expert clinical team
- a link with other health service colleagues (community and hospital)
- support for members of the team
- teachers and trainers
- social work to the hospital and advice to the team
- a weekly review of current practice and longer-term audit.

Administration

Administration of the child protection team requires a skilled secretary who is able to provide suitable support. Requirements include:

- easy, open access to the doctors on the rota by the social services department, police, other health professionals or carers (parents, grandparents and others). Children should be seen by appointment: physically abused children or children at risk of further harm are usually seen the same day. Children thought to have been sexually abused, with the exception of rape victims, may often be seen by arrangement to the advantage of child, parents and professionals. There is little justification for seeing children in the late evening at the convenience of a doctor
- efficient typing and distribution of reports
- support the committee work involved in area child protection committee, training, review of clinical practice (audit) and service development.

Accommodation

The accommodation needed at each district general hospital includes:

- receptionist
- quiet waiting area with toys
- interview/examination room: more than one room is needed if there are angry or upset relatives
- admission to a ward for a few children (see later).

Few health centres are adequately equipped. Children should *not* be examined in police stations; it is clear that there are only rare circumstances in which a child should be seen at a police station (HMSO 1988).

Nursing staff

It is essential to have nursing staff who should be trained (RSCN or nursery nurse) for work in the clinic or on the ward. They are expected to:

- receive and support the child and family
- chaperone the doctor (male or female)
- weigh and measure the child
- collect specimens, e.g. urine, and assist at collection of swabs, e.g. for sexually transmitted diseases, forensic
- support the child during photography.

Equipment

The list of equipment required is not extensive:

- usual examination trolley
- microbiological swabs, etc.
- sexual offences pack (from police)
- good illumination/magnification
- camera/photography service
- access to haematology, biochemistry, radiology
- colposcope, glass rods, etc. (optional)
- domestic refrigerator for appropriate storage of swabs used in STD screen and some forensic specimens.

Hospital beds

Access to hospital beds is needed for admission of injured infants, investigation of infants failing to thrive and occasionally sexually abused children.

Clinical advice

There will be a need for clinical advice from colleagues such as genito-urinary, orthopaedic, paediatric surgical or gynaecological consultants.

Therapeutic service

The requirements for psychological intervention and treatment (see Ch. 15) include:

- child and family psychiatrists and teams which may include play therapists, occupational therapists, dance and art therapy
- child psychologist
- child psychotherapist
- adult service to support caregivers.

Interagency work in child protection

Stages of investigation

There is a sequence of events in the investigation of an individual case and some of these stages overlap. Doctors may be involved at all stages and, rather than using medical skills only during the initial recognition and assessment, children and families may be helped by ongoing paediatric involvement. The doctors involved also need to understand how cases are to be handled (area child protection committee procedures) See Table 14.2.

The six stages, as described in Working Together (1991), are:

- referral and recognition
- immediate protection and planning the investigation
- investigation and initial assessment
- child protection conference and decision-making
- comprehensive assessment and planning
- implementation, review and, where appropriate, deregistration.

Table 14.2 The child protection process (Messages from Research 1995)

Rate of registration on CPR	0.8/1000 Gloucester (1992) 10.0/1000 Southwark
Of total number of children referred ?abuse	75% receive one home visit 25% CPC held 15% placed on CPR
Children registered at CPC	61% (of conferenced children)
Children referred ?abuse who remain within family	96%
Does registration protect?	
Non-accidental injury	25% re-abused within 6 months 2% seriously
Child sexual abuse	43% ('unsafe') 9 months later

Referral and recognition

- Any person who has knowledge of, or a suspicion that, a child is suffering harm or is at risk of significant harm should refer to one of the statutory agencies (social services department, NSPCC or police).
- Referrals may be from the child's family, other members of the public or professionals working with the child and family.
- All professionals working with children and families should be adequately trained to recognise signs of abuse and how to respond.
- Professionals who receive the referral have to balance the need for action to protect the child with the harm which may be caused by unnecessary intervention.
- Except in cases of extreme urgency professionals will discuss referrals with other colleagues in child protection agencies and the referrer before acting. A specialist opinion may be needed here to carry the work on.
- If the child protection agency decides that a formal investigation is not needed the referrer should be informed.

Immediate protection and planning an investigation

- If there is a risk to the life of a child or a likelihood of serious injury, the child's immediate safety must be secured by the statutory agency. Does the child need removing to some other place, either on a voluntary basis or by obtaining an emergency protection order?
- If the child is removed there is a requirement to return the child as soon as it is safe to do so.
- Could the child's safety be secured by the alleged abuser being removed from home or agreeing to leave?
- Are the other children in the home safe?
- The parents should be given appropriate opportunity to participate in the process and efforts made to facilitate contact between the family and child if there is an emergency protection order.
- A strategy discussion between the statutory agencies, usually social services and police, is needed at a very early stage to plan the investigation and the extent to which this will be a joint investigation. If the police are undertaking a parallel investigation which may lead to the prosecution of an alleged abuser there are issues concerning the child and his needs versus legal requirements. Working Together (1991) says very clearly, 'the welfare of the child must be of the first importance'.

There is a danger that the strategy discussion becomes an 'alternative child protection conference' with only selected professionals and no parents present. This may lead to decision-making based on inadequate information leaving children at risk. In the past case discussions were similarly flawed, hence the current insistence on the protocol for the child protection conference.

Investigation and initial assessment

- The social services department have a duty to investigate where there is reason to suspect a child is suffering from or is likely to suffer significant harm. This includes children in a local authority placement (foster-home, residential home, school).
- The four prime tasks are:
  - to establish the facts giving rise to the concern
  - to decide if there are grounds for concern
  - to identify sources and level of risk
  - to decide protective or other action in relation to the child and any others.
- Interviewing of children requires staff who are competent and trained. Investigative interviews should be kept to a minimum. If court proceedings have been started the court's agreement is needed for examinations for the purposes of expert evidence. Interviews should proceed at the child's pace. Recording of the interviews should be accurate and differentiate between fact, hearsay and opinion (see Ch. 9).

- If allegations are found to be unsubstantiated the care givers with parental responsibility, the child (if appropriate) and the referrer should be told in writing, and a suitably worded apology offered which does not leave the investigations open to challenge.

Child protection conference and decision-making

The child protection conference is held following an investigation of an incident of possible abuse. It is convened by the social services department or NSPCC.

> The child protection conference (CPC) provides the prime forum for professionals and the family to share information and concerns, analyse and weigh up the level of risks to children and makes recommendations for action (Working Together, 1991, p 31).

- The conference may decide:
  - if the child's name shall be put on the *child protection register* (see below for further details of the register)
  - which *statutory agency* will carry ongoing child care responsibility and when the child protection review will be (if necessary)
  - to designate *key workers* for the child (social services department or NSPCC).
- Conferences should take place *within 8 working days* of referral (maximum 15 days). Practice has not been able to meet this timing and the average wait is 34 days due to the shortage of suitable Chairs, (The Chair is a senior social worker with appropriate training and experience but from a different agency, e.g. NSPCC, to give impartiality), good accommodation, availability of professionals and also the need to gather adequate information so the child protection conference can reach decisions based on a thorough investigation.
- *Parents or care givers* are expected to be invited to the child protection conference – the only exceptions, which require justification, are if the care giver is violent or has threatened violence, has a significant mental health problem or, in child sexual abuse, a care giver is the alleged abuser and his presence is likely to have an adverse effect on the effectiveness of the child protection conference.
- Sometimes where *teenagers* wish to attend the child protection conference a decision has to be made as to who attends, teenager or care giver, both or both but for different sections? Teenagers should only attend if there is a consensus that this will be in their 'best interest' but, in contrast, they are expected to attend child protection reviews.
- Another development has been the attendance of *solicitors* at child protection conferences. This may be quite threatening to professionals and it is essential that the Chair ensures a solicitor is there to support his or her client, not to cross-examine the potential witnesses.
- *General practitioners* and *health visitors* may have a particularly difficult role; they continue to work with the family after the episode or otherwise, of abuse, when the other agencies have withdrawn and in addition may have the care of the abuser and abused. Therefore, not only does the primary care team have a difficult role, they usually have the least experience and training with 2–3 cases or fewer each year.
- Research shows that on average 10, but up to 16, people attend the child protection conference; only 21% of parents are there for the whole meeting but there is usually a consensus at the end, i.e. whether to register or not (Messages from Research 1995).
- The *duration* of child protection conferences has increased, which also makes for difficulty for professionals with fixed commitments.
- There is an increased emphasis on professionals working in *partnership* with parents but equally parents have responsibility towards their child(ren) and in the final analysis the welfare of the child is paramount (Children Act 1989).
- *All* professionals attending a child protection conference should submit a short, relevant report to the Chair of the CPC. As a point of

good practice, doctors should go through the report with the care givers before the child protection conference.

- If the medical practitioner cannot attend it is imperative that a medical report is available, but the amount of *clinical detail* contained in the report may include a relevant history, and a summary only of the findings with an opinion as to the significance of the physical signs with reference to the 'whole picture'.
- A *full medical report* (see below) should also be available for the court, other doctors or 'second opinions', but experience shows that these reports may be inappropriately interpreted by others present at the child protection conference and unless the author is present the abbreviated form is preferable. This is also better practice if parents receive a copy of the medical report: the child should be afforded some privacy.
- The only *people involved* in a child protection conference should be those who need to know and have a contribution to make: these include the social services department, NSPCC, police, education, paediatrician, general practitioner, health visitor, school nurse, midwife, probation service, voluntary organisations, lawyer (for local authority).
- *Minutes* are distributed to those who attended the child protection conference, but parents should receive, as a minimum, the findings of the child protection conference, who attended and the recommended plan.

Child protection conferences

Initial child protection conference:

- Brings together the family and professionals to exchange information and plan together
- Convened by social services or NSPCC
- Called after an investigation under Section 47 of the Children Act of an incident of or suspicion of abuse
- Decides:
  - level of risk to child(ren)
  - need for registration
  - plans for future
- Key worker appointed (social services or NSPCC) to:
  - fulfil the statutory responsibilities
  - lead interagency work

Child protection review:

- Reviews arrangements for protection of child
- Examines current level of risk
  - Is the child adequately protected?
  - Should registration be continued or ended?

Case reviews (by area child protection committee)

A case review is held whenever a case involves an incident leading to the death of a child where child abuse is confirmed or suspected, or a child protection issue arises that is likely to be of major public concern. There should be an individual review by each agency and a composite review by the area child protection committee.

Doctors involved in case reviews should seek advice from a senior colleague, usually the designated doctor, and professional advice is also available from the Medical Defence Union or the Medical Protection Society. Details of case reviews are found in Working Together (1991).

Clinical review of practice is essential and requires good record-keeping and computerisation to produce accurate statistics. Quality of service as well as numbers should be reviewed to record the service provided and to detect any clinical trends. In-house clinical review of cases by a senior midwife, health visitor and paediatrician is an important way of improving clinical practice and highlighting training needs.

Comprehensive assessment and planning

After registration of a child the initial plan includes a comprehensive assessment in order fully to understand the child and family and so plan further action. This is principally carried out by the social services department but there may be a need for contribution from a paediatrician (failure to thrive, development), psychologist or psychiatrist.

A written child protection plan with the contributions expected of the care givers and professionals is agreed, and the key worker is responsible for coordinating the plan.

Implementation, review and deregistration

The interagency child protection plan requires regular review to ensure that it provides protection from abuse for the child. Reviews are held at a minimum interval of 6 months. The first one is usually held at the end of the child and family assessment where the full child protection plan is produced. Deregistration may only be decided at a child protection review.

Effective practice to protect children

Research into the preconditions needed if practice is to be effective (Messages from Research 1995) suggest:

- a sensitive and informed professional/client relationship, but the researchers concede that even skilled interventions may fail to engage some families constructively.
- an appropriate balance of power between participants: the balance alters during the course of the case, and social work research shows that if parents accept that the intervention is 'fair', there is no undue delay or withholding of information a positive balance more often than not develops.
- a wide perspective on child protection: the ideal outcome is that the child is not re-abused, and that the welfare needs of the child and needs of the parent or caregiver are met – this is assessed as occurring in less than 25% of families.
- effective supervision and training of social workers.
- services which enhance children's general quality of life: no single strategy will be effective in all situations, fostering, adoption, ousting the abuser, specialist therapy and other services may be effective in some situations. However, all that can be said is that outcomes for children 'are generally better . . .' if the above conditions prevail. Some situations are more difficult to work with than others, and examples would be an infant with a severe shaking injury (new and old subdural haematoma) and two care givers 'who never leave him' or the 3-year-old daughter of the local primary school headmaster who alleges sexual abuse by her father and there are equivocal physical signs. The advocated approach is based on the process of Section 47 enquiries and the provision of Section 17 services.

Child protection register (CPR)

A child protection register is kept by social services department in each area. It is not a register of all children who have been abused but of children for whom there are unresolved child protection issues and for whom there is an interagency child protection plan. These plans are reviewed every 6 months.

Professionals concerned about a child can quickly learn of any child protection plan by making enquiries to the child protection register and social services department. Before a child is registered the conference must decide that there is, or is a likelihood of, significant harm leading to the need for a child protection plan. One of the following requirements needs to be satisfied.

- There must be one or more identifiable incidents which can be described as having adversely affected the child. They may be acts of commission or omission. They can be either physical, sexual, emotional or neglectful. It is important to identify a specific occasion or occasions when an incident has occurred.
- Professional judgement is that further incidents are likely or significant harm is expected on the basis of professional judgement of findings of the investigation in this individual case or on research evidence. The conference will need to establish so far as it is possible a cause of the harm or likelihood of harm. This cause could also be applied to siblings or other children living in the same household so as to justify registration of them. Such children

should be categorised according to the area of concern.

Child protection register: summary

- A register is kept in each social services department area
- It lists only children about whom there are unresolved child protection issues and for whom there is an interagency child protection plan
- It is therefore *not* a register of all children who have been abused
- Children are registered only after a child protection conference
- Categories are:
  - neglect
  - physical injury
  - sexual abuse
  - emotional abuse
- Deregistration is considered at each child protection review

Categories of abuse for registration

The following categories should be used for register and for statistical purposes. They are intended to provide definitions as a guide for those using the register. In some instances, more than one category of registration may be appropriate. This needs to be dealt with in the protection plan. The statistical returns will allow for this. Multiple abuse registration should not be used solely to cover all eventualities.

- *Neglect*: The persistent or severe neglect of a child, or the failure to protect a child from exposure to any kind of danger, including cold or starvation, or extreme failure to carry out important aspects of care, resulting in the significant impairment of the child's health or development, including non-organic failure to thrive.
- *Physical injury*: Actual or likely physical injury to a child, or failure to prevent physical injury (or suffering) to a child including deliberate poisoning, suffocation and factitious illness by proxy.
- *Sexual abuse*: Actual or likely sexual exploitation of a child or adolescent. The child may be dependent and/or developmentally immature.
- *Emotional abuse*: Actual or likely severe adverse effect on the emotional and behavioural development of a child caused by persistent or severe emotional ill-treatment or rejection. All abuse involves some emotional ill-treatment. This category should be used where it is the main or sole form of abuse.

Residential care: children's homes, boarding schools, foster homes

> It would not be wise for anyone to approach this Report on the basis that it all happened a long time ago and nothing like it could ever happen again (Andrew Kirkwood QC, Leicestershire Inquiry 1992).

About 200 000 children under the age of 18 years live away from home in England and Wales (see Ch. 16), from a total of 12 million children at any one time:

- 8000 in children's homes in 1995 (40 000 in 1975)
- 35 000 in foster-care
- 110 000 in boarding schools (30 000 in schools for children with disabilities or emotional or behavioural problems, of which half are provided by the local authority and the remainder are independent).

The Children Act 1989 requires independent boarding schools to safeguard and promote the welfare of children and to be available for inspection.

In *People like us: The Utting Report*, Utting (1997) wrote

> The Review was precipitated by the past activities of sexually and physically abusive terrorists in children's homes . . . A single perpetrator is likely in a lifetime's career to abuse hundreds of children, who suffer pain, humiliation and torment, and incur permanent emotional damage . . . They are very dangerous people.

The protective strategy set out by Utting involves:

- a high threshold of entry to paid and voluntary work with children to deter committed abusers
- a vigilant management which protects children and exposes abuse
- effective disciplinary and criminal procedures to deal with offenders
- approved communications concerning known paedophiles on a 'need to know' basis.

Child protection in foster-homes or institutions (see Ch. 16)

Investigation of possible abuse of children in a foster-home or residential setting must be as rigorous as in other circumstances. Similarly, extrafamilial abuse should be referred as for intrafamilial abuse, and child protection issues assessed on their merits.

Where the alleged abuser is a child or younger person, both abused and abuser are investigated.

Organised abuse (see Ch. 13)

Investigation of organised abuse ideally needs a carefully worked-out plan as, by definition, there will be a number of abusers involved and also a number of children and/or young adults. There may be a very tight organisation within the group and investigation will need to be at least as well-organised and sophisticated as that of the group. The type of ring varies: further description is found in Chapter 13.

Working Together (1991) gives some guidelines for the investigation of organised abuse.

- It should be coordinated at a senior level of each agency.
- The timing of the intervention must be planned and agreed by all agencies.
- Media management should be agreed locally (area child protection committee procedures).
- Agreement is necessary over adjoining geographical boundaries.

Hospital attendance of children who may have been abused

Initial admission

Abused and neglected children may be seen in the Accident and Emergency department, out-patients (paediatric medicine, surgery, orthopaedic, orthodontal, therapy, etc.) or on the wards as in-patients. Each department should have appropriate guidelines and close links with the hospital's child protection team for easy access to advice. However, as baseline enquiries the staff (nursing or medical) should feel able to make some checks:

- to the child protection register
- to the social services department (is the child/family known to social services)
- what does the general practitioner, health visitor, or school nurse think.

Involvement of police and social services

The police prefer to be contacted early if a seriously injured child is seen, for example a shaken baby with a serious head injury, subdural haemorrhage, retinal haemorrhages, facial bruising and multiple fractures.

In the event of an apparently seriously injured child presenting at the accident and emergency department the police may want an 'instant diagnosis': this is an indication for a consultant paediatrician to be called in.

Caution is needed before reaching an opinion as the police may want to arrest the alleged abuser and it is essential to be confident in the interpretation of the computed tomography brain scan, skeletal survey, retinal haemorrhages and clotting screen (with the help of colleagues) before giving an opinion. The social services department may also be very concerned to have an early diagnosis because of the need to protect other children in the family. For example, the admission of the baby to the paediatric intensive care unit will add considerably to the stress of a family which may be already dysfunctional.

In serious cases, such as above, with an infant on the paediatric intensive care unit it is helpful to the social services department and the police to have the name of a senior doctor and nurse who is easily available for day-to-day advice and vice versa. This limits the number of telephone calls and aids communication. The police may want to interview the parents: they should be asked to give a time and the hospital should provide a suitable room off the ward where the police (preferably no more than two, non-uniformed officers) may see the parents privately. Even parents who have been charged and may be in custody should usually visit, albeit accompanied by prison officers who may be asked to be discreet; handcuffs must be reserved for exceptional circumstances.

If the child's condition deteriorates the police presence tends to increase and it behoves the hospital to make a room with a telephone available to prevent the disruption and upset which follows if accommodation is not available and the ward is taken over.

- The *police photographer* may be requested by the police to photograph the child; again privacy is needed.
- A *forensic pathologist* may be requested to see a severely injured child, and various forensic swabs may be collected (usually shortly after admission and resuscitation).
- The *coroner* should be informed of any 'suspicious deaths' or unexplained deaths. it is also usual practice to discuss with the coroner before life-support is withdrawn.

If the child does die, parents and siblings are preferably involved in the dying child's care, as is usual practice. This may need explaining to the police.

It is also very important that all the staff who have been involved in the care of the dying child are given the opportunity to talk: it is exceptionally difficult to cope with the 'unnecessary' death of a child.

Role of the Accident and Emergency department

The Accident and Emergency department has an important task in the recognition of abuse and neglect; staff must be aware of hospital guidelines in cases of possible abuse. Increasingly liaison health visitors work in the Accident and Emergency department and social services may arrange for named hospital staff to have direct access to the child protection register and social services department computer from Accident and Emergency. This should facilitate proper use of these utilities, which are very useful but in practice underused because of delays in accessing information.

Ideally the health visitor or school nurse is notified of all attendances of children 0–16 years to the Accident and Emergency department.

Clinically in the Accident and Emergency department points of concern include:

- care givers who take their child to different hospitals, to conceal from staff that the child has repeated injuries
- care givers who regularly take the child to hospital with trivial complaints such as a cold or minor injury – is this neglect, anxious or inadequate parenting? But remember factitious illness too (see Ch. 12)
- facial bruising, or any bruising in infancy
- fractures under 2 years
- 'head injuries' in infants and toddlers: remember shaking or impact injury
- scalds and burns, especially forced immersion scald, burns on the dorsum of foot, hand, buttocks
- repeated ingestions in toddlers
- self-harm or overdose of drugs is associated with child sexual abuse and other abuses
- vaginal bleeding in a pre-pubertal girl
- any genital injury in boys or girls including 'straddle injury'
- allegation of abuse, e.g. on contact weekends with the non-custodial parent.

Indications for hospital admission

Admission for in-patient care is indicated

- for any child who requires medical or surgical treatment as an in-patient, e.g. because of a fractured femur
- for a child with unexplained injuries requiring further investigation, e.g. a skeletal survey
- in severe failure-to-thrive in infancy, but sometimes in older children
- for children who have taken overdoses, have anorexia, or have inappropriate illness behaviour
- occasionally for a general anaesthetic to allow a full examination in a child who may have been sexually abused
- for infants (usually) where there is a history, e.g. of apnoea, which may be factitious – the management is discussed in Chapter 12 and the role of covert video surveillance in the recent Shabde Report (1997).
- for any episode of an apparent life threatening event (ALTE).

Care in hospital

Parents must be kept informed, treated courteously and given necessary privacy and are usually involved in the care of their child.

Visiting by parents and relatives should be discussed by the social worker with them and the ward sister: it is not reasonable for the social services department to ask the nursing staff to supervise the parents where the child is thought to be at risk. The nurses may also provide a good assessment of the child–parent attachment with additional information of the parents' ability to handle and feed their child and the frequency of visiting.

Children should not be cared for in siderooms as further abuse may occur while they are in hospital. All accidents should be properly monitored; children thought to be victims present (with their parents) a particular management problem (Ch. 12).

The nursing staff bear the brunt of the problems associated with the admission of abused children to the ward. Angry and distressed parents shout at the nearest person in authority. They may have many unmet needs themselves, are demanding and may be reluctant to be in hospital. Nursing and medical staff need training to see the child as a child in need and not as 'another social problem'. Attitudes are passed on from medical staff and it is reasonable to expect all paediatricians to be able to care for abused children.

Junior medical staff should be assisted by their colleagues and should never handle a case of abuse alone. A senior house officer should not be 'the paediatrician' in court. Interviewing parents is a skilled art – the most junior doctor may take an initial, non-confronting history, but a senior doctor should be the one to explain why the history does not explain the injuries or other physical signs. Joint interviews with the parents involving the social worker and paediatrician are a very useful method of investigation.

Good communication between the parents, nursing and medical staff and the social worker is essential. The nurse in charge of the ward should know:

- why the child is on the ward and what is the clinical plan of investigation
- what the parents have been told
- if there is any statutory order
- what is the short-term plan (social services department)
- what to do, and who to contact if the child is removed from the ward (tell social services department and after-hours emergency social services department and police)
- that although it is reasonable to try and dissuade the parents from discharge against advice, staff should not become involved in any physical restraint.

Medical notes

Hospital medical notes are the property of the health authority although the contents are 'owned' by the doctor. The courts may order the release of notes and all comments in the records should be capable of later scrutiny and interpretation.

Points to remember

- All medical notes should be clearly written; entries should be dated and signed
- If investigations are requested these should be listed and the results should have been recorded. It is the doctor's responsibility to record results and to ensure that any appropriate information is passed on to parents, general practitioner and others who 'need to know'
- Contemporaneous records (i.e. written at the time of interview or examination) are usual. This leads to maximum accuracy in recall. The court may ask whether notes are contemporaneous
- Notes should be detailed, record verbatim remarks made by the child or adult and be an accurate and objective record of the interview. Persons present at the interview should be identified
- Physical examination should be well described, using diagrams and measurements to explain the clinical picture
- The reasons why a diagnosis is made should be listed, and the differential diagnosis
- The management plan should be clearly recorded; for in-patients include guidance as to what to do if parents do not cooperate. The social worker's name and telephone number should be clearly recorded in the notes
- A summary of the outcome of the child protection conference compiled by the attending doctor is written in the notes
- When the child leaves the clinic or hospital ward the notes should record where he or she went, with whom, and if paediatric follow-up has been arranged
- When parents seek a second opinion, paediatricians may send notes to the selected paediatrician, at the request of the paediatrician. It is not usual to send notes to solicitors unless directed to do so by the court. It is important that all paediatricians recognise that their first duty is to the child and that this overrides all other obligations. Paediatricians may decide to agree to requests by solicitors for reports if they are to be disclosed, that is made available to all parties. In care cases all reports are now 'disclosed' to all parties
- Medical reports and police statements are also written (see p. 359–361)

Second medical opinions

There is a danger that a child may be referred for repeated physical and psychiatric assessments, a practice deplored by the Cleveland Report (Butler-Sloss 1988, p. 245). The Report also states clearly (p. 248)

> Medical Practitioners who have examined a child for suspected sexual abuse and disagree in their findings and conclusions should discuss their reports and resolve their differences where possible; in the absence of agreement identify the areas of dispute, recognising their purpose is to act in the best interests of the child.

In an adversarial system it is unlikely that this will be possible, as doctors may be appointed because of their known clinical perceptions of abuse. Clearly, if professionals are working in the best interest of the child (see Ch. 17):

- all records and reports should be available to the paediatrician or psychiatrist asked for second opinions
- if the doctor wishes to examine the child, photographs or video the interview, the child's consent is needed. The doctor should justify why the child must be seen, rather than making a report from the records
- the guardian *ad litem* (a senior social worker appointed by the court to represent the child's interests) may be the most appropriate person to request second opinions – the child's welfare is his or her sole responsibility
- social work reports and police statements are an essential part of the information needed to provide a thorough second opinion.

Clinical management of possible child abuse

All cases of child abuse are different, but the same clinical skills are used on each occasion. A diagnosis of child abuse means that the doctor's opinion is that abuse has probably occurred. He or she may think it is a highly probable diagnosis but can rarely be 100% certain. The diagnosis is built up, like a jigsaw, in parts. The history, the examination and the results of investigations lead to a provisional diagnosis, which is assessed in the light of investigations by social workers and the police. A child protection conference will further scrutinise all the evidence and a minority of cases will then be heard in court. In care courts the evidence is tested against the 'balance of probability', not 'beyond all reasonable doubt' as in criminal courts. The standard of proof required by care courts is high; necessarily so given their statutory powers to remove children from their families.

Doctors should be aware that non-doctors often do not appreciate that an opinion describes the doctor's conclusion on the basis of received information and is not a certainty. If a doctor diagnoses a myocardial infarction, are they correct in 60%, 70%, 80% of cases? It is difficult to explain this concept, yet the doctor in child abuse cases are expected to get the diagnosis right every time, without appearing to be so arrogant as to suggest they cannot make mistakes.

If the doctor builds up the jigsaw carefully, can justify each piece of the picture and works closely with colleagues from other agencies, the child protection conference and courts become a safety-net to ensure mistakes are recognised. If the standards of proof are too high, children will not be protected, but neither is there a place for inadequate investigation and assessment by doctors, social workers and police which may also lead to children suffering.

Initial management: examples

The examples in Tables 14.3–14.6 suggest how cases might be initially managed. The clinical picture is described in the left-hand column and the management notes on the right, leading up to the time of the child protection conference. There may then be ongoing paediatric involvement and assessment, whether or not a diagnosis of probable child abuse has been made, if the investigation has demonstrated ways in which the child and family could be supported.

Allegations of abuse by professionals

All professionals working with children are at risk of allegations concerning the abuse of children in their care, but professionals may also abuse children. Professionals should question why they are doing their particular job and ensure they do have clear boundaries. It is also necessary to recognise that paedophiles are attracted to jobs which involve child contact and are often 'good with children'. Thus it can be a difficult task for teams of adults working with children – whether teachers, social workers, doctors or voluntary workers – to recognise that colleagues may and do abuse children.

Procedures should be established for each professional group in order to protect children and adults as far as is possible. For doctors this will usually involve forethought when setting up clinics or situations where a child is to be examined. However, if doctors spend time in specialist holiday camps for children, for example, guidelines are as for other residential workers.

Resources are needed to implement these procedures, but the medical defence unions are clear in their advice and on the real possibility of allegations against practitioners. Flexibility is possible when the child is young, the doctor a woman and so on, but sexually abused children in particular may have sexually provocative behaviour and have been damaged by earlier abuse.

Once procedures have been agreed locally the managers of the unit should become responsible for their funding and implementation. It may be necessary to seek advice from the appropriate professional body if a doctor does feel vulnerable (see also Ch. 17).

Table 14.3 Baby 'stopped breathing'

Clinical problem	Management notes
3-month-old infant brought by teenage parents to casualty department – 'stopped breathing' ↓ o/e Pale, quiet baby. Badly bruised chest. Well nourished. Clean. Bilateral retinal haemorrhages. No signs sexual abuse ↓ *Blood test* • blood film normal • clotting normal *Skeletal survey* fracture 5th and 6th ribs bilaterally and shaft of left femur *Photographs* injuries ↓ Opinion: ill baby – needs admission. Probable physical abuse ↓ ADMIT ↓ He needs a CT brain scan. Any evidence bony disorder (copper, osteogenesis imperfecta)? Other differential diagnoses considered	This baby is clearly ill and needs immediate medical evaluation. The first doctor should take a simple history and avoid confrontation. Later a more senior doctor should explore this inadequate history. The parents should be involved and understand the need for medical tests; implied consent is usually considered adequate unless a general anaesthetic is to be given. The need for skeletal survey and photographs should be explained. Parents will usually allow admission, especially when the baby is clearly unwell A senior doctor should become involved at this stage. Social services are contacted, asked to become involved and, in a case of serious physical assault, they will inform the police early in the investigation (strategy discussion). The parents must know that the social services department and, later, the police have been informed. (i) If parents uncooperative re: admission – SSD → EPO → Police (ii) If parents cooperative – SSD → voluntary admission (iii) Strategy meeting – SSD/police (iv) Police/SSD investigation (v) Do the parents/carers need support, childcare, solicitor? (vi) Plan CPC and longer term management (see p. 341–344) (vii) Discharge planned – foster parents, extended term by parents

Table 14.4 Facial bruising

Clinical problem	Management notes
4-year-old child seen in day nursery to have bruised face. ↓ Seen by doctor in health centre, OP clinic, *not* busy casualty department, *never* police station ↓ *History* – child 'wet the bed on purpose, so I hit him' – stepfather ↓ o/e Frightened, thin boy. Height 10 pc, weight < 3 pc. Four parallel bruises left cheek, 'finger-tip' bruises upper arms. Different ages of bruising. Poor language development ↓ *Opinion* Physical assault – slap mark and grip marks Underweight Appears frightened, poor speech needs evaluation Bedwetting – age appropriate ↓ Further medical evaluation needed – growth, development, emotional well-being – but as an outpatient Emotional maltreatment is seen as a central issue Other siblings need assessment too	Officer in charge of day nursery contacts social services department Social worker visits nursery, sees parents and arranges to take the child and parents for paediatric assessment (often with a community paediatrician) Social worker contacts health visitor for up-to-date report Family already known to social services department, marital and financial problems. Previous unexplained bruising 2 months ago Two younger siblings in nursery will need to be examined Is it safe for this boy to go home? Strategy discussion (police and social services department, ± paediatrician) Further social worker investigation needed before a child protection conference within the next week

Table 14.5 Intrafamilial sexual abuse

Clinical problem	Management notes
14-year-old girl tells friend who tells teacher 'I'm fed up with my dad getting into my bed and making me have sex'. Teacher tells girl she cannot keep this 'secret' but will help her Social worker (SW) and police officer (PO) see girl in school Arrange appointment with paediatrician at health centre or OPD (not police station) Examining doctor takes history as appropriate – n.b. date LMP, use of tampons, other sexual activity, vaginal discharge. Full physical examination, finishing with genitalia and anus. Mouth? Are: • pregnancy test needed? • STD swabs needed? • forensic swabs needed? • photographs needed? Physical examination compatible with repeated vaginal intercourse	Schoolteacher accepts initial story, informs educational welfare officer or social services department (child protection agencies). Immediate investigation by social services department of any previous information and strategy discussion that day between social services department, police and education SW and PO visit mother and seek her cooperation. The girl may prefer to see a woman doctor, which should be arranged. Do not make child repeat history unnecessarily Mother usually attends examination, but mother and daughter should give consent. The girl should decide who she wants to have in the examination room. Teenagers often prefer to be seen alone; this is not acceptable, so ask the clinic nurse to stay too Reassure the girl that she is 'normal' anatomically, there is no 'damage', but remember possibility of pregnancy or presence of a sexually transmitted disease Police decide to arrest father from work Will mother protect her daughter? What of other teenage daughters and son, aged 9 years? Child protection conference arranged

Table 14.6 Emotionally disturbed child

Clinical problem	Management notes
School refers 9-year-old boy ('P') to school doctor. He is failing to learn, wets, occasionally soils, and has no friends Seen with mother at school medical. 12 months earlier 'Uncle John' moved into the family. P's behaviour has always been a problem but worse in last 6 months o/e Restless, fidgety child, with a frequent brief smile. Height 75 pc, weight 50 pc. Physical examination normal Follow-up arranged by CMO in 2/12 but as no improvement referred to consultant paediatrician Seen in clinic – findings as above *Opinion* Emotionally disturbed boy – needs further assessment, is this child sexually abused? Seen by clinical psychologist for three sessions P tells mother Uncle John is abusing him – mother tells uncle Referred back to paediatrician – full examination	The school and school nurse should have useful background knowledge on this boy Past records describe an intelligent child, initially did well at school but always problems of concentration, poor peer relationships, gets bullied Educational psychologist confirms that the boy has no specific learning problems and is underachieving Could he have more support in school? School hears child is wandering around the estate until late into the evening Sexually explicit drawings found in his school jotter Paediatrician discusses concern with child abuse coordinator who will gather the known information and review – child's disclosure precipitates an early strategy discussion and investigation by social services department and police Child protection conference arranged

The procedures should have the weight of procedures rather than guidelines.

Abuse by professionals? Avoidance strategies

- Record and witness any injury, e.g. fall on floor
- Record allegations of anything
- Ensure touching is appropriate, as perceived by child too
- Record any inappropriate touch or suggestion by child
- Witness allegations if possible
- Do not physically examine child on your own
- If interviewing child on own for long period consider use of one-way mirror, leave door ajar, etc.
- Do not 'cover up' for a professional colleague
- Before interviewing or examining any child, ensure consent has been obtained from child and parents

CASE HISTORY 14.1

A 12-year-old girl who had severe learning problems had been referred because of sexually provocative behaviour towards male teachers at school. A female paediatrician examined her alone. The child suddenly sat up, flung her arms around the doctor and kissed her passionately on the lips. What would a third party have made of this encounter?

Confidentiality and consent

Doctors are anxious about issues of confidentiality but the General Medical Council in its annual reports of 1987 and 1993 (see earlier) gave unequivocal advice:

> where a doctor believes that the patient may be the victim of abuse or neglect the patient's interests are paramount and will usually require a doctor to disclose information without consent to the statutory agency.

The doctor may feel a responsibility towards the whole family; when there is a conflict of interest between the child and parents, what should the doctor do? The advice again is clear, 'the rights of the child should prevail' (HMSO 1988).

No professional should work in isolation in this field, and inexperienced doctors should all have access to more senior colleagues for advice. Each NHS trust has access to informed legal opinion.

In the USA there is mandatory reporting of possible child abuse cases. All professionals are required to tell the child protection agencies if they have concerns of possible abuse. There are advantages for professionals in that they are obliged to report and the balance is towards early reporting. In the UK doctors will hesitate – can they justify their actions, is enough known, is it really serious? If there are good interagency links, with respect between professionals, a doctor may feel able to ring the local social services office, discuss the case with the child abuse coordinator and work out a plan of investigation. Doctors should share appropriate information as building up a diagnosis of abuse is like putting the pieces of the jigsaw together and other professionals often have information which clarifies the clinical picture. The police too have a legitimate interest in child abuse, and as part of a team will usually work in conjunction with other professionals.

Confidentiality in cooperative work

Confidentiality at child protection conferences is also a legitimate concern. It should be the responsibility of local trainers under the auspices of the area child protection committee to ensure that there is a common ethical code. Information must be shared, but members of the case conference need to be confident that confidentiality will be respected; the degree of confidentiality will be governed by the need to protect the child (Working Together 1991). Written reports are increasingly laid before child protection conferences, and medical reports should be factual considering that later they may be used in court.

If parents attend part or all of a child protection conference care should be taken not to infringe a third party's confidentiality.

Consent: general issues

Consent for medical examination in paediatric practice is often implied. When a parent takes a child to see a doctor because the child has earache, help for the child is being sought. Parents expect the doctor to take a history, to ask the parent and child about symptoms and to examine the child. In this circumstance the examination would involve examining ears, nose, throat and chest, but the examination would depend upon the history. Although it is courteous to ask the child 'Is it all right if I look in your ears?', parents, by their presence, are assumed to be willing for the examination to take place.

Paediatric assessment of children referred because of possible abuse

Although the examination of a child who may have been abused is triggered by the issue of maltreatment, an assessment of the whole child should be included in the examination. Health, growth or developmental problems should be recognised as the examination serves the purpose of a full health check. Consent (usually verbal) is required for this examination as well as for any necessary medical investigations or treatment. The Cleveland Report said 'The child is a person and not an object of concern' (Butler-Sloss 1988). There is also emphasis, later taken up by the Children Act 1989, on listening to children, hearing their views and seeking their (appropriate) consent for medical examination.

Children, except very young children, should always be asked for their permission by the doctor before examination. In practice physical examination is not possible without the child's cooperation. However, depending on the child's age and understanding, the nature and purpose of the examination should be discussed so that the child's consent is informed (see later). The Children Act (1989) considers the child's welfare to be paramount, and the child may be vulnerable when given the choice to consent to or to refuse medical examination in the context of abuse. Abusers recognise this and may pressurise the child to refuse, fearing the consequence of corroboration of the allegations. The Act rightly leaves the consent with the teenager, but adults (parents or professionals) must be careful how they counsel children in these circumstances and should not offload their anxiety on to the child.

Current law

The Children Act is therefore clear that children, depending on their age and ability to understand, should be asked for their consent to examination. Parents must be fully involved in any procedures. Since 1986 and the Gillick ruling, older children have been able to give their own consent to medical treatment. Also, although parents must be involved, this does not mean that they may pressurise older children or insist on being present during the interview with the doctor or at the examination. In 1988 doctors were given clear advice as to the basis for medical consent (HMSO 1988, pp. 13–14). Examination without consent may be held in law to be assault. But for consent to be valid it must be informed, which means that the person must be aware of what he or she is consenting to and the possible consequences. The consent must be freely given without fear, threats, fraud or coercion. By the age of 16 years, children are regarded at law as capable of giving consent. Clearly there are exceptions, for example a child with significant learning difficulties.

Current practice

If a medical appointment has been requested by a parent, social worker or police officer in a case of possible maltreatment, the doctor should formally ask for consent from the person with that authority (usually the parent or child) to talk to the child and examine him or her. Paediatricians usually rely on verbal consent, and this practice is rarely challenged. In contentious cases, practitioners may prefer a signed and witnessed consent to be taken. Police surgeons follow this latter practice.

However, consent is equally valid whether given orally or in writing as long as it is informed and freely given. Consent is needed for any investigation, for example skeletal survey, and written consent is always sought before a general anaesthetic is given. If consent is witnessed by a professional witness it carries greater weight but in many instances there is no such witness, however preferable in law.

Teenagers and older children need a more detailed preparation than younger children with a different level of understanding of the procedure and of the possible consequences of full investigation of any allegation. It should be emphasised, though, that the 'medical evidence' is but a part of the greater 'jigsaw' which includes the social work and the police investigation. The medical should rarely be seen as the final arbiter – 'yes, there has' or 'no, there hasn't' been abuse.

CASE HISTORY 14.2

A concerned mother, on discovering that her 16-year-old nephew had been abusing her 12-year-old daughter for 4 years, wanted her girl examined. The mother was worried about 'damage or infection', and the girl as to whether she was 'normal'. The mother wanted 'proof' and it helped the girl to have medical corroboration of her story. The paediatrician helped with these concerns and referred the girl on for counselling.

Consent in cases such as the above should be informal and is unlikely to be problematic. Photography also requires consent. Photography may cause additional distress but if a colposcope is used (a piece of equipment with a light source, magnification and an integral camera) this may be minimised. Also, good photographs coupled with clear clinical notes and diagrams should make it difficult to justify further medical examinations. This must be in the child's best interest as the child is not submitted to a further examination but a competent second opinion may be provided nonetheless.

Other issues of consent

- Rarely, doctors will examine children without consent, but this is limited to emergencies of life or limb.
- If children are living at home, in the care of their parents and the children are too young to decide for themselves, the parent has the power to consent to medical treatment.
- When parents have delegated the care of their child to others they can also delegate their power to consent to medical treatment.
- When a local authority has parental responsibility for a child, it may, in appropriate cases, delegate the power to consent to medical treatment to others, for example the care givers. In most cases where a local authority has parental responsibility. It is obviously important that in these circumstances the local authority and the parents discuss medical consent, covering various contingencies, before it becomes needed.

Notes have been prepared for doctors (DoH 1991a) which advise them to consider before medical examination:

- Who has the right to consent to this examination or assessment?
- Is the child subject to a court order?
- What are the directions of the court, if any, in relation to the order? Has the court sanctioned the medical examination?
- Who has parental responsibility?
- Will the assessment be used in court proceedings?
- What are the views of the child, and has a guardian *ad litem* been appointed?
- Does the child have any difficulty in communicating for which special arrangements need to be made?

All the above questions must be addressed – if in doubt ask a lawyer. The British Agencies for Adoption and Fostering have produced a useful leaflet for practice which refers to children placed by local authorities and adoption agencies (BAAF 1991). All care givers (persons providing day-to-day care) need to know what to do in an emergency, for prophylactic or other care.

Summary

Children should never be denied emergency treatment because of the lack of formal consent. However, some forethought is needed when children are with care givers other than their parents to ensure that the care giver has authority to consent to examination and treatment when a child becomes less acutely ill. Consent for other medical examinations, for example an assessment concerning neglect and possible other abuse, may be problematical. Who has parental responsibility? What does the court authorise?

Tread warily! Do not be in contempt of court, and remember that courts may refuse to accept medical reports from examinations they have not authorised.

Some special cases

- *Emergency protection order*. Once proceedings have been started always ask the court's permission for medical examination; the applicant of the emergency protection has parental responsibility as long as the order lasts and may consent for emergency treatment, although this should be discussed where practicable with the parents

- *Child assessment order*. The court authorises medical examination
- *Care order*. The local authority has parental responsibility and may give consent. This power may be delegated to caregivers in certain circumstances. The parent(s) also hold parental responsibility but the local authority may determine the extent to which they exercise this. However, older children in care may also give consent or refuse as for other teenagers who understand the issues
- *Children in local authority accommodation* under Section 20 of the Children Act. The local authority has no power to consent to medical treatment unless this has been delegated by the parent or other person with parental responsibility
- *Children placed for adoption*. Birth parents retain parental responsibility for children of any age placed under the adoption agencies until they have been freed for adoption. The degree to which the parents are able to exercise this responsibility varies with the legal status of the child, arrangements made with the parent and any Section 8 order which is in effect. Clearly it is essential to plan with the birth parent if they would prefer to withdraw from this responsibility and the adopters need to be given delegated responsibility as long as they inform the agency of any treatment. Once children have been adopted they differ from foster-children in that all parental responsibilities are transferred to the adopters
- *Wards of court* differ in that the High Court has the right and power to consent to medical treatment and directions must be sought on the ward's behalf. Under the Children Act, children will no longer be made wards of court

Medical reports

Medical reports are written for a variety of purposes and their format will vary (Figure 14.3). If a child is seen because of possible abuse a report should automatically be written and sent to other agencies on a 'need to know' basis. This usually means the child's general practitioner, local social services department and child health (community). The written report will confirm the findings which will have been discussed earlier with the family and their social worker and others. It is important that a written report is available at the child protection conference, compiled by the paediatricians, clinical medical officer or police surgeon who examined the child.

Only if there is good communication will children at risk be protected, and doctors need to establish an efficient practice for provision of reports.

Types of report are:

- initial medical report
- full medical report
- affidavit/affirmation
- police statement.

Initial medical report

If an emergency protection order is sought from the court, for example if parents are threatening to remove a 6-week-old baby with multiple fractures from the ward, a short report may be written just to confirm the injuries and state that a provisional diagnosis of physical abuse has been made. The social worker can present this at court as 'evidence of harm', and that, given the age of the child, 'significant (further) harm' is likely, and so satisfy the conditions for the order. This report should be dated and have the name, date of birth and address of the child and professional address, name, signature and degrees of the doctor. It should be followed up by a more complete medical report. This is a legal document, and all opinions will be open to scrutiny later.

Full medical report

A medical report should be written to be available at the child protection conference on each child. There will be occasions, for example complex cases of failure to thrive or emotional abuse, when a longer, more detailed report is needed and the doctor needs more time to gain all the relevant information. In these circumstances an interim report should be written and an additional report written later.

In cases of child abuse it is not usual for the doctor to wait to write a report until asked to do so by the local authority's solicitor. This would cause unnecessary delays and difficulty for the child protection conference. In other situations a solicitor, representing the child (on behalf of the guardian *ad litem*) or the parents, may ask for a second opinion. This may be a paper exercise – that is, commenting on reports and notes – or the child and family may be seen. The medical report will state which papers the doctor has had made available to him and then comment on the findings and the interpretation of these findings. This should be an objective comment, remembering that the child's welfare is the main responsibility, not the protection of adults or vilification of colleagues.

A sample medical report is shown in Fig. 14.3.

- The *presentation* of the report should be clear – typed double-spaced with wide margins and headed 'medical report: private and confidential'.
- The *purpose* of the report should be remembered; also that it is to be read by non-medical professionals. What does the doctor think and why? The doctor does not have to be 100% certain, and can rarely be so, but can give an assessment of probability. Courts interested in child welfare have a different standard of proof based on 'the balance of probabilities', as compared with criminal courts where the standard of proof has to be 'beyond reasonable doubt' (Criminal Justice Act). In criminal cases the terms 'consistent' and 'not consistent' are used as opposed to 'probable' (HMSO 1988, p 39).
- The *content* includes:
  - Brief, relevant history, including circumstances and explanation of the injury. Only significant past medical history is included.
  - Description of the physical examination to include the child's demeanour, height, weight, cleanliness. All lesions (bruises, lacerations, burns, scars) described by size (cm), colour, depth, etc. Systems examination including genitalia and anus.
  - Investigations and results (dated).
  - Any further spontaneous comments by child during examination, e.g. 'Kenny stuck me with a knife'.
  - Opinion as to what has happened and why. The injury may be unexplained – in a baby of 3 months is this probably abuse, or is abuse unlikely? Discuss the findings in the light of the other information, build up the 'jigsaw' which has led to your opinion so that you are able to justify it at the child protection conference or in court.
  - The professional address of the doctor, qualifications, and maybe also a list of experience with children or child abuse: this will be confirmed if the case goes to court. Always date reports and sign the top copy for court.
  - Distribution to family general practitioner, local social services department, child health service and others as appropriate, such as other paediatricians, NSPCC, local authority solicitor.
- Always keep a copy of the medical report; it may be appropriate to have a separate secure filing cabinet for 'abuse notes'. In these circumstances it is important that other relevant records (hospital notes, child health notes, general practice notes) contain a copy of the report for reference. The report may later be used in various courts and made available to lawyers representing the child, local authority or parents.
- Think before circulating the report: inexperienced doctors are well advised to discuss the contents with a colleague. If still in doubt, contact the NHS trust lawyer. If the case goes to court the medical report may or may not be agreed by the various parties; if it is contested the author will be asked to attend court.
- Note that in some circumstances the child's address should be withheld, e.g. in foster-care where there may be a risk of removal.

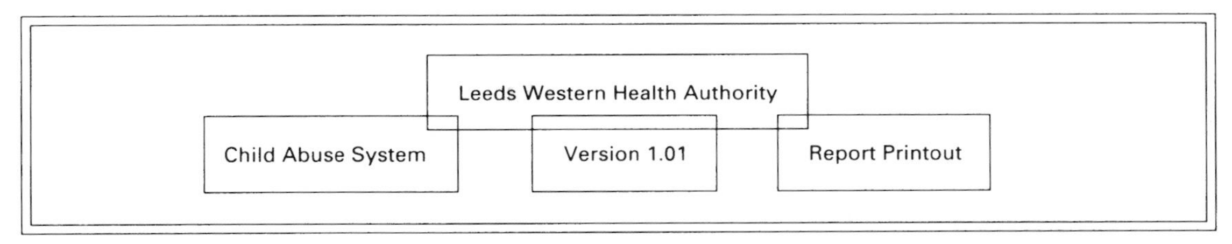

Department of Community Paediatrics
Leeds General Infirmary
Leeds
LS2 9NS
Tel: LEEDS 432799 — ext: 2152

Date: 12/04/90

PRIVATE AND CONFIDENTIAL

Name: SNOW, JOHN
Date of Birth: 06:06:87
Address: 12 ICE STREET
LEEDS 30
YORKSHIRE
Telephone:

Alias:
Gender: M

GP: DR. BLOB
Address: 122 BLOOMER ROAD
LEEDS 30

Social Worker: SUSAN WRIGHT
Telephone:

Social Service: BUCKSHAW ROAD
Telephone:

Health Visitor: JUNE SMITH
Telephone:

Consultant: DR BLANK

School: BELMONT PARK NURSERY

Police: NOT APPLICABLE
Telephone:

History: I examined John aged 2 years on 3.3.90 at .... Hospital at the request of .... Social Services Department. He was brought to the hospital by his mother Ms. Snow and S. W. Susan Wright.

Ms. Snow told me that she had gone out to Bingo the previous evening leaving John in the care of a 16-year-old girl baby-sitter. John was asleep on her return and it was not until the following morning she found he had two black eyes and bruising around his face. She immediately contacted her Health Visitor who referred him on to S.S.D.

The family are not previously known to S.S.D.

There is no past medical history of note.

Immunisation — complete.

Examine: Well cared for boy, nutrition good. Height 90 cm (50 pc) weight 14 kg (> 50 pc) Lively and playful.
Injuries
1. Left black eye with red-purple bruising extending 4 cm × 1 cm below eye, associated with some swelling.

Fig. 14.3 Sample medical report.

2. Right black eye with red-purple bruising extending 4 cm × 0.5 cm below eye
3. Left angle of jaw a row of red-purple bruises 4 × 0.5 cm
4. Anterior aspect both shins × 3 0.3 cm yellowing bruises

Heart: Heart sounds I & II nil added
Chest: clear
Abdomen: soft
Genitalia: normal
testes descended
Anus: normal
Investigations — Blood film normal
Clotting screens normal
Photographs were taken

Opinion: Physical abuse.

The bruises around the face are recent and likely to have been caused within the previous 48 hours. The two black eyes are consistent with blows from a fist and the bruises below the jaw finger marks (grip.) Considerable force has been used and accidental injury is improbable given two black eyes, and the site of bruising below the jaw which is rare in accidental injury. There are three discreet areas of injury, all likely to have been caused at the same time.

The bruises on the shins are as seen in ordinary play.

John's general care, growth and development appears normal.
The blood test shows that John does not have an unusual tendency to bleed.

Signature: JOHN BLANK CONSULTANT COMMUNITY PAEDIATRICIAN

C.C. G.P.:
Social Services: local office
NSPCC
Mr. Barnett, Sweet Street (Child Protection Coordinator)
Dr. Robertshaw, Child Health
Miss M A P Carlton, Child Health (Nursing)
Dr. C J Hobbs if Western Child/Dr. J Wynne if Eastern Child

Fig. 14.3 *Continued.*

Affidavit/affirmation

An affidavit is a written report which is a statement of evidence and is set out in a standard way, although exhibits to the affidavit may include, for example, earlier medical reports. A solicitor will usually set out the affidavit which then must be sworn or declared before a commissioner for oaths or other authorised officer. In practice, a solicitor (acting as an authorised officer) usually does this for a small fee, payable by the requesting solicitor.

The affidavit is made available to the judge and all parties to the case. If it is agreed the witness may not be called to give evidence. Oral evidence is given when the evidence is not agreed but may be limited to the reports, for cross-examination.

More usually in proceedings under the Children Act 1989, the professional will be asked to sign a statement on the understanding it will be placed before the court.

Police statement

Police statements differ in their presentation from medical reports (see example, Fig. 14.4). The investigating police officer will request that a statement is written and doctors will often prefer to write their own statement rather than sign one written in the police officer's language. Statements are written on a form provided by the police; each sheet should be signed at the bottom and copies always kept. A fee is payable for the statement.

STATEMENT OF WTINESS

(C.J. Act, 1967, s 9, M.C. Act, 1980, s 102, M.C. Rules, 1981, r 70)

STATEMENT OF: ....
AGE/Date of Birth: JOHN L BROWN OCCUPATION: ....
ADDRESS: Over 21 Paediatrician
Belmont House, Belmont Grove,
Leeds General Infirmary POSTCODE: ....

This statement (consisiting of ______ pages signed by me) is true to the best of my knowledge and belief and I make it knowing that, if it is tendered in evidence, I shall be liable to prosecution if I have stated in it anything which I know to be false or do not believe to be true.

Dated the _____ day of __________ , 19 John Brown

re: TRACEY Y. d.o.b. 9.9.80 5, Green Sweet, Leeds 34.
I am Dr John L Brown, my degrees are Mb ChB MRCP. My current post is Consultant Community Paediatrician, at Leeds General Infirmary. I was appointed in 1984. I have an interest in Child Abuse, and have examined abused children over the last ten years.

I examined Tracey Y, aged 10 years, at 3.00 pm on 7.7.90 at the request of West Yorkshire Police. She was brought to Leeds General Infirmary by her mother, Mrs Y. and Policewoman Z.

I had been asked to examine Tracey following an allegation that she had been sexually abused.

ON EXAMINATION: Well, co-operative child. Ht 140 cm (75 pc). Wt 35 kg. (75 pc). Pre-pubertal. Became very anxious when genitalia examined.
Heart — normal
Lungs — normal
Abdomen — soft. Genitalia. Minimal but uniform reddening of vulva.
Hymenal opening gaping, 1.5 cm horizontally and 1.5 cm vertically, thin rim of hymen remaining with irregularities at 5 pm and 9 pm.
No discharge, scarring or tears.
Anus — normal.
Investigations — Forensic swabs not taken, last alleged assault 3 weeks earlier.
— Bacteriological swabs taken 7.7.90 and initial report negative 9.7.90.

Mrs Y told me that Tracey had told her Aunt Susan that her father had been putting his fingers into her tuppence. Tracey had complained that he had hurt her and it had started when she was 7 years old, on her birthday. It happened about once a week.

Policewoman Z had already taken a Statement from Tracey and confirmed this history.

OPINION: The physical examination is consistent with digital penetration of the hymen. The hymenal opening is wide for a pre-pubertal girl, only a thin rim persists, there are no definite tears but I note two irregularities which may represent healed tears.

I note the history of alleged painful digital penetration over a period of 3 years. The signs are consistent with this history.

The reddening of the vulva is a non-specific sign. The swab was negative, showing no evidence of bacterial infection.

Statement taken by:

Given a clear disclosure by the child, physical signs which are consistent with the child's description, the probability is that she has been sexually abused.

JOHN L BROWN — Paediatrician

Fig. 14.4 Sample police statement.

Criminal proceedings take place at the direction of the Crown Prosecution Service. For a guilty verdict the case must be 'proved beyond all reasonable doubt' and, given the difficulty for children to give evidence, even with video links, the percentage of successful prosecutions, especially of child sexual abuse, is low (less than 5% of all alleged child sexual abuse).

Police statements differ from medical reports in that the court will only hear factual information and not hearsay.

The format of a police statement

- Name, date of birth and address of child
- Name, professional address, degrees and current post of examining doctor with short statement of relevant clinical experience
- Why the medical was requested, e.g. 'following an allegation by the child that she had been sexually abused'
- Where the child was seen, who brought him or her, who was present to give a history, present during the examination (what time of day and how long the examination took may be asked in court)
- Describe the child's demeanour during the examination and the details of the examination in full
- Record simply any history given, and say by whom
- Describe any relevant symptoms such as pain, vaginal bleeding
- Record if photographs were taken and by whom
- Record if blood tests, radiographs, microbiological investigations were performed, and results if available
- Forensic tests:
  - record which tests were carried out
  - who the specimens were handed on to
  - label, date, sign and seal all samples (see details, p. 262)
- *Opinion*
- Are the physical signs consistent with the history?
- Was the physical examination normal, as might be consistent with an allegation of oral sex?
- Is the probability of abuse very high, as for example would be the case if the child has gonorrhoea?
- Is it possible to give a time-scale to the abuse (albeit roughly)?
- Are there signs to suggest recent or chronic abuse, or both?

- *Note:* Always check a police statement with a senior doctor before dispatch

Forensic evidence

Forensic medicine seeks to explain the relevance of clinical signs, such as bruising, in a legal context. Any doctor who presents evidence of a physical assault to a court is giving forensic evidence. There is clearly overlap between forensic medicine and pathology; some practitioners are involved in both fields.

Although most children's doctors will feel confident to examine children who may have been physically abused or neglected, extra training is needed in the collection of certain specimens, for example in a case of recent rape. There has been considerable debate as to the role of paediatricians and police surgeons. Some paediatricians have been adequately trained to collect specimens but few police surgeons will feel confident to care for the child and his or her family paediatrically and will ask for a joint examination. It is likely in the future that, as for physical abuse, paediatricians will undertake the bulk of all child abuse work, calling on specialist police surgeon colleagues for help in appropriate cases. The appointment of women as police surgeons solely to examine women and children who may have been sexually assaulted is a welcome initiative as long as there is close cooperation with paediatricians in child cases, and children are not examined in a police station.

This section concentrates on evidence which may be found in cases of sexual abuse; interpretation of bruising and other injuries is discussed in Chapter 4, and Fig. 14.5 is an outline approach to medical and forensic investigation of child sexual abuse.

Forensic tests

All forensic tests are based on Locard's principle which states 'every contact leaves a trace'. For example, if an abuser has ejaculated over the

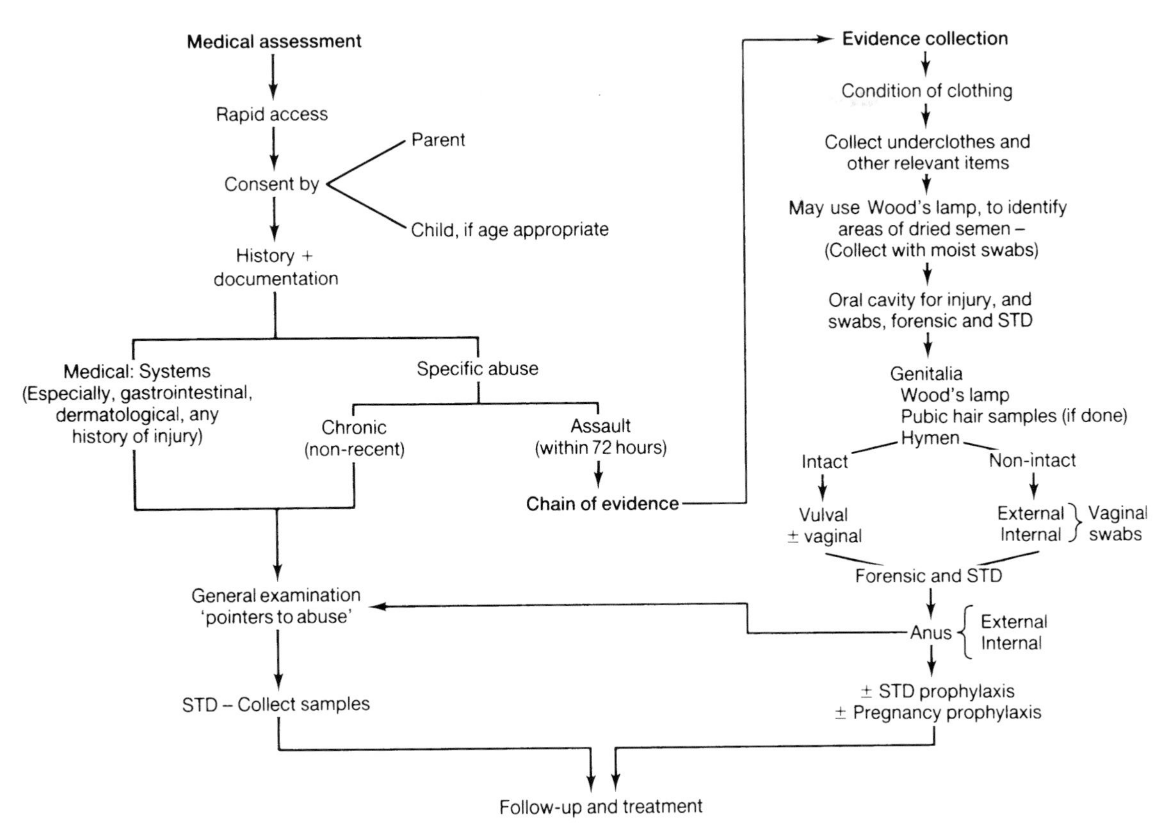

Fig. 14.5 Outline approach to medical and forensic investigation of child sexual abuse (Jenkins & Lewington 1997).

child, semen stains may be found on the child's body or clothes. If the child has scratched an assailant, blood may be found on either party. Fibres from the clothes worn by the child or assailant may be found on the other, and so on.

Clearly, the evidence which is obtained and its relevance depends on the type of abuse, where it occurred and how long ago. In practice, positive laboratory forensic tests are found in few victims of child sexual abuse. This is because most child sexual abuse is intrafamilial and ongoing. The child may disclose at any time following the most recent assault, which may have occurred days, months or years earlier. This will allow healing to occur and the physical examination may be entirely normal. Detection of semen varies with time too. Ideally swabs are taken from the mouth, vagina and anus within 24 hours of the assault. Spermatozoa have been identified in the mouth after 12–14 hours, the anus after 3 days, the vagina after 6 days and the skin after 24 hours (Gabby et al 1992, RCP 1997; Table 14.7). If the child has bathed, changed clothes or had a bowel movement evidence will have been destroyed. Even semen stains on the child's bedclothes may be explained – 'I slept in his bed because he was frightened after a nightmare'. Transfer of fibres within a household is inevitable owing to contact between people and furniture (Table 14.8).

Table 14.7 Time limits for the detection of spermatozoa and seminal fluid (RCP 1991, 1997)

	Spermatozoa	Seminal fluid
Vagina	6 days	12–18 hours
Anus	3 days	3 hours
Mouth	12–14 hours	3 hours
Clothing/bedding	Until washed	Until washed

Table 14.8 Forensic investigations (after DHSS 1988, McLay 1990, Jenkins and Lewington 1991, 1997)

Sample	To identify	Container	Comment
Clothing – as appropriate	Stain, pubic hair, debris	Paper/polythene bags	Open if wet/damp
Urine	Drug/alcohol assay	Sodium flouride bottle	
Blood – as appropriate	Drug/alcohol/solvent DNA (frozen)	Sodium flouride & Potassium oxalate bottle EDTA plastic syringe	Record time taken
Saliva	Semen	Plain bottle	Difficult†
Mouth swab	Semen	Plain sterile swabs	
Skin swab	Lubricant, blood, saliva, semen	Plain sterile swab, dampen with tap water	
External vaginal swab and internal vaginal swab	Lubricant, blood, saliva, semen	Plain sterile swab	External then internal (if possible penetration)
External anal and internal anal swab	Lubricant, blood, saliva, semen	Plain sterile swab	External then internal – dampen with tap water
Penile swab – external	Lubricant, saliva, semen	Plain sterile swab	Not urethral – unless ?STD
Matted hair	Semen	Polythene bag	Cut matted hair
Pubic hair – loose	Alien hair	polythene bag	
Storage Freeze as directed – blood group, DNA	Freeze: specimens for semen, sperm, alcohol, solvent	Refrigerate: urine for drugs, hair, clothes	Microscopy: sperm in saliva, anal, genital, skin swabs
* Preferably use 'rape kit' – provided by police, read instructions!	* Swabs to screen for sexually transmitted diseases (STD) – local hospital laboratory	* Unless the assault has been recent 'forensic tests' on sofa, bedding, carpet > positive tests	* HIV screen – see protocol Ch. 11
* Pregnancy test	* Follow-up examination if ?infection or treated STD	Timing of tests: see p. 363	
* 'Morning after pill' – up to 72 hours after assault Shearing PC 4 – 2 tabs start, 2 tabs 12 hours later IUD may be useful – 5 days but, caution if STD	* Prophylactic treatment Ciprofloxacin 500mg start doxycycline 100mg bd for 7 days		

* *NB Ensure 'chain of evidence', need to date, time, sign containers/labels,*
† *It is difficult for a child to collect saliva – may give the child bottle at beginning of the examination*

Forensic samples

Samples are examined in a forensic science laboratory: they may be *evidential samples* or *control samples* (blood and saliva) for comparison purposes.

Stains may include:

- blood
- semen
- saliva
- lubricant
- vaginal fluid
- faeces.

Plain cotton wool swabs (dampened with water if necessary) are used to remove stains.

The other evidential trace material is loose material or debris, and forceps or swabs are used to remove this. Clothing is inspected by the forensic scientist and may reveal fibres or particulate debris, but pubic hair may be recovered from the child's body.

Examination of unwashed clothing, bedding, carpets, chair covers, or objects used to assault the child is more likely to give evidence than examination of the child.

Materials such as textiles, head hair, paint or wood fragments are unlikely to be evidentially important when the abuser is known to the child and family.

Forensic examination

The forensic investigation depends on the clinical situation. The complete examination which is appropriate for an adult woman who has been

Taking of samples

- Use sampling materials and containers from a sexual assault pack (provided by police)
- Store samples as instructed, e.g. in a refrigerator or freezer (Table 14.8)
- Label each specimen with
  - child's name
  - date taken
  - person taking sample
  - type of sample
- Attach a 'Criminal Justice Label' to container or outer wrapping
  - complete the label with type of sample, sample number and signature of all who handle the sample until it gets to court
  - the sample number consists of the doctor's initials and the number of the sample, e.g. JMW/1 saliva sample, JMW/2 urine sample
  - usually the numbering starts again with each examination; the only exception is if two or more children are examined as part of the same enquiry – label consecutively
- Seal all samples with clear adhesive tape over the signed label, use freezer tape for specimens which are to be put in the refrigerator or freezer. Wind the tape completely around the top of bottles and turn the top of bags over twice and seal
- Samples to be taken are listed in Table 14.8.

raped on waste ground differs in many respects from the more limited examination needed of a 4-year-old girl who has been indecently assaulted by her older brother at home. A 'sexual offences form' should be available with kits and is a useful aide-mémoire and means of record.

The examination, which is part of a medicolegal investigation, should be described carefully. Points to remember include the following.

- Write legible notes, date and sign them, use professional address.
- Include the child's full name and address, date of birth and who accompanied him and gave consent; why, where and when the examination took place.
- Record a full history and detailed examination with diagrams if useful.
- Note if photographs are taken and by whom.
- Use a forensic check list to record specimens taken and where dispatched (sexual offences form).
- Use appropriate containers and swabs (in forensic kit supplied by police).
- Write a police statement as requested, keep a copy and usually complete a medical report for social services department, general practitioner and child health.

The examination of the assailant is not described (McLay 1990).

DNA profiling

In the past, by using conventional blood grouping (ABO and rhesus) techniques, it was possible only to exclude a man from paternity or show that his blood was not that found on a victim. By including secretor status and less-common blood groupings, the ability to demonstrate the reverse increases, i.e. the likelihood of paternity increases with the number of matched additional systems. The specificity of testing has been greatly enhanced by DNA profiling.

DNA profiles may be obtained from blood, semen and hair roots, but there is little DNA in saliva. Likewise in bloodstains there is little DNA as the DNA is found in the nuclei of white blood cells. Thus DNA profiling is a less sensitive technique when applied to bloodstains than conventional grouping. Semen is rich in DNA: for semen stains or vaginal swabs DNA profiling is more sensitive than conventional grouping.

Calculations show that an individual has a 1 in 4 chance of having a band in a given position. DNA profiles yield about 11 bands and, if all match, the chance of obtaining that particular profile in the general population is 1 in 2 700 000; if there are 14 bands the chance occurrence is 1 in 15510. If the specimen is small and the amount of DNA limited, fewer bands may be obtained; however, four bands reduce the chance occurrence to 1 in 200, better than conventional grouping methods. Conventional grouping methods continue to have uses in excluding suspects and testing bloodstains and saliva specimens.

Summary

1. Local guidelines, provided by the Area Child Protection Committee in line with Working Together (1989) and the Children Act (1986), should underpin all multi-agency practice.
2. Investigation of a case of possible child abuse should be logical and considered (Figs 14.1 and 14.2).
3. Doctors have a responsibility to recognise possible child abuse and to work together with other professionals in order to protect children.
4. Child protection teams based on each district general hospital enable doctors and other professionals to work together, share expertise, give support, teach, research and audit practice.
5. Child protection work spans community and hospital practice and should be well coordinated. Resources are needed to improve all aspects of practice.
6. Clinical management is often complex and should not be the sole responsibility of junior medical staff.
7. Allegations of abuse by professionals must be considered and procedures are needed to protect children and professionals.
8. The welfare of children usually overrides issues of confidentiality where child abuse is concerned.
9. Consent is necessary before any medical examination.
10. Adequate training is needed for all doctors undertaking child protection work – paediatrically and forensically. Co-working with colleagues (police surgeons) is indicated where a paediatrician is not experienced in collection of forensic samples.

REFERENCES

Access to Health Records 1990 A guide for the NHS. NHSME HSSG (91)16

American Academy of Pediatrics 1991 Guidelines for the evaluation of sexual abuse of children. Pediatrics 87(2):254–260

BAAF 1991 Consent to medical treatment for children. Practice Note 23. British Association for Adoption and Fostering, 11 Southwark Street, London SE1 1RQ

Birchall E, Hallett C 1995 Working together in Child Protection. HMSO, London

Butler-Sloss E 1988 Report of the Inquiry into Child Abuse in Cleveland 1987. HMSO, London

de la Haye Davis H 1987 Protocol for the forensic medical examination of a sexually abused child. The Police Surgeon 32

DHSS 1988 Sexually abused children – the sensitive medical examination and management. Royal Society of Medicine, London, pp 40–43

DoH 1988 Working Together. A guide or social workers undertaking a comprehensive assessment. HMSO, London

DoH 1991a An introductory guide for the NHS: the Children Act 1989. HMSO, London

DoH 1991b Child abuse: a study of inquiry reports 1980–1989. HMSO, London

DoH 1997 Child protection: medical responsibility. HMSO, London

Gabby T, Winkleby M A, Boyce W T, Fisher D L, Lancaster A, Sensabaugh G F 1992 Sexual abuse of children. The detection of semen on the skin. American Journal of Diseases of Childhood 146(6):700–703

Gibbons J, Conroy S, Bell C 1995 Operating the child protection system: a study of child protection practices in English local authorities. HMSO, London

Gillick v. West Norfolk and Wisbech Health Authority 1986 AC112

GMC 1987: Annual Report 1987, General Medical Council, London, p 15

Hallett C, Birchall E 1992 Coordination and child protection: a review of the literature. HMSO, London

HMSO 1988 Diagnosis of child sexual abuse: guidance for doctors. HMSO, London

Hobbs C J, Wynne J M 1987 Management of sexual abuse. Archives of Diseases of Childhood 62:1182–1187

Home Office 1992 Memorandum of good practice on video recorded interviews and child witnesses for criminal proceedings. Home Office and Department of Health, London

Jenkins D, Lewington F 1991 Forensic evidence. In: Physical signs of sexual abuse in children. Royal College of Physicians, London, Chapter 9.

Jenkins D, Lewington F 1997 The significance of forensic medical samples which may be taken in suspected CSA. In: Physical signs of sexual abuse in children. Royal College of Physicians, London, Chapter

Kolvin I (Chairman) 1988 Child sexual abuse: principles of good practice. British Journal of Hospital Medicine 39:54–62

McLay W D S 1990 Rape. In: The new police surgeon. Association of Police Surgeons of Great Britain, pp 82–111

Messages from Research 1995 Child protection: messages from research. HMSO, London
RCP 1991 Physical signs of sexual abuse in children. Royal College of Physicians, London
Shabde N 1997 The role of covert video surveillance. In: The management of induced illness syndrome. Report of a Working Group, Northern Yorkshire NHS Executive
Smith M, Penney B, Heverin A, Nobes G 1995 Parental control within the family: the nature and extent of parental violence to children. Messages from research. HMSO, London
Thorburn J, Lewis A, Shemmings D 1995 Paternalism or partnership? Family involvement in the child protection process. HMSO, London
Utting Report 1997 People like us. The review of safeguards for children living away from home. HMSO, London
Working Together 1988 Working together: a guide to arrangements for inter-agency cooperation for the protection of children from abuse. HMSO, London
Working Together 1991 Working together under the Children Act 1989. A guide to arrangements for inter-agency cooperation for the protection of children from abuse. HMSO, London

FURTHER READING

Bentovim et al 1988 Annual Report of Council (BMA) 1989–90 DNA Profiling. HOFSL
Jones D P H, McQuiston M G 1988 Interviewing the sexually abused child. Gaskell Royal College of Psychiatrists, London
McMurray J 1989 Case conferences. In: ABC of Child Protection. Meadow S R (ed) British Medical Journal London 57–64
Wilson K, James A (eds) 1995 The Child Protection Handbook. Baillere Tindall, London

15

Psychological intervention and treatment

During the last three decades much has been written about the way in which the cycle of abuse might be broken and how the psychological consequences can be understood and possibly treated. The need for better-trained therapists and support staff working with children who have been maltreated is vital, though with poor resources available it is left behind to the detriment of children and future generations.

Considerable advances have been made in the treatment area and these advances have been based on well-developed techniques, particularly of child offenders and victim treatments. This chapter, after an overview of the needs of the children, provides a guide to the major therapies and the theories on which they are based, and then proceeds to what has been learnt about how to treat children and their families.

Professionals working in the area of child abuse are not left in any doubt that abuse or maltreatment has consequences for the child in both the short and long term (Kempe & Kempe 1984, McFarlane & Waterman 1986, Bentovim et al 1988, Browne et al 1988, Sgroi 1988, Wyatt & Powell 1988, Cicchetti & Carlson 1989, Sgroi 1989, Adcock et al 1991, Bentovim 1992, Calder et al 1997).

The needs of the child

Depending on the maltreatment of the child, a number of psychological interventions can be used. The needs of any particular child will be influenced by the age and developmental stage of the child, the form of abuse, whether the abuse has occurred inside or outside the family, and in what way the maltreatment is recognised by those caring for the child and the authorities. All of these aspects should play a part in the decision process as to how to proceed in the selection of help offered and be considered in assessing the child's needs. The range of interventions is wide and while a considerable number of children, even when they have been maltreated in some form or other, will reach an acceptable level of personal development because of the growing up process itself, or because of help from friends, teachers, or non-maltreating parents, for a much larger number of children who have been maltreated the outlook is poor and their special circumstances need to be addressed (Hotaling et al 1988, Wyatt & Powell 1988, Briere 1992).

Not all, but many of the maltreated children need help of a professional kind so that their distorted development does not remain forever stuck and does not impede their own emotional growth as well as that of the children they may have in the future. The children and their families will be the central point of discussion.

What help and when

The question is always, 'how do we know when help is appropriate?' Some children are evidently distressed, but for others the memories of the abusive experience may be repressed, lie dormant and as if invisible to the outside world until something triggers the expression of the emotional turmoil. For children who have been badly abused the disturbed behaviour and emotional distress is apparent, not only by how the children are perceived by others but also by how difficult it is to care for them when they are in foster-care or with a non-abusing parent.

The trigger for the teenager may be a first close emotional relationship; for the adult it may be when they get married or have their first child. Here one may see the emergence of an intergenerational pattern with poor parenting skills being a main component for further abuse in the next generation. It is now better understood that the experiences of maltreatment in childhood – whether the abuse was physical, emotional, sexual, failure to thrive or other forms of maltreatment – have consequences which present themselves at the time and re-emerge in the teenage years and in adulthood particularly during times of stress.

One common consequence is that the future parent may lack experience and understanding of how to care for the children in the next generation. For others the emotional consequences simply make it impossible for them to provide appropriate affectionate care.

The increasing numbers of adults who have come for therapy over the last decade indicate that much maltreatment is ignored for a long time despite often severe symptoms and distress. Disturbances in behaviour, ill health or distress are being attributed to 'nerves', instead of acknowledging the antecedents of the childhood problems. It is well understood that the effects of abuse will re-emerge through the children's developmental stages, from childhood to old age.

Child abuse and its treatment cannot be discussed without thinking about families, parents, siblings, foster-parents and care givers in institutions. Nor should the stress that accompanies this kind of work for professionals go unmentioned.

As indicated in previous chapters, child maltreatment presents in a combination of abusive behaviours, and the jigsaw mentioned in Chapter 9 can give a clear picture of the interaction between various factors surrounding the abuse. The child, the circumstances, as well as the details of the maltreatment need to be assessed and recognised as a first step towards psychological treatment. For children who have been sexually or ritually abused a separate dimension has to be thought of which relates to the fact that many children are unable to disclose what has happened to them. All children who have been maltreated, in whatever way, need to have the opportunity to disclose but often the physical marks or neglect are sufficient and telling and make it easier for the child to say what has been happening.

The story of abuse unfolds like a jigsaw and the issue of treatment has its own corner in the jigsaw with a particularly intricate and complex pattern and fit. Putting this corner together can take a long time and often it looks as if a piece of information, memory or emotion does not fit.

The story, like a difficult piece, has to be turned this way and that before it does make sense, both to the child, the carers and professionals. Reder et al (1993) conducted reviews into reports of 37 fatal child abuse cases and have given insight into the dynamics of these tragedies.

Assessment

The chapters discussing specific forms of child abuse (physical, emotional, failure to thrive, etc.) have incorporated strategies for assessment and these can be usefully followed when making decisions about therapy. However, there are aspects of the child and adult which need to be specifically attended to in choosing psychological treatment.

The severity of the abuse will need to be assessed separately (Reder & Lucey 1995), and physical as well as psychological evidence is to be taken into account. Stratton & Hanks (1991) have proposed a model – broad questions which need consideration:

- how did the child or adult perceive the maltreatment?
- do they feel to blame for the maltreatment?
- how anxious is the child/adult?
- are they depressed, phobic?
- what are the behavioural difficulties?
- are they underachieving or overachieving?

When a child has been sexually abused the impact of this abuse needs to be assessed:

- what sense did the child make of the abuse?
- what perception have they of themselves?
- was the child coerced or forced?
- did the child 'cooperate' or 'accommodate' (Summit 1983) so that the abuse could continue?
- when did the abuse start?
- how long did it go on for?
- was it kept hidden from the outside world?
- note the different forms of maltreatment.
- note other important life events for the child (e.g. parents' illness, death, etc.).
- any other trauma in the child's life.

Developmental issues must also be borne in mind:

- the child's age when abuse began
- the length of time abused
- at what stage did the sexual abuse become intrusive?
- was the abuse kept a secret?
- was there a disclosure, if so to whom and what was the response?
- how was the child treated after disclosure?

Sgroi (1988, 1989) in her two volumes on child sexual abuse has described different forms of assessment in more detail. This section is aimed to help the reader think about the issues involved in making decisions and giving advice (treating the information as a guideline). Procedures, treatments and strategies for understanding abused children and adults are developing at a steady pace. Practitioners need to be mindful of the different laws, procedures in their agency as well of the developments in therapeutic techniques. Bentovim (1992) discusses the trauma organised systems when physical and sexual abuse have occurred in families.

Types of psychological treatment

We now examine how the major therapies and treatments may help a child and his or her family when child abuse has occurred. A brief discussion about what therapy is in principle is followed by a description of the four major theoretical frameworks which are most influential in underpinning psychological therapies practised all over the world. We then continue by describing a number of interventions and therapies which may follow the discovery that a child has been abused. Hunter (1995) in his edited book gives insight into the provisions for treatment with child victims and perpetrators of child sexual abuse. Wilson & James (1995) have a good section by different authors on interventions in child abuse cases. Briere (1992) discusses the theory and treatment of abusive trauma.

What is psychotherapy?

Principally psychotherapy it is a 'talking cure' but it may also include behavioural interventions and active participation. In the various psychotherapies both the client/patient and the therapist use conversation and language as a means of communicating with each other. Even in play therapy with very small children who have not acquired language in the fullest sense some words and sounds pass between the participants. Psychotherapies are distinct from physical treatments and should only be carried out by trained professionals. Many specific psychotherapies have been developed. Therapies are based on psychological theory and currently there are four major approaches to psychotherapy which form the basis for many subgroups and divisions which developed from one or other theoretical model.

Behaviour psychotherapy

Behaviour psychotherapy is based on learning theory and was developed from Pavlov's conditioning principles. It focuses on the maladaptive behaviour as such and, broadly speaking, attempts to change such behaviours by using positive or negative reinforcers in order to extinguish or inhibit certain behaviours. So, for instance, when a child wets or soils, the therapy concentrates on eliminating this behaviour. The reason why the behaviour may have occurred is not explored – the effort is spent on modifying the undesirable behaviour. Many specific treatment procedures exist under this umbrella, e.g. *desensitisation techniques* for reducing excessive emotional reactions such as fears, *aversion therapy* to reduce overdependence on specific gratifications, *token economy* programmes, *assertiveness training*, etc. Skinner (1953) developed techniques on the principles of learning theory which are used to manipulate deviant or maladaptive behaviours towards a goal. Behaviour therapy may also be used to get a symptom under control so that other therapies can be used.

Cognitive psychotherapy

Cognitive psychotherapy is based on the individual's perceptions and thinking and was first developed around the issues of depression. The psychotherapist actively modifies the patient's way of thinking and attempts to change the negative outlook of the patient into a more positive one. *Non-directive psychotherapies* also developed from a cognitive model. *Rational–emotive therapy* is another cognitive therapy which centres on people's belief systems and the fact that the beliefs can be distorted in their thinking, causing them psychological difficulties. These difficulties, whether in terms of people's cognitions or behaviour, can be modified by this therapy.

More recently behavioural and cognitive psychotherapies have been used together; new specific ways of working within this framework have been developed under the umbrella of *cognitive–behavioural therapy*. This combination of therapies has been found to be effective in alleviating many problems of individuals. Cognitive therapy has also made links with analytic theory and *cognitive–analytic theory* is now an accepted way of proceeding.

Psychodynamic psychotherapy

Psychodynamic psychotherapy is based on theories of motivation and drive in human beings and the interaction between them. It relies on understanding the developmental history of the patient – what effects upbringing and relationships in early childhood have on psychological well-being and disturbances in the child and what the effects on later development may be. The therapist pays attention not only to the dynamics in the patient's outside world, particularly the family, but also to what happens inside the session. Much of what patients express in the session will make it possible to understand their functioning and malfunctioning. The story told by the patient – adult or child – will often represent the antecedents to the disturbance. The relationship between therapist and patient is one of the most important tools in this therapy. Brown & Pedder (1978) and Clarkson & Pokorny (1994) provide clear introductions to the field.

Psychoanalysis

Psychoanalysis belongs in a category of its own.

Psychodynamic and analytic psychotherapy are both derived from psychoanalytic principles. Since psychoanalysis as such is rarely available on the NHS the reader is referred to a dictionary such as Rycroft (1968) for a full definition.

Systemic therapy

One of the more recent forms of therapy, systemic therapy, was developed particularly for helping families and individuals. All behaviour, whether functional or not, is regarded as an attempt by the individual to cope with the systems in which they function. This approach avoids interpreting symptoms and other behaviours as caused by characteristics of the individual, but sees them rather as the outcome of the history of the person and of their attempts to cope with the situations to which they have been exposed. The systems in which interpersonal relationships play a major role are regarded as the most important. The systemic approach has a particular value in helping the therapist to understand the adjustments that an abused child and other family members will make in an attempt to survive physically and psychologically in an abusive environment (Stratton & Hanks 1991, Reder et al 1993). It has also been found useful because other therapeutic approaches can be used and coordinated within a general systemic perspective. It therefore makes it easier for professionals with different training to find common ground and work together productively.

Other psychotherapies

There are many different types of schools of psychotherapy (e.g. the humanistic–existential school, gestalt therapy, drama therapy) which will not be discussed here. However, the applicability of *psychodrama* and *play therapy* relevant to children will be explored subsequently. The choice of therapy depends not only on the age of the child and the form of the abuse but also on the stage of the process the child has reached.

Who should be included in the therapy?

The common model of treatment for an adult or child who is not well or is having difficulties is to treat this adult or child. A child may have been admitted with injuries and treated satisfactorily in hospital. Intervention and/or collaborative and supportive work with the parents and other professionals needs to take place, otherwise this child will be back in the same position of risk, having received further injuries and the cycle will simply be repeated. Assessment of the situation with the caretakers, and possibly other siblings is essential (Reder & Lucey 1995). The range of people to be included in therapy when a child has been abused is indicated in Table 15.1. There may be other combinations which make up the specific group receiving help; the table is not meant to give the impression that therapy can only be offered with a rigid framework in mind. More than one type of therapy may be helpful at any one given time and this will be discussed further. As an example, the family may come for

Table 15.1 People who may be involved together in therapy when a child has been abused

Individual	The child alone
Dyad	Mother and child
Triad	Mother, father and child
Family	Including all who live in the household, possibly also grandparents
Sibling group	Particularly when the children of the family are together without their parent(s)
Foster-parents	With the specific child or all the children in the family Support for foster-parents
Therapeutic groups	Children and teenagers, mothers, fathers, perpetrators
Groups for perpetrators	Men, women, adolescents, boys and girls
Marital couple	Mother and father
Community programmes	As proposed by Henry Giaretto
Educational programmes	As proposed by KIDSCAPE
Staff in institutions	Consultations to children's homes
Staff	One-to-one supervision, or group supervision on casework, group work or family work Stress management and support

family therapy but one child may also be seen in individual therapy in order that specific emotional and behavioural aspects can be attended to. A parent who has been abused as a child may also need individual help.

It is important to fit the therapy to the needs of the individual child and family but often this is not possible because services may not be available in a given area. Careful planning and matching of needs and available services is essential when assessing which treatment to recommend. Most small children would benefit from their parent(s) or carers being actively involved in the therapeutic process, if not actually present. However, there are instances when it is beneficial even for very small children to be given time on their own. This is particularly so if a child is being hurt, neglected or sexually abused. An example would be if the care givers of this child are in a frame of mind that would not allow them to acknowledge their behaviour towards the child. In such circumstances they would, simply by their presence, be most likely to intimidate the child and not allow him or her to voice what is causing distress. There may be many reasons for this, not least that the child needs to be keeping his or her 'secrets' and not telling on the abusing adult. The child left alone with a therapist might tell about these experiences, but a careful assessment of this situation has to be made in advance. Not every child who tells can be thought of as being safe on return home after a disclosure. Summit (1983), with his concept of the accommodation syndrome, emphasises this point only too well. Bentovim et al (1995) discuss the facilitating process of interviewing children who have been sexually abused in the light of the Memorandum of Good Practice (Home Office 1992) and highlight important issues which need to be considered.

CASE HISTORY 15.1

A mother and her two children had been coming for therapy because of what was termed 'difficult behaviour of the children'. In the fourth session one of the children made a spontaneous disclosure and the other child drew a picture saying 'this is what is happening to us both'. The children were describing sexual contact with an adult. When the mother asked them who this grown-up was, the children became anxious and only after some coaxing from the mother did they tell her that it was their father. This mother had considerable difficulties believing that her husband could harm her children. On the other hand, she was convinced that if he knew what had been said he would become extremely angry with all of them. When she telephoned him to say that she would not come home today but had gone to stay with her parents he threatened her and the children with a 'good hiding' if they did not come home. It was only after the conversation with her husband that she could believe that the children needed protection, and maybe so did she.

Talking with children who have been abused

Children often make unexpected, spontaneous disclosures if they have been abused because the therapeutic situation, whether in the medical or psychotherapeutic environment, invites exploration of causes of their illness or behaviour and provides an atmosphere in which the child and adult are offered trust. When an ordinary consultation or therapy session turns into a disclosure session this can bring about considerable problems, not least for the children. The professionals in such a situation need to be as clear as possible what the immediate future holds. Vizard & Tranter (1988), Davies (1991), Vizard (1991), Bentovim et al (1995), Fry et al (1996), Jones (1996) discuss the interviewing process in situations when the protection of the child is the immediate issue. Professionals should have acquainted themselves with the procedures and be aware of who to contact in the professional network if such a situation occurs. The Memorandum of Good Practice (Home Office 1992) and Working together (1991), to be rewritten, are good guideline material.

Would an abused child benefit from therapy on his or her own, or would it be better if they were seen with some other family member? Table 15.2 provides a simple indication of which

Table 15.2 Would an abused child benefit from therapy individually, with others and/or in groups?

Therapy	Type of abuse				
	Physical	Neglect	Emotional	FTT	Sexual
Individual	B	C	A	C	A
Mother+child	A	B	B	A	A[a]
Parents+child	A	C	C	B	A[a]
Family	A	A	B	B	C[a]
Siblings	C	C	C	D	C[a]
Foster-parents	B	B	B	A	A[a]
Marital couple	C	D	D	D	C
Group	C	C	C	C	B

A, Method of choice, likely to be essential; B, often useful; C, sometimes useful; D, rarely useful
[a] Treatment with non-abusing adults.

groups it is usually appropriate to treat, this short section by no means reflecting the amount written on the subject. In considering these various possibilities it became clear that most forms of abuse can be treated in most groupings, so that there will rarely be any need to assume that only one form of treatment is worth considering. However, another implication of the table is how important it is to construct an individual case profile and base decisions on that. This would take full account of the age of the child, his or her home circumstances, the willingness and motivation of all to participate and a professional judgement of what would most benefit the child. The immediate response once abuse has been identified will inevitably have implications for all family members and will usually be more effective if they are all actively involved (Bentovim et al 1988, Sgroi 1988, 1989). Helpful information on this matter can also be found in Messages from Research (1995). Monteleone & Brodeur (1994) give an interesting perspective on interviews with children when they have been abused.

Supporting the family when abuse has occurred

A child or teenager who has taken the courageous step to tell about his or her abuse or has been found to have been abused because of injuries or what they have 'inadvertently' said or done needs help to follow swiftly. The child or teenager is usually not in a position to cope with the disclosure situation alone.

Equally, when child abuse has been recognised and a diagnosis formulated by professionals, the next step is usually to think of help in the form of interventions and/or treatment. For the child who has been sexually or ritually abused and has made a disclosure to an adult, care giver and/or professional, special and careful preparations should be made for the child to go to the next step. This next step may involve the police and social workers instigating a disclosure interview in accordance with their procedures (see above and Ch. 14 and 17). Following this, further assessment by professionals should lead to interventions appropriate for the child.

The help that follows can take many forms and some of these are discussed briefly below. Help can consist of therapeutic work and/or much more practical support which will benefit children and families. Porter (1984) addressed the role of self-help groups and alternative support networks, emphasising that they play an important part in dealing with the problem of child sexual abuse. The same can be said for other forms of abuse too.

The list of therapies mentioned below includes community programmes as an attempt to counteract child abuse in society as a whole. In Britain such programmes have not taken off but in the USA Giaretto's (1977) model has been evaluated and shown to be effective. Bagley & King (1990) have also described their research which includes descriptions of how whole communities can be educated and given information about how to counteract child abuse in their neighbourhood.

Educational programmes for children have figured largely in the area of child sexual abuse and in Britain the lead has been taken by KIDSCAPE with Michelle Elliott in developing such programmes. Brassard et al (1983) have produced video material which can be used to help children understand about child sexual abuse.

Crisis intervention

Crisis intervention is applicable for many problems, in response to an acute crisis which has overwhelmed the person(s). The main aim is to give reassurance, support and guidance. In most cases the aims are set in terms of short-term work with the client. In cases of child abuse there may be an initial telephone helpline but most often there is face-to-face contact with those involved in the abusive situation. Generally, as well as in abuse cases, this form of intervention focuses on the acute, present situation. A drop-in centre could be the vehicle for crisis intervention, but most often it involves a professional intervening quickly, concerned with the child's safety as a priority.

Telephone helplines

Telephone helplines have been found to be useful in the past, particularly when parents and care givers reached the end of their tether and felt they would hurt a child in their care. The National Society for the Prevention of Cruelty to Children (NSPCC) provides such a service in some areas. More recently, and with the acknowledgement that sexual abuse exists, such telephone helplines have also been made available for children. *Childline* is probably the best known nationally, but there are many more local telephone lines which are set up by either the NSPCC or NCH (National Children's Homes). It has been established that these telephone lines are being used extensively; evaluation of such services is in progress (Browne & Saqi 1988).

Nurseries

A nursery is an invaluable resource when small children have been abused. It can provide care and safety for the child who has been abused on the one hand, and a break from the child for the carer, mother and/or father, on the other. Often nursery staff are trained to help parents gain vital skills such as how to care for the child, feed the child, play with the child, etc. They may provide a model of childcare which has not been hitherto accessible for the parent(s) and for some parent(s) this contact can be sufficient to change the way they treat their children. The NSPCC nurseries are particularly geared to help parents learn different parenting skills and provide both education and therapy.

There are further support services available in various parts of the country and family aides are amongst them. They are usually women who are employed (by social services) from the community and neighbourhood, who may support a family who have difficulties and abusing or neglecting patterns in the home. They can participate with the parent(s) in tasks such as cooking, feeding the children, bathing the children, playing with them, etc. Family service units provide nursery facilities and can make interventions which include therapy.

Most interventions, though, rely on the child and family receiving therapeutic help in some form or other over a period of time. As indicated, voluntary help can be very useful but most of the time a trained counsellor or therapist is needed to help the child and family develop.

Therapies with longer-term objectives

Once the immediate crisis, usually after disclosure, has passed, the task of planning for longer-term therapeutic objectives arises. In most cases, a range of choices exists, and the information acquired during the first stages of intervention will help guide the choice. The purpose of this chapter is to provide a picture of what can be expected from the major therapeutic approaches and is there to help make decisions about how to proceed therapeutically. The basic choice is whether psychological treatment should be offered to the family (whole or part), to the child in a group setting, or to the child individually. In some cases more than one form of therapy may be desirable and practicable, while in others it may be judged that one form of intervention should be tried and evaluated before others are considered.

The advantages and limitations of three groups of therapies are reviewed after they have been described, but a preliminary orientation is worthwhile. Family work will be chosen when it is clear that:

- the future welfare of the child requires changes in the attitudes and behaviours of other family members

- the psychological problems that the abuse has created for the child will best be resolved within the matrix of the family relationships.

Treatment outside the family may be necessary if the child has to be removed (or in the case of older children when they remove themselves) from the family. It may also be useful, for instance in conjunction with family work, to give the child some space and distance from the pressures of the family in which they can make their own adjustment to what has happened. Group therapy has the advantage of reducing the sense of isolation so common in children and adults who have been abused. This work can be more cost effective but assessment for group work, as for other therapies, is essential because the motivation, psychological capacity to work in therapy, and the timing in terms of the state of mind and emotion of the person are important milestones to be considered. Individual work can be more focused on the needs of the individual child and may be important if the child is young, handicapped, or unable to work within any kind of group setting.

The position of the perpetrator is of course crucial. Research has so far indicated that family therapy with perpetrators is extremely difficult and in many cases simply not successful. Family work with non-abusing family members has a much greater potential to achieve positive and lasting changes.

Patterns of maltreating families

Crittenden & Ainsworth (1989) distinguished between families who physically abused, neglecting families, and families who both physically abused their children and neglected them. They found characteristics which differed between the parent groups and showed how important it is to recognise into which pattern the parents fit. This does not have to be done at the referral stage, but early on in the therapeutic work and during assessment. Furniss et al (1984), Bentovim et al (1988), Patton (1991), Bentovim (1992), Hanks & Stratton (1988, 1995) and Wilson & James (1995) are amongst those who have researched how the pattern of family functioning can be understood when sexual abuse has occurred and what implications this has for therapy.

Physically abusing families

Crittenden & Ainsworth (1989) found that the prognosis for the physically abusing families once they entered therapy was very good. They found that most of the time the parents were motivated to change but that their coping strategies were poor. Their need to use power over others and dominate wherever possible was paramount. For instance the mothers in this group use punishment as the only means of discipline in order to control and teach their offspring.

Neglecting families

The characteristics of the neglecting families differed significantly in that these parents' coping strategies relied on withdrawal from difficult situations rather than control. Disciplining the children seemed not to be an option. The mothers always felt that others knew better and rarely finished tasks they had begun. The parents had no plans or expectations for themselves, let alone their families, and their children were particularly passive in infancy. The treatment for these families has to be quite different from the above group because these mothers are not easily motivated and often have little understanding of why any change is needed in the way they care for their children.

Abusing and neglecting families

The pattern for the abusing and neglecting families is different again. The research showed that when considering the issue of interventions for this group it became clear that only for some can change be predicted, and then only when long-term support was available. To break the cycle of abuse in these families proved much more difficult than in the other two groups. Members of such families feel that they have no control over their lives and that the possibility for change is beyond their reach. In these families parental coping strategies oscillate from sullen withdrawal to violent outbursts. The children are not treated consistently and all are inclined to feel both utter frustration and helplessness. The children are often out of control and resist control while the parents' expectations of them are either very high or they have no expectations of their children at all.

Sexually abusing families

When Furniss et al (1984) investigated families where sexual abuse had occurred they found a pattern which showed that the emotional and sexual relationship between the parents was poor and tension-laden, despite outward appearances to the contrary. The relationship between the mother and her abused children was distant. The child was brought up to act as both peer and partner to the father and became trapped in what Summit (1983) calls the 'accommodation syndrome' which includes secrecy and denial. Furniss et al (1984), Furniss (1991) and Bentovim et al (1988) indicated that the strength of this pattern varies between families and that they can, along a continuum, be grouped into either conflict-avoiding families or conflict-regulating families (Furniss 1985). The first type of family avoids looking at the issues and is afraid of being discovered. They are often described as moralistic and rigid. The second type of family shows a more disorganised and quarrelsome pattern of interaction. Here more actual disturbance can be visible, the boundaries between adult roles and those of the children are blurred or non-existent, and violence is used when frustration and confusion reach a peak (see also Patton 1991).

Describing such family patterns, however briefly, illustrates the interactions that take place in the abusive families and it shows why treating one member of such a system is not likely to break the cycle of abuse. Some of the more widely used therapies available are discussed below, and sources of research and practice are indicated.

Women who sexually abuse children

Our understanding about the fact that women too abuse children sexually has increased. Elliott (1993) edited an important work on this subject. Sgroi & Sargent (1993) discussed the impact and treatment issues for children and adults who have been sexually abused by female perpetrators. Matthews (1993) described her work with female sexual abusers. Saradjian in association with Hanks (1996) described the research conducted around women who sexually abused. Many of these women were mothers and the victims of their abuse were their own children. Wolfers (1993) addressed the paradox of this form of abuse and linked it to the position of power and powerlessness in the public and private sphere.

It is extremely difficult to identify women who sexually abuse their own children, but they are not all that uncommon in paediatric clinics. Confronting these mothers is often not a way forward and will end up in withdrawal rather than beginning to break the cycle of abuse. It is easy to get enmeshed because the scenario seems so improbable and many of the women are otherwise very ordinary, likeable people of whom one would not expect abuse. However, these women are no more able to break the abusive cycle on their own than are male perpetrators of sexual abuse, and the children may need to be protected and taken out of the relationship before any work with the women and children can begin. It is not clear whether women manage to overcome this kind of behaviour towards children, and more research is needed before commenting conclusively on the matter.

Children are at risk of becoming very distressed and disturbed by this form of abuse; they need to be put at the centre of any deliberation and plans. Women may abuse very small children (sometimes infants of only a few weeks old). The women may be on their own with several children in the family but only one child sought out as the victim. They may sexually

When may women abuse sexually?

- When they live on their own with their children
- Within a married relationship
- Together with men who are their short-term partners or casual acquaintances
- Within prostitution (being paid)
- Within a lesbian relationship
- When they have a handicapped child (usually an older boy)

abuse their children, both male and female, in conjunction with men. Saradjian (1996) has developed a specific therapeutic stance in helping those women who feel sufficiently motivated to break the cycle.

There is now more understanding and written work available about female sexual abuse, and the reader is guided to this more specialised area via the references given.

Family therapy

When a child is maltreated at least two people are directly involved, and if the maltreatment takes place within the family it is most often a parent who is doing something to the child. Once such a dyad exists within the family it usually affects the other members of the family too. They become disturbed or worried by what they see, or hear, and have to keep out of the way lest they get involved. In the case of another adult they may find it too painful to acknowledge and therefore have 'to look the other way'. Crittenden & Ainsworth's (1989) work shows the complex interactions that may occur within the different families.

Family therapy takes as its basis the assumption that what people do is largely determined by the contexts in which they find themselves. For most people, and particularly for children, the family contains the most important relationships in their lives. To bring about major change in a person's life, it will often be useful, or even essential, to bring together their family, so that repeating patterns can be exposed, and relationships renegotiated. This theoretical position has given rise to a body of practical techniques for bringing about change in families. Hoffman (1981) provides an excellent general overview of the work of the pioneers of family therapy; De Shazar (1986) offers a useful account of why family therapy practice takes the form it now does; Burnham (1986) is a sound and readable survey of the field; and Stratton et al (1990) have attempted to provide a highly practical manual which shows what family therapists do, and why. Bentovim et al (1982) explore the applicability of systemic family therapy to all kinds of family problems.

Family therapy is practised most often by a team working together, with a therapist in the room with the family and the rest of the team behind a one-way mirror to observe the family and give help to them from a perspective where they can quietly listen and form helpful interventions for the family. Because families and their interactions are very complex, a team helping the therapist to help the family has been proven to be of considerable value (Campbell & Draper 1985, Stratton et al 1990, Reimers & Treacher 1995).

Developments in the field of child sexual abuse produced further, more specific, work with families: Furniss (1983), Furniss et al (1984), Bentovim et al (1988), Glaser & Frosh (1988), Hanks & Stratton (1988) and Bentovim (1992) all describe ways in which families can be conceptualised and worked with when sexual abuse has occurred.

Families where physical maltreatment to a child or children has occurred need to work together on change and the case described here illustrates several of the most important issues.

CASE HISTORY 15.6

John, aged 2 years 6 months, was referred to the hospital because his mother had said that if the child was not placed in hospital she could not guarantee that he would not be hurt again. John's mother had suffered from depression on and off since his birth, she had injured John previously and the social worker involved with the case was concerned not only for John but for his two older brothers, aged

6 and 9, as well as the mother and father. This was a well-off family, with father a professional in a large organisation. John was not a planned baby, unlike the other two. Mother had just started a career and felt that she could not continue, that it was her duty to look after him.

Mother came with John for therapy and it became very clear that there were many problems which had developed. John had simply no language, and would only point. He continually tried to have physical contact with his mother but she could not bear it and pushed him away time and again. At the same time she was as deeply distressed as John. The house was immaculate, nothing was out of place. After some sessions of therapy together with his mother John began to play with some toys – an aeroplane, bricks, cars – and interact with the therapist. Mother moved away into the furthest corner and watched. Encouraged by the therapist John began to play, make noises, move the toys around, etc. Mother watched for many sessions as John progressed in his play and began to speak, naming the toys and even the colours. Mother said she knew that he could understand many things, but that he simply did not speak at home. By this time mother had moved her chair much closer and began to watch John's play with a little more interest.

The other two children joined mother and John in the sessions and it became clear that they too were at times distressed and hit very hard or put into bathwater that was far too hot. Mother had told them not to tell anyone but the children could not help but play out the upset they felt and what they had experienced. The therapist interpreted their play not only in terms of their psychological hurt but also by exploring the realities of the situation and what had happened. Through drawing, playing and talking, the children and mother began a conversation and at that point father, who had been very reluctant to become involved, attended the sessions as well.

Over a considerable number of sessions the situation eased. Father took much more responsibility for the day-to-day care of his children. John went to nursery for two mornings a week at the age of 3 years and mother found some work which she could do during this time. This brought her into contact with other people and her social life improved.

Alongside therapy there occurred of course monitoring by social services, visits to the paediatrician and contact between the different systems. All of these processes should be regarded as part of the intervention.

Equally, in cases of failure to thrive a family therapy approach can be most helpful because children often fail to thrive because of emotional difficulties in, and between, members of the family. Some of the therapeutic interventions are described in Chapter 3. In cases of failure to thrive it has been found to be more productive to offer therapy for the mother and child or for the whole family. Food is one of the most emotionally laden aspects of family life and withholding or refusing food is an intensely powerful communication. The children can become barometers of how the rest of the family are coping by their weight gains or losses. This can include the child being frightened because of physical or emotional harm coming to them and not being able to eat, or a mother becoming depressed about the loss of a parent, the husband's health, or her own weight. It can of course also be because there is poor bonding between mother and child resulting from resentment. Winnicott (1964) described in detail his observations of mother and baby feeding at a very early stage in the child's life and how the relationship between family members can influence this.

Family therapy when sexual abuse has occurred

Family therapy may be indicated when sexual abuse has occurred, particularly when the abuse has been perpetrated by someone outside the nuclear family:

- a stranger
- a friend of the family
- a relation of the family (aunt, uncle, cousin, etc.)
- a grandparent.

The primary issue here is that the child is, in principle at least, believed, and that the parent(s) are motivated and committed to protect their child(ren). Many families are devastated when one of their children has been sexually abused and have the greatest fears about the consequences for these children. They naturally worry about how to approach the subject with the child, whether the other siblings 'know', and also quite often feel that their child has been tainted with something immoral from which neither the child nor they themselves will ever properly recover. A considerable number of these children end up rejected and misunderstood, miserable and uncared for.

Equally, if the abuse has been within the family but the abusing family member has left the family and the non-abusing parent is committed to protect the child(ren), family therapy may be of considerable benefit, especially in dealing with the unexpressed guilt and resentment that are such a common aftermath to the disclosure of intrafamilial abuse.

When the sexual abuse is perpetrated within the nuclear family, family therapy can be appropriate with:

- the non-abusing parent and child(ren)
- the above group plus a social worker
- the above group plus grandparents
- the children plus foster-parent(s).

When children are not supported or believed by their parents but have for instance been taken into care, family therapy can be very helpful in doing important work with the siblings. One of the most important aspects is that it helps each of them to examine their perceptions of each other and themselves. Family therapy helps also to preserve a sense of the family, albeit as a subsystem, and can give tremendous support to the individual and the sibling group.

Family therapy can also be appropriate, though within considerable constraints and with legal back-up, when the abusing parent is joining the family after having been in prison or ending a period of probation. It is not possible to discuss this issue in this chapter and the reader is directed to Hotaling et al (1988) and Salter (1988).

Bentovim et al (1988), Glaser & Frosh (1988) and Furniss (1991) are some of the authors who have described in detail those interventions using family therapy which may contribute to change when sexual abuse has occurred.

Group therapy for children and adults

It has long been understood that groups of people, at whatever age, working together in therapy can be most productive and bring about change in the individual. Self-help groups are of immense importance for families and individuals but will not be discussed here. There are many forms of group therapy, broadly divided into behavioural, humanistic, analytic, psychodynamic, and cognitive schools of thought and theory. The theories guiding group therapies are in essence the same as those used in individual therapy but the main emphasis is on the problems between individuals rather than within the person alone. Group work in Great Britain developed during and after the Second World War, with Bion (1961) and Foulkes (1964) and later Yalom in the USA pioneering the work. Rogers (1961) and Yalom in the USA (1975) developed group therapies away from the analytic model. Peled & Davies (1995) have manualised their approach on group work with children of battered women.

Essential criteria for group therapy are:

- professional leadership
- consistent attendance
- that the experience is therapeutic.

The therapist's role is:

- to monitor the individual's progress and needs
- to facilitate the group process
- to formulate appropriate interventions
- to avoid injury to members of the group.

For children and adults who have been abused or are abusing, group therapy has been found to be of immense value. The aim of this section is to describe different ways of selecting groups for specific patients and explain why it might be useful for individuals to experience sharing and examining problems in the presence of others. Here we concentrate on the difficulties group members have when they attempt to relate to each other, rather than discussing the differences of technique and theory related to therapeutic groups.

Formation of groups

For children, the groups are usually formed on a peer group basis; groups for adults can function with a considerable age span between members. Therapeutic groups generally do not have to be constructed of people who have the same or similar problems. It is thought that most often people learn from each other because of their differences, not because of their sameness. However, in order to deal with a specific aspect of people's lives, it can be useful to form groups with adults or children who have the same basic complaint. Groups based on a common problem have a particular advantage in changing the belief that the individual is alone in their experience. Issues of child sexual abuse have particularly highlighted this aspect of therapeutic group work (Glaser & Frosh 1988, Hildebrand 1988, Sgroi 1988, 1989).

Groups for parents

There are possibilities for mothers and fathers to come together into a group and learn about parenting their children, how to control their impulses and how to understand that their own background may have contributed largely to how they are behaving today in a family setting. They may recognise why they cannot bear a demanding child. But most of all they may begin, in company and in the safety of a group led by a trained therapist, to change their behaviour. Talking with others about difficulties that these parents and children are experiencing is often the first opportunity group members have to discuss the details surrounding the maltreatment.

Groups for parents who have a child or children who have been abused usually have specific aims and a fixed number of sessions, with time and space being the same for every session. The frequency of meetings is set, and the group lasts for a specific time (usually 1½ hours). The group therapist and group members leave at the end of the therapeutic time. Groups are most often time-limited and meet on a weekly basis, but they can also be ongoing and open-ended. Whether the membership of the group can be added to (an open group) or whether the group is closed (a fixed number of people) will have been decided by the group leader(s) or therapist(s) in advance. The members of the group will be informed of all of these particulars and this information will be necessary to help them make choices. An assessment as to whether they would benefit from the group and the group from them is always carried out before they can be accepted.

Mothers are almost always at the centre of child abuse. The children are more often in her care than in the father's and even if it is not the mother who abused the child, she is the one who did not manage to protect. This is a difficult area and many mothers blame themselves terribly, while others feel helpless or deny that they could have been more aware and protecting. Mothers are also the ones who, unless they divorce themselves from what has happened to their child(ren), pick up the pieces and have to provide ongoing care. The mother's well-being is paramount and a group may provide a place and time where she can express her emotions, share her ideas and worries, and learn both from other members of the group and from the leadership and the interactions between all of them.

Many of the parents have experienced emotional deprivation in their own childhood and this may make them resentful and ambivalent about understanding their children's needs. Many such parents base their ideas of child-rearing on what their own needs are rather than the needs of the children. Cognitive change under such circumstances can prove difficult because there is often a direct contradiction to what the mother's/parents' own needs are: for example not hitting the child when he or she has done something the mother has forbidden, despite the mother's feelings of frustration.

For these parents the experience in which the idea originated must somehow be revived enough to be recognised and understood, so that they can bring reason to bear. Otherwise they are apt to talk wisely in their groups about what to do with their children, but then at home, perhaps after a brief attempt to do what seems 'not really right', revert to their own practices, convinced that these are the only ones that work for their particular children (Kempe & Kempe 1978, p. 106).

Groups for mothers whose children are failing to thrive

Groups may have specific topics which they aim to cover. For instance, a group for mothers who have children who fail to thrive will discuss not only the children's behavioural patterns but also the role of food, feeding and the preparation of food. Mothers' ideas about weight and dieting can be on the agenda, not only for the children but also for themselves. Sharing with other women the problem of having a child who is very thin and not developing can lessen the feelings of isolation and guilt. It can also help to end the denial about the failure to thrive and bring about an acceptance that something different needs to be done to help the child to grow.

The way in which interventions can be planned when children are failing to thrive is discussed in more detail in Chapter 3. Research (Hanks et al 1987) with this patient group has shown that mothers working with each other on some very practical things – like cooking, shopping, where to find information about resources available to them, how to fill in forms in order to get assistance, how to speak to officials as well as developing the courage to ask for things – were all issues that could usefully be shared once the mothers met in groups. These groups can be formed either on the basis of self-help groups or led by a health visitor or social worker, psychologist or psychiatrist. These groups will have very specific aims and the leader will have to make clear where his or her competence lies and what will be undertaken. However, it must also be stressed that mothers and fathers of children who fail to thrive often have psychological difficulties which contribute to the child's failure to grow. Kempe & Kempe (1978) described a mother who is typical of parents who abuse. They showed the difficulties many mothers have in helping their children to individuate – to see them as other than an extension of themselves. Kempe & Kempe (1978) quoted a mother as saying, 'No, I am sure the baby doesn't need to be fed yet; I'm not hungry yet.' She was quite unable to distinguish between her own body needs and his.

Because of the abusing parent's own, often appalling experiences in childhood, they have few inner resources to care adequately for their children. A group may be of help, particularly when it can become cohesive and begin to acknowledge that there may be differences in how children are being cared for. Kempe & Kempe (1978, p. 106) pointed out that one characteristic of abusing parents relates to their distorted views about what to expect of their children; they 'often cling to those ideas tenaciously, in the face of all kinds of professional persuasions'. Discussing such issues with fellow mothers or fathers can make different ideas more acceptable and may make it possible for them to learn how to imagine themselves to be in the child's position, recognising the child's needs rather than their own. Seeing and experiencing in a group how other mothers/parents achieve such changes in their perceptions can make it more acceptable for the others.

Groups for mothers/parents of children who have been physically abused

Groups for mothers when the child has been physically abused by her or her husband/partner offer a particular opportunity to work with what has happened. Violence is a very tricky subject and many women would not be able to discuss the issues of their and their children's battering by their husbands in front of the husbands/partners. For this reason alone it is important to have clear assessment criteria. During the assessment and selection period for a group such issues can be addressed in advance by gaining a clear history of the group member's past and present. Only after it has been established what the mother and/or father experienced, and how they have abused their children or have not been able to protect the children, can a decision be made about what would be most helpful. In many cases this leads squarely into the area of families and the interaction between family members.

This is not to say that groups of parents meeting to work on their children's maltreatment cannot be helpful. However, much is known through research about families and parenting in maltreating families (Browne et al 1988, Hotaling et al 1988, Cicchetti & Carlson 1989), and this knowledge can assist in the development of specific group work and in setting the goal and aims.

We have found that groups of mothers and toddlers coming for therapy have a strengthening effect on the relationship between the mother and her toddler, and that this sometimes generalises to other children and partners. These mother and toddler groups are focused on everyday problems which the mother can discuss and thereby learn about different ways of caring for her children. Such groups may also give the mother a chance to have a therapeutic experience which gives her confidence to mobilise her positive characteristics and competencies, first in the safe environment of the group and later outside the group. It may also become a stepping stone towards accepting that therapy for her is a way forward. Many men and women in abusive situations are quite frightened of therapy. Many professionals may join them in their fear, particularly when they have witnessed others becoming distressed during therapy. This is sometimes thought to be 'the fault' of the therapy rather than a reaction to the abuse that has been experienced. Therapy is a tool to help people come to terms with what they have experienced in their lives, and this includes taking responsibility for their own behaviours and reactions.

It seems that for other forms of abuse the family model of therapy can provide a useful framework for change, particularly when small and dependent children are involved, though it is quite different in the area of child sexual abuse.

Groups for sexually abused children, adolescents and adults

Research and practice has concentrated on groups for sexually abused children, adolescents (DeLuca et al 1997) and adults as well as for perpetrators of sexual abuse, both men and women.

Groups have been formed for:

- women who have been sexually abused in childhood
- men who have been sexually abused in childhood
- mixed groups of men and women sexually abused in childhood
- adolescent females who have been sexually abused
- adolescent males who have been sexually abused
- children of various age bands who have been sexually abused
- children under the age of 5 years who have been sexually abused
- men who have sexually abused children
- women who have sexually abused children
- adolescents who have sexually abused children (this work is more often with male offenders).

Groups for sexually abused children

Working in groups with sexually abused children shows benefits, and the pioneering work was carried out in the USA. Gottlieb & Dean (1981) and Giaretto (1981) were amongst the first to recognise the value of group work with children who had been sexually abused. Reeker et al (1997) undertook an outcome study of group treatment for sexually abused children and concluded that group treatment for these children is effective.

Glaser & Frosh (1988, p. 133) indicate that groups for sexually abused children should be for about 8–10 members and that the children are most helped if they are placed in groups reflecting their age and maturity. Age bands could be for 4–6-year-olds, 7–9-year-olds, 10–12-year-olds, 13–15-year-olds and 16–18-year-olds. The pros and cons of putting children into therapeutic groups are not only age-dependent but also relate to 'the nature of the children's respective relationship with the abuser and with each other'; Glaser & Frosh advise that it is important to include more than one child with a specific experience, so that none of the children should feel that their experience has been one which no one else has gone through. This highlights one of the central issues for children and adults alike, namely the isolation that so many feel, an isolation which can become a crippling aspect of people's development. Hildebrand (1988) describes very clearly the work carried out at the Hospital for Sick Children, London, based on the work of Giaretto (1981) and Berliner & Stevens (1982).

Porter (1986) also reported on early treatment for young male victims of sexual assault and indicated that

> group and family therapy are the two most important modalities for treatment of young male victims of sexual abuse. The peer group is the preferred and most productive mode of group treatment. The preferred number of group members is 8, no less than 4, and no more than 10. Though developmental as well as chronological age must be considered, generally the younger the children, the narrower the age spacing.

Berliner & Ernst (1984) described group work with young children who had been sexually abused. Nelki & Watters (1989) also described a group programme with girls aged between 4 and 8 years using Summit's (1983) accommodation syndrome as a basis for their focused work. They paid particular attention to issues such as

> meeting strangers, safe touching, secrets, telling someone, anger and punishment, fault and responsibility and helping the children to understand that their body belonged to them.

Such work has been found to help the children develop more adequately, increase their confidence and help them to distinguish between abusive and non-abusive situations more clearly.

Furniss et al (1988) reported the work of a goal-directed group for adolescent girls, one of the first of such groups set up in Britain. This group work was undertaken to offer the girls help in their own right and was added to the family therapy sessions that they were already involved in with other members of their families. Furniss et al (1988) reported that:

> the therapists used a number of methods. Firstly, interpretation was used, centring on the processes both within the group and between the girls and the therapists (Bion 1961).

Because it was anticipated that these children would show considerable disturbance during the treatment, including the group, the therapists

> were prepared to intervene actively, if required, even going so far as to restrain the girls physically in situations of extreme and potentially dangerous acting out.

This work is of particular importance because it describes the process of the group step by step and shows the tremendous emotional distress the children experience in their attempts to make sense of what has happened to them.

Groups for adults who have been sexually abused as children

It is not possible to discuss in detail here the group work which is being carried out for adult victims of child sexual abuse. Many of the women and men who have been abused benefit from individual and group therapy. Sometimes it is important that the abused person speaks to a therapist individually at first. In this one-to-one situation she may begin the work of reconstructing the events, distinguishing between what she thought happened and her recollection of what actually did happen. Many women and men are aware that they had only been able to keep in their conscious thoughts some of the events. Some realise that they have entirely blocked the experiences of their childhood and need the one-to-one relationship in therapy to work out what happened and when. However, in many therapies it becomes clear that talking to other people is a step many patients do not think they can ever take. Looking for help from close relatives or friends therefore remains a closed option. Working on such issues in a therapeutic group where people learn to speak out in the presence of more than one other is invaluable to most. Group work facilitates changes in the patient which are not as easily achieved in individual or family therapy.

These groups can be long-term in duration, but it has also been found useful to have groups with limited sessions and very specific aims which are shared between the therapists and patients: for instance working on relationship issues or difficulties surrounding childcare. Furniss et al (1988), Barnett et al (1989) and Sgroi (1989) described in detail the work of a goal-oriented group for sexually abused adolescent girls and adults. They found that after follow-up considerable improvements had been achieved by these young people on a number of indicators in their present life.

The short-term aims relate to the difficulties these women and men experience in the present: the tensions in their relationships, the confusions in their struggle to communicate their needs in relationships. Many patients have become socially isolated and can be burdened with phobias or depression which limit their lifestyle considerably. Their relationship with their children is only too often distorted and causes problems not only for the children but also for the adults. Valente and Shuttleworth (1997) described group work with women survivors of sexual abuse where they not only drew on the their experience to create boundaries, safety and listening but also incorporated laughter and humour at an appropriate level. They felt that 'frivolity has a place in this most serious work'. This is not often discussed in child abuse work, though the humour in therapy is not entirely a new concept.

Long-term group work with people who have been abused as children can be very beneficial and is usually conducted on group therapy principles (Yalom 1975, Sgroi 1989). It has been found to help these patients, in some cases, to make profound changes in their adult lives.

The adult sex offender and treatment

Groups for male abusers

Work with male perpetrators has been developing with some speed, particularly in the USA. Salter (1988) Clark & Erooga (1994) have given a clear practical guide to the treatment available. Group treatment is a valuable tool, but has also shown the enormity of the problem and the difficulties which emerge for the perpetrators and those who are attempting to help them change their sexually abusive behaviours towards children. This must be viewed in the context of the behaviours known to be part of the perpetrator's repertoire. Wolf (1988) described the patterns in which perpetrators 'groom' and prepare their child victims for abuse and how they keep control over their victims. Wolf (1988) and Bremer (1991) describe the denial by perpetrators of the abuse and point out that it persists far into treatment, whether this be in individual therapy or in groups. Wolf describes the Northwest Treatment Associates of Seattle programme for sex offenders and quotes from their work, saying that 'offenders will only tell 25% of the sexual abuse they have committed'. Salter (1988) describes the same programme and other treatments in detail. This includes the perpetrator's acknowledgement of the sexual abuse he has committed. It demands that all the sexual maltreatments are spoken of, and how sexual impulses and inappropriate behaviours in the present are coped with. These groups are very different from those conducted for children or adults who have been sexually abused, and behavioural cognitive theories are the underpinning of the work. Vizard (personal communication, 1990) confirms the structure of groups with perpetrators of sexual abuse to be as described above, even if the group members are motivated to change. McGarvey & Lenaghan (1996) described a structured approach to group work with adolescent perpetrators. They too advocate that group work with such a patient group is effective alongside other more individual treatment programmes.

Salter (1988) has provided an excellent and comprehensive overview of how to identify, assess and treat perpetrators of sexual abuse of children. She also describes how men come to sexually abuse children and distinguishes between the activities of paedophiles and those men who are not paedophiles but who sexually abuse children. Bremer (1991) writes about how adolescents and adults abuse sexually and 'groom' or prepare children for abusive activities. Wolf (1988) discussed the 'sex offender's search for a child' and described the pattern which sex offenders report they have adopted when offending against the child. Wolf, like Salter, believes that treatment can be effective for a number of such offenders. The programme developed by the Northwest Treatment Associates of Seattle, Washington, has been operating since 1977 and treats up to 200 offenders at any given time. Group therapy, covert sensitisation, behavioural therapy, social skills training, sex education and cognitive restructuring are all aspects of the treatments allocated to the individual. Salter concludes that

> The insight-oriented therapist who wishes to treat sex offenders must accept the fact that compulsive behaviours respond first and foremost to cognitive/behavioural techniques.

Vizard (1990) described the East London Sex Offenders Group's work with adult sex offenders which she and her colleagues are undertaking and confirms that, in a therapeutic group, confronting the denial and taking responsibility for the abuse are a first step towards change in the abusive behaviour. Sexual offending against children has been discussed in detail by Morrison et al (1994), Calder (1997) wrote an excellent paper on children and juveniles who sexually abuse.

Groups for female abusers

There is considerable resistance to acknowledging that women can and do sexually abuse their own and other children. However, the literature and research on this topic are increasing and a greater understanding is developing. Welldon (1988) gave a clear description of women who sexually abused their own children and those of others. Faller (1987) described her findings about women abusers and Mathews et al (1989) carried out a thorough study in an attempt to understand the psychological mechanisms of women who abuse children sexually. The outcome of the therapeutic intervention reported in the latter study shows that, unlike men, women do not seem to have the same 'criminal personality' characteristics and that treatment can be more effective. The women viewed as 'caring and non-judgemental, showed that the direct treatment modality was most helpful in creating change'. In this study many of them did change, as measured by a number of criteria including their insight into the sexual abuse. Barnett et al (1989) described their group work with women who had been abusing children sexually and concluded that the distorted beliefs held by these women to justify their abuse of children were reduced by the majority. They acknowledged that outcome studies must rely on long-term follow-up before such group treatment can be shown to be effective.

Groups for adolescent abusers

Working with adolescents who have been abused and become abusers in their turn poses specific difficulties. However, changes have been shown to be possible with this group. A number of treatment programmes exist in the USA and Bremer (1989) said

> The sexual assault cycle provides an understanding of how the youth gives himself permission to hurt others, how the victim is selected and identifies what must change to develop a non-abusive lifestyle. Denial is the sex offender's first line of defence

and this is no different for adolescents. Confronting this denial is a necessary process which must be undertaken continuously until change has taken place. The work carried out by Bremer and others in the Hennepin County Home School, Minnetonka, USA, includes working in groups. Bremer also outlined specific characteristics shown by juvenile sex offenders. They include:

- a distorted understanding about the self in relation to others
- irrational thinking
- sexualisation of non-sexual needs
- compulsivity
- poor impulse control
- mood disorders
- dysfunctional patterns of family functioning.

Providing a safe and secure environment away from the victim of the abuse is one of the most important aspects of treatment with this group – only then can the denial, history and other specific characteristics be addressed.

Though it should be stressed that individual work, during or after the ending of the group, is in almost all cases an essential component of any offender's programme with adolescents, group work is an integral part of the treatment. It is not possible here to describe the treatments that are thought helpful for adolescent offenders, except to say that the work in the USA indicates that treatment with adolescent offenders has more long-lasting effects than treatment for adults who have been in the habit of sexually abusing children for many years.

Individual therapy

As already discussed above, individual psychotherapy involves two people – a trained therapist and a patient – who together attempt to work through life experiences and, as in child abuse cases, through the traumatic events experienced. The aim of psychotherapy is to relieve troubling symptoms and achieve changes in personality in the child or adult (Bloch 1979, Brown & Pedder 1978). The reader is referred to these and other references for further information about what psychotherapy is. The complexities and the dynamics which are part of the therapeutic relationship are not discussed here. Many references already given in this chapter will lead the reader to an explanation of therapy, but Brown & Pedder (1978), Bloch (1979), Boston & Szur (1983) and Walker et al (1988) provide further answers, including case material. In this section the treatment for the abused child and adolescent is discussed, and a description of 'play therapy' for the very young child is also included.

Briere (1992) gave one of the most insightful and comprehensive account of the theory and treatment of the lasting effects of child abuse and trauma. Monck (1997) evaluated the therapeutic work undertaken in community-based programmes. When the people (including mothers) who informed a professional of the child's sexual abuse were asked to rate the children's behaviour and their symptoms, many of the children were thought to be either in the 'clinical' or 'borderline' range of severity. The evaluation found 'some hopeful signs of improvement' but also commented on a surprisingly high number of children who did not reach the end of their planned treatment.

Individual therapy is almost always concerned with the entire person, adult or child; their experiences in all areas of life need to be considered. This applies even when a very specific problem such as child abuse has been part of the person's history. Therapists using behaviour therapy as a means to bring about change prefer to concentrate on the symptoms and their manifestation, rather than on the history and dynamics of a person, adult or child. However, in cases of child abuse the history and origin as well as the relationships and context in which the abuse occurs need to be understood by the therapist and often by the patient before change can take place. Exploration of the abuse – who was involved, when and where it took place – can lead, at least in part, to the patient's understanding the role of symptoms they might carry. What has most often been found in cases of child sexual abuse is that the children at times need behavioural treatments in order to change some of the behaviours, for instance very sexualised behaviours which have become habitual, as well as insight and psychodynamic understanding. It is no paradox that these children need to have established firm boundaries, be allowed to think in a clear and undenying manner and at the same time become flexible and more at ease. Their vulnerability and strength need to be understood. The flexibility of therapeutic interventions with these children can be taxing but also rewarding (Boston & Szur 1983, Copley & Forryan 1987, Bentovim et al 1988, Glaser and Frosh 1988, Wiehe 1997, Aldridge & Wood 1997).

CASE HISTORY 15.3

A 16-year-old girl came to the clinic with epileptic fits for which the doctors could find no organic cause. All manner of tests had been carried out but nothing was found. She was on medication to alleviate the fits but was also referred for therapy because she had become very distressed.

As therapy began she realised that the first fit occurred just after she had been hit hard on the head by one of her parents and she had fallen, hitting her head against a wall. The parent who had not hit her felt devastated and protective towards the daughter ever afterwards and would recall this event frequently. The patient then began to speak of the frequency of the fits and made the connection that they always occurred when she was in a potentially argumentative or aggressive situation. While talking about this she realised that the arguments usually stopped once she started a fit, whether it happened at school or at home. Once she fitted, people paid attention to her and cared for her instead of continuing their argument either with her or with a third party. She said she felt bad about that at times and that family and friends had told her that they dared not be cross with her because they knew this would always bring on a fit.

After she recognised these connections – arguments, being hit on the head, falling, being comforted, etc. – the fits disappeared but the patient became very sad and depressed. At that point the therapy began to address the maltreatment this young girl had experienced throughout her life, how she had developed and as a consequence learnt to behave towards others. In this case the girl having recognised some of the underlying reasons for her behaviour, namely the neglect and maltreatment she had experienced, had no difficulties in:

- acknowledging her sadness and depression over this lack of care,
- recognising her anger and her consequent bullying behaviour towards others,
- seeing that the 'fits' were part of her attempt to be cared for rather than neglected, and
- beginning to think of how to do things differently.

Not all therapy patients can unravel their difficulties in this way, let alone work out resolutions to their problems. The therapy cannot be described in more detail here but it may be worth pointing out what Winnicott (1965) highlighted so clearly. He recognised that much antisocial or illness behaviour of children who have been neglected by parental figures and the environment is in fact a plea for help. Boston & Szur (1983), in their descriptions of children in psychotherapy, come to the same conclusion; the reader is referred for detailed case studies to these authors.

As discussed in the section on groups, sometimes it is relevant to focus only on the very specific issues of the abuse, but most often the person/child as a whole needs to be considered. Long-term analytic therapy has been shown to be beneficial in many cases. Anna Freud (1981) said about a child's sexual abuse that:

> . . . he [the child] is also experiencing a type of stimulation for which, developmentally, he is wholly unprepared. Nevertheless, he cannot avoid being physically aroused and this experience disastrously disrupts the normal sequence in his sex organisation. He is forced into premature phallic or genital development while his legitimate developmental needs and their accompanying mental expressions are by-passed and short-circuited. (pp. 33–4)

For other patients more focused, goal-directed therapeutic work has also been found to be helpful, particularly as the number of people who come forward speaking of their abuse in childhood is rising steadily and resources are scarce. It may be useful to consider once more the continuum along which the consequences of all child abuse can occur:

short-term consequences ⟶ death.

There has been evidence (Finkelhor 1986, Bagley & King 1990) that some people suffer considerably less than others in the long term when they have been abused as children. This depends largely on the parenting the children receive and the environment they have grown up in. Some children and adults can become well-adjusted, particularly if the abuse has not been denied and if they have been protected, believed and respected as individuals with rights to emotional well-being, rights to grow, rights to physical health and rights to develop sexually. If this is granted to the child in an appropriate way, then indeed development can progress largely unhindered. However, this is a difficult state to achieve when the abuse of a child has continued undetected over many years or if those parenting the child were in collusion with the abuser, or denied it altogether (Kempe & Kempe 1978, 1984, Wolfe 1987; Walker et al 1988). The consequences in such cases are usually far more serious and can span the life of the individual and even affect future generations. The abuse can lead to scars and injuries never healed, permanent handicap, brain damage, learning difficulties, stunted growth and failure to thrive. Emotionally the consequences can range from difficult behaviours, nightmares, aggression and relationship problems, through to depression, apathy and self-mutilation, and to the child or adult becoming mute, showing psychosomatic illnesses such as paralysis, or becoming schizoid and mentally ill. At the end of the continuum is death itself.

For many small children who have been abused therapeutic help is most appropriate when the non-abusing parents, a foster-parent or care giver can partake in the process and learn along with the child to interact in a different way and understand each other so that the child can give up behaviours that contribute to, or are a consequence of, the abuse. Wetting and soiling, nightmares, destructive behaviours, not eating, not being able to sleep, hurting themselves or others are just some of these behaviours. Not all adults are capable of that change and in such situations it is essential that an assessment of this capacity, motivation and willingness for change is carried out before the therapeutic process can begin. When children have been sexually abused by one or by both of their parents the picture changes. When both parents have been involved in their child's sexual maltreatment it will not be appropriate to involve them in therapy with the child. Also, when the non-abusing parent is denying the abuse the child may need space and the experience of an adult who can be more accepting of the child's experience and help the child to express this. Because of the almost addictive quality of behaviour in adults when they have sexually abused a child, it will simply not be safe for the child to be in the abusive parent's presence until major changes have occurred in the abusing adult's life.

Individual therapy with the child means that an adult and child work together on forming a close therapeutic relationship which may last over a long time, sometimes years. It is necessary to match the therapy to the child in a way that is appropriate for the child's age and development; this process should be carefully assessed. With some children it is important to realise that after some therapeutic work has been done the therapy may have to stop for a while and allow the child to grow. At a later stage, possibly around the age of 10–12 years or during adolescence, further therapeutic work may be undertaken in order to build on the child's earlier experience in therapy. In this way children may be helped to continue to grow, making sense of their lives and particularly helping them to form relationships. The work with the child focuses not only on the abuse itself but also on all the other experiences, good and bad, which the child has had – what their relationships have been like and with whom, and what they feel about themselves. Many abused children feel they are to blame for whatever maltreatment they received. This has been particularly highlighted when therapists attempted to treat sexually abused children.

Children who have been physically abused and neglected often need therapeutic help in their own right, and a plan for such therapy may develop out of the children's and families' needs rather than out of something that is dictated from the beginning, as the case below illustrates. At the assessment stage it was very clear that this family needed to be seen together and that they could not be separated abruptly without leaving them all feeling insecure and possibly anxious about what each was going to say about the other in their session. Parents quite naturally find it threatening when their children are taken into individual therapy where they might say things or describe the parents in a way that is unacceptable to the parents. Winnicott (1982) describes with superb clarity and detail the therapeutic work he undertook with children and how be negotiated the interactions between parents and child so that the therapy should strengthen their relationships rather than weaken them. Axline (1964), Copley & Forryan (1987) and Boston & Szur (1983) provide excellent accounts with details of individual therapy with children who are disturbed, often as a consequence of their maltreatment by adults.

CASE HISTORY 15.4

Zoe, aged 7, and her brother Lee, aged 5, came for therapy with their mother because both children were failing to thrive and their mother had found no other way of 'controlling the children' than by hitting them hard, sometimes with her hands, sometimes with objects. In the session the children would cower in a corner whenever the mother said anything to them, but once mother became engrossed in telling her story to the therapist the children became giggly and restless, breaking toys, drawing on the furniture and being generally difficult. Mother would then shout and the children would return to their cowering positions. At neither the cowering nor the excitable stage did they play constructively. It soon became clear that the children were in a constant state of alert, watching mother's every move. If mother left they would become quiet and cry but not attempt to follow her until she said they could. Neither of them would speak except in whispers to each other which frustrated the mother.

Their drawings consisted of scribbles and resembled drawings of children aged 3 rather than 5 and 7 years. How well the children draw is of course not the issue, what is important is that their drawings are seen as a communication revealing some of their inner state. To acknowledge this communication in an appropriate way, neither too effusively pleased nor dismissive, is the job of the adult. This is a fine and important balance for the therapist, parental figures, or other professionals.

The children, in their attempt to anticipate mother's moves and protect each other from her behaviours, became locked in an almost symbiotic relationship. Therapeutic work on their individuation from each other was one important goal which led to them having therapy individually as well as with their mother. It was in the individual sessions that age-appropriate developmental tasks could be worked through; the children's fear for each other and themselves that mother would hurt them or leave them could also be tackled, and their anger and frustration dealt with. The children both became more relaxed and managed to concentrate on their play in a more developmentally appropriate way. The change for Zoe was particularly visible. She began to work at school and after a couple of months was reading like the other children in her class. She had also stopped wetting, and was able to separate from her brother more securely.

Therapy with the sexually abused child

Jones (1986) pointed out that

> The child's experience has to be understood by the therapist in order to provide treatment. . . . In particular, the predicament of the sexually abused child, the impact of abuse upon thinking, attitude, self-view, sexuality and making relationships with other people, as well as the effects of sexual abuse on behaviour, have proved useful bases for treatment.

Jones found that children in individual therapy move through three specific phases of treatment. The starting phase is particularly concerned with the child getting a sense of the task ahead, the working through of his or her feelings and emotions and letting them become visible, so to speak. The middle phase can persist for a considerable time and consists of the main body of therapy. This phase includes the child and therapist becoming aware of the child's guilt about what has happened and this is also linked to the threats that may have been made to the child. Often angry and frightening feelings come to the surface during this phase and children can become aggressive, usually copying what has been done to them. The child may be most ambivalent about meeting the therapist at this stage. This is followed by a period where the child becomes acutely aware of the lack of care received from parental figures and of the lack of emotional warmth and security, leading to another stage of dissociation – dissociating oneself from physical and psychological pain. It is during this phase in particular that a secure home with cooperation from those who look after the child is of importance. The 'closing phase' is another powerful experience for the child, particularly when endings and separations have always been abrupt and without preparation. This phase of therapy often leads to the children reflecting on the difficult times in their lives and it leaves them wondering how the therapist will 'make goodbye happen'. The children will have become somewhat dependent on the therapist and trust him or her with very difficult feelings. Discussing the ending with children well in advance, helping to express what they think might happen and what they would like to happen can be explored in detail during this phase. Reviewing the path therapy has taken, and what happened during this time, both inside and outside the sessions, can be used to help children bring together parts of their life in a meaningful way. The other professionals involved may also have to be contacted specifically to let them know about the significance of this stage in therapy. Professionals and parental figures involved with the children need to be informed about the ending and understand how important the proper resolution of this phase is. Now more than ever is it important that the children actually get to the sessions, and on time.

CASE HISTORY 15.5

For 5-year-old Katy therapy had reached the 'closing phase' and five more sessions had been arranged for her. An extra session had been arranged where Katy and the therapist told her mother about the plan. Katy's mother had said she was pleased about that. For the fourth session Katy was brought almost 20 minutes late; the mother was distraught and said she thought she would 'never manage to get to the hospital for the appointment'. She had thought that the therapist would have given up on her and the session was spent on working through the different anxieties that this incident had brought to a head. The following session Katy did not come at all and mother telephoned after the session saying that Katy had been at a birthday party enjoying herself and she did not want to spoil her fun; she also thought that Katy was so much better that it 'would not have mattered if she missed a session'. The therapist repeated that it was very important for mother to bring Katy for her sessions and on time. Two difficult sessions followed with Katy being very unsettled and angry, not only outside the session and with her mother but also inside the session and with the therapist. However, the ending did come about as arranged and Katy was able to leave her therapy as planned.

The reason for bringing this vignette to the reader's attention is to illustrate that therapy with adults and children is different from other interventions. A commitment to this work in children has also to be undertaken by the adults who support the child while in therapy. If this commitment is not present the therapy may cause the child more distress, bringing up feelings of disloyalty amongst other difficulties. MacFarlane & Waterman (1986) discuss therapy for very young children in detail and throw light on many of the difficulties that surround therapy for the sexually abused child.

Play therapy

Play therapy is a technique devised particularly for very young children who are not quite able to let the adult world know in words what they wish to communicate. They are usually well able to communicate in other forms; dolls, animals, doll's houses, doll's house furniture, sand, water, plasticine and other play materials are used with the children to make it easier for them to tell their story to the adults. This technique is useful for all forms of child abuse. Doyle (1987) paid particular attention to showing how this form of therapy might be applied with children who have been sexually abused.

Individual therapy for the adolescent

For the adolescent individual therapy can be particularly helpful, though, as seen from the discussion in the section on group treatment, the two types of therapy may be tailored to the child's needs and a third, family therapy, also considered. Older boys and girls who have been sexually abused over a number of years will have to address their many deeply disturbing feelings, including their sense of guilt, their feeling of it all having been their fault, their ambivalence, their feeling of worthlessness and their feelings of being rejected or of being worth rejecting. Sinason (1988) discussed some of the issues that children in individual therapy have to work through when they have been sexually abused and, though the child she describes was aged 5 years, older children also experience very similar feelings during therapy.

McCarthy (1988) examines the consequences for children once they have disclosed. He brings to our attention that

> Incest victims frequently exhibit very strong and even overwhelming feelings of hate. For them, managing this hate is a major task.

The disclosure interview for the sexually abused child

When children have been sexually abused they are almost always interviewed or prepared to make a disclosure statement about their abuse. It is not possible to go into specific detail of how to conduct such interviews, but Jones & McQuiston (1988) have concentrated on the specific issues. Though disclosure work with children does not constitute therapy, all such interviews have to be therapeutic in essence and provide the child with understanding of their situation and support. The legal requirements need to be addressed when preparing for such interviews and the 1989 Children Act has to be adhered to. Jones & McQuiston point out that

> Great care needs to be taken to remain open and honest throughout the interviewing process as in any constructive, supportive interaction with children. The style of this relationship may be quite different from the usual experience of the abused child with adults and can pave the way for future interviews. Although it is a natural tendency to attempt to protect children from pain and disappointment, it will harm them if they are told that 'everything will be okay don't worry'. The child will quickly see through this, and see no reason to trust another in a long line of disappointing adults. (p. 16)

Glaser (1995) commented on videotaping children's evidence in child abuse cases and concluded that children were left unprotected from the effects of the legal system when they were involved in court action. Davies et al (1995) reported on videotaping children's evidence and what use was made of these tapes. It also looked at the children's reactions.

Bentovim et al (1997) discuss how interviews with children who may have been sexually abused need to be conducted and facilitated. Monteleone & Brodeur (1994) detailed the different stages of the interview with the child and how to engage the child in conversation in an age-appropriate way and have provided a format which may be thought about when talking to children. See also Vizard's (1993) excellent chapter on interviewing children when they have been sexually abused and is linked to the memory and false memory debate.

The issue of recovered memories (labelled in advance by some writers as a 'false memory syndrome') remains contentious and unresolved. The best hope for a resolution would seem to come from a thorough understanding of the functioning of memory in relation to extreme emotional events. The Royal College of Psychiatry (Brandon et al 1998) and the British Psychological Society (1995) have issued thoughtful reports on the matter. Andrews et al (1995) and Andrews (1997) have written about implications on clinical work when the recovery of memory is addressed. Dale & Allen (1998) have researched into the issue. Many publications have appeared which cannot be discussed here.

Therapy for sexually abused children and adults with learning difficulties

More recently professionals have become alert to the many abused children and adults who have learning difficulties. Again it is not possible to enter into a discussion about the difficulties and complexities of this work, let alone consider the person who has learning difficulties.

Workers from the USA and Britain have made a concerted effort to bring to notice the plight of this group of people. Sinason (1990) described her therapeutic work with patients with learning difficulties and has highlighted some very important findings. The most outstanding finding seems to be that many people with learning difficulties have their condition made far worse by the abuse and present as more severely handicapped than their potential level. Sinason (1990) has carried out psychodynamic psychotherapy with such individuals and found a remarkable improvement following resolution of inner conflicts related to the abuse. Group therapy does not always benefit these children and adults. Because of their very individual difficulties they need the attention of a one-to-one relationship in order to come to an understanding about what has happened to them. Family therapy can be helpful as an additional form of therapy if the family members are cooperative. It is during such family therapy sessions that family members, often for the first time, see their child as operating at a far higher level than they had up until then believed possible. Ordinary members of the family often take more convincing that the level of functioning of the person with learning difficulties could be heightened.

Training and supervision for professionals

Training and supervision for professionals working in the area of child abuse has been a continuing undertaking. The emotional impact on all those working with child abuse was discussed by Morrison who highlighted the relationship between training and being able to cope with the task. The Department of Health issued two HMSO publications in 1991 (Working Together under the Children Act 1989 and it's Addendum and Working with Child Sexual Abuse: Guidelines for trainers and managers in Social Services Departments). Wilson & Jones (1995) have discussed issues relating particularly to social workers but their thinking is equally valuable for other profesionals.

It is important to recognise that people from all walks of life are able to contribute in a positive way to alleviating some of the problems of child abuse. Training and supervision and support will be necessary almost at every level, from government departments making resources available, to parental figures and professionals making decisions about the children's daily lives when child abuse has taken place. For instance, foster-parents, who do a vital job, need more formal training but definitely need some introduction to the topic of child abuse and they will require far more support than they are at present allocated. The successful placement of a child depends on the strength the foster-parent(s) can continue to put into the job of caring for the child and understanding, training and support will be a vital part of this. It is probably fair to say that for judges, on the other hand, who have the immense responsibility of making decisions about the children's lives, training is more important than ongoing support.

Each person in this network will bring to the situation their own professional training but, because some of the issues in child abuse are so new to all, much sharing of facts and information about the subject and interprofessional training is essential. The emotional impact on those working in the area can at times feel overwhelming. Burn-out has increased amongst many professionals. The denial and scapegoating that can ensue has been shown to be a powerful aspect of many cases. Psychotherapists with a systemic and dynamic theoretical framework have had some insight into this because of their thera

Summary

1. Support and therapy is an important part of a child's recovery when he or she has been abused.
2. Different forms of therapy and supportive work are available.
3. Assessment of the individual child's need – linked to the form of abuse they have experienced – is vital for a planned therapeutic programme.
4. The needs of the child and the resources available in any given area have to be matched to the child.
5. It is important that both professionals and parents/carers cooperate, in the child's best interest, when therapy is made available.
6. Children will find it impossible to make emotional progress if they find themselves in an opposing position to those they depend on.

-peutic work in general and are therefore well placed in supporting others in this area.

Child abuse demands a response which is imaginative, based on clear knowledge and which sometimes demands courage in confronting our own or others' emotional reactions. This chapter has concentrated on the kinds of external help that might be provided for abused children and their families. Professionals too need outside help to provide them with a perspective on what is happening to them, and to help free them to take the action that is needed.

REFERENCES

Adcock M, White R, & Hollows A 1991 Significant Publications, London

Andrews B, Morton J, Bekerian D A, Brewin C R, Davies G M, Mollon P 1995 The recovery of memories in clinical practice The Psychologist 8:209–214

Andrews B 1997 Forms of memory recovery among adults in therapy In: Read & Lindsay (eds) Recollection of Trauma: scientific research and clinical practice.Plenum, New York

Axline V 1964 Dibs: in search of self. Penguin, Harmondsworth

Bagley C, King K 1990 Child sexual abuse. Tavistock/Routledge, London

Barnett S, Corder F, Jehu D 1989 Group treatment for women sex offenders. Practice 2:118–159

Bentovim A, Gorrel Barnes G, Cooklin A (eds) 1982 Contents of family therapy, Vol 2. Grune & Stratton, London

Bentovim A, Elton A, Hildebrand J, Tranter M, Vizard E 1988 Child sexual abuse within the family. Wright, London

Bentovim A 1992 Trauma Organised Systems. Karnak Books, London

Bentovim A, Bentovim M, Vizard E, Wiseman 1995 Fascilitating interviews with children who may have been sexually abused. Child Abuse Review 4:246–262

Berliner L, Stevens D L 1982 Clinical issues in child sexual abuse. In: Conte J R, Shope D (eds) Social work and child sexual abuse. Hawarth, New York

Berliner L, Ernst E 1984 Group work with preadolescent sexual assault victims. In: Stuart I R, Greer J G (eds) Victims of sexual aggression: Treatment of children, women and men. Van Nostrand Reinhold, New York

Bion W R 1961 Experiences in groups. Tavistock, London

Bloch S 1979 An introduction to the psychotherapies. Oxford University Press, Oxford

Boston M, Szur R 1983 Psychotherapy with severely deprived children. RKP, London

Brandon S, Boakes J, Glaser D, Green 1998 Recovered memories of childhood sexual abuse. Brit J of Psych 172:296–307

Brassard M R, Tyler A H, Kehle T J 1983 School programs to prevent intrafamilial child sexual abuse. Child Abuse and Neglect 7:214–245

Bremer J 1989 Sex offender specific treatment with juveniles: critical components. Presented at a conference on Child Abuse and Neglect, Breaking the Cycle, Leeds University

Bremer J 1991 Intervention with the juvenile sex offender. Human Systems Journal of Systemic Consultation and Management 2(3–4):235–246

Briere J N 1992 Child Abuse Trauma. Sage Publications, Newbury Park

Brown D, Pedder J 1978 Introduction to psychotherapy. Tavistock, London

Browne K, Saqi S 1988 Approaches to screening for child abuse and neglect. In: Browne K, Davies C, Stratton P (eds) Early prediction and prevention of child abuse. Wiley, Chichester

Browne K, Davies C, Stratton P (eds) 1988 Early prediction and prevention of child abuse. J Wiley, Chichester

Burnham J B 1986 Family therapy. Tavistock, London

Calder M C 1997 Juveniles and Children who Sexually Abuse. Russell House publishing Ltd, Lyme Regis

Campbell D, Draper R (eds) 1985 Applications of systemic family therapy. Grune & Stratton, London
Cicchetti D, Carlson V 1989 Child maltreatment. Cambridge University Press, Cambridge
Clarkson P, Pokorny M, 1994 The Handbook of Psychotherapy. Routledge, London
Copley B, Forryan B 1987 Therapeutic work with children and young people. Robert Royce, London
Crittenden P 1988 Family and dyadic patterns of functioning in maltreating families. In: Browne K, Davies Stratton P (eds) Early prediction and prevention of child abuse. Wiley, Chichester
Crittenden P, Ainsworth M D S 1989 Child maltreatment and attachment theory. In: Cicchetti D, Carlson V (eds) Child maltreatment. Cambridge University Press, Cambridge
Dale P, Allen J 1998 On memories of childhood abuse: a phenomenological study. J of Child Abuse & Neglect. 22:799–812
Davies G, Wilson C, Mitchell R, Milson J (1995) Videotaping children's evidence: an evaluation. Home Office, London
Department of health 1991a Working together under the Children Act 1998, London
Department of Health Working with Child Sexual Abuse: Guidelines for Trainers and Managers in Social Services Departments. London, HMSO
De Shazar S 1986 Keys to solution in brief family therapy. W W Norton, London
Doyle C 1987 Sexual abuse: giving help to the children. Children and Society 3:210–223
Faller K 1987 Women who sexually abuse children. Violence and Victims 2(4):263–276
Finkelhor D 1986 A sourcebook on child sexual abuse. Sage, Beverly Hills, CA
Foulkes S J 1964 Therapeutic group analysis. Maresfield Reprint, London
Freud A 1981 A psychoanalyst's view of sexual abuse by parents. In: Mrazek P B, Kempe C H (eds) Sexually abused children and their families. Pergamon Press, Oxford
Furniss T 1983 Mutual influence and interlocking professional–family processes in the treatment of child sexual abuse and incest. Child Abuse and Neglect 7:207–223
Furniss T 1985 Conflict-avoiding and conflict-regulating patterns in incest and child sexual abuse. Acta Paedopsichiatrica 50:299–313
Furniss T 1991 The multi-professional handbook of child abuse. Routledge, London
Furniss T, Bingley-Miller L, Bentovim A 1984 Therapeutic approach to sexual abuse. Archives of Disease in Childhood 59(9):865–870
Furniss T, Bingley-Miller L, Van Elburg A 1988 Goal-oriented group treatment for sexually abused adolescent girls. British Journal of Psychiatry 152:97–106
Giaretto H 1977 Humanistic treatment of father–daughter incest. Child Abuse and Neglect 1:411–426
Giaretto H 1981 A comprehensive child sexual abuse treatment program. In: Mrazek P B, Kempe C H (eds) Sexually abused children and their families. Pergamon Press, Oxford
Glaser D, Frosh S 1988 Child sexual abuse. Macmillan Education, London
Gottlieb B, Dean J 1981 The co-therapy relationship in group treatment of sexually mistreated adolescent girls. In: Mrazek P B, Kempe C H (eds) Sexually abused children and their families. Pergamon Press, Oxford
Hanks H, Stratton P 1988 Family perspectives of early sexual abuse. In: Browne K, Davies C, Stratton P (eds) Early prediction and prevention of child abuse. J Wiley, Chichester
Hanks H, Hobbs C, Seymore D, Stratton P 1987 Infants who fail to thrive: an intervention for poor feeding practices. Journal of Reproductive and Infant Psychology 6(2):101–111
Hanks H G I, Stratton P M 1995 The effects of child abuse: signs and symptoms In: Wilson & James (eds) The Child Protection Handbook
Hildebrand J 1988 Use of groupwork in treating child sexual abuse. In: Bentovin A, Elton A, Hildebrand J, Tranter M, Vizard E (eds) 1988 Child sexual abuse within the family. Wright, London
Hoffman L 1981 Foundations of family therapy. Basic Books, New York
Home Office 1992 Memorandum of good practice on video recorded interviews and child witnesses for criminal proceedings. Home Office and Department of Health, London
Hotaling G T, Finkelhor D, Kirkpatrick J T, Straus M A (eds) 1988 Family violence. Sage, London
Jones D 1986 Individual psychotherapy for the sexually abused child. Child Abuse and Neglect 10:377–385
Jones D P H, McQuiston M G 1988 Interviewing the sexually abused child. Gaskell Royal College of Psychiatrists, London
Kempe R S, Kempe C H 1978 Child abuse. Fontana Books, London
Kempe R S, Kempe C H 1984 The common secret: sexual abuse of children and adolescents. W H Freeman, New York
McCarthy B 1988 Are incest victims hated? Psychoanalytic Psychotherapy 3(2):113–120
MacFarlane K, Waterman J 1986 Sexual abuse of young children. Holt, Rinehart & Winston, London
Mathews R, Matthews J K, Speltz K 1989 Female sexual offenders. Safer Society, Orwell, MA
Messages from Research 1995 Child protection: messages from research. HMSO, London
Nelki J S, Watters J 1989 A group for sexually abused young children: unravelling the web. Child Abuse and Neglect 13(3):369–378
Patton M Q 1991 Family Sexual Abuse. Sage Publications, Newbury Park
Porter E 1986 Treating the young male victim of sexual abuse. Safer Society, Syracuse, NY
Porter R (ed.) 1984 Child sexual abuse within the family. Ciba Foundation/Tavistock Publications, London
Reder P, Duncan S, Gray M 1993 Beyond Blame. Routledge, London
Reder P, Lucey C 1995 Assessment of Parenting. Routledge, London
Rogers J 1961 A therapist's view of psychotherapy. Constable, London
Rycroft C 1968 A critical dictionary of psychoanalysis. Penguin, Harmondsworth

Salter A C 1988 Treating child sex offenders and victims. Sage, Newbury Park, CA
Sgroi S 1988 Vulnerable populations, Vol. 1. Lexington Books, Lexington, MA
Sgroi S 1989 Vulnerable populations, Vol. 2. Lexington Books, Lexington, MA
Sinason V 1988 Smiling, swallowing and stupefying: the effect of sexual abuse on the child. Psychoanalytic Psychotherapy 3(2): 97–111
Sinason V 1990 Presentation at ACPP Conference, Research and Child Abuse, Cardiff
Skinner B F 1953 Science and human behaviour. Macmillan, New York
Stratton P, Hanks H 1991 Incorporating circularity in defining and classifying child maltreatment. Human Systems Journal of Systemic Consultation and Management 2(3–4):181–200
Stratton P, Preston-Shoot M, Hanks H 1990 Family therapy. Venture Press, Birmingham
Summit R C 1983 The child sexual abuse accommodation syndrome. Journal of Child Abuse and Neglect 7:177–193
Vizard E 1990 Presentation at Child Abuse Practice in the 1990's conference, July
Walker C E, Bonner B L, Kaufman K L 1988 The psychologically and sexually abused child. Pergamon Press, Oxford
Welldon E V 1988 Mother, madonna, whore. Free Association Books, London
Wilson K, James A 1995 The Child Protection Handbook. Bailliere Tindall, London
Wilson K, Jones J 1995 Specific issues in training for child protection practice. In: The child protection handbook. Wilson & James (eds) Bailliere Tindall London
Winnicott D W 1964 The child, the family and the outside world. Penguin, Harmondsworth
Winnicott R W 1965 The maturational process and facilitating environment. Hogarth, London
Winnicott D W 1982 Through paediatrics to psycho-analysis. Hogarth, London
Wolf S C 1988 The sex offender's search for the child. Presented at SRIP Conference on Child Abuse and Neglect, Breaking the Cycle, Leeds University
Wolfe D A 1987 Child abuse; implications for child development and psychology. Sage, Newbury Park, CA
Working Together 1991 Working together under the Children Act 1989. A guide to arrangements for inter-agency co-operation for the protection of children from abuse. HMSO, London
Wyatt G E, Powell G J (eds) 1988 Lasting effects of child sexual abuse. Sage, London
Yalom I D 1975 The theory and practice of group psychotherapy. Basic Books, New York

16

Out-of-home care for the abused or neglected child: listen to the child

The emphasis in child and family policy following the Children Act 1989 is on the importance of the natural family and the duty of the local authority to support 'children in need' and their families. Practice has been evolving to provide short-term residential placements or foster-homes where the abused child can receive skilled alternative care at times of family stress and where good links are maintained with the family throughout with the expectation of early return home. The alternative approach has been 'rescue and fresh start' ideally through adoption, but there have many difficulties in practice and outcome has been uncertain (Thorburn 1995). The care of teenagers is difficult, as shown by the numbers who are 'thrown out' of the family home or run away. Different strategies are needed for this group (Newman 1989).

Clearly a balance has to be struck and the Department of Health in introducing the Children Act advised

> The Act seeks to protect children both from the harm which can arise from failures within the family and the harm which can be caused by unwarranted intervention in their family life (DoH 1989).

The wish to 'rescue' children in the 1970s and 1980s has been tempered by an acknowledgement of the inherent problems in providing good long-term care to damaged, vulnerable children who need more care than is available in an average home and where there is a chronic lack of psychological and psychiatric services to all children, families and carers.

Accommodating children

Children who are provided with accommodation are said to be 'looked after' by the social services. The term includes children who are subject to compulsory care orders as well as voluntary arrangements. The social services must provide accommodation if:

- there is no person with parental responsibility
- the child is lost or abandoned
- the person who has been providing care for the child has been prevented from doing so
- they consider the welfare of a child over 16 years is likely to be prejudiced without accommodation.

When planning for or reviewing a child's case, social services must have regard for: (Child Health in the Community 1996)

- the child's state of health
- the child's health history
- the effect of these on the child's development
- arrangements for the child's health surveillance and treatment
- the child's special educational needs.

Children's homes (Table 16.1, 16.2)

Children's homes, where the most vulnerable children are 'looked after', are staffed by residential workers of whom 50% are still untrained. In the past abuse appears to have been endemic in residential schools and homes, where very vulnerable children are easily targeted.

Foster-care

'Fostering is in crisis' (Warren 1997), there are not enough places for the children in need of a home who are '. . . increasingly older, more troubled, and more traumatised' (Brindle 1997). There is pressure to develop a professional, trained, and paid service to provide good foster-care for them. As a group (on 31 March 1995), 45% of foster-children were aged 9–15 years and many were in long-term placements, unable to go home because the harm they had suffered or were at risk of suffering. This research was important because it had been assumed that most placements in foster-care were of younger children who returned home quickly.

The Curtis report (1946) and the Warner Committee (Warner 1992) described the emotional deprivation of children in residential homes, but recent research of abuse in foster-homes (Hobbs et al 1997) shows the lack of safeguards there too. Well-publicised cases such as that of Roger Saint (Guardian 1997) a paedophile foster-father who abused children over 16 years, demonstrate the need for adequate vetting. Mr Saint had a conviction in 1972 for indecently assaulting a 12-year-old boy but he went on to foster 20 boys from 10 local authorities. Ongoing evaluation of every placement and foster-carer is essential.

Number of children in care

In 1995 there were 49 000 children looked after (in care) in England, of whom 65% were fostered: in 1991 there were 60 000 children in care of whom 58% were fostered. There were 8200 children in residential care in 1995, 5700 in community homes and 1400 in private or voluntary homes. Adoption peaked in 1968, with 25 000 adoptions of whom 12 500 were infants. The position had changed by 1991 when only 7000 children were adopted of whom only 900 were infants.

In a 5-year follow-up, 2% of adoptive placements and 51% of long-term fostering placements were disrupted (Holloway 1976). Disruption was related to age at placement and not special needs, previous disruption or being placed with siblings. In another study in Scotland of permanent placement, the disruption rate over 2 years of age was 21% and over 8 years it rose to 38%. A second Scottish study showed even higher levels of disruption, as much as 66% at the age of 12–16 years at the time of permanent placement (Tables 16.1 and 16.2).

Table 16.1 Main types of placement (Rowe et al 1989)

Age (years)	Foster-home	Adoptions	Residential
0–4	77%	8%	6%
5–10	65%	1%	25%
11+	15%	0%	62%

Table 16.2 Breakdown in placement (Thorburn 1990, DOH 1991)

Placement at home[a]		25–49%
Short-term fostering		20%
Professional fostering of adolescents		38–53%
Long-term fostering at 5 years		20–41%
Adoption in infancy		Few
Adoption 3 years +		20%
Adoption adolescents		30–50%
Residential care moves		21%
Children with special needs		25–40%
	<10 yrs	10%
	>10 yrs	15–20%
	15 yrs	50%

[a] *1 in 4 'home on trial' neglected or reabused.*

Placements: key messages

The key messages (after Thorburn 1990, Holloway 1997, Howe 1998) are:

- few babies are available for adoption but infant adoption does not usually break down.
- almost all children under 4 years placed for permanence remain with the new family.
- over 50% of the 'permanent' family placements of children over 7 years old are disrupted and teenagers have an even higher breakdown rate.
- more preventive work is needed and support for families: disruption is not more likely if the child has special needs or medical problems, two situations where the family receive more support (O'Hara 1991, Triseliotis 1991a).
- 20% of children are unlikely to go home after an initial period away from home and of those that do 38% suffer a further breakdown, and the chances of rehabilitation decrease with each failed attempt. By the age of 8 years the rate of foster-care breakdown is 1 in 4, by 12 years 1 in 2, and for 15–16-year-old teenagers running away from care, 1 in 2–3.
- inter-country adoption requires the same thorough assessment of the would-be parents as for national adoption. Caution is also needed as the medical screening of the baby may be incomplete and later there may be problems of identity for the child in adolescence. Examples of poor screening are a baby of an HIV positive mother where the infants' status is unknown, a baby found to be a hepatitis B carrier and another baby with severe microcephaly.
- children may be 'looked after' at the request of their parents: this is voluntary care or 'accommodation', but with time the local authority will assume parental responsibility for many (about 40%).
- about 40% of the total of children in care have been admitted following statutory proceedings (care orders). Abused and neglected children may be in care because of proven 'harm' or under the guise of other social problems such as maternal illness, housing problems, abandonment, parental imprisonment.
- the family background of children in care compared with the general population showed that: 6 times as many had a single parent, 5 times as many families were on income support, 3 times as many were in rented accommodation. The usual picture is therefore one of poverty, unemployment, large families and single parents (OPCS General Household Survey 1985).

Adoption regulations

The adoption regulations (in England and Wales) were changed in 1997 and made changes to the composition of adoption panels and made their work more accountable. The changes are in conjunction with the 1977 and 1983 Regulations. Overseas adoptions are difficult with complex ethical considerations. Paedophiles may also seek a child from overseas to avoid SSD assessment (Trigeliotis 1993b).

Physical and mental health of 'looked after' children

Children who have been abused and/or neglected and live away from home have a greater than average number of health problems.

Bamford & Wolkind (1988) summarised the physical and mental health of children in care. As a group they have a higher risk for psychiatric ill health and social deviance than any other easily identifiable group in our society.

Payne (1996a,b) reported on 151 children referred for adoption medical examinations.

- 28 were less than 12 months of whom 14 had special needs, including individual disability, family history of schizophrenia or an older sibling with disability.
- Of the total group, 64 (56%) had a medical, behavioural or learning problem or a substantially adverse family history (incest, schizophrenia, neurofibromatosis).
- Breakdown of placement was rare in infancy, but 10–20% of adoptions of older children failed.

Holloway (1997), as mentioned earlier, did a retrospective 5-year study to describe the outcome of permanent placements (adoption or fostering).

- Disruption was related closely to age at placement (96% of disruptions occurred at 9 years of older).
- Factors not associated with breakdown were special needs, sex of the child, sibling group and previous disruption.
- It is assumed that behavioural and emotional problems were the cause of the disruption, but details are not given. However, the age at disruption (9–16 years) is not surprising given the expected conflicts in adolescence on top of an unsatisfactory and often emotionally damaging earlier childhood.

Lawrenson (1996) in a review of the literature wrote of the complex health needs of children in care and the difficulty in meeting these needs. He looked at a group of children in residential care to assess the children's physical and mental health needs. The children were aged 10–16 years and placed in mixed gender children's homes. The social services department in Leeds is committed to foster care preferentially and uses residential care when fostering fails. These children were by definition 'hard to place'.

- Physical needs were met – for example dental appointments and immunisation – but there was a high incidence of behavioural problems and school difficulties.
- Sexualised behaviour and acts of abuse were highlighted as particularly difficult behaviours to manage.
- 17/17 had been abused at home
- 4 had also been abused in care
- 5 (all boys) were perpetrators of child sexual abuse
- 4 girls had sexualised behaviour
- 12 children had emotional and behavioural problems
- 5 had moderate or severe learning problems
- 6 children were excluded from school
- 3 were in special school because of learning problems
- 3 were in special school because of emotional and behavioural disorders
- 5 children were in mainstream school, 3 doing badly.

In an OFSTED report (DoH 1995):

- 20% of children in care had an educational statement, half for emotional and behavioural difficulties. (Statements are drawn up when a child has special needs which cannot be met out of the school's usual resources: 1–2% of children in the general population have such needs)
- 10% of children attended special school
- 12% did not attend school regularly (25% of older children).

It is hardly surprising that over half the children in care leave school with no qualifications: those that do best are girls in more stable foster care (Biehal et al 1995) and employment prospects are poor (Stein & Carey 1986).

The sexualised behaviour of the children in Lawrenson's paper is important. In a study in Leeds (Mulcahy & Lacey 1987) of residents of a girls' home, aged 12–16 years

- 53% were sexually active
- 22% were prostituted
- 37% had a sexually transmitted disease (14% gonorrhoea).

Stein (1996) wrote that children involved with street projects and safe houses do not readily disclose to being prostituted but 20% are (see Ch. 13). Teenage pregnancy is common in girls leaving care: nearly 50% are pregnant by the age of 19 years, compared with a rate of 5% in the general population of 15–19-year-old girls. Although most of these young mothers cope, in 25% there are significant child protection issues.

Other reports also suggest high levels of cigarette smoking and abuse of alcohol, drugs and substances. Polnay et al (1996) noted inadequacy of health provision to children's homes and proposed a multidisciplinary team approach. He quoted the Children Act 1989 and the requirement for children in need to have an individual health care plan which would highlight problems wanting attention. The Health of the Nation report (DoH 1992) targets teenage pregnancy, STD, cigarette smoking, suicide and poor diet – teenagers in care should be a prime target for health promotion. However, unless emotional needs are met, and the poverty and homelessness of teenagers leaving care is addressed, progress will be slow (Stein 1994).

Most looked after younger children are cared for by foster-parents and over the last 10 years it has been recognised that children with special needs may be fostered successfully rather than given placements within large institutions (Argent 1997). Adoption of children with special needs has been unexpectedly successful, and perhaps reflects the adopters and also, importantly, the support they receive (O'Hara 1991, Triseliotis 1991a).

Local authorities are under-resourced for the tasks demanded of them: many of their residential staff are untrained, jeopardising the effectiveness of shared or respite care, and the health service is unable to provide a comprehensive psychological/psychiatric service.

Why take a child into care?

The reasons necessitating the removal of a child from his or her home should be compelling. The problems of providing good alternative care, especially as the child grows older, are great, but leaving a child at home who wants to leave has consequences too.

Children taken into care are often unhappy and emotionally disturbed; they may have been abused. Does the foster-home have the strength and support to care for them or will they be moved from foster-home to foster-home to children's home? Will they be abused in care? Will they run away?

The origins of poor parenting need to be addressed if the cycle of deprivation is to be altered. Prevention will involve education, real support of families in need and the alleviation of child poverty. Poverty is a major stress and a significant factor in the final break-up of already disadvantaged families. Child-rearing patterns are changing in other ways with an increased divorce rate and numbers of reconstituted and lone-parent families. As the shape of society changes it is children who are affected most by insecurity and disruption.

When children are received into care, it is generally the case that the younger the child the better the outcome, as long as subsequent care is good. Nonetheless, it is now recognised that early emotional damage may have effects lasting for life. It is also evident that repeated accommodation in care, whether voluntary (on the part of the carer) or by court order and/or frequent change of foster-home, is damaging. Being left in a poor home is no solution; children who leave care for continuing abuse or neglect at home also do badly especially in terms of emotional development.

Consequences of a neglectful or abusive childhood

The summary indicates that the consequences for the child of a neglectful or abusive childhood

Consequences for the child: summary

- Failure to grow
  - physically
  - intellectually
  - emotionally
- Development of difficult behaviours
- Persistent medical problems
  - deafness
  - squint
  - under-treated asthma
  - unimmunised
- Present to carers
  - small thin child
  - overweight adolescent (more girls)
  - poor social habits, e.g. blowing nose, use of WC
  - wetting, soiling, feeding, sleep problems
  - depressed, withdrawn, 'blank'
  - angry, aggressive, 'conduct disorder'
  - wander, fail to distinguish stranger from family or friend, over-friendly, shallow relationship
  - sexually precocious
  - school failure

are many and serious. Some of the problems arising for carers are shown in Table 16.3.

It is evident that foster-parents or residential case workers are often given an extraordinarily difficult task, caring for disturbed children who will only learn if given time, patience and skilled handling. Carers are not given adequate training, support and resources to do this, and the spread of provision is poor. The situation for carers has become even more difficult, with the increased recognition of child sexual abuse; sexually abused children are often very disturbed and their sexualised behaviours difficult to tolerate.

Children in care do not need (and do not deserve) 'good enough' care – they need better than average parenting to help heal the wounds and scars resulting from previous poor care and maltreatment. Much good, caring work is done and many children succeed but there is an unacceptable 'failure' rate. Too many children move from home to home, continue to fail and finally leave care with few skills and nowhere to go. The Children Act 1989 states

> An order should only be made if the court is also satisfied that the order it is considering will positively contribute to the child's well being and be in his best interests.

This puts a burden on all professionals and carers to ensure that the child is doing better in foster-care – otherwise why is he or she there?

The situation for children and carers is made much more difficult by uncertainty and delay in making long-term plans. Contact with parents is essential for most, but is destructive for some children. We have already seen that children who do best in the care system are those who are adopted at a young age, although there is a breakdown rate here too. Children do not handle

Table 16.3 Consequences for carers

Problem	Result or actions needed
Emotional	
Feeding (in 50–60%)	Each mealtime disrupted
Wetting, soiling, withdrawn	Endless patience and time needed, upset to rest of family
Angry, destructive	Time needed for child, other children upset, frightened, toys broken
Wandering	Anxiety
Poor social habits	Patience and teaching – upset to other family members
Learning/school problems (occur in >10%)	Attendance at clinic, e.g. speech therapy, educational psychology Involvement of carers in therapeutic programmes
Medical problems or psychological disorder	Attend clinics, become involved in therapy, family sessions
Antisocial behaviours: theft, lies, smoking, running away	Involvement with other agencies, e.g. police, school but disruption to family life too. Attend court, police stations, etc.
Sexually precocious behaviour or abusive or provocative behaviour (towards carers or children)	Education, support, therapy (as for medical problems) Educate carers and their children Appropriate care/advice
Pregnancy/STD	

conflict well (as is also shown in studies of children of divorced parents) and security is essential for emotional well-being and growth.

It is evident that long-term planning is needed whether the child is accommodated voluntarily with parental responsibility continuing (the majority) or has been taken into care. The child's wishes should be known and they should be given due consideration. It is important to take the child seriously but not to give inappropriate responsibility. Research shows that children usually felt that coming into care was the best option at the time (Kufeldt 1987), but 10% did not agree. Most children realised that they were in care because of their parents' problems, older children recognising parent–child difficulties. Children must know as soon as possible what their future holds: where they will live, which school they are to attend, what arrangements will be made about seeing their friends, their pets and their 'family'. Children should be helped to understand their changing situation and be involved in an age-appropriate way, with ongoing decision-making concerning their own lives and futures.

The role of health professionals

Paediatricians, psychologists and psychiatrists have not met the challenge of children in care. There has been little research into the physical health of children in care in the UK, but their mental health has been examined in some detail and summarised in a review (Bamford & Wolkind 1988). Although the emotional needs of children in care have been evaluated, there is much to do if they are to be met. Studies in the USA suggest that many foster-children have physical as well as emotional problems.

Growth problems are common, but cardiovascular abnormality and poor dentition occur too (Hochstadt et al 1987). This is at variance with Lawrenson (1996), possibly because of the better primary care service in the UK. Growth problems are related to emotional deprivation and persists if emotional needs are not met, whether at home or care.

Table 16.4 outlines tasks for paediatricians, whether working in the community or hospital.

The Boarding-Out Regulations

The Boarding-Out Regulations (1988) (Fig. 16.1) were introduced in an attempt to repair the deficiencies in the medical support given to children in care. The local authority has thereby a responsibility to arrange examinations and obtain a written assessment of the state of health of the child, the need for medical and dental care and to review the welfare and progress of the child. Appropriate forms have been supplied by the British Agency for Adoption and Fostering (BAAF) which allow necessary detail to be collected.

Service specification

A service specification has been published for the 'medical advice for children requiring substitute care' (Payne 1996) and the BAAF Model Business Plan includes figures of time to meet these duties (BAAF 1996). The plan should ensure that:

Boarding-Out Regulations: requirements of medical examination

- 'Baseline' assessment of growth, development and emotional state, diagnose any specific medical disorder
- Provide child's carers with relevant medical information, e.g. past illnesses, immunisation status, allergies, current health needs
- Listen to child's and carers' worries
- Complete 'My Health Passport' if provided (see text)
- Refer for appropriate investigation or treatment (after discussion with general practitioner)
- Provide a written report to general practitioner, social services, child health department to include:
  - review of child's health
  - physical developmental, emotional growth
  - progress (i.e. at subsequent visits)

Table 16.4 Tasks for the community paediatrician

At home	In care[a]
Recognise abuse early	Recognise abuse in care
Recognise neglect	Monitor growth, development and emotional well-being
Work with parents, child and primary care team:	Assess any special needs (educationally)
• support use of local resources	Work with carers, social worker closely, especially on management problems
• facilitate services for e.g. squint, glue ear, immunisation	Arrange appropriate medical, psychological, psychiatric treatment
• ensure parents understand professional concern	Work with child's natural family if appropriate
• advise on behaviour problems	Be prepared to say if the placement is failing
Be prepared to give evidence in court	Advise social services/adoption panel
Advise social services	

[a] *For whatever reason – voluntary or on order.*

- medical reports are available which give an assessment of the state of the child's health and need of health care
- professional advice is available to social services to interpret the report and assist in health care decisions
- child health surveillance is provided
- good practice on confidentiality, i.e. sharing medical information with social services as it proves in the child's interest
- there are clear policies on consent to examination or treatment of accommodated children, with regard to 'Gillick competent' children
- children with special needs are not overlooked.

BAAF have also produced 'My Health Passport' for children in care. It is designed for older children (8 years upwards) who, it is suggested, can complete sections themselves. The passport is intended to encourage awareness of health issues but also gives information to the child about his or her own medical history. It will also help, if kept up-to-date, when children move placement and there is an inevitable time lag as the general practitioner's records follow on behind. If the Boarding-Out Regulations also work properly the social worker should have an up-to-date medical dossier in the social work file.

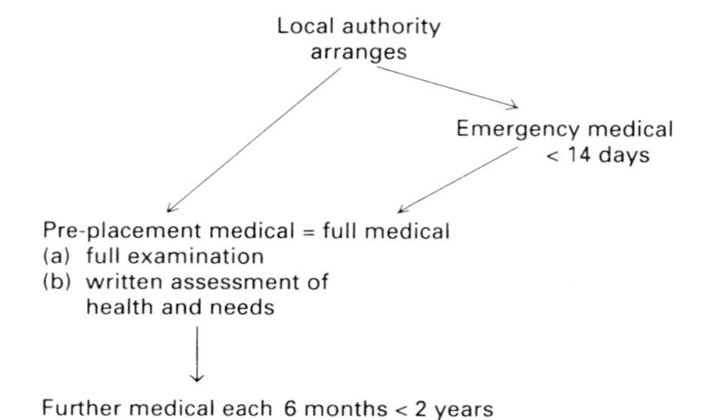

Fig. 16.1 Boarding-Out Regulations 1988 (replacing 1955 regulations).

For the medical service to work in the children's best interest the doctors must be trained and ideally offer a continuity of service. The old 'army medical' approach is simplistic and unhelpful. Although the child will need to be weighed and measured, the physical examination should be completed as appears appropriate. Older children should give consent and, in practice, listening to the child and hearing his or her concerns is likely to be more fruitful than regular physical check-ups. Emotional problems are common – if the doctor does show interest, teenagers usually are ready to talk.

It is also essential to give time to listen to the carers and take note of their worries and concerns, advising or referring on as necessary. There are considerable resource implications if this work is to be done well, but it could be truly preventive medicine.

The outlook for children in care has traditionally been poor and earlier recognition of problems may help in the long term. It is often alleged that 'care' itself causes all the problems, but this is clearly simplistic. Almost all of the children in care have had an impoverished childhood, if not an abusive one, before moving to alternative care: they frequently enter care emotionally and intellectually delayed or damaged. The 'system' should thus be geared to the needs of infants through to teenagers. Young children may do well in foster-care and then go home; some families subsequently cope, but others fail again. Children may continue to be damaged: of children returned home after care, the percentage experiencing problems increases with age. Medical surveillance for these children who may now be 'out of care' or at home on various orders should continue (Tizard & Hodges 1989, 1990, Stein 1990).

The consequence of poor care in childhood, emotional retardation, leads to the formation of shallow relationships, and antisocial behaviour becomes conduct disorder (Bamford & Wolkind 1988). As a result young men who have been in care are over-represented in the prison population. This high percentage has a negative correlation with the time in care – the longer the boy was in care the fewer the convictions.

Children who are adopted in the long term do better than those who are fostered, who do little better than those left at home. However, those in good foster-homes with continuity and consequent security do better than those teenagers brought up at home who are 'out of control' and then are inappropriately cared for in under-resourced, large children's homes or other institutions (DOH 1995). Current research has, however, challenged the fostering versus adoption debate, and the indications are that long-term fostering may have a more positive outcome than adoption of older children.

Girls who have received poor parenting and care tend to drift into pregnancy and transient relationships which fail. As teenage mothers their babies are often small, the mother–child interaction is poor and by the time the child goes to school he or she is likely to have behaviour problems. Thus the cycle of disadvantage repeats itself (Janus et al 1987, Bamford & Wolkind 1988).

The reasons why some children in care do better than others are not fully understood, but there are clearly several factors involved. Some children just appear to be more resilient to life's adversities. Children of schizophrenic parents are over-represented in care. Children in care tend to be of lower birthweight – what are the effects of intrauterine growth retardation (including cigarettes, drugs and alcohol abuse)? Yet environmental factors are the most important when considering the reasons why children are in care. These children often come from large, poor, stressed families where problems and disharmony lead to eventual family breakdown and care. This pattern may alter with current changes in family structure. The care experience may then compound the poor start offered the child. The care system itself is not the sole reason for the poor outcome, but the system has failed to meet children's needs. Research shows that, overall, adopted children have fewer long-term problems in ordinary living as well as a lower rate of psychiatric disorder. Inadequate foster-care or residential care or staying in poor, abusive homes will continue to offer children an impoverished lifestyle. 'Keeping them out of care' as an answer to the ills of the care system is not a solution, although it is superficially attractive to those with money to save.

Abuse in care

It has recently been recognised that abuse is as commonly found in foster homes as children's homes (Hobbs 1998). Table 16.5 outlines the background information in this retrospective study. Ideas as to prevention of abuse and promotion of good health in accommodated children are:

- evaluation and further research into the adequacy of care and level of abuse in foster homes and children's homes
- prevention of abuse on contact and ongoing assessment of the benefits to the child or, any negative attributes from ongoing access

Table 16.5 Summary of child abuse and 'accommodated children' (Hobbs 1998)

From 1990–1996 158 children were referred to paediatricians	Foster care	Children's home
Number of children, Gender Age: mean/range in months	133, 59 boys and 74 girls 80 months/12–14 months	25, 17 boys and 8 girls Mean age 12.5 years
Abuser: Foster parent/staff in home Parent/relative i.e. on Contact	29 NAI 22 CSA 8 NAI and CSA (41% of total incidents) 11 NAI 24 CSA 6 NAI and CSA (23% of total incidents)	Staff member: 8 children NAI Other children in home: 4 children 2 NA and 2 CSA
Other child (sibling, other accommodated child, child of foster family	4 NAI 24 CSA 1 NAI and CSA (20% of total incidents)	Child outside home: 13 children 4 NAI and 9 CSA
Unknown	2 NAI 7 CSA 1 NAI and CSA	
Abuse prior to care in 80% of children	45 NAI, 72 CSA, 15 Emotional, 33 Neglect, 9 FTT, 5 Abandoned, 12 Mother ill, 20 Unknown	In majority
Behaviour difficulty: reported to paediatrician in 57% (foster care)	Total with behaviour difficulty 78 includes: 'problems' 58 sexualized behaviour 37 sees mental health professional 17	In majority
Learning problem/disability	35	> half
Abused in care	42 NAI, 76 CSA*, 15 NAI and CSA	12 NAI*, 6 CSA, 6 NAI and CSA
Type of abuse and gender	60% CSA involved girls 60% NAI involved boys	4 girls CSA, 4 girls NAI 8 boys CSA, 8 boys NAI
Presentation of abuse	32% disclosure, usually to social worker 22% Behaviours 22% Injury 15% Symptoms e.g. 'soreness'. Also – concern from school, abuse of other child	
Management	10 Contact – increased supervision 18 Returned home 8 Other foster home 14 To children's home 26 Plan to move ?where 43 Plan not known 8 Child Protection Conference 6 Foster families – > 1 report (4 had 2 reports, 1 had 3, 1 on contact)	Not available
Number of placements	59 in 1st, 39 in 2nd, or 3rd, 14 in 4th or more (cf. national statistics)	
Rate of abuse reported by paediatricians: General population 3.9/1000 children 0–17 years	In foster care 29.5/1000 children	In children homes 23.3/1000 children

Notes: some children were abused more than once and in different ways before and after being in care. The data is incomplete but gives an overall view – some of the NAI was a central finding with one death (shaking by a foster mother of a 2-year-old), 8 burns, 72 children had NAI with bruising but no fractures. Of the CSA, 39 children had abnormal genital signs, 18/39 consistent with penetration; 53 had abnormal anal signs, 34/53 consistent with penetration. The sexually abused children had the highest level of disturbed behaviour, i.e. 62% but 55% of the NAI group were also categorised as disturbed.

- careful paediatric assessment for all children to ensure health, growth, emotional well-being, behaviour and any abuse/neglect is recognised
- an understanding by all professionals of the risk of abuse, even in tried and tested placements. Ensure case has an allocated SW for the child and a different one for the foster parents. Planned reviews
- support and training for carers – wetting, soiling, antisocial behaviours are difficult within a 'family' setting and sexualised play/behaviours may be the 'final' insult

- more therapeutic services for child, to include foster parents and staff
- planning, attention to detail (Lamming 1996) and *listen to the child*
- thorough investigation of allegations of abuse, mandatory Child Protection Conferences
- audit all staff, keep all allegations and thoroughly investigate
- implement Warner Report 1992 – on employment of paid or voluntary staff.

There is an urgent need to provide for the needs of teenagers in long term care, particularly in children's homes. The cumulative effects of poor care at home and then care (some have been in 20–30 placements) results in:

- 25% of teenagers do not go to school; 75% leave school with no qualifications
- four times the risk of a mental health problem compared with other teenagers
- poor general health, poor compliance and diagnosis of chronic disorders e.g. asthma, vision and hearing
- 30% of homeless have been in care
- 40% of young prisoners have been in care
- 70–80% of those leaving care become unemployed.

The high number of runaways demonstrates the failure of parenting and the care system of the 1980s. Recent work has highlighted the level of institutional abuse; American research shows 39 per 1000 children in care report abuse but only 1 in 5 incidents are officially reported (Westcott 1992). See also the Utting Report (1997, Ch. 14).

Frequently abuse in care is not adequately investigated even when reported, although authorities are now instituting more appropriate procedures (Working Together 1991). Paediatricians and child psychiatrists must be aware of abuse in residential settings, involving staff or peers, recognise warning signs and act on behalf of individual children. The abuse may be institutionalised and part of the 'treatment of disturbed children', as in 'pin-down' where the report documented 132 cases of solitary confinement in Staffordshire homes in 1983–89 (Westcott 1992). However, unless residential staff are adequately trained, supervised and paid as skilled professionals the standard of care will remain inadequate for many emotionally disturbed children. Closing down all the children's homes is not an acceptable alternative to attempting to raise standards and meet children's needs.

Runaways – teenage homelessness

The rapidly rising numbers of teenagers running away from unhappy or abusive homes or inadequate local authority care (Abrahams & Mungall 1992) should point the way to more imaginative initiatives to meet the needs of this distressed and disadvantaged group. Much published research into teenage runaways is from the USA but there is an increasing body of information in the UK which is providing a similar and worrying picture, with an estimated 75 000–90 000 young people running away each year. Rees (1993) in a population study (in the UK) found that 1 in 7 children under 16 years gave a history that they had run away overnight or, a rough incidence of 12/1000 children each year compared to the reported incidence of 6/1000 children each year. Features of the children include (Rees 1993, Stein 1990, Lawrenson 1997):

- most episodes are 'one off', the child does not go far, and is usually alone
- many have a history of truancy
- for some children there is a progression as running away escalates (to escape abuse or rejection), truancy inevitably increases, and the child is gradually dissociated from home, school and any social support.

There is often a history of substitute care:

- the home background is often poor and the family is reconstituted
- around 10% of runaways are under 11 years
- over half the children sleep rough, i.e. this is a serious statement by the child, yet their parents may not report them missing
- a sub-group of children develop a pattern of running from home which may continue in

substitute care. Frequent runaways are over-represented in police statistics; 30% overall have run away from care, mainly children's homes
- it is vital that each episode of running is taken at face value: was it temper, unhappiness or abuse that caused the child to run?
- chronic running may lead to homelessness, crime and increased morbidity (see later).

The London safe house

The Children's Society have researched young runaways using the safe house in London, the first in the UK (Newman 1989). Of the one-third of the children who ran away because of problems at home, the usual complaint was of constant arguments and breakdown in communications. Many had been thrown out of the parental home or had left because of violence (Table 16. 6).

- Of the total sample of 532 young people, 98 said they had been sexually abused at some time, that is 18% of the group or 29% females and 6% males
- 25% of those admitted to the house had run away from care.

The paper notes the unhappiness of children placed in secure units – young people whose only 'crime' was running away. As others have written (Heany 1989), it is a lottery whether the often abused runaway is helped or punished. Others were unhappy in children's homes, foster home or assessment centre. Several had been bullied and physically abused in residential care. Many felt that in care they were not appropriately involved in the planning of their own future, and that their own opinion was not considered. This has been well expressed:

> When I was in care I felt that no-one had the time to talk to me as an individual to find out what I wanted and how I felt. I felt no-one cared for me so I got hurt and bitter and then I fought out and was labelled a problem and locked away (Heany 1989).

On the streets of our cities are children of 8–9 years upwards, absent from school and wanderers, who eventually go home but may be at considerable risk nonetheless. These children are often involved in shoplifting, may drift into prostitution (boys and girls, especially if sexually abused previously), smoke, abuse drugs, alcohol and solvents. Other older children run and run, and eventually may stay away. The reality of running away and subsequent homelessness is described (Newman 1989) as a national problem which needs urgent attention by 'providing appropriate care and resources to which young runaways should have a right'.

Homelessness exists in all our cities and a description of homeless adults looked at the origins and morbidity of the adults, which again reflects the urgent need to help the teenager (*Lancet* 1989). Medical problems develop alongside homelessness with the teenager at risk with a high morbidity for accidents, physical illness, psychiatric disorder, poor nutrition, untreated infections, drug and alcohol abuse and sexually transmitted disease. These children need a lot of skilled support, not punishment or locking up.

Table 16.6 Reasons for leaving home and care (1985–87). This information was available for 84% admitted into the safe house (Newman 1989)

Reasons for leaving	%
Problems at home	33
Problems in care	25
General unhappiness	16
More specific problems	13
Problems at school	6
(non-runaways)	5
Total	98

Problems of adolescent runaways

The abuse of adolescents in the USA is well documented. In spite of a general view that child maltreatment is the major problem, family violence does not stop at the end of childhood and may increase (Powers & Eckenrode 1988). The association of maltreatment at home with runaway and homeless youth has been looked at in more detail (Powers et al 1990). The characteristics of runaways in the USA are summarised in Table 16.7. In general most runaways are in their mid-teens and give a long history of emotional

Table 16.7 Characteristics of runaways (Kufeldt and Nimmo 1987, Lancet 1989, Abrahams and Mungall 1992)

Gender	More boys pushed out More girls run away Approximately equal numbers
Age	Peak 15–17 years Range 12–18 years (66% are 14–16 but 7% under 11 years)
Family	25% lived with both parents (cf. 68% general population), >33% single parent, more from single, broken, divorced homes. Afro-Caribbean and Asian children are over-represented
Care	33–50% (96% from residential homes)
Recurrence	Most run more than once 30% run five times or more
Mood	Depressed Poor self-image >50% Suicidal
School	Average 2 years behind peers, school problems 25%, learning problems 7%
Antisocial behaviour	Delinquency 15%, drug/alcohol abuse 20%
Maltreatment	30–70% – may be more than one type Physical abuse 20–40% Sexual abuse 5–12% Neglect 20–42% Emotional abuse? 100%
Referral	< 10% had told welfare agencies of abuse
Where do they run?	98% of runaways stay within a few miles of home To friends, relatives and many return voluntarily
How long do they stay?	Most stay away a few days 2% were away longer than 2 weeks
Why did they run?	Arguments with parents Abuse

conflict and abuse. Boys are more likely to be pushed out (thrown out) of home and so become homeless, whereas girls, especially sexually abused girls, run away. They are an unhappy group as a whole, at real risk of suicide, especially those who have been sexually abused. They have often failed at school, although before running only 15% have a history of delinquency. Once on the street, 70% of a sample (Powers et al 1990) were approached with offers of illegal activities.

For the teenager on the streets there is a continuation of the spiral of abuse, neglect and exploitation (Powers et al 1990). 'Running away to sea' used to be considered a normal expression of adolescent behaviour and the separation process, but the picture has changed and these 'throw-away children' are a reflection of current familial and societal pathology (Powers et al 1990). These teenagers are unhappy; they run because of social and environmental determinates. The families are dysfunctional and emotionally abusive. The runners come from all sections of UK society. There may have been physical or sexual abuse. The children may have been pushed out and cannot return. The tragedy is that they are not running *to* anything which offers promise but *away* from an intolerable situation. These teenagers sacrifice their adolescence, growth and development by running to another hostile, stressful environment without real hope of a better future. The challenge is an urgent one.

'Safe houses' offer emergency care to a small proportion of teenagers, but only if this large group are seen as victims rather than villains will realistic proposals be made. Given the lack of legitimate provisions – that is, housing, training, jobs – many will inevitably drift into criminal activity, prostitution, drug abuse or early parenthood. This will cost them years of their life (or life itself) and society will have to bear the cost of inappropriate imprisonment and the effects of another generation of deprived babies.

Summary

1. Children who are cared for away from home have particular emotional needs; these needs may not be recognised or met. Many have been abused.
2. Children and young people in care (and their families) are required to be involved in care planning and management of their health needs (DoH 1995).
3. Children who have been or are in care have a higher risk of mental ill health and social deviance than any other easily identifiable group in our society.
4. The numbers of children accommodated by the local authority have fallen markedly in recent years; foster-care is usually preferred but 8600 children were in children's homes in England in 1996.

5. Children may be abused in foster-homes, adoptive homes and institutions (see Utting Report 1997, Ch. 14). They need a voice (Heary 1989).
6. In general, younger children who are adopted have the best long-term outlook.
7. Adoption of children with physical or learning disability is successful in many instances. The adoption of children damaged by abuse or neglect is less successful.
8. An increasing number of children run away from home and care each year. More local support, for child, parents and carers is advocated (Abrahams & Mungall 1992). Safe houses are urgently needed. Streets are dangerous, more than one in seven runaways trade sex for money, 25% are abused (sexually and/or physically) whilst running, and many self-harm and an increasing number abuse drugs (Lee 1995, Linehan 1997).
9. Doctors have an important task: to recognise the physical and emotional needs of children in care and to offer advice and support to carers whilst arranging appropriate treatment or therapy for children (Table 16.4).
10. Specialist doctors also advise social services and adoption panels.

REFERENCES

Abrahams C, Mungall R 1992 Runaways: exploding the myths. National Children's Home, 85 Highbury Park, London N5 1H, p 10

Argent H 1997 The placement of children with disabilities. Practice Note 34, BAAF, London

Bamford F, Wolkind S N 1988 The physical and mental health of children in care. Economic and Social Research Council, London

Biehal N, Clayden J, Stein M 1995 Moving on. Young people and leaving care schemes. HMSO London

Boarding-Out Regulations 1988 New Regulations and Associated Guidance: Boarding-out of children (foster placement) Regulations 1988; Accommodation of children (charge and control) Regulations 1988. Local Authority Circular LAC (89)4. DoH, London

Brindle D 1997 Paying for the best. Guardian, London, 21 May 1997

Butler I, Payne H 1997 The health of children looked after by the local authority. Adoption and Fostering 21(2):28–35

Curtis Report 1946 Report of the Care of Children Committee. HMSO, London

DoH 1989 Introduction to Children Act 1989. HMSO, London

DoH 1991 Patterns and outcomes in child placement. HMSO, London.

DoH 1992 Health of the Nation. HMSO, London

DoH 1995 Looking after children – good parenting, good outcomes. HMSO, London

DoH 1996 Children looked after by local authorities. Year ending 31 May 1995. Department of Health, London

Guardian 1997 Leader. An inevitable scandal. Guardian, London, 24 May 1997

Heany A 1989 A number not a name. A voice for the child in care. VCC paper no 4, London

Hobbs G, Hobbs C J, Wynne J M 1997 Child abuse in foster care. In press

Hochstadt N et al 1987 The medical and social needs of children entering foster care. Child Abuse and Neglect 11(1):53

Holloway J S 1997 Outcome in placements for adoption or longterm fostering. Archives of Diseases of Childhood 76:227–230

Howe D 1998 Adoption outcome research and practical judgement. Adoption and fostering 22(2):6–15

Janus M et al 1987 Adolescent runaways: causes and consequences. Lexingham Books, Lexingham, MA

Kufeldt K, Nimmo M 1987 Youth on the street: abuse and neglect in the 80s. Child Abuse and Neglect 11:531–543

Lancet 1989 Homelessness (leader). Lancet ii:778

Lamming H 1998 Facing the future. HMSO, London

Lawrenson F J 1996 The health of looked after children. MMedSci dissertation, Leeds University

Lawrenson F J 1997 Runaway children: whose problem? BMJ 314:1064

Lee M,O'Brien R 1995 The game's up: Redefining child prostitution Childrens Society, London

Mulcahy F M, Lacey C J 1987 Sexually transmitted infections in adolescent girls. Genitourinary Medicine 63:119–121

Newman C 1989 Young runaways . . . finds from Britain's first safe house. Children's Society, London

NHS Executive 1996 Child health in the community: a guide to good practice HMSO, London

O'Hara G 1991 Placing children with special needs – outcomes and implications for practice. Adoption and Fostering 15(4):46

Payne H 1996a Medical advice for children requiring substitute care: service specification. Adoption and Fostering 20(1):57–58

Payne H 1996b Medical problems in adoption and the implications for post-placement support. Adoption and Fostering 20(2):65–66

Polnay L, Glaser A, Rao V 1996 Better health for children in resident care. Arch Dis Child 75(3):263–265

Powers J L, Eckenrode B 1988 The maltreatment of adolescents. Child Abuse and Neglect 12:189–199

Powers J L, Eckenrode B, Jaklitsch 1990 Maltreatment among runaway and homeless youth. Child Abuse and Neglect 14:87–98

Rees G 1993 Hidden truths: Young people's experience of running away. Childrens Society, London

Rowe J, Hundleby M, Garnett L 1989 Child care now. Research Series 6, BAAF, London
Stein M 1990 Living out of care. Barnado's, London
Stein M, Carey K 1986 Leaving care. Basil Blackwell, Oxford
Stein M, Rees G, Frost N 1993 Running the risk. Children's Society, London
Thorburn J 1990 Inter-departmental review of adoption law. Background Paper no 2. Review of research relating to adoption. DoH, London
Thorburn J 1995 Out of home care for the abused or neglected child: research, planning and practice. In: Wilson K, James A (eds) The child protection handbook. Balliére Tindall, London, Chapter 24
Tizard B, Hodges J 1989 IQ and behavioural adjustments of ex-institutional adolescents. Social and family relationships of ex-institutional adolescents. Journal of Child Psychology and Psychiatry 30:53–75, 77–97
Tizard B, Hodges J 1990 Ex-institutional children: a follow-up study to age 16. Adoption and Fostering 14(1)
Triseliotis J 1991a Perceptions of permanence. Adoption and Fostering 15(4):6
Triseliotis J 1991b Inter-country adoption: a brief overview of research. Adoption and Fostering 15(4):46
Utting Report 1997 People like us. The review of safeguards for children living away from home. HMSO, London
Warner N 1992 Choosing with care – the report of the Committee of Enquiry into the selection, development and management of staff in children's homes. HMSO, London
Warren D 1997 Foster care in crisis. National Foster Care Association, London
Westcott H 1992 Institutional abuse of children – from research to policy. NSPCC, London
Working Together 1991 Working together under the Children Act 1989. A guide to arrangements for inter-agency co-operation for the protection of children from abuse. HMSO, London

ADDRESSES

British Agency for Adoption and Fostering (BAAF) 11 Southwark Street, London SE1 1RQ
The Children's Society, Edward Rudolf House, Margery Street, London WC1X 0JL

17

Legal aspects of child abuse work

Courts

Doctors who recognise child abuse will inevitably become involved in civil cases and care proceedings. Much less commonly will they be asked to give evidence in criminal proceedings (Table 17.1). This is because of the difficulties in collecting evidence, particularly when young children are involved. The Crown Prosecution Service (CPS) in England and Wales makes the decision whether to

Table 17.1 Which court?

Court	
Criminal Court (Magistrate's Court, Crown Court)	Police statement is basis of evidence, given orally if not agreed Proof needed 'beyond all reasonable doubt' No hearsay evidence Videolink and screens may be used if witness under 14 years old Public and Press present Child's identity may not be disclosed[a]
'Family Proceedings Court' (Magistrate's Court, County Court, High Court)[b]	Evidence may be oral, written or both if not agreed[c, d] Proof needed 'on balance of probability' Hearsay evidence allowed Videoed evidence may be allowed Judge or Magistrate gives reason for decisions made No public present Press allowed but reporting restricted and child may not be identified[a]

[a] *The Cleveland Inquiry commented on the need to protect children from identification by the media (Butler-Sloss 1988, p 253).*
[b] *Divorce and other civil matters included as well as child abuse cases.*
[c] *Medical report usually available to Magistrate and all involved parties.*
[d] *Affidavits in High Court, oral evidence may be restricted to elucidation of points in affidavit only.*

bring a criminal case and will do so only if the crime is serious, if it is in the public interest and if there is a real possibility of a successful prosecution. Prosecutions are mounted more often when the defendant has pleaded guilty and hence the child and professional witnesses are unlikely to be called to give evidence. The number of cases which are eventually heard in criminal proceedings is low and so successful prosecutions are few, and appear to be falling: from around 10% in 1989 to less than 5% in 1991 (West Yorkshire Police 1992), where it remained in 1997. This should be seen in the context that of women complaining of rape in England and Wales in 1996 there were convictions in only 8% of the cases.

Giving evidence

Few doctors enjoy giving evidence in court. Doctors tend to be hesitant about appearing and when they do they expect the proceedings to be 'fair' and the court to hear what they have to say. In practice the court often feels more like a battleground, with more concern for the law and the demolition of the witness than for the child.

Professional witnesses may become frustrated when they feel they are not able to share with the court their full knowledge of the child. The rules of evidence differ in criminal and civil courts and the professional witness needs to understand in particular about hearsay evidence. *Hearsay evidence* is information which the doctor has learned second-hand: for example, if the child said to the social worker '. . . my Dad hit me' and the social worker passed this information on to the doctor. The doctor should describe his or her examination of the child and state an opinion as to the causation; this may be 'an unexplained injury' or 'not any ordinary accident'. The CPS may prefer the doctor in this situation to include in the police statement that 'I examined [the child] at the request of Leeds Social Services because of an allegation of physical assault . . .' and conclude '. . . the injury is consistent with a hard blow from an outstretched hand'. The CPS may write back and put several explanations to the doctor, and ask for a further opinion. The doctor is then giving expert opinion rather than professional evidence and should be careful to keep within his or her own expertise and support an opinion with reference to the medical literature. Medicine is not an exact science: bruises may start to go yellow after 18 hours or fractures develop soft callus at 10–14 days (Ch. 4), but doctors should resist the exactitude often requested to date injuries within tight time-bands.

Expert witnesses and the use of expert testimony under the Children Act 1989 differs from criminal cases. In criminal courts the rules of evidence are adhered to strictly with no hearsay evidence allowed, which is at least straightforward. Also a defendant may only be convicted if the case has been 'proved beyond all reasonable doubt'.

In courts concerned with the welfare of children the position is different. The court wants to hear from the child and it may only be through third parties, for example the guardian *ad litem*, the parents, social worker or a doctor, that all the collected evidence may be presented. In care proceedings, the laws of evidence were therefore changed to allow the whole picture to emerge and hearsay evidence was made admissible. The case must be proved 'on the balance of probability', this being a lower burden of proof but still an exacting one. In addition a recent ruling made it clear that when considering the probability that, for example, the child had been raped, the court required a higher standard of proof (or probability) than for a lesser sexual assault.

Giving evidence clearly is a skill which doctors working with abused children must acquire, but it does take considerable time to feel confident in court. Giving evidence is never easy.

A paediatrician who examines a child who has allegedly been physically abused may be called as a professional witness to give evidence of fact, that is to describe the examination of the child. The court will expect the paediatrician to explain the child's injuries in the light of the available history but also with a view to the child's development, and any medical disorder. Criminal courts may wish to hear of first-hand evidence the paediatrician has of neglect, whereas care courts will usually explore growth and development in a much more general way, allowing third party information too.

Other doctors may be called as professional witnesses to give evidence of, for example, physical assault. Unless the doctor is trained appropriately and can demonstrate the necessary experience he or she should be careful to keep to the brief and not include any opinion outwith that expertise: lawyers are generally sharp and appear to delight in demolishing professional witnesses.

The paediatrician uses contemporaneous notes (i.e. notes made during and immediately after the examination) diagrams, radiographs and scans (a paediatric radiologist or neuroradiologist would usually present these in complex cases), photographs, other laboratory results, and increasingly may be expected to discuss the findings in the context of the relevant literature, referring to published work. Anecdotal stories in the context of 25 years of practise are interesting but not always compelling. The paediatrician may give expert testimony and the distinction between a professional and expert witness is not always clear-cut. An expert witness may be called who has not seen the child but who can interpret the case for the court using specialised knowledge. It may be necessary (from the point of view of payment) for the doctor to talk to the CPS solicitor before the trial to establish his or her status and fee.

Expert witnesses and the Children Act 1989

Civil proceeding concerning children are based on the following propositions (Wall 1997)

- confidentiality
- non-adversarial nature of proceedings
- avoidance of delay.

The Expert Witness Pack (Family Law 1997) has been published to assist in proceedings concerning children.

Expert witnesses

- Are instructed by an advocate after permission by the court has been gained, i.e. to ensure that this is an appropriately qualified doctor
- Should have appropriate clinical experience
- Should be up-to-date, and usually in clinical practice
- Should write a 'wholly objective report' in the child's best interest
- Their report should be disclosed in civil cases
- Are encouraged to meet and define areas of agreement and disagreement
- If experts are in agreement a joint statement may avoid attendance at court
- Should allow the court knows their availability; judges will often allow their evidence to be 'interposed'
- The level of appropriate fees is contentious and should be agreed pre-trial and approved by the Legal Aid Board

It is evident that a doctor should give evidence in a way in which the court can use it most effectively. This means speaking clearly, not too fast, not too quietly, in layman's terms so that the evidence can be understood by all in the court – not just the judge, but the jury members, defendants and parents as well as the lawyers.

As in any clinical presentation the doctor should be able to justify all he or she says and avoid exaggeration or dogmatism. a witness who is impartial is much more credible. To give evidence in a calm, collected way requires careful preparation, including a pre-court conference with the lawyers. The lawyers may help by explaining the legal aspects of the case to the doctor who can in turn ensure that the medical opinion is understood.

Giving evidence

- Be well prepared – talk to lawyers before coming to court
- Take all relevant notes, radiographs, reports and statements to court
- Be on time
- Give evidence clearly, slowly, avoid jargon
- Expect to justify your medical opinion
- Be impartial – the child's welfare is paramount
- Say if you do not understand a question
- Say if you do not know the answer

- Answer the question which is put
- Try to be succinct, only agree to 'yes' or 'no' if appropriate, but do not give unnecessary detail
- Only comment on topics on which you are informed

However, lawyers may also attack the witness. Courts are more of a battlefield than a cricket-field. Table 17.2 gives a doctor's view of this: the summary below is taken from a lawyer's guide to cross-examination.

How to unsettle a doctor as a witness (a lawyer's guide)

- Generally avoid frontal attack
- Conduct a positive cross-examination, at least initially
- Raise doubt about the expert in a subtle way:
  - use leading questions
  - limit expert's opportunity to explain opinion
  - hide the ball
- Undermine the expert's assumption
- Raise the possibility of bias or partiality
- As a last resort use other ammunition – sexist, political, personal attack

Practical points

- Courts will try and be flexible in terms of the timing of the doctor's evidence – even though timing frequently goes awry.
- In criminal cases the paediatrician is usually the 'prosecution's witness'. After receiving a 'court warning', write a detailed note of your availability to the court clerk and follow this up with a telephone call: there may in addition be a helpful police officer coordinating witnesses. Note: a court warning for 10 a.m. on the first day of the trial will almost always find several disgruntled witnesses sitting outside the court, and they may sit there for hours or even days.
- Only limited negotiation is possible once the case has started, and the witness may be compelled to attend.
- Take only the relevant clinical notes to court.
- In civil cases planning court attendance is usually more successful, although the doctor may be asked to be available over 2 weeks this is unreasonable and the requesting advocate will usually negotiate for a mutually convenient half-day.
- Preferably meet the advocates pre-trial.
- Arrive at court in good time, tidily dressed (although wedding/funeral suits are not compulsory!)

Court procedure

The doctor will initially be sworn, or affirmed, by the court clerk and then invited to sit or stand. In care proceedings, where attempts are being made to make the court less threatening, the chairman of the bench will often invite the wit-

Table 17.2 How to unsettle a doctor as a witness (a doctor's view; after Anderson 1990)

Question	Reply
How many cases have you seen like this, Dr?	Give direct reply
Have you been trained in this work specifically, Dr?	Give direct reply
What work in this field have you had published, Dr?	Give direct reply
Why have you altered the date in the notes?	You may not remember – say so
Why is the medical report dated differently in various copies?	Has the computer print-out done this automatically?
Why have you changed pen?	Demonstrate different pens in your possession
Why have you written on the back of an investigation mount sheet, Dr?	Convenience
Complex question with several subsidiary queries	Ask to repeat question, and insist on answering each question separately
Ask to discuss a hypothetical but unlikely scenario	Comment logically and say it is unlikely, if it is
Are you 100% certain, Dr?	Explain cannot be 100% certain but highly probable, or unlikely, etc.
Question each injury, even the most minor, in order to destroy the whole	Explain the importance of pattern recognition – and acknowledge if there are accidental injuries

ness to sit. In other courts where the witness is more comfortable sitting or has a lot of papers it may be more practicable to sit, with the judge's permission. The advocate may stand or sit, and replies are directed to the judge or chairman of the bench, and not to the questioner. Forms of address are given in Table 17.3.

The witness will first be led through his or her evidence, in a straightforward way, by the advocate for the prosecution in criminal cases or the lawyers representing the local authority (or the instructing lawyer) in care cases; then the witness is cross-examined. It is usually during the cross-examination that the doctor will be tested most. There is usually a reasonable dialogue which often allows the doctor to make points missed in his evidence-in-chief. However, more time may be spent (or so it seems to the witness) in examining his or her curriculum vitae than the evidence. This is an increasing trend, but if the doctor keeps calm the threatening lawyer will appear bullying rather than the doctor incompetent. If the doctor does become angry the lawyer has succeeded: an emotionally wrought witness gains little credibility and will be dismissed as emotionally involved in the case and therefore biased (Butler-Sloss 1988, pp. 202–252).

For a witness who does feel threatened and is losing confidence, it is useful to take a deep breath and avoid eye contact with the lawyer: avoidance of eye contact is achieved more easily when sitting, and distances the lawyer. It is also possible to regain composure by politely asking the advocate to repeat the question: this buys time, and with luck the advocate will have forgotten what he or she asked.

Always remember, a children's doctor knows more about children than any lawyer (almost) and if the doctor 'sticks to his last' that knowledge will become apparent. Do not assume a high level of understanding of child health issues in court or a sophisticated appreciation of children's needs. A paediatrician is an expert and can explain to the court the fundamentals of good childcare.

However, a well-prepared witness must be aware of the legal system and its rules:

> The medical profession needs to appreciate the legal implications of and their responsibility for the evidential requirements of their work (Butler-Sloss 1988, p. 252).

Table 17.3 Forms of address

Personal	Court	Address
Magistrate	Magistrates Court	Sir or Madam
Circuit Judge, Recorder	Crown or County Court	Your Honour
High Court Judge	High Court	My Lord or My Lady
Lords Justice	Court of Appeal	My Lord or My Lady
Lords of Appeal	House of Lords	My Lord or My Lady

Court procedure: summary

- Know your way about the courtroom (see Figs 17.1 and 17.2)
- Wait outside court – do not discuss evidence with other witnesses
- Stand and bow with the court as judge or magistrates enter or leave court
- If the court is already sitting, bow to judge or bench from witness box on arrival and departure
- The court clerk will administer the oath or affirmation
- Stand or sit to give evidence (see text)
- Expert witnesses may sit by the lawyer to listen to all the evidence. Do not whisper or cause distraction
- At the end of your evidence the court will usually release you – your instructing lawyer will ask permission

Planning a court appearance

Witness summons

The courts are aware that doctors may only give evidence at the expense of other work and are usually accommodating about the timing of a doctor's appearance to avoid inconveniencing patients, for example in an outpatient clinic. The instructing lawyer should plan a rough timetable with the other lawyers so that the doctor is able

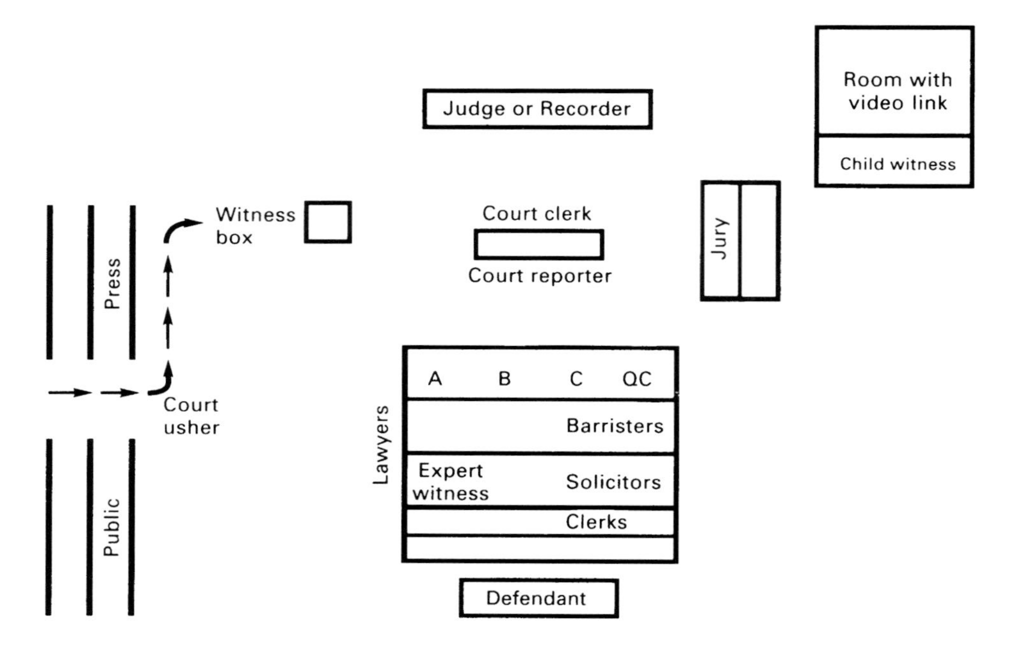

Fig. 17.1 Layout of Crown or County Court. In criminal proceedings, A represents the prosecutor and B the defence lawyer. In care proceedings, A represents the local authority, B the child's lawyer (instructed by the guardian *ad litem*), C the parents' lawyer. Wigs and gowns are worn in criminal proceedings only.

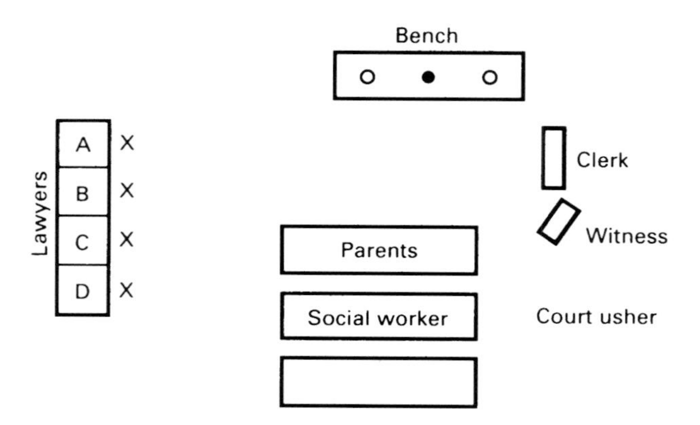

Fig. 17.2 Layout of Magistrates' Court (care court).
○, magistrate; ●, chair of bench; A, lawyer for local authority (usually); B, lawyer for child (instructed by guardian *ad litem*); C, lawyer for father; D, lawyer for mother; X, expert witness (for A, B, C or D).

to set aside a half-day in which to give evidence. This is usually adequate in child abuse cases but inevitably timing is often inexact. Expert witnesses may choose to sit for days on end in court. Each individual doctor must consider where his or her priorities lie in court work.

A doctor who is called to give evidence usually accepts this as part of his or her professional duty, hence a witness summons is unnecessary. Courts have powers to compel the attendance of a witness, and Magistrate's High Courts and County Courts may also order the doctor to produce relevant documents or notes. If the court feels the doctor has evidence which is relevant, for example in a criminal case, the witness really has no choice and may be arrested for failure to attend. In other circumstances, such as the defendant pleading guilty or if medical reports are agreed, the doctor may not be called.

Lawyers often seem to come to decisions at the last minute, and the case is suddenly settled when lawyers representing all parties meet in the courtroom. The attending doctor can only attempt to smile benignly and go away and put in a bill (library and training funds may at least benefit).

Children's evidence

Interviewing children

The interviewing of children has been much researched and the consensus remains

> . . . contrary to the traditional view, recent research shows that untruthful child witnesses are comparatively uncommon, and like their adult counterparts they act out of identifiable motives (Home Office 1989).

More recent work has supported this view (Spencer & Flin 1993, Watson 1995). Working Together (1991) gave guidance as to good practice, drawing on the Cleveland Report (Butler-Sloss 1988):

- Interviewers are to be of acknowledged competence.
- Interviews should be conducted under area child protection committee procedures.
- The number of investigative interviews should be kept to a minimum.
- Interviewers should retain an open mind.
- The interview should focus on the needs of the child, be at an appropriate pace and level and enable the child to talk.
- Recording of interviews should be accurate and differentiate fact, hearsay and opinion.

Interviews may be audio- or videotaped. These tapes may be used in family proceedings where there is no restriction on hearsay and in certain circumstances in criminal proceedings (see later). The 1992 Memorandum of Good Practice (Home Office 1992), which is voluntary guidance as to the management of video-interviewing for criminal proceedings, has been used as 'the rules' required for interviewing.

There has not been in practice the necessary flexibility needed for interviewing very young, disabled or frightened children, even by very skilled interviewers. As a consequence the aim of the Memorandum:

> Children have a right to justice and their evidence is essential if society is to protect their interests and deal effectively with those who would harm them (Home Office 1992)

has not in many cases been met. In 1994 further guidance looked at the implementation of the Memorandum (SSI 1994) with the requirement for video facilities, training, specialist police and social workers and support for the interviewers. The report was critical of the selection of children to interview, too many videos were made and few were used in court. An evaluation of videotaping and trials involving child witnesses (Davies et al 1995) showed:

- cases took on average 17 weeks to come to trial
- over 70% of witnesses were girls
- the average age was 12 years (range 3–18 years)
- within the study period 15 000 tapes were made, 5000 were referred to the CPS, 100 cases went to trial, 79 with tapes.

Details of interviewing children are given in Chapter 9.

Children giving evidence

In 1989 the Pigot Committee proposed radical changes to the rules governing the evidence of children in criminal proceedings (Pigot Report 1989). An emasculated version of these proposals appeared in the Criminal Justice Act 1991 (Spencer 1991). However, Spencer acknowledges that there are important changes in the Act:

- At committal proceedings the defence no longer have the right to call the child to give live evidence and must make do with a written statement (hence the child is not cross-examined twice).
- The Director of Public Prosecutions may serve 'notice of transfer' in child abuse cases and bypass the committal stage altogether.
- Competency: children under the age of 14 years shall give unsworn evidence.

In effect, the judge may continue to rule a witness incompetent and advise the jury to ignore the child's evidence if he or she is incoherent or fails to communicate in a way that makes sense. It is currently unclear whether the court will also disqualify children who do not understand the duty to tell the truth, which was the hurdle felt by many to be inappropriate for young witnesses and hence the advice of Pigot that the competence requirement should be dispensed with.

The Children Act 1991 makes young children competent in civil cases.

Cross-examination of the child has altered in that an unrepresented defendant loses the right to cross-examine the child him- or herself. But the trauma of a cross-examination of an abused child, up to 2 years after the initial interview, remains.

The Pigot Committee proposed a scheme where the child would first have been examined by a trained expert and the interview videotaped. The defence would see the tape and if the case was contested the defence would cross-examine the child before a judge in chambers at a pre-trial hearing and this too would be videotaped. At trial the first tape would have replaced the child's live examination in chief, the second the child's cross-examination. The child would therefore have given initial evidence in less formal circumstances and have dropped out of the trial at an early stage.

The Home Office's scheme has prevailed and although an initial videotape of an interview with a child becomes admissible, as a new exception to the hearsay rule, it is only on condition that the child attends court to be cross-examined there (Spencer 1991a,b).

In order to attempt to relieve some of the stress on the child, early trial dates are to be sought and children may give evidence on 'live-link' video apparatus or be screened from the defendant in court (for children under 14 years).

The failure to implement Pigot's scheme means that few children will give evidence, and fewer still will give evidence successfully, breaking down under cross-examination, traumatised by the abuse and then by the legal process (Spencer et al 1990). In court

> '. . . over half of the children showed signs of tension and one third were very unhappy . . .' (Davies 1995).

Davies & Noon (1991) found that 25% of questioning was not age-appropriate, and 17% of defence barristers consistently used inappropriate language. The Royal Commission on Criminal Justice 1993 recommended that judges be 'particularly vigilant to check unfair and intimidatory cross-examination by counsel of distressed or vulnerable witnesses'. Perhaps this needs stating at each court before any trial begins?

Children may be prepared by going to the court pre-trial and having a private place to wait, the judge and lawyers may remove their wigs, screens or a videolink may be used, but still many children will not be heard, as the low successful prosecution rate testifies.

Parents and professionals also remain anxious about the short- and longer-term effects of giving evidence. Children show anxiety before going to court (and trials may be delayed as long as 2 years) and it is at least a further 12 months after the trial before their anxiety symptoms are comparable with those of abused children who did not give evidence. If the alleged abuser is convicted this may be therapeutic but if the abuser is acquitted, for whatever reason, the child may feel he or she has been publicly shown to be a liar.

Therapy for the child may start before the trial if necessary but the CPS should be informed and the nature of the therapy explained. This may lead to 'contamination of the evidence' as viewed by the court, but it is increasingly accepted that the welfare of the child is the most important consideration.

Other evidence

Pre-recorded videos have been used for several years already, particularly in wardship courts. This use has caused controversy, especially when child psychiatrists have videotaped sessions as part of usual practice and the disclosure of abuse has been made during a therapeutic rather than an investigative interview. This has led to criticism in courts of technique, particularly the use of leading questions and more complex hypothetical questions. Doubt has also been expressed as to the amount of pressure put on children during sessions. It has, though, to be acknowledged that some adults put a lot of pressure on children not to talk, with threats of violence, even death, and therapists may be confronted with a silent 'frozen' child who will only be helped by unburdening him- or herself; in such a case simple questioning is not enough.

Protocols have been written and different techniques are used by those interviewing children in different circumstances. For example, a social worker and a police officer taking part in a routine child abuse investigation will not use the techniques necessary for the sophisticated interview of the frozen child disclosing abuse after years of silence, conducted by a child psychiatrist or psychologist with a particular interest in child abuse.

In the future it may be appropriate to have a video camera available in all rooms where possible abused children are interviewed and examined. Children not infrequently disclose during or after a physical examination, and the spontaneity of such a disclosure makes it particularly valuable.

Techniques of interviewing are not described in detail here but authoritative works are those of Jones & McQuiston (1988) and the chapters on interviewing and assessment of sexually abused children in a description of the work of the Great Ormond Street Sexual Abuse Team (Bentovim et al 1988), and Furniss (1991) on the preparation for disclosure and the management of disclosure of child sexual abuse.

The Recommendations of the Report into Child Abuse in Cleveland 1987 includes the paragraph:

> Children should not be subjected to repeated interviews nor to the probing and confrontational type of 'disclosure' interview for the same purpose, for it in itself can be damaging and harmful to them (Butler-Sloss 1988, p. 245).

This advice has been taken into account by investigators – there is a place for straightforward interviews of the type many social workers and police officers (from Child Abuse Units) do routinely. It is also clear from recent complex cases in the UK that more highly trained interviewers are also needed and workers skilled in more specialised techniques are required to undertake this work. Such interviewers are likely to be social workers, psychologists or psychiatrists who have developed a particular interest in this aspect of child abuse. Poorly conducted interviews will hinder rather than help child protection.

The Cleveland Report also states.

> Children should not be subjected to repeated medical examinations, solely for evidential purposes (Butler-Sloss 1988, p. 245).

This puts a burden on the doctor to ensure that not only must the initial medical examination be thorough, but it must also be properly recorded. Children do not like being physically examined, yet in order to protect them the examination should yield as much information as possible. Clearly written medical notes with a good description of physical signs, annotated diagrams and clinical photographs should provide such a record and obviate the need for further examinations. A further medical opinion may be obtained from scrutinising the notes rather than the child. If interviews are taped, children may also be spared repeated questioning.

Child abuse and the criminal injuries compensation scheme

A scheme for compensating victims of violent crime was first established in the UK in 1964. The Criminal Injuries Compensation Board considers claims where the applicant has sustained 'personal injury directly attributable to a crime of violence'. Physical assault and sexual abuse are both considered crimes of violence whether the child sexual abuse is indecent assault or rape, incest or buggery. The injury may also be psychological trauma due to the crime of violence.

There is a time limit of 2 years from the time of the assault to make the claim, but 'we adopt a sympathetic attitude towards late claims made within a reasonable time of reaching age 18 (Stationery Office 1997). No claims are valid for events that occurred before 1979.

The tariff of injuries is from level 1 to level 16 (£1000–17 500), although this is negotiable. The lowest level is for 'minor abuse – bruising beyond ordinary chastisement' or 'minor indecent assault – non-penetrative indecent physical act over clothing' (CICA 1996).

It is not necessary that the offender has been convicted before an award is made. The Board has to 'be satisfied on the balance of probability that the event alleged actually occurred' and this will be much easier of the police have been informed.

If the alleged offender abuser lives in the same household the Board has to be satisfied that he or she will not benefit from the award.

The claim is made on behalf of children up to the age of 18 years by the adults who have parental rights. This may be the child's parents or, if the child has been abused at home, the director of social services, or, for a ward, the court. Enquiries are made by the Board of police, doctors and social workers to gain information on the full circumstances of the assault, the extent of the injury and the prognosis. The payment is assessed on the same basis as damages in the civil courts and is usually awarded as a lump sum.

Application forms and further details are available from the Board. Although doctors are not in a position to claim for a child they may suggest to a parent or social worker that a claim is in order, as most children are still not compensated. Doctors will also be asked to fill in the inquiry forms, for a small fee.

The law – the Children Act 1989

The Children Act 1989 is a comprehensive piece of legislation which integrates and simplifies the law regarding children. It was implemented in October 1991. In terms of child protection the Act seeks to strike a balance between family in-dependence and the protection of children, recognising that the welfare of the child is paramount whilst ensuring fairness for parents and emphasising family upbringing (Shepherd 1991).

Main points of the Children Act 1989 (child protection aspects)

- The Act is comprehensive, and consolidates earlier law dealing with children
- It was implemented in October 1991
- It seeks to be 'user-friendly', i.e. comprehensible
- The upbringing of children is primarily the responsibility of parents
- A balance between child protection and undue interference in family life is sought
- Child protection is improved by the introduction of Child Assessment Orders and lower threshold for Emergency Protection Orders
- Emergency Protection Order may be challenged in court after 72 hours by parents
- In courts 'the child's welfare is paramount'
- A court order should not be made unless it is better for the child than not making an order
- A timetable will be set by the court to avoid undue delay

The impetus for change came from the recognition that the law was unnecessarily complex, parents felt they had inadequate rights when social services departments thought their children were at risk, and social services departments felt they had inadequate powers to intervene effectively when children were at risk (DoH 1991).

The Children Act does not alter the adversarial system in English courts which many childcare professionals find destructive to the overall management of cases of child abuse, often causing an unnecessary degree of polarisation of children, families and professionals.

Public and private law relating to children are brought together under the Children Act.

- *Public law* deals with those areas where society intervenes in the action of individuals (such as care proceedings).
- *Private law* addresses the behaviour of adults towards each other (such as with whom the children should live following divorce).

The main principles of the Children Act 1989 are (Home Office 1991):

- The welfare of the child is the paramount consideration in court proceedings.
- Wherever possible children should be brought up and cared for within their own family.
- Children should be safe and protected by effective intervention if they are in danger.
- When dealing with children, courts should ensure that delay is avoided, and may only make an order if to do so is better than making no order at all.
- Children should be kept informed about what happens to them, and should participate when decisions are made about their future.
- Parents continue to have parental responsibility for their children, even when their children are no longer living with them. They should be kept informed about their children and participate when decisions are made about their children's future.
- Parents with children in need should be helped to bring up their children themselves.
- This help should be provided as a service to the child and his or her family, and should:
  - be provided in partnership with the parents
  - meet each child's identified needs
  - be appropriate to the child's race, culture, religion and language
  - be open to effective, independent representations and complaints procedures
  - draw upon effective partnership between the local authority and other agencies, including voluntary agencies.

Child protection

The Children Act 1989 contains a new framework for the care and protection of children. It introduces new orders for use when children are at risk of significant harm. Care and supervision orders remain, but the grounds have been rationalised. There are new provisions to enable local education authorities to take action where children are not receiving proper education.

Significant harm

Under the Children Act 1989, harm is defined as ill-treatment or impairment of health or development. Ill-treatment may be physical, sexual or emotional ill-treatment of the child. The Children Act requires the court to be satisfied as to the occurrence of significant harm, or the likelihood of it, and its causes before making a care or supervision order (Hobbs 1991). Courts will define over the next few years what is meant by significant harm (see later).

Figure 17.3 (White 1991) illustrates the criteria used in assessing harm. The court will then find if the 'threshold criteria' (of significant harm) have been met, but this does not mean that a care or supervision order will necessarily be made. Other orders, for example under section 8 of the Act may be made (see below).

- Ill-treatment of the child is sufficient in itself to satisfy the criteria.
- It is not necessary to show that impairment of health or development follows the ill-treatment.

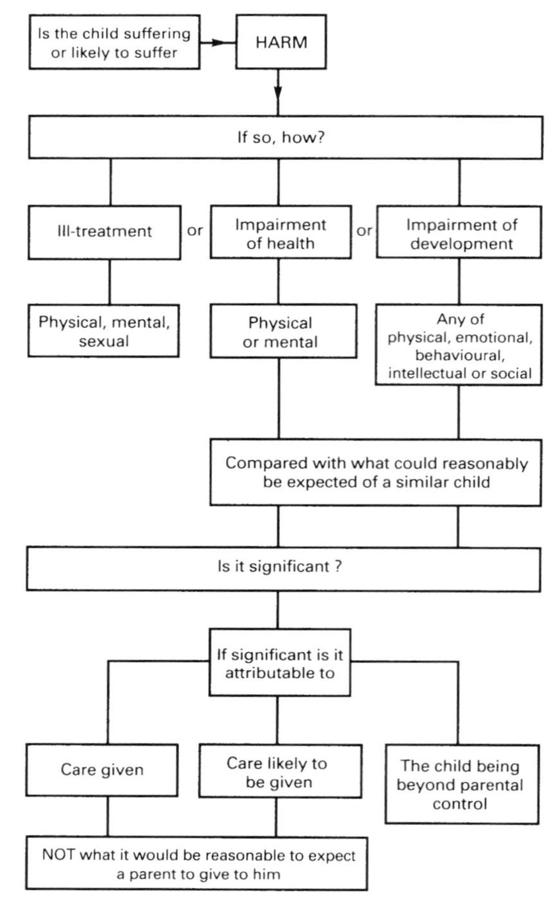

Fig. 17.3 Significant harm criteria (White 1991).

- The court may wish to identify who ill-treated the child – did the carer harm the child or fail to prevent harm?
- Impairment of development includes physical, intellectual, emotional or behavioural development.
- Significant harm is thought to mean considerable or important (case law will elucidate this further).
- Existence of past harm is not in itself sufficient to meet the criteria, although it may be relevant as to whether further harm is likely.
- Probability of further harm is not yet defined but means a risk greater than a possibility – that which on the balance of probability is likely (White 1991).
- The court also has to find that the harm is attributable to the care given, or likely to be given (by the carers).
- The care which the court expects parents to give is that standard which reasonable parents could be expected to provide (with appropriate support from community-wide services).
- The care expected may not be of a lower standard because the parents are unintelligent, alcoholic, drug abusers or otherwise disadvantaged.
- If the child has particular needs because of behaviour or handicap the court may require a higher standard of care than for an average child.

The paediatrician's assessment of significant harm

The contribution of the paediatrician in an individual case will vary (Lynch 1991). The evidence of harm (Fig. 17.3) caused by:

- ill-treatment (physical, mental, sexual)
- impairment of health (physical or mental)
- impairment of development (physical, emotional, behavioural, intellectual or social)

may be assessed by a paediatrician with skills in the recognition of:
  - child abuse (physical, sexual)
  - manifestations of child neglect and emotional deprivation
  - growth failure
  - developmental disorders.

The law wants evidence that:

- the child is suffering or likely to suffer significant harm
- the harm is attributable to care given or likely to be given to the child
- the making of an order is better for the child than making no order.

A paediatrician should be in a position to give an overall view of the child, the abuse and the child's needs. The court wishes to obtain from the paediatrician:

- the assessment of the child's condition
- an opinion as to the reason or reasons for that condition
- advice on a management plan
- the likely prognosis.

Hobbs (1991) makes the important point that the severity of injury does not necessarily correlate with the seriousness of harm and it is the psychological component of a child's care which is the central issue. An abused child may not grow, develop intellectually or learn to love, and an assessment of the child's past and current condition (growth charts, developmental progress, emotional/behavioural state) gives a multifaceted view.

Harm and abuse may be well hidden, particularly in child sexual abuse; because a child appears to be doing well at school, and the family is not apparently dysfunctional, does not mean that the child is not suffering. It means, though, that the harm from abuse must be balanced with the effect of an intervention in the family.

The courts

Family Courts with a non-adversarial and an inquisitorial ethos, which many feel would be the next appropriate development in child and family matters, are not established. The Act creates 'the court' which includes the High Court, the County Court and the Magistrates Court. The High Court already has a Family Division and in the lower courts Family Proceedings Courts are also now established.

All applications for care and supervision orders will start at the Magistrates Court, and most will be heard there. If, however, there is reason to transfer the case to the County or High Court, an order is made to that effect. Depending on their complexity or seriousness cases may move within 'the court'. Access to the wardship jurisdiction of the High Court will be restricted to those truly exceptional cases which cannot be accommodated in the lower courts.

The child

The main principle of the Children Act 1989 is that the child's welfare must be the paramount consideration of the court. The court must ensure that the child's wishes and feelings are known before coming to any decision. Consideration must also be given to the child's racial origin and cultural and linguistic background.

An order should not be made, even if the grounds are established in care proceedings, unless this is better for the child than not making an order. It is also acknowledged that delay in making decisions about a child's upbringing is likely to prejudice the child's welfare.

A 'welfare check list' sets out the relevant factors to be taken into account by the court when considering care proceedings and contested family proceedings. Children's lives will be determined by four additional types of order available in family proceedings (Section 8 orders; Table 17.4) as well as case and supervision orders.

The court's welfare checklist

- The wishes of the child
- The child's physical, emotional and educational needs
- The likely effect on the child of any change in circumstances
- The child's age, sex, background and any characteristic the court considers relevant
- Any harm the child has suffered or is at risk of suffering
- How capable are the parents or any other potential carers

The parents

Parents are responsible for looking after their children, and local authorities have a duty to support them. The concept of parental responsibility is used instead of parental rights. Children are individuals and parents are expected to meet

Table 17.4 Orders under Section 8 of the Children Act 1989

Residence Order	Where children will live
Contact Order	Who will have access
Specific Steps Order	Determining parental responsibility
Prohibited Steps Order	Steps not to be taken without the leave of the court

their child's needs whether moral, physical or emotional. Separated parents continue to share this responsibility, and unmarried fathers will find it easier to share parental responsibility under the Act.

The care which parents are expected to provide for their children is that of a 'reasonable parent'. The standard of care which is reasonable for a normal, healthy child may not be reasonable if the child has special needs, for example cystic fibrosis. That a parent is physically disabled or intellectually slow is not relevant as long as the child receives reasonable care. However, if a disabled parent by virtue of disability cannot cope, whether the parent seeks or accepts help or not, this is unreasonable and grounds for an order.

When children are living away from home because their parents cannot care for them properly this is preferably a voluntary arrangement. The parents then retain responsibility and act as partners with the local authority. If a child is under a care order the local authority has parental responsibility and the power to prescribe the parents' responsibility but only as far as is necessary whilst safeguarding the child's welfare. The local authority shares parental responsibility with any parents or guardian as far as possible.

The local authority

The local authority has a duty to safeguard and promote the welfare of children 'in need' in its area and promote their upbringing by their families. The social services may ask for help from housing, health and education authorities, with the expectation that they will receive it.

Children's services plans are now a statutory requirement of the Department of Health (England and Wales 1997) with respect to services for children in need. The focus has shifted away from crisis-led intervention to needs-led intervention (where possible). Examples are:

- educational needs of looked-after children
- children with diabetes (a register should be maintained)
- mental health services
- drugs action team
- children living in poverty.

Child protection

The Act aims to protect children from harm, which may be from failure or abuse within the family or the harm which can be caused by 'unwarranted intervention in family life' (Fig. 17.4).

Before a court will make an order it must be satisfied of certain preconditions:

- that the child is suffering or is likely to suffer significant harm which is attributable to the care he is receiving from his parents, or
- that the child is beyond parental control.

The definition of harm includes physical or sexual abuse as well as other forms of maltreatment which do not cause physical injury.

What is significant harm?

- Compare the child's health and development with that of a similar child
- The care given by the parents should be what might reasonably be expected
- Minor shortcomings in care or deficits in development may have a cumulative effect which results in significant harm

However, the court will also consider, in making an order, whether it will be in the child's best interests and positively contribute to his or her well-being.

The courts have discretion, subject to the above preconditions, to:

- order the assessment of a child
- order the removal or retention of a child in an emergency
- order that a child be put under local authority care or supervision pending a full investigation and hearing of the proceedings
- order that the child be put under the longer-term supervision of a local authority
- make private law orders altering the arrangements about with whom the child

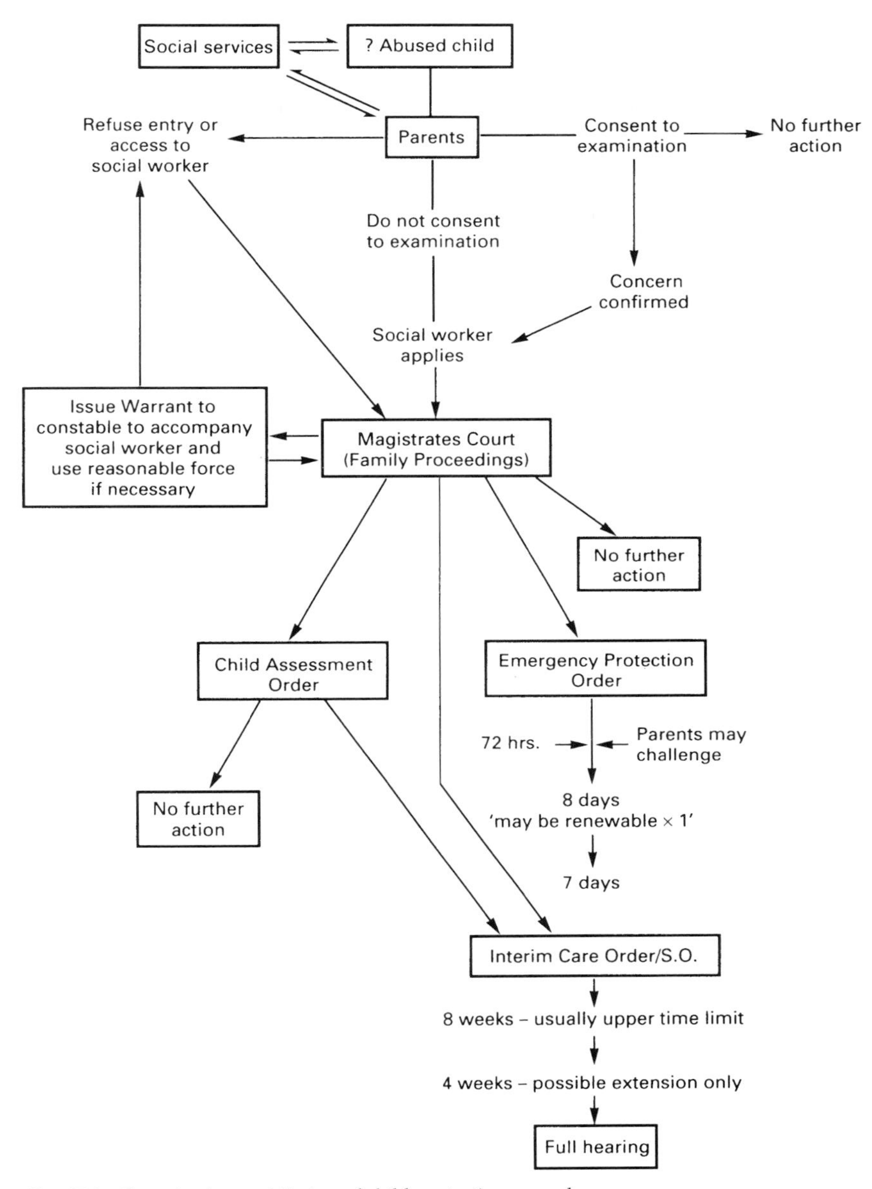

Fig. 17.4 Organisation and timing of child protection procedures.

lives, regulating the child's contact with other people, determining any particular matter relating to the child's upbringing and prohibiting any particular step being taken in respect of him or her.

Court orders which may be made

Emergency Protection Orders

The precondition of an Emergency Protection Order is that there is reasonable cause to believe that the child is likely to suffer significant harm unless

- the child is removed from where he or she is to another place
- the child is kept where he or she is
- the parents unreasonably withhold access to the child and there is reason to believe that access is required as a matter of urgency.

The order may last for 8 days, and can be extended once for a period of 7 days. It may be challenged at 72 hours by the parents if they were not present at the initial hearing. There is a presumption of reasonable parental access during this period and if the social worker becomes satisfied that the child would be safe he or she should go home.

Any person may apply to the court for an Emergency Protection Order although it would usually be a social worker employed by the local authority.

Child Assessment Order

A Child Assessment Order is used when the parents are uncooperative and there is a need to decide whether significant harm is likely but there is not an emergency. Notice is given to all those involved and a full hearing takes place so that all sides can be represented.

If an order is made, it lasts 7 days; it does not give parental responsibility to the holder and the court directs what the assessment should be. It is acknowledged that 7 days may not be long enough to complete a full multidisciplinary assessment but after this period enough should be known to enable decisions to be made as to further action, if any.

An application may be made by a local authority or NSPCC social worker.

Interim Care and Supervision Order

The preconditions for making an Interim Care or Supervision Order are as for a Care Order, except that the court only has to conclude that there are reasonable grounds for believing the circumstances fulfil the conditions rather than being satisfied on the balance of probabilities that they do (see previously for the grounds).

A first Interim Care Order or Supervision order may last for 8 weeks but subsequent orders may not last more than 4 weeks. The court may also, when making an Interim Care Order, make an order regarding contact or a medical examination. It is expected that the final hearing will be held within 12 weeks.

Care and Supervision Orders

The preconditions for these orders have been given previously. Supervision Orders last 12 months in the first instance but may be renewed for a period of up to 3 years in total.

Non-attendance at school is no longer in itself grounds for a Care Order – the usual grounds must exist. The local education authority may, however, apply for an Educational Supervision Order. The supervising education officer has powers to give directions to children and parents to ensure the child receives a proper education. Committing offences is no longer grounds for care but if the child is already subject to a Supervision Order the court may require him to live away from home for a period of 6 months.

Before a Care Order is made the court must consider the proposed arrangements for contact (access) and all the parties' views on these arrangements.

When *young people leave care* the local authorities have increased duties and powers to prepare, advise and assist them. The duty to advise and assist extends until the age of 21 years.

Guardians ad litem are appointed in almost all care and related proceedings but also in applications for Emergency Protection or Child Assessment Orders.

Evidence and procedural matters

The Children Act gave the Lord Chancellor power to provide by order for hearsay evidence to be admissible in civil proceedings relating to children. From March 1990 hearsay evidence was allowed in Juvenile Court or civil proceedings. The Act also enables the court to hear the unsworn evidence of a child in all civil proceedings if the child understands the duty to speak the truth and has sufficient understanding to justify his or her evidence being heard.

The rules of privacy have been altered under the Act in that a Magistrates Court may sit in private in the same way as the High and County Courts already do. It is an offence for television and radio as well as newspapers to publish material which will allow a child to be identified.

Implications of the Children Act for health authorities

Children's doctors will need to have knowledge of the Children Act whether they work with children with special needs, abused children or children in care, adoption of children or other children living away from home. An excellent summary of the Act has been published (HMSO 1989), the full Act with interpretation (White et al 1990), and training advice (Training Together 1990, DoH 1991).

The major issues are:

- working together – interagency cooperation
- medical input – examination, assessment, treatment
- care of children by health authorities
- training (Butler-Sloss 1988, p. 252).

Working together

As has been discussed previously, all agencies involved in child protection must work together, but this is equally true for children with special needs and their families. This is emphasised in the Act.

Medical input

Medical and psychiatric examinations, assessment and treatment may be directed by the court from the earliest stage of the proceedings, that is if a child is subject to an Emergency Protection Order, an Interim Care Order or Child Assessment Order.

Care of children by health authorities

The Act also seeks to protect the welfare of children who spend long periods in health or education authority or private homes or hospitals. The local authority must be informed of such children by the health authority or owner of private establishments. The local authority is then required to see not only that the child's welfare needs are met but to promote contact with his family and to rehabilitate home if appropriate.

Training

Training is needed not only by individual agencies but also by multidisciplinary groups to ensure that policy in each district develops along sound lines.

Consent

- The situation for consent is clarified in that, once a child is the subject of a court order, parental responsibility and hence the right to give consent goes to the applicant (usually the social services department).
- Emergency treatment is much as previously – a carer who does not have parental responsibility may 'do what is reasonable in the circumstances for the purpose of safeguarding or promoting the child's welfare'. The carer could be anyone caring for the child, and indeed in life-threatening circumstances a doctor would act immediately without consent.
- If parents unreasonably refuse an examination, and the grounds are met, a Child Assessment Order may be made and the court directs the examination.
- If parents – both having parental responsibility for the child and whether married, unmarried, separated or divorced – cannot agree whether to consent to examination or treatment the court could make a Specific Issues Order to determine the matter.
- The child's consent is necessary for psychiatric or medical examination, if he has

sufficient understanding to make an informed decision. A child who refuses to give consent may not be overruled by his or her parents or the court.

Consent

- Who has the right to consent?
- Is the child subject to a court order?
- What are the directions of the court?
- Who has parental responsibility?
- Will the assessment be used in court proceedings?
- What are the views of the child? Has a guardian *ad litem* been appointed?
- Does the child have any difficulty in communicating for which special arrangements need to be made?

Court orders

- The courts have increased powers to authorise the medical or psychiatric examination of children either at the time the order is made or during the course of Emergency Protection Orders, Child Assessment Orders or Interim Care Orders. The court may also prohibit medical examination or assessment of the child. This should stop unnecessary examination once an adequate assessment has been carried out.
- Many children will be examined with parental consent before an Emergency Protection Order is made but if this examination is likely to be controversial the applicant for the order may ask for court directions. Similarly, the initial examination may make it clear that a more detailed assessment is needed and this may also be directed by the court when making the order.
- The Child Assessment Order allows for 'a multidisciplinary assessment in a non-emergency situation' over 7 days. This will allow information to be gathered to enable further decision-making to occur: are the concerns confirmed or refuted? Longer periods of assessment, including full psychiatric and family assessments, are likely to take place during Interim Care or Supervision Orders.
- Treatment Orders can only be made by the court on the advice of a registered medical practitioner or psychiatrist registered under the Mental Health Act, and if the child consents and if satisfactory arrangements can be made. Any change in treatment plan should be referred back to the court.

Timing

The Act recognises that delays may be detrimental to the child, and courts will set timetables (see Fig. 17.4). There are clear resource implications involved in the courts directing that medical and psychiatric assessments are to be completed. If priority is given to the orders even less preventative work will be done with children and families. Similarly, if professionals spend longer periods in court they will have less time with their other patients.

Summary

1. The legal system in the UK continues to serve the requirements of adults rather than those of children.
2. Children will not be 'heard' in the criminal justice system until the rules of cross examination are radically revised.

3. The age of criminal responsibility, (10-years-old in England and Wales, eight-years-old in Scotland) is lower in the UK than the rest of Europe. The withdrawal of '*doli incapax*', which gave partial protection to children aged between 10 and 13-years-old denies what is evident – that a child, by definition, is immature and many children who commit crimes are 'in need' and require a therapeutic and educational programme that may allow them to progress, whereas punishment further damages and retards social responsibility.
4. Most doctors dislike giving evidence – good preparation is essential – and remember – don't get angry! You know much more about children than your protagonists.

REFERENCES

Anderson L C 1990 Physician expert testimony. In: Wissow L S (ed) Child advocacy for the clinician. Williams & Wilkins, Baltimore

Bentovim A, Elton A, Hildebrant J, Tranter M, Vizard E 1988 Child sexual abuse within the family: assessment and treatment. Wright, London

Butler-Sloss E 1988 Report of the Inquiry into Child Abuse in Cleveland 1987. HMSO, London

CICA 1996 Victims of crimes of violence, Issue 1, April 1996. Criminal Injuries Compensation Board, Glasgow

Davies G, Noon E 1991 An evaluation of the live link for child witnesses. Home Office, London

Davies G, Wilson C, Mitchell R, Milsom J 1995 Videotaping children's evidence: an evaluation. Home Office, London

DoH 1991 The Children Act 1989: an introductory guide for the NHS. Department of Health, London

Family Law 1997 The Expert Witness Pack. Jordan, Bristol

Furniss T 1991 The multiprofessional handbook on child sexual abuse. Routledge, London

HMSO 1989 An introduction to the Children Act 1989. HMSO, London

Hobbs C J 1991 Significant harm. Paper in Conference Report no. 6. Michael Sieff Foundation, London

Home Office 1989 Report of the Advisory Group on Video Evidence. HMSO, London

Jones D P H, McQuiston M G 1988 Interviewing the sexually abused child. Gaskell, London

Lynch 1991 Significant harm: the paediatric contribution. In: Adcock M et al (eds) Significant harm. Significant Publications, London

Pigot Report 1989 Advisory Group on Video Evidence (Pigot Report) 1989. HMSO, London

Plotnikoff J, Woolfson R 1995 Prosecuting Child Abuse. An evaluation of the Governments' speedy progress policies. Blackstone, London

Shepherd S 1991 Aspects of the Children Act – a medical perspective. Health Trends 23(2)

Spencer J 1991a Reformers despair. New Law Journal June 7 1991:787(b)

Spencer J 1991b Children's evidence and the Criminal Justice Act: a lost opportunity. The Magistrate Nov 1991:181–182(a)

Spencer J, Flin R 1993 The evidence of children: the law and psychology. Blackstone, London

Spencer J, Nicholson G, Flin I R, Bull R 1990 Children's evidence in legal proceedings. Law Faculty, University of Cambridge

SSI 1994 The child, the court and the video. Social Services Inspectorate, Department of Health, London

Stationery Office 1997 TS 10 April 1997

Training Together 1990 The Children Act 1989: training together. Family and Child Care Law Training Group, London

Vizard E 1991 Interviewing children suspected of being sexually abused. in: Hollin C R, Howell K (eds) Clinical approaches to sex offenders and their victims. J Wiley, Chichester

Vizard E 1997 The work of the Expert Witness Group. Child Psychology and Psychiatry Review 2(3):131

Wall N 1997 Judicial attitudes to expert evidence in children's cases. Archives of Disease in Childhood 76(6):485–486

Wattam C 1995 The investigative process. in: Wilson K, James A(eds) The child protection handbook. Balliére Tindall, London

West Yorkshire Police 1992 Child Abuse Statistics. Report 1989/1990/1991

White R 1991 Significant harm: its management and outcome. In: Adcock M et al (eds) Significant harm. Significant Publications, London

White R, Carr P, Lowe N 1990 A guide to the Children Act 1989. Butterworths, London

Working Together 1991 Working Together under the Children Act 1989: a guide to the arrangements for interagency cooperation for the protection of children from abuse. DHSS and Welsh Office. HMSO, London

ADDRESS

Criminal Injuries Compensation Board, Whittington House, 19 Alfred Place, London WC1E 7LG: Tel 0171 636 9501; Blythswood House, 200 West Regent Street, Glasgow G2 4SW: Tel 0141 221 0945

18

Fatal child abuse

There is plenty of historical evidence that the practice of infanticide was a widespread form of disposal of unwanted children over the ages. Accounts of children being exposed on mountain tops, thrown into pools to see if they would float, or being actively killed are all well known. Illegitimate children who would bring disgrace upon the mother and handicapped children who might pass on their defects if allowed to live were especially vulnerable. It is also likely that many more children died from starvation and neglect as their parents did not have the means to support the numbers of children to which even a moderately healthy woman can give birth in her reproductive life.

In modern times death from child abuse and neglect remains a major cause of mortality. Controversy continues to surround this area and this is reflected in the debate over the epidemiology of fatal child abuse.

Child homicide and fatal abuse

Various authors suggest that child homicide and fatal abuse are distinct entities (Greenland 1987, Gelles 1991, Browne & Lynch 1995) Homicide is seen as 'usually the result of a single fatal assault' whereas a death from child abuse 'usually occurs in association with assault and neglect over a much longer period' (Falkov 1996). There is likely to be overlap between the two.

In this chapter the two terms are used interchangeably.

Epidemiology of fatal child abuse

An increasing number of people are being murdered by strangers. The most common method of murder is strangulation of women and stabbing of men, and the most vulnerable group to be murdered are babies under the age of 1 year (Rose 1990). Murder of people of all ages has become more common in society, figures rising from around 250 deliberate killings per year in the 1950s to around 750 per year in England, Scotland and Wales at the present time. This is only a fraction of the annual total for the USA. There, child homicide accounts for about 5% of all child deaths (aged 1–17) and 1% of deaths in those aged 18 or over (Wissow 1990).

In England and Wales between 11 and 25% of homicide victims are children and in the majority of cases the perpetrator is a parent. Although much feared and widely publicised, abduction and murder by a stranger is relatively rare. In 1984–93, 57 children were murdered by strangers – between 5 and 6 per year (Browne & Lynch 1995). In fact more child murders occur in the home. 42% of all murders and manslaughters at all ages are related to domestic disputes.

Approximate figures for child abuse deaths are (Central Statistical Office 1994):

- USA: 5 children per day killed by care givers
- UK: 1–2 children per week killed by care givers

From the figures that are available, it appears that infant and child homicide deaths have remained stable over the last 20 years (Home Office 1994, Creighton 1995), although there are fluctuations in rate from year to year. In 1991, newspaper reports identified 99 children (44% boys, 56% girls) under 16 years who died of non-accidental injury in England, Wales and Scotland (*Independent on Sunday* 1992). The majority of perpetrators were related to their victim (Table 18.1). The risk of death increases with diminishing age, as shown in Table 18.2.

Table 18.1 Perpetrators of domestic and child homicides (Browne et al 1995)

Fathers and stepfathers	49%
Mothers	33%
Brothers and sisters	4%
Boyfriends and girlfriends	4%
Unrelated to the child	17%
Males	65%
Females	35%
Single perpetrator	94%
Strangled, suffocated or smothered	41%
Committed in family home	64%
Assailants committed suicide after the murder	16%
Children under 5 years	59%

Table 18.2 UK child homicides in 1992

Age group	Total	Number of offences per million children
Infants (under 1 year)	38	48
Toddlers (1–4)	25	8
Children (5–15)	40	5
Total children (<16)	103	61

Infanticide is legally defined as

> the killing of a child under the age of 12 months by the child's mother when the balance of her mind is disturbed because she had not fully recovered from the effect of childbirth or lactation (Infanticide Act 1938).

Filicide refers to killing of a child by either parent. The law is much more lenient in its handling of mothers who kill their children than fathers. Most mothers convicted of infanticide are given a probation order with a psychiatric treatment recommendation. Fathers are more likely to receive custodial sentences.

What are the factors which lead parents to kill their children?

Wilczynski (1995) classified filicide into various categories of motive, based on the perpetrators' statements to the police:

- *Retaliation*: usually displaced anger on to the child, often meant for the person's partner. These killings occurred in a background of severe marital conflict including domestic violence.

- *Jealousy* of, or *rejection* by the child. Men usually committed these killings. The man felt resentful because it was not his child, or the child received too much attention from the mother, or the child appeared rejecting of the perpetrator.
- *Unwanted child*: usually involve the mother. The child was unplanned or unwanted from conception. Includes neonaticides. Handicapped children may be among the older unwanted children with feelings of rejection developing after birth.
- *Discipline killings* follow attempts to discipline the child for behaviour which the parent finds irritating.
- *Altruistic killings*: of children who are suffering, or with parents who have distorted perceptions of themselves.
- *Psychotic parents.*
- *Factitious illness by proxy* (see Ch. 12).
- *Sexual, ritual or organised abuse.*
- *Self-defence*: obviously very uncommon.

Falkov (1996) found that parental psychiatric morbidity was common in fatal or near fatal child abuse. Part 8 of Working Together (1991) reports that, out of 100 cases, evidence of psychiatric illness in the parent who killed or in their partner was found in 32 reviews (25 perpetrators, 10 partners). The majority in both groups were mothers. Four out of five of these 'psychiatric' cases had pre-existing child protection concerns and in two-thirds there had been a child protection conference. The primary psychiatric diagnosis in order of frequency was:

- psychosis (40%)
- depression (20%)
- personality disorder (20%)
- factitious illness by proxy (8%).

There was a noteworthy lack of puerperal psychosis (one case) and alcohol-related problems.

Drug dependence was more common. Children of all ages appear to have been killed where there was parental mental illness.

The findings of this study underline the need for cooperation to develop between adult mental health services and childcare agencies. There is only a limited tradition of this in the UK.

Under-reporting of deaths from child abuse

Official figures are likely to underestimate the true scale of fatal child abuse; in cases where the findings are in any way doubtful the parents will be given the benefit of the doubt because of the tragic circumstances which accompany the death of a child.

Deaths from child abuse are notoriously difficult to quantify. There has been a long debate over the incidence of fatal child abuse. Jobling (1976) wrote

> estimates of children who die each year from their injuries range from 100 to 750. What the exact numbers might be has now become a controversial guessing game, some arguing that these figures are almost certainly an underestimate whereas others believe that the lower estimates are nearer the mark.

An analysis for 1974–83 of the International Classification of Disease (ICD) codes

- E904 hunger, thirst, exposure, neglect
- E960–969 homicide and injury purposely inflicted by other persons (includes E967 child battering and other maltreatment)
- E980–989 injury undetermined, whether accidentally or purposely inflicted,

revealed that on average over this period there were 138 deaths per year and an additional 50 deaths where violence played a part but death was recorded as from natural causes. Adjusting for the fact that 68% of deaths were caused by parents or care givers (although in another 20% by someone well known to the child), and allowing for 12 missed diagnoses, the figure of 156 deaths per year from child abuse or neglect at the hands of the parents was arrived at. The figure of three per week was adopted by the NSPCC in its publicity in the 1980s (Creighton 1984).

As in the USA, the rates for fatal abuse fall with age. In 1987 in the USA the rate was 6.15 per 100 000 under 1 year of age, 2.09 from 14 and 0.67 from 59. The rate was 1.24 from 10–14, and for 15–19 it rose dramatically to 8.32, reflecting the heightened vulnerability of teenagers (Wissow 1990).

The National Commission of Inquiry into the Prevention of Child Abuse noted that the situation with regard to information about deaths from child abuse remains as difficult as ever. Sources of information for child deaths from abuse come from various sources:

- criminal statistics
- Office of National Statistics
- child abuse death inquiries (Part 8 of Working Together 1991)
- confidential inquiries into stillbirths and deaths in infancy
- local studies.

> The problems of collating these statistics and the reluctance of professionals to make a diagnosis of death by abuse, results in an under-representation of such deaths in official statistics (Childhood Matters 1996).

In the USA others have started to explore further the links between abuse and neglect and child death. McClain et al (1993) used death certificate data to define six coding categories:

- explicitly child abuse and neglect deaths
- homicides
- injury deaths of undetermined intentionality (60–84%)
- accidental injury deaths (7–27%)
- sudden infant death syndrome (SIDS) fatalities (1.3%)
- natural cause deaths (6.1%).

Research studies and crime data were used to estimate the proportion of deaths that were actually due to abuse and neglect (figures in parentheses).

- Deaths from abuse and neglect showed estimated annual rates over the 10 years of up to 1814 in the age group 0–4 years, and 2022 in the age group 0–17 years.
- Around 90% of child abuse and neglect deaths occurred in children aged under 5 years, and 41% in infants, i.e. up to the first birthday.
- About 85% of deaths thought to be due to child abuse and neglect were not recorded as such, i.e. the overt component was only 15%.

This study confirms that officially reported child abuse and neglect deaths grossly underestimate the true occurrence. Death certificates are collected and recorded for a variety of legal and social purposes, not primarily for research. McClain et al (1993) point out that

> failure to suspect child abuse and neglect, uncertainty about definitions, and fear of recriminations may result in vague descriptions on death certificates leading in turn to miscoding of child abuse and neglect deaths as deaths due to natural causes, accidents, or injuries of undetermined intentionality.

In the USA a statewide system of child fatality review panels is developing. In Missouri (Ewigman et al 1993) in 4 years, 121 deaths from definite child abuse and neglect were identified, 25 from probable and 109 possible maltreatment. Only 47.9% of the definite cases could be identified from the ICD9 code on the death certificate. The other 63 cases were coded as accidents (27), SIDS (6), natural causes (14) and undetermined whether accidental or purposely inflicted injuries (16). The authors comment on the alarming under-reporting of maltreatment, a lack of basic skills in the investigators, failure to communicate findings to others and lack of access to other professionals' records as common findings. They also comment how easily maltreatment can be concealed, how the lack of a clear accepted definition of maltreatment and no uniformity of data collection and reporting procedures among health, social services and law enforcement agencies can influence acknowledgement of this problem.

Recognition of fatal child abuse

Clinical presentation of fatal child abuse

- Severely battered infant or child
- Unexpected death where occult injury is found
- Cot death presentation (death due to suffocation)
- Accidents where neglect is a major factor – child deliberately or passively left in dangerous situation e.g. drowning, house fire
- Deliberate poisoning
- Recurrent unexplained deaths
- Child death associated with sexual assault

Severely battered infant or child

The medical cause of deaths from severe battering is usually obvious and many of these cases have been the subject of public inquiries. In England, Maria Colwell, Kimberley Carlile, Jasmine Beckford and Tyra Henry are examples (DoH 1991). This form of lethal abuse has perhaps been studied more than any other. The picture that has emerged has been of the violent besieged family often in touch with but avoiding professional intervention, which frequently was unable to address the danger of the family situation for the child. More recently, Reder et al (1993) found that some children are accorded particular psychological meaning which places them at greater risk of severe maltreatment or death. Further, studies of these deaths indicates that many of the children were already known to child protection agencies and that the parents were young, poor and socially isolated (Greenland 1980). Warning signals and help-seeking behaviour had not been interpreted by child protection workers who lacked experience or appropriate training and whose practice could be characterised as showing an absence of assessment, goal-setting and effective communication with other professionals (Greenland 1980). These deaths have in many ways fuelled changes in the law as well as in professional practice.

Unexpected death where occult injury is found

Christoffel et al (1985) reviewed deaths at a paediatric teaching hospital in Chicago over 2 years. They identified 43 unexpected deaths (defined as deaths occurring before arrival at the hospital or within 10 days of hospitalisation in children past the first month of life and unrelated to any previously known congenital anomaly or medical condition). Of these, 27 were due to natural causes but nine were thought to be due to child abuse or neglect. In three of these cases injury was only discovered at autopsy. Deaths due to suspected child abuse and neglect were so categorised:

- if the child demonstrated inflicted or unexplained trauma
- if there had been inadequate supervision
- if there was probable delay in seeking care.

Two factors – dead on arrival and 1 year of age or less – had predictive value for child abuse.

The finding of an injury such as a fractured rib in an infant dying unexpectedly raises serious concerns if there is no obvious explanation for it.

Cot death presentation (suffocation)

Awareness of the reality of suffocation as a lethal form of child abuse has been sharpened by the use of covert videotaping of children being smothered in hospital by a parent (Southall et al 1987). A group of children who usually presented acutely to accident and emergency departments moribund or cyanosed, and who would recover with resuscitation or spontaneously, were called 'near miss cot deaths' or 'children with apparent life-threatening event' (ALTE). After admission to hospital such events would in some cases be observed on the ward, in others they might cease. It was with similar cases that videotaping demonstrated the smothering taking place.

CASE HISTORY 18.1

A 19-year-old mother became pregnant to a violent alcoholic boyfriend who had beaten her up. When her own family found out about the pregnancy they abandoned her although later there was some reconciliation. The mother herself had a history of failing to thrive as a child, of sexual abuse by an uncle as a teenager, and she was admitted to a children's home with behaviour problems at the age of 13. During early pregnancy she suffered from serious depression and was admitted to hospital at 32 weeks with vaginal bleeding. There were difficulties with accommodation and several moves. At 3 weeks of age the baby was admitted to hospital with a history of going blue. His mother said that he had become limp and floppy, and she needed to resuscitate him. During the admission the mother reported two further episodes but nothing untoward was noticed either on this or any subsequent occasion by the staff. The mother was described as anxious and found it difficult not to keep picking him up. She gave a history that her sister had recently had a cot death. She was discharged, but the baby was re-admitted at 8 weeks of age with further apnoeic attacks. Further investigation failed to reveal an adequate cause. The child was discharged; 3 days later he was admitted moribund and subsequently died. The infant had been monitored at home with an apnoea alarm, and this apparently had sounded as the mother entered the room. The history given was that the baby's face was blotchy and discoloured immediately the mother picked him up. The sequel to this tragic case was that the mother attempted suicide and required long-term psychiatric care. This case had a sense of inevitability about the outcome which staff looking after the mother and child expressed as a grave concern. In such cases there appears to be an open warning by the mother of impending disaster and the need is for support and acknowledgement of the risk.

There are links between this kind of abuse and factitious illness by proxy. Meadow (1990) reviewed 27 young children who, using strict criteria (confession, prosecution or video observation), were thought likely to have been suffocated. 18 children survived and 9 died. The important features included:

- sudden and unexpected deaths in previous siblings
- excess of boys in index and sibling groups
- near-miss cot death presentation
- petechiae on face or mouth, bruises to neck in a minority
- survival with handicap a possibility
- recurring attacks which failed to reveal a cause on extensive investigation
- pillow, pad of material or hand used
- many children outside the usual range for true SIDS cases, i.e. >6 months.

The concern that some infants found dead in their cots might have died from abuse due to suffocation has been raised from time to time. Historically one of the earliest published series of unexpected deaths in infants in the UK was by Templeman, a police surgeon from Dundee. He reported 258 cases, many of whom probably had features in common with today's cot deaths (Templeman 1892). He attributed these deaths to overlaying and the causes as:

- ignorance and carelessness of mothers
- drunkenness
- overcrowding
- according to some observers, illegitimacy and the (life) insurance of infants.

The association of sudden death in infancy and child abuse has always been a powerful issue affecting practice and research in this area. The association has been the subject of various recent reviews (Emery 1993, Reece 1993, AAP 1994). It is always important that clinical rigour is applied in making the diagnosis of sudden infant death syndrome (SIDS). In the US, the Committee on Child Abuse and Neglect of the American Academy of Pediatrics (AAP 1994) indicated that a death should only be ruled as due to SIDS when:

- a complete autopsy is done, including cranium and contents, and autopsy findings are compatible with SIDS
- there is no gross or microscopic evidence of head trauma, intracranial injury, cerebral

oedema, cervical cord injury, retinal haemorrhage, or mechanical asphyxia

- there is no evidence of trauma on skeletal survey
- other causes of death are adequately ruled out, including meningitis, sepsis, aspiration, pneumonia, myocarditis, abdominal trauma dehydration, fluid and electrolyte imbalance, significant congenital lesions, inborn metabolic disorders, carbon monoxide asphyxia, drowning or burns
- there is no evidence of current alcohol, drug, or toxic exposure.

The National Institute of Child Health and Human Development in the US has suggested an extended definition of SIDS to include a requirement for a scene of death examination and a review of the case history. This recommendation makes good sense in all cases of SIDS if the environment surrounding the child is thought to be of importance.

The establishment of the diagnostic category of SIDS has done a great deal to absolve parents and physicians alike from all sense of guilt, and has enabled bereavement care programmes to be established and funds to be obtained for research into the cause(s) of SIDS (Emery 1992). Emery also points out that SIDS as an entity does not exist and that there are many patterns of causes. As mentioned above, filicide is defined as child death caused by a parent and differs from infanticide which relates only to the mother and has a specific meaning in law. Emery (1985) estimated that filicide as the probable mechanism of death in unexplained, unexpected deaths could be as high as 1 in 10 or as low as 1 in 50 where the deaths were looked at on a more superficial level. This of course means that the majority of such deaths are not due to filicide.

Further evidence of an association between cot death and child abuse comes from the finding that the SIDS rate for siblings of children on the child abuse register in South Derbyshire was 15.6 per thousand births, whereas the national rate for SIDS was 2.0 and the local rate 3.1 (Newlands & Emery 1991). Detailed and long-term studies in another part of England of known abusive and neglectful families and kinships (Oliver 1983) revealed that, out of 147 families studied over 21 years, of 560 children, 41 had died (26 in the first year of life). In only three cases was there a criminal conviction and many cases would have fitted the SIDS category, had it then been in existence. More recently Hobbs et al (1995) found that issues of child abuse and neglect were common findings in unexpected deaths in infancy. Results of detailed local inquiry into 37 unexpected deaths, of which 28 were diagnosed as SIDS, revealed issues of abuse and neglect in 27 of which it was the major issue in 10. It was suggested that in order to facilitate diagnosis, a detailed jigsaw should be constructed (Table 18.3).

Accidents where neglect is a major factor

Childhood injury is now the major cause of mortality after infancy. Use of the term 'accident' has been criticised because it may imply an act of God rather that an event which arises out of a set of circumstances that may be modifiable or preventable. An 'injury event' may be a better term, inviting analysis of the factors responsible for its occurrence.

A notable example of the link between neglect and child death is seen in children dying in fires, either at home or in cars. Many children who die in these situations have been left alone in the house, including those of pre-school age. Gill (1984) reported the deaths of seven pre-school children left alone in conflagrations in 10 cars: seven other children who were burned survived. Interestingly, in conclusion Gill suggests that parents should be advised against leaving pre-school children alone in cars, as though this might otherwise be seen as reasonable childcare practice. Up to one-third or more children who die or are injured in house fires have been left alone at the time.

The law is more specific with regard to leaving young children unattended in the home. In an earlier study in London which looked at 24 child deaths in house fires, 10 children had been left alone or with other children in the house at the time. Because many parents in such situations are seen as victims of their own inadequacy,

Table 18.3 Jigsaw of fatal abuse in infancy (Reece 1993, Committee on Child Abuse & Neglect 1994) (permission required from John Wiley and Sons Ltd, *Child Abuse Review*)

Events around death	Death scene investigation	Other deaths	Post-mortem
How long child alone Parent reaction Delay in summoning help Unusual childcare practices Thermal environment Temperature control	Blood, clothing, bedding Signs of struggle Living conditions: • signs of neglect • reactions by carers • hostility • discord • accusations	Unexplained deaths in siblings, infant deaths in extended family	Time of death Injury, occult fractures on radiology Unrecognised illness Signs of neglect Suffocation Unusual chemistry Toxicology Failure to thrive
Family patterns	**Mother**	**Father**	**Parents' relationship**
Family dysfunction, incest, violence Multiple problems Poverty and not coping, Stresses ++ Frequent moves of address	Victim of abuse/neglect in care as child Difficulty with relationships, many partners, psychiatric history Unsupported as mother	Paternity unknown or unstated (?incest) Violent, in prison Main carer or absent, distant and uninvolved, unsupportive	Brief, unstable, violent, no room for child – threatens relationship
Child	**Attachment**	**Pregnancy**	**Siblings**
Unplanned, unwanted, wrong gender, one too many Doubtful paternity Seen as difficult, e.g. cries too much, ill or handicapped	Poor mother–child relationship Attachment insecure, anxious or ambivalent	Unplanned, late ante-natal booking Poor ante-natal care Birth outside hospital Concealment	Abuse/neglect, on child protection register Concerns re growth and development Previous death(s) Previous unexplained illness
Bereavement	**Social services**	**Police**	**Substance abuse**
Unusual response to the death	Previous case conference Children on child protection register Previous involvement	Criminal record Violence Parent is Schedule 1 offender	Major addiction in parent(s) Smoking, alcohol Self-abuse, suicide attempts

limited intellectual ability, poverty or other seemingly unavoidable factors, such deaths will officially be reported as accidental to spare the parents further suffering.

Safety neglect is defined as a situation where an injury occurs because of a gross lack of supervision (Schmitt 1981). It can be difficult to diagnose as there may be other factors responsible for behaviour which on the face of it might seem seriously neglectful. Single mothers with several children may have little option but to leave them alone briefly, particularly if an unexpected situation arises. In neglect it is the establishment of a regular pattern of inadequate parenting which is characteristic. Repeated accidents should be a warning sign that the child is at risk and be acted upon.

Another way in which neglect may be a major factor in child death is through a failure to seek appropriate medical care for an ill child. A well-known situation is that of the Jehovah's Witness family who, believing that blood transfusion is against the laws of God, prevent their child from having a life-saving transfusion. A much more commonly encountered situation is where a common illness in a neglected and weakened child (e.g. failing to thrive) is not adequately attended to, becomes serious, treatment is delayed and the child is admitted in a moribund state perhaps too late to avert disaster.

CASE HISTORY 18.2

An 11-month-old child died at home from measles. There had been long-standing concerns about this child and the other three older children because of failure to thrive, including delayed development thought to be the result of inadequate parenting.

Various agencies were involved in helping the family. Shortly before the youngest child died, the family moved area without letting the professional agencies know and into accommodation which was cold and sparsely furnished, in the middle of winter. The child was discovered dead in bed. Post-mortem showed advanced measles bronchopneumonia.

Deliberate poisoning (see Chapter 12)

Non-accidental poisoning as a form of child abuse has been recognised for some time (Kempe et al 1962, Rogers et al 1976). In a review of the literature (Dine & McGovern 1982) of 48 children intentionally poisoned, eight died (17%). These cases present in a variety of ways, making diagnosis a challenge. The fatal cases included the use of such diverse substances as pepper, which induced apnoea, table salt, phenformin and barbiturates. Paracetamol poisoning may induce fatal acute liver necrosis; because of the delay in onset, by the time the child is admitted to hospital there may only be therapeutic serum levels of the drug present and differentiation from other possible causes of acute liver necrosis may be impossible. Links with factitious illness by proxy are also described.

Recurrent unexplained deaths

Families in which two or more cot deaths occurred were reviewed by Emery (1986). Out of 12 families with two or more cot deaths, in two the care was seriously at fault and could have contributed to death, and in five filicide was probable.

More recently, Wolkind et al (1993) studied 57 deaths from 27 families, including three who had experienced 3 deaths.

- 31 (55%) were probably the result of actions by one of the parents (filicide).
- Only five (9%) were considered to be true or idiopathic SIDS.
- In two-thirds of the families there was a history of psychiatric illness in one or both parents.
- 18% of the families lived in situations of serious social deprivation.
- Other identifiable factors were present in a majority of the other cases, e.g. in half of the deaths in the first month of life, metabolic abnormality was found.
- 20% were thought to be due to accidental suffocation.

The risk of a cot death in the population at large is about 1 in 500; the risk of a second one is estimated at about 1 in 150. Recurrences appear to increase the likelihood that abuse has been responsible. In one well-known case in the USA over a period of 14 years two parents, Mary Beth and Joseph Tinning, buried their nine children. Until the last child died, the authorities never suspected or acted (Wallace 1986). Sometimes parents will fail to reveal details of these deaths at a later date. The lack of prosecution or conviction hampers the protection of future children.

CASE HISTORY 18.3

An infant of 2 months was dead on arrival at hospital. Intubation and ventilation was attempted but there was no response. The mother said that the child had fallen about 14 inches from a settee on to a linoleum-covered floor. Half an hour after this the baby stopped breathing. There was bruising to the back of the head and buttocks, and at necropsy a single but extensive skull fracture, four old healing rib fractures and a healing clavicular fracture were found. The cause of death was said to be the inhalation of vomit. Although some concern was expressed, the mother was given the benefit of the doubt and no prosecution was taken. Two years later, the same mother was left to mind a friend's 4-year-old child while the child's mother went away for a weekend, causing anxiety to the social service worker who knew of the arrangement but was powerless to prevent it. On the mother's return, severe bruising to the child's face was found and reported to the police. During the course of interviewing the woman an admission was made that she had injured the child and also that she had violently thrown her own baby, hitting his head on a hearth and thereby causing his death.

Child death associated with sexual assault

The association of battering and sexual abuse has been described (Reinhardt 1987, Hobbs & Wynne 1990). Violence is frequently a part of the sexual assault; in addition it can be used as a means to threaten or silence the child. If the abuser is threatened or frightened of exposure by the child, violence may escalate and ultimately the child's life may be at risk. Out of a total of 130 children identified where evidence of physical injury and sexual assault coincided, there were four deaths. The ages ranged from 0.4 to 13.8 years. Other cases have been provided by colleagues elsewhere. Case history 18.4 was supplied by Dr Arnon Bentovim.

CASE HISTORY 18.4

A 2-year-old boy died as a result of injuries thought to be non-accidental. There was fresh and old bruising to the forehead, retinal haemorrhages and deep bruising to the retroperitoneal tissues at the lower end of the aorta anterior to the lumbar spine. In addition there was fresh bruising around the penis with the appearances of a bite mark. Death was related to a large subdural haematoma. There were also bite marks on the cheek and the back of the thigh. The anus was normal.

CASE HISTORY 18.5

A 14-month-old infant was brought in dead to the Accident and Emergency department. The stepfather who accompanied the child said he had left her briefly in the bath and on returning found her face down in the water. Bruising was noted around the mouth and her hair was dry although he later told the police that he had given her mouth-to-mouth resuscitation and put her in front of the fire which had dried her hair. At post-mortem examination the lungs were dry; the cause of death was consistent with asphyxia but the following were noted: old healing midshaft fracture of femur, several fingertip bruises around both knees, a grossly gaping and dilated anus (noted on arrival at hospital) and weight below the third centile. Two surviving siblings were removed into foster-care and a case conference was held at which further information became available:

- The dead child's weight had progressed reasonably well until the mother married the new stepfather, when it had fallen significantly below the third centile.
- The fractured femur had allegedly occurred when the child had fallen over and as the child had not been too upset she was not taken to hospital.
- The bruises had allegedly occurred from crawling on a stone floor.
- Shortly after the stepfather joined the family the 2-year-old sibling sustained a burn on the back of the hand from a clothes iron. The mother failed to take the child to hospital as advised by the general practitioner, and the health visitor no longer felt welcome at the house.

Both siblings in foster-care began to disclose of oral and anal abuse by the stepfather. There was no prosecution although care orders were made in the juvenile court on the surviving children.

The danger to older children who are being sexually abused also needs to be stressed. Hobbs & Wynne (1990) describe the case of a 13-year-old girl who was abused by her stepfather. The abuse involved aggressive and sadistic acts. Attempts were made to protect the girl, with apparent co-operation from the mother. The stepfather became aware that the authorities were increasingly involved. The girl, who had been staying away with a friend, returned home where she was murdered along with her mother. The stepfather committed suicide.

Abduction and murder of children by strangers frequently involves a sexual motive. Jones & Krugman (1986) describe the case of a 3-year-old child who was sexually and physically assaulted and left for dead, but who survived and gave evidence.

Investigation of suspicious death

- Necropsy should preferably be performed by a pathologist who has training in both forensic and paediatric pathology.
- Necropsy may be unrevealing in cases of suspected abuse in young children.

- Smothering and drowning cannot always be excluded.
- Medical and social history play a major role in the interpretation of the necropsy findings.
- Severe head trauma can occur without fractures.
- Previous deaths, injuries, abuse or admissions to care may be covered up by the parents.
- Current crises should be sought in the parents' personal lives.
- The need for toxicology or electrolyte samples to check for inappropriate drug or salt ingestion should be considered. Samples of vitreous humour, blood, urine, stomach contents and various tissues can be sent for analysis.
- Site of death examination may involve police, pathologist and forensic scientist.
- Post-mortem radiographs may reveal occult bony injury.
- A confidential professional inquiry to share information concerning a child's death may conclude that factors were present in the care of the child which contributed to the death of the child. Such information may assist professional agencies in providing care to the family if a further child is born.

Summary

1. Fatal child abuse is often not recognised and reported. Statistics can therefore be misleading.
2. The observation that death due to abuse is particularly high in the first year of life reflects the burden of unwanted pregnancies and the vulnerability of infancy.
3. Teenagers, especially if homeless or unsupported, are especially at risk both of abuse and of abusing their own infant.
4. Links with all forms of abuse are evident.
5. Patterns of unexplained infant and childhood deaths are recognised in abusive families and kinships.
6. Clinical recognition depends on confidential information-sharing, skilled pathology and an appreciation of the social issues for the family.
7. A link exists between a sub-group of cot deaths and child abuse.

REFERENCES

AAP 1994 Committee on Child Abuse and Neglect Distinguishing sudden infant death syndrome from child abuse fatalities. Pediatrics 94(1):124–126

Browne K D, Lynch M A 1995 The nature and extent of child homicide and fatal abuse. Editorial. Child Abuse Review 4:309–316

Browne K D, Hamilton C, Oakes 1995 Domestic and child homicides in the UK. Journal of Interpersonal Violence

Child Abuse 1991 A study of inquiry reports 1980–1989. Department of Health. HMSO, London

Childhood Matters 1996 The National Commission of Inquiry into the Prevention of Child Abuse. Stationery Office, London

Christoffel K K, Zeiserl E J, Chiaramonte J 1985 Should child abuse and neglect be considered when a child dies unexpectedly? American Journal of Diseases in Children 139:876–880

Creighton S J 1984 Trends in child abuse. NSPCC, London

Creighton S J 1992 Child abuse trends in England and Wales 1988–1990. NSPCC, London, pp 14–16

Creighton S J 1996 Fatal child abuse – how preventable is it? Child Abuse Review 4:318–328

Dine M S, McGovern M E 1982 Intentional poisoning of children – an overlooked category of child abuse: report of seven cases and review of literature. Pediatrics 70:32–35

Emery J L 1985 Infanticide, filicide and cot death. Archives of Disease in Childhood 60:505–507

Emery J L 1986 Families in which two or more cot deaths have occurred. Lancet i:313–315

Emery J L 1993 Cot death and child abuse. In: Hobbs C J, Wynne J M (eds) Bailliére's Clinical Paediatics. Bailliére Tindall, London

Ewigman B, Kivlahan C, Land G 1993. The Missouri child fatality study: Under reporting of maltreatment fatalities among children younger than five years of age 1983 through 1986. Pediatrics 91(2):330–337

Falkov A 1996 Fatal child abuse and parental psychiatric disorder. ACPC series report no 1. Department of Health, London

Gill D G 1984 Conflagration of children in cars. British Medical Journal 288:973

Greenland C 1980 Lethal family situations: an international comparison of deaths from child abuse. In: Anthony E J, Chiland C C (eds). The child in his family, vol 6. J Wiley, New York, pp 389–408

Hobbs C J, Wynne J M 1990 The sexually abused battered child. Archives of Disease in Childhood 65:423–437

Hobbs C J, Wynne J M, Gelletlie R 1995 Leeds inquiry into infant deaths: the importance of abuse and neglect in sudden infant death. Child Abuse Review 4:329–339

Home Office 1994 Criminal statistics for England and Wales 1993. CMND 2680, HMSO, London

Independent on Sunday 1992. Independent on Sunday, London, 12 January 1992.

Jobling M 1976 The abused child. National Children's Bureau, London

Jones D P H, Krugman R 1986 Can a three-year-old child bear witness to her sexual assault and attempted murder? Child Abuse and Neglect 10:253–258

Kempe C H, Silverman F N, Steele B F, Droegmueller W, Silver H K 1962 The battered child syndrome. Journal of American Medical Association 181:17–24

McClain P W, Sacks J J, Froelke R G, Ewigman B G 1993. Estimates of fatal child abuse and neglect, United States 1979 through 1988. Pediatrics 91(2):338–343

Meadow R 1990 Suffocation, recurrent apnea, and sudden death. Journal of Pediatrics 117:351–357

Newlands M, Emery J L 1991 Child abuse and cot deaths. Child Abuse and Neglect 15:275–278

Oliver J E 1983 Dead children from problem families in NE Wiltshire. British Medical Journal 286:115–117

Reder P, Duncan S, Gray M 1993 Beyond blame: child abuse tragedies revisited. Routledge, London

Reece R M 1993 Fatal child abuse and sudden infant death syndrome: a critical diagnostic decision. Pediatrics 91(2):423–429

Reinhardt M A 1987 Sexual abuse of battered young children. Pediatric Emergency Care 3:36–38

Rogers D, Tripp J, Bentovim A, Robinson A, Berry D, Goulding R 1976 Non-accidental poisoning: an extended syndrome of child abuse. British Medical Journal 1:793–796

Rose D 1990 Murder in Britain. Guardian, London, 1 January 1990

Schmitt B D 1981 Child neglect. In: Ellerstein N S (ed) Child abuse and neglect. A medical reference. J Wiley, New York

Southall D P, Stebbens V A, Rees S V, Lang M H, Warner J O, Shinebourne E A 1978 Apnoeic episodes induced by smothering: two cases identified by covert video surveillance. British Medical Journal 294:1637–1641

Templeman 1892 Edinburgh Medical Journal

Wallace A 1986 After 9 deaths in 14 years, mother arrested. New York Times, 8 February 1986, p 1

Wissow L S 1990 Fatal maltreatment. In: Child advocacy for the clinician. Williams & Wilkins, Baltimore, pp 172–184

Wolkind S, Taylor E M, Waite A J, Dalton M, Emery J L 1993 Recurrence of unexpected infant death. Acta Paediatrica 82:873–876

Working Together 1991 Working Together under the Children Act 1989: a guide to the arrangements for interagency cooperation for the protection of children from abuse DHSS and Welsh Office. HMSO, London

Appendix to Chapter 11

Table 11.2 Consecutive referrals to a community paediatric clinic

Mother/socially	Past history	Drug history	Baby
Single 32 years First pregnancy No partner Foster-care 7 weeks Remains on drugs	Anorexia Depression Self-harm – 60 overdoses	Cigarettes Nitrazepam Amitryptiline Diazepam	Term 2.34kg ECS fetal distress 'Screamer' Development 8 weeks
Single 15 years Second pregnancy No partner In foster-care ?social drug user	'out of control' boyfriend 26, 37 years In foster-care	Cigarettes, 20/day Ecstasy LSD Cannabis No alcohol	Term 3.2kg Growth good Development = 7 months
Single 24 years Second pregnancy Partner currently withdrawal of drugs	Partner previous heroin abuse 2 year-old child	Heroin, 12 months Methadone in pregnancy	Term 2.8kg Day 3 symptoms
Single 16 years First pregnancy Partner in foster-care Mother-baby unit Home-partner's mother Stopped drugs	Foster-care 8 years physical and emotional abuse 15 years heroin/prostitution/pimp drug dealer	Cigarettes Heroin Amphetamines Cocaine Cannabis	39 weeks 3.34kg Day 3 symptoms Day 17 discharge
Single 17 years First pregnancy No partner Mother-baby unit Home with grandma Later, prison due to theft Stopped drugs	Glue sniffer 15 years	Cigarettes Alcohol Cocaine Methadone	Term 3.37kg Day 3 symptoms Day 36 discharge Development = 8 months
Single 24 years First pregnancy Partner drug abuser Home-grandma, foster-care when reabused drugs	Drugs from 16 years Casual re-abuse of drugs	Cigarettes Heroin Methadone	Term 3.38kg Day 3 symptoms Day 36 discharge Development = 6 months

Single 18 years First pregnancy Home-grandma Re-abused drugs	Cigarettes Opiates DF 118	Cigarettes Opiates DF 118	Term 3.31kg Day 3 symptoms Day 40 days Development = 7 months
Single 19 years First pregnancy Home FTA follow-up	Heroin DF 118	Heroin DF 118 Social user	Term 2.95kg Well as neonate Discharged 3 days
Single 25 years Fourth child Foster-care-home	Cigarettes Wine, bottle/day	Cigarettes Wine, bottle/day Friends all drink in each others homes	38 weeks 2.3kg Emergency CS – fetal distress Failure to thrive Language delay

Index

Numbers in *italic* refer to boxes or tables
Numbers in **bold** refer to case histories